DIFFERENTIAL DIAGNOSIS IN PRIMARY CARE

FIFTH EDITION

R. Douglas Collins, MD, FACP
Senior FAA Medical Examiner
Former Associate Professor of Medicine
Medical University of South Carolina
Former Associate Clinical Professor of Medicine
University of Florida School of Medicine
Chatsworth, California

 Wolters Kluwer | Lippincott Williams & Wilkins
Health
Philadelphia · Baltimore · New York · London
Buenos Aires · Hong Kong · Sydney · Tokyo

Acquisitions Editor: Sonya Seigafuse
Product Manager: Kerry Barrett
Production Manager: Alicia Jackson
Senior Manufacturing Manager: Benjamin Rivera
Marketing Manager: Kim Schonberger
Design Coordinator: Holly McLaughlin
Production Service: SPi Global

Printed in China

Library of Congress Cataloging-in-Publication Data
Collins, R. Douglas.
  Differential diagnosis in primary care / R. Douglas Collins. — 5th ed.
      p. ; cm.
  Includes index.
  ISBN 978-1-4511-1825-4
  1. Diagnosis, Differential. I. Title.
  [DNLM: 1. Diagnosis, Differential. 2. Primary Health Care. WB 141.5]
  RC71.5.C62   2012
  616.07'5—dc23

                                                                  2011020563

Care has been taken to confirm the accuracy of the information presented and to describe
generally accepted practices. However, the authors, editors, and publisher are not responsible
for errors or omissions or for any consequences from application of the information in this
book and make no warranty, expressed or implied, with respect to the currency, completeness,
or accuracy of the contents of the publication. Application of the information in a particular
situation remains the professional responsibility of the practitioner.

The authors, editors, and publisher have exerted every effort to ensure that drug selection
and dosage set forth in this text are in accordance with current recommendations and practice
at the time of publication. However, in view of ongoing research, changes in government
regulations, and the constant flow of information relating to drug therapy and drug reactions,
the reader is urged to check the package insert for each drug for any change in indications
and dosage and for added warnings and precautions. This is particularly important when the
recommended agent is a new or infrequently employed drug.

Some drugs and medical devices presented in the publication have Food and Drug
Administration (FDA) clearance for limited use in restricted research settings. It is the
responsibility of the health care provider to ascertain the FDA status of each drug or
device planned for use in their clinical practice.

To purchase additional copies of this book, call our customer service department at (800) 638-
3030 or fax orders to (301) 223-2320. International customers should call (301) 223-2300.

Visit Lippincott Williams & Wilkins on the Internet: at LWW.com. Lippincott Williams &
Wilkins customer service representatives are available from 8:30 am to 6 pm, EST.

10 9 8 7 6 5 4 3 2 1

To my wife, Norie

Over 30 years ago, I embarked on a mission to share with students and clinicians everywhere my approach to differential diagnosis. Today, I'm happy to say that for many of you out there that mission has been fulfilled.

The fifth edition should be even more useful to you in the diagnosis of common symptoms and signs. I have divided this edition into three sections. Section One is devoted to the history and physical examination, particularly special examination techniques for common symptoms and signs. Section Two applies my method of differential diagnosis to an exhaustive list of symptoms and signs, as in previous editions. I have carefully revised this section to include up-to-date diagnostic tests and expanded the list of diagnostic possibilities where appropriate. Section Three is I believe unique to textbooks of differential diagnosis. Here, I have explored common diseases that may be a symptom of many other diseases. For example, you want to consult this section when you have a case of diabetes mellitus or congestive heart failure that is not responding to treatment.

Acknowledgments

I want to thank my wife, Norie, and her sister, Mildred Mendoza, for the excellent job of typing this manuscript. I am grateful to Kerry Barrett, Product Manager, and Sonya Seigafuse, Acquisitions Editor, for their diligent efforts in making the finished product possible.

Finally, I thank the good Lord for the strength and wisdom he has provided me to complete this project and look forward to writing the next edition.

Contents

SECTION THREE: Diseases that are Symptoms of Other Diseases 449

PART A

The Routine History and Physical Examination

After 50 years of practicing medicine, the author has discovered many productive and time-saving methods in taking a history and performing a physical examination. He believes these techniques are worth passing on to younger clinicians.

THE HISTORY

This section will examine each part of the history and demonstrate how to obtain the most information in the shortest period of time.

● Development of the Chief Complaint

The physician begins this portion of the history by visualizing a strength, duration graph (Figure 1). It is important to know the following:

- The intensity of a symptom, when and how it began, and its duration.
- If the symptom onset was sudden or insidious.
- If the symptom is steady, progressive, or intermittent.
- The exact location of the symptom and whether it radiates to other areas of the body.
- What other symptoms are associated with it and what precipitates it, aggravates it, and relieves it.

Chest pain can be used as an example. Depending on the information the physician gathers about the chest pain, he or she may reach different conclusions about it. This is graphically displayed in Figure 1.

- If it is severe, think myocardial infarction or pneumothorax.
- If it is mild to moderate, think Tietze syndrome, pleurisy, or pericarditis.
- If it is intermittent, think angina pectoris or Tietze syndrome.
- If it is steady, think pleurisy, myocardial infarction, fracture, pericarditis, or pneumothorax.
- If it radiates to the jaw or the left upper extremity, think coronary artery disease.
- If it is associated with dysphagia, think reflux esophagitis.
- If it is precipitated by exercise, think angina pectoris.
- If there is associated diaphoresis, think myocardial infarction or some other form of coronary artery disease.

- If it is associated with fever and chills, think pleurisy, pneumonia, and pericarditis (strong possibilities).
- If it is relieved by an antacid or lidocaine (Xylocaine) viscous, it is probably reflux esophagitis.
- If it is relieved by nitroglycerin, it is probably angina pectoris. (Remember, nitroglycerin can also relieve esophagitis.)

The principles demonstrated by this example of chest pain can be applied to almost any symptom.

● Past History

The clinician should always ask if there have been previous **accidents**, **operations**, or **hospitalizations**. He or she would also want to know if there is a history of contagious disease such as hepatitis, tuberculosis, recurrent pneumonia, gonorrhea, human immunodeficiency virus (HIV), or syphilis. To make the past history inquiry more complete, it is important to remember the following pearl: ask if the patient has ever had any eye disease, ear–nose–throat (ENT) disease, lung disease, liver disease, kidney disease, skin disease, blood disease, bone disease, or endocrine disease. In other words, take each internal organ from head to toe and ask if the patient has a history of disease of that organ. This will not only result in a more thorough past history inquiry but almost certainly save an enormous amount of time.

● Review of Systems

Here is another area where the physician can use a unique method to cover the entire body in an organized way, thus saving a lot of time. Because symptoms are organized into five categories, as emphasized subsequently in this book, one simply asks the following questions:

- Do you have any pain anywhere in your body?
- Do you have any lumps or bumps anywhere in your body?
- Have you had any bleeding from any body orifice (mouth, nose, ear, rectum, vagina, urethra), or have you coughed up blood, vomited up blood, urinated blood, or had bloody diarrhea?
- Have you had a nonbloody discharge from any body orifice?
- Have you had difficulty with any body function? Especially, have you had difficulty hearing, seeing, breathing, swallowing, moving your bowels, urinating, walking, talking, or performing your job?

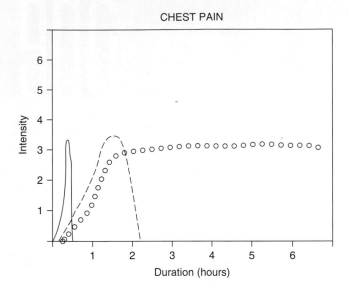

CHEST PAIN

● **FIGURE 1** Chest pain. *Solid line* is typical of angina pectoris. *Dashed line* is typical of coronary insufficiency or unstable angina. *Line of small circles* is more typical of a myocardial infarction.

● Family History

No doubt the clinician will ask about diseases that affected the patient's mother and father. However, it is important to include the grandparents on both sides of the family as well as brothers, sisters, and children. (Remember, mental disease is hereditary! You can get it from your children).

● Habits

The physician should not forget to ask about the use of caffeinated beverages in addition to cigarettes, alcohol, and illegal drugs. In the author's opinion, caffeine is more dangerous than nicotine.

● Social and Sexual History

The clinician should be sure to ask about multiple partners of the same and opposite sex, even though it may be embarrassing. And it is necessary to ask about arrests, anxiety, depression, and suicidal reaction or attempts. Do not forget to ask about anal sex, as this is a significant way that HIV and hepatitis are spread.

THE PHYSICAL EXAMINATION

Here are some useful pearls to keep in mind during the routine physical examination. (Part B will contain pearls to use in your examination of patients with the most common symptoms and signs.)

First, it is essential to take a good look at the whole patient. Determine whether he or she is fat or slim; tall or short; pale or ruddy; or depressed, anxious, or happy. Assess whether he or she is positive or negative when interacting with the physician or distant and almost sorry to be in the office.

1. It is necessary to conduct an eye examination, including an examination of the eye grounds. The physician can detect at least 30 diseases with a careful ophthalmoscopic examination. Open the examination room door a crack, turn the lights off, and have the patient focus on his or her outstretched thumb (give the patient something to look at). Now, focus the ophthalmoscope on the cornea and pupil at about 10 inches away and then move into the fundus at about 1 to 2 inches away. Do not tilt your head; this may block the patient's other eye from seeing his or her thumb. If need be, practice this examination on a nurse or other person in the office until it is routine. If it is still difficult to see the fundus, dilate the pupil with a short-acting sympathomimetic compound.

   Most physicians perform an adequate ENT examination. Two points require emphasis. If the ear drums are blocked with wax or other debris, remove it by irrigation and then reexamine the ears. Alternatively, perform a whisper test of each ear at 3 feet, although this is not as good. However, if there is middle or inner ear pathology, the physician will realize it because of the significant hearing loss.

2. If the clinician moves directly to the heart and lungs from the ENT examination, he or she misses a lot of pathology. It is essential to examine the neck next. Palpate for a thyroid nodule or enlarged thyroid, enlarged lymph nodes, other masses, and tracheal deviation. Look for jugular vein distention. Check that the range of motion is full and there is no nuchal rigidity, especially in a child with fever. Listen for bruits.

3. Now for examination of the lungs. It is necessary to listen over the right middle lobe and the trachea. The physician frequently bypasses percussion these days, but he or she should not. If there are rales, see if they clear on coughing.

4. Moving to the heart, the clinician routinely checks for irregular rhythm, cardiomegaly, and murmurs, but it is just as important to listen carefully to the heart sounds. This is the best way to tell if a systolic or diastolic murmur is present and what valve is involved. For example, if there is a systolic murmur and the second heart sound is diminished or absent, it is most likely aortic stenosis. If A2 is greater than P2, hypertension is very likely. (If one is unsure of how to interpret the heart sounds or a little rusty, it is necessary to obtain assistance from a cardiologist.)

5. There is not much to remind a physician about examination of the abdomen. Certainly, check if the liver, spleen, or kidneys are palpable. And check for an unexpected mass. When presented with a patient with abdominal pain, it is important not to forget to check for rebound tenderness and resonance over the liver (indicating air under the diaphragm). Retraction of one or both testicles may indicate peritoneal irritation from a ruptured viscus. The routine physical examination requires an examination of the external genitalia and rectal and vaginal examination. The clinician should not skip it. Some women state that they just had their annual Papanicolaou (Pap) smear, but if they have come for a complete physical examination, it is necessary to do at least a manual examination. Besides, the gynecologist may not have

completed a thorough manual examination when doing the Pap smear. For an obese woman in whom one cannot palpate the adnexa adequately, it is necessary to order an ultrasonic examination.

6. The physician must also examine the skin and nails. It is possible to detect many diseases by looking at the nails, such as the clubbing in congenital heart disease, chronic obstructive pulmonary disease, and bronchiectasis; the thickening in hypothyroidism; and the spoon nails in iron deficiency anemia.

7. Most physicians rely on nurses and other health-care professionals to take blood pressure. Unless these nurses have received your instructions about the auscultatory gap, this is not a good idea. The author teaches health-care professionals in his office to take blood pressure with the radial pulse first before applying the stethoscope. That way they almost always obtain an accurate systolic pressure. It is necessary to use a large cuff in obese patients.

   The clinician should not forget to check for axillary and inguinal adenopathy and peripheral pulses. If the dorsal pedis and posterior tibial pulses are absent, he or she needs to check the femoral arteries for absent pulses or bruits. The patient may have a Leriche syndrome.

8. Unless a clinician is a neurologist, he or she is not going to perform a thorough neurologic examination during the routine physical examination unless the patient's complaints are definitely neurological. Here is an abbreviated examination that may be useful if there is simply no time to do a thorough examination:
   - Check coordination by having the patient pat the physician's hand with each of his or her hands and feet in rapid succession. Have the patient stand with his or her feet together and close his or her eyes. Check the patient's gait.
   - Now, check for weakness or hemiparesis by having the patient grip the physician's fingers with each hand and dorsiflex and plantar flex his or her feet against resistance.
   - Check sensation in all four extremities with a tuning fork, preferably a 128-cps one. Also, use a cotton applicator on all four. Check for simultaneous stimulation by seeing if the patient can recognize the physician's fingers on one or both extremities at the same time.
   - Check the cranial nerves, beginning with the funduscopic examination (which you have already done); have the patient follow a light; and check the gross visual field by confrontation, pupillary equality, and response to light. Check facial nerve function by telling the patient to close his or her eyes and whistle and then watch to see if the patient can extend his or her tongue in the midline. Finally, check for nuchal rigidity. The examination is not finished until the physician has checked for the symmetry of the physiologic reflexes on all four extremities and plantar responses on the feet.

The author realizes that this still seems like a lot; however, there are no other shortcuts to a good neurologic examination.

If the readers have any pearls that they would like to share, they are encouraged to write to the author (care of Wolters Kluwer Health/Lippincott Williams and Wilkins) so they can be included in the next edition.

PART B

Special Clinical Examination Techniques for Common Symptoms and Signs

The routine history and physical examination demonstrated above is all well and good when the patient is asymptomatic; however, it is grossly inadequate when a patient presents with certain common symptoms and signs. Additional clinical techniques for evaluation of patients with many common symptoms and signs will be discussed here. They are the result of the author's many years of experience in clinical practice as well as reviewing a host of textbooks on physical diagnosis. Although some of these techniques will be familiar to the reader, many will not.

Note that these symptoms and signs are organized into the five categories used in the review of systems: pain, lumps and bumps, bloody discharge, nonbloody discharge, and functional changes. The author hopes that the reader enjoys this fresh approach to the physical examination.

PAIN

● Abdominal Pain

The purpose here is not to enter into a thorough discussion of inspection, palpation, percussion, and auscultation of the abdomen but to emphasize portions of a good examination that are often overlooked.

No matter what portion of the abdomen is involved in the complaint, the physician must look for rebound tenderness. If present, it is a clear indication of peritonitis or a ruptured viscus. One applies pressure to the abdomen where the pain is located and then suddenly releases it. If the patient winces, there is rebound tenderness and a serious abdominal condition. Guarding and rigidity usually indicate the same thing.

It is necessary to listen for bowel sounds for at least 3 minutes. If they are absent, there may be peritonitis or paralytic ileus. If they are hyperactive and high-pitched, there may be a bowel obstruction. In male patients, look for retraction of the testicles. If the right testicle is retracted, there is a possibility of a ruptured appendix. When both testicles are retracted, peritonitis from a perforated peptic ulcer or pancreatitis is likely.

One should look for Murphy sign. Place your thumb under the right subcostal margin and have the patient take a deep breath. If the patient winces, the sign is present. Do not forget to check for inguinal and femoral hernias as well as umbilical and incisional hernias. A rectal and pelvic examination must be done in any case of abdominal pain. They are essential in diagnosing a pelvic appendix, ruptured ectopic pregnancy, pelvic inflammatory disease

(PID), and endometriosis. The finding of occult blood in the stool may point to intussusception or mesenteric infarct, as well as peptic ulcer disease and neoplasm.

If appendicitis is suspected, it is essential to look for a Rovsing sign. Applying pressure in the left lower quadrant causes pain in the right lower quadrant. Do not forget to look for psoas sign.

● Arm and Hand Pain

The patient presenting with acute arm and hand pain should usually be no problem. A fracture dislocation, cellulitis, or even "tennis elbow" is obvious. Perhaps the clinician will miss referred pain from acute coronary insufficiency, but this is not likely. It is chronic recurrent pain in the arm and hand that often confounds the clinician. First, palpate the joints for the various forms of arthritis. Next, look for tenderness of the radial–humeral joint (tennis elbow) and lateral epicondyle (golfer elbow). If these techniques fail to reveal the diagnosis, it is time to look for the neurological causes of the pain in four places:

- Begin by palpating the cervical roots and performing a cervical compression test and Spurling test.
- Next, perform Adson tests for the various types of thoracic outlet syndrome.
- Now, tap the ulnar groove in the elbow for ulnar entrapment. Sensation to touch and pain should be reduced in the little finger and the lateral one half of the ring finger if this is present. In some cases, the hypothenar eminence and interossei muscles are atrophied.
- Finally, tap the medial surface of the wrist (Tinel sign), and flex the wrist for 3 minutes (Phalen test) to pin down the diagnosis of carpal tunnel syndrome. Sensation to touch and pain will be diminished in the first three fingers and the medial one half of the ring finger if this is present. In advanced cases, there may be atrophy of the thenar eminence.

Obviously, a neurologist will perform a more detailed examination, but a primary care physician should be able to pick up most causes of chronic arm or hand pain using these techniques.

● Chest Pain

The author has no doubt that the reader will do an adequate job of auscultation and percussion of the heart and lungs in cases of chest pain. But what about remembering to check for tracheal deviation? The author recently had a case of carcinoma of the lung where the only clinical sign was tracheal deviation to the side of the lesion. In addition, remember to

- Palpate the costochondral junctions to rule out Tietze syndrome.
- Look for a dermatomal rash in case the patient has herpes zoster.
- Check the axillary and cervical lymph nodes for metastasis.

Above all, it is essential to remember to check the lower extremities for signs of thrombophlebitis such as a positive Homan sign.

● Dysuria

Many cases of dysuria are associated with a urethral or vaginal discharge, so the techniques used to evaluate these complaints apply here (see pages 10 and 9). In male patients presenting with dysuria alone, the physician will want to massage the prostate to determine if there is chronic prostatitis. If a discharge is produced by this procedure, even a small amount, the patient probably has prostatitis. One can confirm the diagnosis by putting a drop on a slide and examining for white blood cells under the microscope. Examine for flank tenderness (Murphy sign) in both male and female patients because there may be pyelonephritis.

In females presenting with dysuria, a thorough pelvic examination is clearly indicated. A uterine mass, PID, or ectopic pregnancy may be the cause of the dysuria.

In both males and females, the physician should be alert for congenital anomalies of the genitourinary tract (e.g., hypospadias) on examination. Catheterization for residual urine may be the only way of picking up a neurogenic bladder or bladder neck obstruction.

● Headache

The patient who presents with headache is a special challenge. There are several things the physician can do while examining the patient when the headache is occurring:

- Occlude the superficial temporal arteries for 1 to 2 minutes. If there is relief of the headache, the patient has a vascular headache, most likely migraine. If the blood pressure is elevated during an attack, think of pheochromocytoma. If there is nuchal rigidity, quite naturally one thinks of meningitis or subarachnoid hemorrhage.
- It is absolutely imperative to do a funduscopic examination to look for papilledema and hypertensive retinopathy. If pressure on the jugular veins relieves the headache, the patient may have a postspinal tap headache.
- Marked tenderness of the superficial temporal artery on one side should suggest temporal arteritis. Transilluminate the sinuses to look for sinusitis. If a pseudoephedrine spray (Neo-Synephrine) relieves the headache, the patient may have allergic or vasomotor rhinitis. Finally, sumatriptan relieves both migraine and cluster headaches and is therefore useful in the diagnosis.

If the physician sees the patient when the headaches are not occurring, a nitroglycerin tablet under the tongue assists in the diagnosis. If this precipitates the headache, the patient may have migraine. Histamine sulfate subcutaneously may precipitate a headache in both patients with migraine and in those with cluster headaches.

An injection of lidocaine 1% into the occipital nerve roots may relieve tension headaches. Note that many patients with so-called tension headache actually have common migraine.

● Hip Pain

When examining a patient with a history of trauma, the physician will undoubtedly obtain an x-ray of the hips before proceeding with an extensive clinical examination. If there is no evidence of fracture, he or she may proceed with an examination of the range of motion (extension and flexion, internal and external rotation) and palpation for point tenderness. Greater trochanter bursitis is a common cause of hip pain and is easily diagnosed by palpation over the greater trochanter bursa and subsequent relief of the pain by injecting the bursa with 1% to 2% lidocaine. Range of motion is restricted, and Patrick test (pain on external rotation of the hip) is positive in both osteoarthritis (and other forms of arthritis) and greater trochanter bursitis.

It is wise to do a femoral stretch test and straight leg raising test to be sure one is not missing a herniated lumbar disc in these patients.

The clinician must palpate the sacroiliac joints. The patient with sacroiliitis may present with "hip" pain.

● Knee Pain

Once again, the physician should obtain an x-ray to rule out fracture in most cases of acute knee pain before proceeding with an extensive clinical evaluation. This evaluation includes range of motion (extension and flexion) and palpation. Test for loose collateral ligaments by fully extending the joint at the knee and attempting to move the tibia, medially and laterally. Next, perform a McMurray test. Flex the knee on the thigh and with the foot rotated first internally and then externally slowly extend the knee. If a "pop" or locking of the joint is heard, the test is positive for a torn meniscus, and a referral to an orthopedic surgeon is necessary. Finally, use the drawer test to check for anterior or posterior cruciate ligament tears or rupture. With the foot dangling over the examination table, attempt to pull the tibia forward and backward on the femur. If there is significant movement one way or the other, the test is positive. Examine the knee for fluid by pressing the patella distally and feeling for ballottement (the patella bobs up and down on pressure).

There are several bursa around the knee. It is worthwhile to inject them with 1% to 2% lidocaine to see if significant relief of knee pain is achieved.

Here again, one must examine the patient for a possible herniated lumbar disc. Look for hip pathology as well.

● Leg, Foot, and Toe Pain

No doubt the reader does not need instruction in performing inspection and palpation of the lower extremities for cellulitis, hematoma, or other mass lesion. The author also does not think it is necessary to discuss the examination of the bones and joints for inflammation or fracture dislocations.

However, the physician should not forget to perform a test for Homan sign to rule out thrombophlebitis and palpate for diminished pulses, not just the dorsalis pedis and tibial pulses, but also the popliteal and femoral pulses. Also, listen for bruits over the femoral arteries to detect significant occlusion of the femoral arteries or terminal aorta (Leriche syndrome).

One thing that many clinicians neglect to do is measure the calves. Often, this is the only way to detect unilateral swelling (in thrombophlebitis) or atrophy (in a herniated lumbar disc syndrome). A clinician should keep a tape measure on his or her person or in his or her bag at all times.

One should perform a straight leg raising test to rule out radiculopathy and external rotation of the hip joint (Patrick test) to rule out hip pathology. Finally, a good sensory examination does not just help diagnose radiculopathy or polyneuropathy but also rules out tarsal tunnel syndrome or Morton neuroma.

● Low Back Pain

In cases of both acute and chronic low back pain, the physician's main consideration is to rule out a herniated disc once he or she has ruled out a fracture with plain films. Perform a straight leg raising test, look for Lasègue sign (flexing the leg at both the hip and the knee and gradually straightening the leg), and check for a reduced ankle jerk (on the side of the pain) in L4–L5 and L5–S1 disc herniations. Also check for loss of pain and touch in the big toe (in L4–L5 disc herniations) and the lateral surface of the foot and little toe (in L5–S1 disc herniations). A foot drop or weakness of dorsiflexion of the big toe is a sign of L5 radiculopathy (or an L4–L5 disc herniation). In cases of chronic low back pain, measure the circumference of the calves and thighs because there is usually wasting on the side of the lesion.

A clinician will miss a disc herniation at L3–L4 or L2–L3 if he or she stops the examination at this point. Continue by performing a femoral stretch test. With the patient stretched out in the prone position, raise the lower leg and flex it onto the thigh. At 100 degrees or less, the patient resists further movement if an L3–L4 herniation is present. The knee jerk is diminished on the side of the lesion in most cases. In addition, there is often loss of sensation in the L3 or L4 dermatome.

No back examination is complete without examining for sacrospinalis (paraspinous) muscle spasm. With the patient standing in the "at ease" position (relaxed with feet 12 inches apart), one should palpate the paraspinous muscles and compare one side with the other. Normally, they should both feel doughy. When one is more tense than the other, a lumbosacral sprain or disc herniation is likely, although many other pathologic conditions of the lumbosacral spine may also be the cause. Anyway, significant spasm is a clear indication for a computed tomography (CT) or magnetic resonance imaging (MRI) scan of the lumbosacral spine.

The physician should not forget to check for tenderness of the sacrosciatic notches. A rectal examination is important to check for sphincter tone and control, which may be lost in a cauda equina syndrome. As mentioned on page XX, many cases of low back pain are due to a short leg syndrome, so measure the leg length.

When there are no objective findings, it is necessary to look for malingering. Certain signs are a clear indication of this condition. First of all, there is secondary gain (e.g., workman compensation). Next, if there is sensory loss, it is nondermatomal. Weakness and muscle wasting are also diffused. Ask the patient to bend over as far as he or she can. If there is malingering, he or she will not bend very far. Now hold onto the patient's hips and ask him or her to rotate the shoulders right and left. If rotation is limited, the patient with low back pain is probably malingering because rotation of the spine is a function primarily of the thoracic spine. Now rotate the whole spine at the hip. If the patient says this duplicates the pain, he or she does not have back pathology. Many patients who are malingering are schooled in resisting the straight leg raising test and thus have a false-positive result; however, if the physician has them sit on the examination table with their legs dangling and creates a distraction, it is possible to straighten their legs without resistance if they are malingering.

● Neck Pain

When reviewing hospital charts, the author finds that the results of the neck examination are rarely listed, so he wonders if this part of the physical examination is often skipped. In a patient presenting with neck pain, the first thing to do is palpate for point tenderness. That way, the physician will not miss a subacute thyroiditis, occipital neuralgia, tender lymph nodes, or brachial plexus neuralgia.

Next, one must check the range of motion in all planes—anterior, posterior, adduction right and left, and rotation to the right and left. The patient should be able to extend 45 degrees, flex 65 degrees (so that the chin touches the chest), adduct 45 degrees right and left, and rotate 60 degrees right and left. Any major deviation from these norms suggests cervical spondylosis, herniated disc, fracture, or other pathology. If there is a herniated disc or significant osteoarthritic spurs, cervical compression or Spurling test precipitates radicular pain down the upper extremity. Tender cervical lymph nodes suggest inflammation in the throat, salivary glands, teeth, or sinuses.

It is necessary to look for Horner syndrome in patients with cervical pain because this may indicate a thoracic outlet syndrome, brachial plexus neuralgia, or mediastinal lesion. Cervical pain is associated with a mass in Ludwig angina, Zenker diverticulum, thyroiditis, and metastatic neoplasms. The pain may occasionally be referred from coronary insufficiency, cholecystitis, or intrathoracic pathology.

● Shoulder Pain

If there is no obvious deformity, the first thing to do with a patient who presents with shoulder pain is to palpate the subacromial bursa, the biceps tendons, and the glenohumeral and acromioclavicular joints. Then it is necessary to test active and passive abduction of the shoulder joint. If the patient has limited active abduction, but the physician can get full or almost full abduction of the joint, the patient very likely has a subacromial bursitis or impingement syndrome. If there is both active and passive limitation of abduction of the joint, the patient has some form of arthritis (e.g., gout, osteoarthritis) unless the shoulder pain is acute, in which case a fracture or dislocation must be considered. A frozen shoulder or adhesive capsulitis must also be considered as well as sympathetic dystrophy. In these cases, it is necessary to look for possible lung or cardiovascular pathology as well. If there is tenderness of the biceps tendon, one should confirm the presence of tenosynovitis of the long head of the biceps by having the patient flex the biceps against resistance.

Finally, it is necessary to inject the bursa, joint, around a tendon, or maybe a trigger point in the shoulder with 1% lidocaine to confirm the diagnosis. Remember, pain in the shoulder can be referred from a cholecystitis, subphrenic abscess, or other systemic pathology.

● Testicular Pain

If there is a mass associated with the pain, the physician should refer to page XX. But what if there is no mass? In these cases, it is necessary to check the size of the inguinal rings and have the patient cough to rule out a sliding inguinal hernia. If the pain is steady, it may be due to L2 or L3 radiculopathy from a herniated lumbar disc or spinal cord tumor. If it is intermittent, one should consider the possibility of a renal calculus. A dermatomal rash would suggest herpes zoster. If the cremasteric reflex is absent on the side of the pain, consider the possibility of torsion of the testicle.

LUMPS AND BUMPS

● Abdominal Masses

(Hepatomegaly and splenomegaly will be considered in subsequent sections.)

The kidneys are not usually palpable, but they may be felt in polycystic kidney disease, hydronephrosis, and hypernephroma. Flank tenderness (Murphy sign) may help verify that the mass is a large kidney, especially if there is an associated urinary tract infection. An aortic aneurysm is in the midline position, and there is most certainly a bruit present on auscultation. It is not possible to feel most carcinomas and other tumors of the intestinal tract until they are advanced significantly. This is true of carcinoma of the head of the pancreas. One probably will not feel it before there is significant bile duct obstruction and jaundice. By that time, there will be significant wasting and generalized pruritus.

The clinician can distinguish a hypogastric mass from a distended bladder simply by inserting a catheter into the bladder. Final definition of a suspected abdominal mass relies on a CT scan of the abdomen or ultrasonography.

● Breast Mass

The techniques used to differentiate a breast mass are in many ways similar to those used in differentiating a neck mass. Transillumination helps differentiate a breast cyst from a benign fibroadenoma or malignant neoplasm. A freely movable mass is more likely benign, whereas a mass that is fixed to the skin or chest wall is more likely malignant. An "orange peel" appearance of the skin over the mass or retraction of the skin means the mass is malignant. Nontender axillary adenopathy on the side of the lesion points to malignancy, whereas tender axillary adenopathy suggests a breast abscess.

A nipple discharge associated with the mass helps further in the differential diagnosis. A bloody discharge points to malignancy. A purulent discharge suggests a breast abscess. A clear or milky discharge points to prolactinemia or pregnancy.

● Edema

The first thing to do is distinguish pitting edema from non-pitting edema. Nonpitting edema should prompt a search for focal or generalized lymphadenopathy and hypothyroidism. For hypothyroidism, the physician looks for thickening of the nails and hair and carotinemia (orange hue to the skin). Lymphedema is usually confined to the legs in filariasis and Milroy disease.

With pitting edema, it is necessary to look for signs of congestive heart failure (hepatomegaly, jugular venous distension, and crepitant rales at the right base), cirrhosis (hepatomegaly, ascites, spider angiomata, caput medusae, splenomegaly, and jaundice), and nephrosis (periorbital and facial edema, albuminuria). Locally, look for varicose veins and thrombophlebitis. In females, exclude a pelvic mass. Remember to look for presacral edema in patients who are bedridden (e.g., nursing home patients).

● Facial and Periorbital Edema

Looking for jugular vein distention helps differentiate a superior vena cava syndrome and congestive heart failure from the most likely cause of this condition, namely acute glomerulonephritis or nephrosis. Also in congestive heart failure, there are usually crepitant rales at the right lung base. If there is fever and chemosis, the physician should be alert to the possibility of cavernous sinus thrombosis.

● Groin Mass

Three masses are frequently found in the groin: a hernia (either femoral or inguinal), a saphenous varix, and enlarged inguinal lymph nodes. The hernia and saphenous varix are usually reducible, whereas the inguinal lymph node is not. Unless there is generalized lymphadenopathy from a systemic condition, an enlarged lymph node in the groin is associated with a lesion of the genitalia. As such, it will most invariably be tender as well.

● Hepatomegaly

Differentiating the causes of hepatomegaly begins with the character of the liver edge. A firm nontender liver edge suggests cirrhosis, whereas a smooth tender liver edge suggests hepatitis or congestive heart failure. A nodular liver surface may indicate metastatic cancer or cirrhosis.

The physician needs to palpate for an enlarged gallbladder. A large nontender gallbladder is often indicative of gallbladder hydrops (due to a cystic duct stone) or an obstructed common duct by a neoplasm (Courvoisier gallbladder). In the latter instance, there is always jaundice, whereas in the former instance, there is not. A tender gallbladder suggests cholecystitis and cholelithiasis.

Now, it is necessary to look for systemic signs of cirrhosis (spider angiomata, palmar erythema, gynecomastia, testicular atrophy, ascites, caput medusae, and hemorrhoids). Most importantly, look for splenomegaly.

One should be sure to look for the Kayser–Fleisher ring in the cornea in Wilson disease and the bronze skin in hemochromatosis, not to mention xanthelasma and tendon xanthoma in biliary cirrhosis induced by hyperlipemia.

● Neck Mass

Differentiating a neck mass that is thyroid tissue from an enlarged lymph node or other mass is no problem. The thyroid mass moves when the patient swallows. A diffuse thyroid mass can be further identified as Graves disease by looking for tremor, tachycardia, and exophthalmos. A toxic adenoma can be differentiated from a nontoxic nodule in a like manner, except the exophthalmos is not as pronounced. In Graves disease, there may be a bruit over the thyroid as well. Another neck mass that moves when the patient swallows is the thyroglossal duct cyst, but it is always in the midline. It is possible to distinguish a Zenker diverticulum by noting the increase in size when the patient swallows liquid.

The experienced clinician knows that a metastatic neoplasm of the cervical lymph nodes can be differentiated from Hodgkin disease by the fact that the metastatic neoplasm is hard whereas the lymph node hypertrophy of Hodgkin lymphoma is softer and rubbery. Transillumination may be used to help differentiate a colloid cyst of the thyroid and a thyroglossal cyst, but a negative result does not rule out either condition.

● Scrotal Mass

Transillumination is extremely useful in distinguishing a hydrocele from a hernia or testicular tumor. It is necessary to use a strong light. A varicocele can be distinguished by the fact that it disappears when the scrotum is raised above the abdomen. A hernia can be diagnosed by the fact that it is reducible unless it is incarcerated. One other sign of a hernia is that the physician cannot "get above" the swelling (i.e., feel the upper border of it) as he or she can with tumors or orchitis. Torsion of the testicle can be differentiated from orchitis by the relief of pain on elevating the testicle in torsion. Also, the cremasteric reflex is absent on the side of the torsion.

● Splenomegaly

Massive splenomegaly is typical of three conditions: kala azar, chronic myelogenous leukemia, and myeloid metaplasia. The best way to examine for an enlarged spleen is to have the patient lie on his or her right side with knees flexed almost onto the abdomen, place the fingers of one's left hand under the subcostal margin, and have the patient take deep breaths. It may be necessary to have the patient take several breaths before the physician is sure that he or she is feeling the splenic margin. Another way to verify clinically that a patient has an enlarged spleen is to do a tourniquet test because there is often a thrombocytopenia. Also, look for hepatomegaly because hepatosplenomegaly is common in many diseases (e.g., cirrhosis, reticuloendotheliosis).

BLOODY DISCHARGE

● Epistaxis

A simple nosebleed is rarely a problem. Most of these are related to bleeding from the Little area in the anterior nasal septum, and packing or cautery is a simple solution. However, when a patient experiences recurrent attacks of epistaxis, the examination must be more thorough and extensive.

The physician should check the blood pressure and eye grounds for evidence of hypertension. Check the lungs for asthma or emphysema. Careful examination of the nasal passages for allergic rhinitis, a granuloma, or neoplasm is important. Perhaps nasopharyngoscopy is necessary. Look for other sites of bleeding and perform a Rumpel–Leede test. Be sure to question the patient thoroughly about drug use and abuse.

● Hematemesis and Melena

Surely a physician is going to consult a gastroenterologist and prepare the patient with hematemesis and/or melena for endoscopy; however, one can help the gastroenterologist by looking for signs of cirrhosis such as caput medusae, hemorrhoids, ascites, jaundice, hepatosplenomegaly, spider angiomata, palmar erythema, and so on. In addition, look for signs of hereditary telangiectasia on the tongue and mucous membranes. Here again a tourniquet test should be a part of the clinical evaluation.

● Hematuria

Careful examination of the flanks for a mass (neoplasm, hydronephrosis, polycystic kidney disease) or tenderness (pyelonephritis or renal calculus) is important. It should go without saying that a thorough pelvic and rectal examination must be done. The physician should look for signs of bleeding elsewhere, and in addition to ordering a coagulation profile, he or she should not forget to do a Rumpel–Leede test. In children, one should look for other possible signs of child abuse.

● Hemoptysis

Of course, the clinical examination in cases of hemoptysis includes inspection, palpation, percussion, and auscultation of the lungs and heart. If these techniques fail to yield the answer, the physician examines the nasal passages for the source. Direct or indirect laryngoscopy may be necessary. Examining the extremities for clubbing (carcinoma of the lung, bronchiectasis, cyanotic heart disease) and edema (congestive heart failure) may be worthwhile. Finally, as in all cases of bleeding from the various body orifices, one should perform a Rumpel–Leede test before continuing the workup in the laboratory or x-ray department.

● Rectal Bleeding

No clinician would skip a rectal examination when a patient presents with this symptom, but he or she often avoids visual inspection of the anus and surrounding area because of the embarrassment. Females should have a vaginal examination as well. When the examination is negative, anoscopy should be done before proceeding with sigmoidoscopy or colonoscopy. If hemorrhoids are suspected, be sure and look for other signs of cirrhosis (e.g., hepatomegaly, spider angiomata). Look for petechiae or ecchymosis of the skin and signs of bleeding elsewhere. Once again, one should perform a Rumpel–Leede test along with a coagulation profile when a local cause for the bleeding is not found.

● Vaginal Bleeding

Usually, the physician finds the cause of vaginal bleeding by a careful history and pelvic examination; however, a rectovaginal examination is almost always necessary to check for a mass or blood in the cul-de-sac, especially if a routine examination is negative. Look for petechiae, ecchymosis, splenomegaly, and signs of bleeding elsewhere. In children, look for other signs of child abuse.

NONBLOODY DISCHARGE

● Ear Discharge

Naturally, the first thing the physician does is examine for a foreign body, wax, or pus in the external canal with an otoscope. If one of these substances is apparent, carefully remove it with a curette (plastic is best) or alligator forceps. Irrigation with a water pick after first softening the cerumen with Debrox is also possible. If one suspects otitis media, test for drum mobility with insufflation through an otoscope with a tight-fitting speculum. This can be achieved by wrapping a rubber band around the end of the speculum. An exudative otitis media is obvious, but the drum is almost normal looking with a serous otitis media. The easiest way to diagnose fluid behind the drum is to test the hearing by whispering numbers first in one ear and then the other. If there is no fluid in the inner ear, the patient can hear the whispered numbers at the same distance in both ears, or at least the hearing will be equal in both. It is also possible to use the Weber and Rinne test to detect otitis media (conductive loss on the side of the otitis media). This will be discussed on page XX. Ultimately, a tympanogram may need to be performed, and it reveals a flat line tracing with increasing pressure on the drum with otitis media, where normally there is a curved line.

● Nasal Discharge

If the discharge is purulent, the author suggests that the physician look carefully for bacterial sinusitis, most likely maxillary sinusitis, especially if it is unilateral. It may be possible to spot the discharge coming from the meatus with an otoscope using a large speculum, but transillumination is the best way to spot a maxillary or frontal sinusitis clinically. If one does not have a sinus transilluminator, use a powerful pin light with the patient in a dark room. Place the light in the mouth and compare the illumination in both maxillary sinuses. Alternatively, one can place the pin light in the orbit and examine for light coming through the palate with the mouth open.

If the discharge is clear, the turbinates will be swollen and bluish with a thin layer of mucus in allergic rhinitis. If the patient has rhinitis medicamentosum from excessive use of nasal sprays, the turbinates will be swollen, but in addition, there will be small pustules on the mucosa. With cocaine abuse, septal perforation may be apparent. In long-standing allergic rhinitis, mucous polyps are evident. In children, be sure to look for foreign bodies. Also, remember that a chronic clear nasal discharge may indicate cerebrospinal rhinorrhea.

(This may seem gross, but here is a little trick one might use to decide what type of discharge there is: have the patient blow into a tissue and examine it!)

● Rectal Discharge

A purulent rectal discharge is almost always due to a perirectal abscess. Nevertheless, the physician should examine the base of the spine and skin over the coccyx for a pilonidal sinus or abscess. On rectal examination, pinch the anal tissue between the thumb and forefinger at 3, 6, 9, and 12 o'clock positions and see if he or she obtains exudates. If the fluid is clear, there is probably a fistula in the anus. Patients with hemorrhoids often complain of a brown discharge, which is simply feces. Of course, the discharge with hemorrhoids is usually bloody and noticed after a bowel movement. The best tool for diagnosis of hemorrhoids, rectal fissures, and fistulae in the anus is an anoscope.

● Urethral Discharge

In patients with gonorrhea, the discharge is purulent, but it is almost always clear with chlamydia and balanitis. The physician must massage the prostate to diagnose the discharge in chronic prostatitis. Be sure to have the patient milk the penis down after the massage. Then one collects a drop or two of the discharge and examines it under a microscope for white blood cells. It should not be necessary to do this in cases of acute prostatitis (and indeed is ill-advised) because this can easily be diagnosed by the swollen boggy feel of the prostate. Do not forget that patients may mislead a clinician by calling a chancre or chancroid a "discharge."

● Vaginal Discharge

The physician should have no problem in differentiating the discharge of candidiasis from trichomonas because of the cheesy white appearance of the former compared with the frothy yellow appearance of the latter. He or she can do a wet saline "prep" and potassium hydroxide (KOH) "prep" as a further means of differentiating the two. One can use a Gram stain to diagnose gonorrhea or bacterial vaginitis, but culture and diagnosis by exclusion are the usual means of diagnosis. More recently, it has been possible to diagnose gonorrhea and chlamydia by sending a sample of urine to the laboratory.

One should be sure to check for infection of the Skene and Bartholin glands. Also, remember that a clear or milky white discharge is often due to chronic cervicitis, which is obvious if one uses a strong light to examine the cervix. The best way to do that is with a fiberoptic vaginoscope.

Not infrequently, a urethral discharge is the cause of the "vaginal" discharge, so be sure to milk the urethra. If the cervix is soft to palpation, the discharge may be due to pregnancy. Finally, a brownish discharge may be due to a rectovaginal fistula due to carcinoma or Crohn disease. Of course, this is a rare condition today.

FUNCTIONAL CHANGES

● Coma

In a patient presenting with coma, the physician begins the examination by looking for bruises (signifying a head injury), fractures (also signifying a head injury or fat embolism), and tongue lacerations (suggesting epilepsy). Smell the breath for evidence of alcohol intoxication, diabetic acidosis (a sweet odor), or organophosphate intoxication (garlic odor). Obviously, the vital signs may indicate the cause such as significant hypertension (hypertensive encephalopathy), rapid, irregular pulse (atrial fibrillation and a cerebral embolism), or fever (meningitis or other infectious disease).

In addition, it is necessary to do the following:

- Check the pupils. If both are constricted, consider narcotic intoxication or a pontine hemorrhage. If both are dilated, the patient may have some other form of drug intoxication. A unilateral dilated pupil suggests a ruptured cerebral aneurysm or herniation from a space-occupying lesion (hematoma, abscess, or tumor).
- Check for nuchal rigidity. If this is present, the patient probably has meningitis or subarachnoid hemorrhage. One should not neglect to perform a funduscopic examination because it may show papilledema (indicating a space-occupying lesion or hypertensive encephalopathy) or hemorrhages (suggesting a ruptured cerebral aneurysm or diabetic coma).
- Do not forget to check the skin for petechiae (suggesting subacute bacterial endocarditis) or ecchymosis (suggesting meningococcemia or trauma).
- Be alert for cherry red lips, a clear sign of carbon monoxide poisoning. Needle tracts are a tip-off for heroin addiction and a possible overdose. Listen for murmurs (suggesting the possibility of subacute bacterial endocarditis) and cardiac arrhythmias (atrial fibrillation with a cerebral embolism or Stokes–Adams syncope).
- Finally, conduct a neurologic examination to determine if there are focal neurologic signs to suggest a

space-occupying lesion or stroke (embolism, thrombosis, or hemorrhage). If there is resistance to eye opening, consider the possibility of malingering. The author had a case like this when he was a resident. Shortly after he began talking to the patient as if the man was not in a coma, he "woke up."

● Cough

When confronted with a patient complaining of cough, it is important to start with vital signs and percussion and auscultation of the chest and heart. If these examination techniques are normal, what else can one do? First of all, do a thorough ENT examination to look for rhinitis, sinusitis, and a postnasal drip. Use transillumination of the sinuses and indirect laryngoscopy to aid in this examination. Check the neck for jugular vein distention, a mass, and tracheal deviation. Check the abdomen for hepatomegaly (suggesting congestive heart failure) and the extremities for pedal edema. This is not a lot, but occasionally these examinations are rewarding.

● Diarrhea

This discussion will focus on the physical findings of chronic diarrhea, because acute diarrhea is usually due to an infectious disease and is often self-limited.

The physician looks for an enlarged thyroid (hyperthyroidism) as well as hyperpigmentation of the skin and mucous membranes (Addison disease). Flushing of the face is indicative of a carcinoid tumor. Sometimes a malignancy of the intestinal tract presents with diarrhea, so one should look for an abdominal mass. A rectal examination is essential not just to look for carcinoma or occult blood but to rule out a fecal impaction that may be the cause of diarrhea, especially in the elderly. A smooth tongue and cheilitis may suggest malabsorption syndrome as may a foaming stool that floats to the top in the commode.

Bloody diarrhea suggests ulcerative or granulomatous colitis but may be seen in colon carcinoma and diverticulitis. An enlarged liver may be a sign of metastatic carcinoma from a pancreatic or colon primary.

● Dizziness

The examination of a patient presenting with dizziness begins with an otoscope examination to rule out impacted cerumen, otitis media, drum perforation, and other middle ear pathology. The physician tests the hearing by whispering in the ear. Be sure to perform a Weber and Rinne test as well.

Next, it is necessary to determine if there are any blood pressure abnormalities such as hypertension (particularly postural hypertension) or hypotension. Obviously, the next important step is to look for cardiac arrhythmias or murmurs. Follow that with a more thorough neurological examination than one usually performs in a routine physical examination. Look for pale nails and conjunctiva or smooth tongue to rule out anemia.

Finally, perform the Hallpike maneuvers. Have the patient sit with the lower extremities extended on the examination table. After turning the patient's head to one side at least 45 degrees, abruptly lower it until it hangs over the end of the examination table and keep it there for at least 1 to 2 minutes. If one observes nystagmus or the patient experiences significant dizziness or nausea, the test is positive for benign positional vertigo. Repeat the maneuver with the head in the neutral position and then to the opposite side.

● Nausea and Vomiting

In cases of acute nausea and vomiting, especially with diarrhea and fever, the patient most likely has viral or bacterial gastroenteritis. This section does not concern these cases, nor does it concern cases of nausea and vomiting with abdominal pain. Evaluation of these cases is addressed under "Abdominal Pain" (see page XX).

Physical examination of patients with chronic nausea and/or vomiting without abdominal pain begins with looking for hepatomegaly, an abdominal mass, or focal abdominal tenderness. A rectal examination is performed, primarily to rule out melena. Obviously, a vaginal examination needs to be done in females to rule out pregnancy, a uterine fibroid, an ovarian cyst, or other gynecologic pathology.

Next, one should do a funduscopy to rule out papilledema and intracranial pathology. Also, perform an ENT examination to rule out otitis media and inner ear pathology. Check for nystagmus and do the Hallpike maneuvers to rule out benign positional vertigo.

It may be necessary to consider giving the patient sublingual nitroglycerin to see if that precipitates an attack, which would point to abdominal migraine as the cause. When all these examinations are unrewarding, the physician relies on the history and diagnostic tests to get a diagnosis.

● Numbness and Tingling of the Extremities

If the complaint is in the upper extremities, it is necessary for the physician to begin the examination by performing examinations for Tinel sign, at the wrist, and Phalen test. If these are positive, the patient may have carpal tunnel syndrome. Next, check for Tinel sign at the elbow. This is positive in ulnar neuropathy, which is usually associated with loss of sensation in the fifth finger and lateral one-half of the fourth finger. Check for a thoracic outlet syndrome by performing Adson tests (see page XX). Check for cervical radiculopathy by performing cervical compression and Spurling tests. Check the reflexes, power, and sensation to all modalities in the upper and lower extremities. If the reflexes are symmetrically depressed, consider the possibility of a polyneuropathy. If they are depressed in one or both upper extremities and increased in the lower, consider the possibility of a lesion of the cervical spinal cord.

If there are cranial nerve signs, there may be a lesion in the brain stem or cerebral cortex. Numbness and tingling and/or weakness of one side of the body usually means there is a lesion of the opposite cerebral hemisphere such as a stroke or space-occupying lesion. If the onset of the hemihypesthesia and hemihypalgesia is acute, the reflexes

on the side of the numbness and tingling will be depressed. If the onset is insidious, the reflexes will be hyperactive. In both situations, there will usually be pathological reflexes.

If the numbness or tingling is in the lower extremities, one should begin by performing a straight leg raising test and/or a femoral stretch test to rule out a herniated lumbar disc. If there is loss of sensation in a dermatomal distribution, that would also be consistent with a herniated disc or other lesion of the lumbosacral nerve roots. Always do a rectal examination to determine tone and control of the rectal sphincter and a pelvic examination to look for a uterine or ovarian mass that may be compressing the sacral plexus. Stocking hypesthesia and hypalgesia suggests a polyneuropathy but may also be seen in the subacute combined degeneration of the spinal cord associated with pernicious anemia. If the reflexes are hyperactive and there are pathological reflexes, suspect a cord tumor or multiple sclerosis. Look for a steppage gait. This is consistent with polyneuropathy, whereas a spastic gait would be consistent with multiple sclerosis or a thoracic cord lesion.

It is necessary to check the pulses in the lower extremities, not just the dorsalis pedis and posterior tibial pulses, but the popliteal and femoral pulses as well. If these are diminished, they may represent peripheral arteriosclerosis or Leriche syndrome.

If the numbness and tingling are present in only the feet, consider the possibility of tarsal tunnel syndrome or Morton neuroma, provided that the peripheral pulses are good. Rarely, numbness and tingling of the feet are due to a parasagittal meningioma.

● Palpitations

Outside of examining the heart for an arrhythmia or murmur, there are a few additional things a physician should do. First, it is necessary to check for an enlarged thyroid, exophthalmos, tremor, and diaphoresis—all findings that would point to hyperthyroidism. Remember, ingesting large amounts of caffeinated beverages can also produce tachycardia, diaphoresis, and tremor.

Next, the clinician should take the blood pressure in the recumbent and upright position to rule out postural hypotension before initiating an expensive diagnostic workup with Holter monitoring or psychometric testing. The author recommends that the patient obtain an inexpensive electronic sphygmomanometer and check the blood pressure and pulses twice daily at home for a week; this might pick up a pheochromocytoma or cardiac arrhythmia.

● Seizures

Suppose a clinician is called to the emergency department to examine a patient who has just had a grand mal seizure. What does he or she look for? All readers know that a good history is most important in establishing the diagnosis of a seizure disorder, but important steps in the physical examination are often overlooked.

First of all, the physician wants to determine if the seizure was real. Look for evidence of trauma, lacerations of the tongue, and incontinence. Also, look for postictal somnolence and hemiparesis (e.g., positive Babinski sign).

Next, rule out causes of symptomatic epilepsy. Is there an unusual odor to the breath (e.g., from alcohol, diabetic acidosis)? Is there a unilateral dilated pupil or papilledema suggesting a space-occupying lesion, aneurysm, or herniation?

Are there focal neurologic signs such as hemiparesis, cranial nerve palsies, or mental changes suggesting a stroke or space-occupying lesion? To further evaluate for a stroke, one must check the carotid artery for bruits and listen to the heart for murmurs of arrhythmias. Is there nuchal rigidity? If so, consider meningitis or a subarachnoid hemorrhage in the differential diagnosis.

Finally, it is necessary to look for skin lesions such as petechiae (suggesting subacute bacterial endocarditis), adenoma sebaceum (indicating tuberous sclerosis), fibromas (suggesting neurofibromatosis), or a port wine stain of the face (suggesting Sturge–Weber syndrome).

● Tremor

The examination of a patient presenting with tremor begins by looking for a thyroid mass, diaphoresis, exophthalmos, and tachycardia. After all, this is something the physician can "cure." Then one looks for cogwheel rigidity, a short-stepped gait, mask facies, and monotonous speech, which are all signs of parkinsonism. If a tremor is absent at rest and occurs primarily in motion or during a finger-to-nose test, it is most likely familial. Tremor on one side of the body associated with hemianalgesia and hemihypesthesia is due to a thalamic syndrome (occlusion of the thalamogeniculate artery). Look for hepatomegaly and a Kayser–Fleischer ring in the cornea in younger people with tremor to rule out Wilson disease. A unilateral intention tremor associated with ataxia may indicate a cerebellar tumor.

● Weakness or Fatigue

It is necessary to begin with a good general physical examination. Particularly, the physician should look for signs of weight loss, a thyroid or abdominal mass, hepatosplenomegaly, and lymphadenopathy. Look for other signs of hypothyroidism (e.g., tremor, diaphoresis, exophthalmos), hyperthyroidism (nonpitting edema, coarse thick nails), and Addison disease (hyperpigmentation of the skin and buccal mucosa). Clubbing may be a sign of carcinoma of the lung or cyanotic heart disease. A smooth tongue may indicate avitaminosis or pernicious anemia. Do not forget to perform a neurologic examination to exclude peripheral neuropathy, dementia, and other degenerative neurologic diseases. Recent weight gain, acne, hirsutism, and purple striae may indicate Cushing syndrome. Although many of these cases wind up in the psychiatrist's or psychologist's office, one should not give up on them too easily.

● Weight Loss

The examination of a patient with weight loss demands a thorough routine physical examination (see page XX). Look for signs of an overactive thyroid (enlarged thyroid, tremor, tachycardia, and diaphoresis). Also, look for hyperpigmentation of the skin and buccal mucosa (signs of Addison disease). One wants to examine, in particular, for hepatomegaly, splenomegaly, an abdominal mass, rectal or prostatic mass, pelvic mass, and lymphadenopathy. Look for jaundice, pale conjunctiva, smooth tongue, and clubbing. The neurologic examination should focus on the possibility of a peripheral neuropathy, muscular dystrophy, or amyotrophic lateral sclerosis. Type 1 diabetes begins with significant weight loss, so check the urine for sugar. If there is marked polyuria, think of diabetes insipidus.

INTRODUCTION

The mission of this section, which is the main body of the text, is twofold. The first part of the mission is to provide a quick reference for the busy physician who needs a list of common diseases that will explain the patient's symptoms and signs. To accomplish this, the author has listed symptoms and signs alphabetically so that they can be found without searching through the index. Then, as the clinician locates the symptoms and signs, he or she will find an illustration of the differential diagnosis for the symptom or sign. Also, in most cases, he or she will find a table listing many diseases that should be considered in the differential. Then, in the text associated with each symptom and sign, the clinician will find the laboratory tests and other diagnostic procedures that will be included in the workup of that symptom and sign. In the appendix, he or she will find the workup of specific diseases in the differential. The clinician can sharpen his or her skills by reading the case histories in each section and developing a differential diagnosis. The answers will be found in Appendix B.

The second part of the mission is to teach the clinician or student of differential diagnosis how to arrive at a list of diagnostic possibilities without referring to a textbook of differential diagnosis. After all, in the course of a busy practice, it is not usually practical to look up a differential diagnosis while interviewing or working up the patient. There has to be another way, and the author believes he has found it.

The first step is to group symptoms and signs into one or more of the following categories:

1. Pain
2. Mass
3. Bloody discharge
4. Nonbloody discharge
5. Functional changes
6. Abnormal laboratory results

Now, the basic sciences of anatomy, physiology, histology, biochemistry, and pathophysiology can be applied to each of these categories to develop a differential diagnosis. This is done as follows.

● Pain

Developing a list of causes of pain anywhere in the body is best achieved by first visualizing the *anatomy* of the area. For example, a 50-year-old man presents with chest pain of 2 hours duration. The physician visualizes the chest and sees the lung, the heart, the esophagus, the mediastinum, the aorta, ribs, and the spine. With his or her

knowledge of what is common, the physician can develop a useful list of the causes of the patient's acute chest pain as follows:

1. Lungs: Pulmonary infarction, pneumothorax
2. Heart: Myocardial infarct, coronary insufficiency, pericarditis
3. Esophagus: Reflux esophagitis or Mallory–Weiss syndrome
4. Mediastinum: Mediastinitis
5. Aorta: Dissecting aneurysm
6. Ribs: Fracture, costochondritis
7. Spine: Osteoarthritis, herniated disc, fracture

The astute clinician who is not in a hurry may want to go to a second step. This involves a more thorough consideration of the etiologies that may affect each organ. It is helpful to have a mnemonic to help recall the etiologic categories. Any one will do, but the author has found the mnemonic **VINDICATE** very useful in the differential diagnosis of pain. Applying this mnemonic to the causes of acute chest pain will provide the following possibilities:

V—Vascular suggests myocardial infarction, coronary insufficiency, pulmonary infarct, or dissecting aneurysm.

I—Inflammation suggests pericarditis or pleurisy.

N—Neoplasm might prompt the recall of a neoplasm affecting the pleura or pericardium such as mesothelioma, carcinoma of the lung, or carcinoma of the esophagus.

D—Degenerative diseases do not usually cause pain so this would not suggest any possibilities.

I—Intoxication might suggest uremic pericarditis.

C—Congenital anomalies are not usually associated with pain in the chest either; however, Marfan syndrome is associated with a dissecting aneurysm.

A—Autoimmune diseases would prompt the diagnosis of lupus pleuritis.

T—Trauma would suggest contusion or hemorrhage of the chest wall or pericardium or fracture of the spine.

E—Endocrinopathies would bring to mind a substernal thyroiditis.

Now, by combining the first and second steps in this process, one can make a very useful table of the differential diagnosis of chest pain. This is the system. Although it may seem cumbersome at first, it can become automatic and second nature with use. The benefit of this system is that one can develop this list of possibilities while interviewing the patient and begin asking meaningful questions to eliminate some of these possibilities prior to the workup. That makes it cost-effective.

● Mass

With few exceptions, anatomy and histology are the basic sciences that are most useful in developing a differential diagnosis of a mass or swelling. It works as follows:

A 38-year-old white woman presents with a history of a right upper quadrant mass. Visualizing the anatomy in the right upper quadrant, we see the gallbladder, colon, liver, duodenum, pancreas, and kidney.

By simply thinking of what is common, one can arrive at the following list of possibilities:

1. Gallbladder: Carcinoma, hydrops
2. Colon: Carcinoma
3. Liver: Hepatoma, metastatic neoplasm, cirrhosis, hepatitis
4. Duodenum: A neoplasm of the ampulla of Vater would rarely present as a right upper quadrant mass
5. Pancreas: Pancreatic neoplasm, pseudocyst of the pancreas
6. Kidney: Hypernephroma, hydronephrosis, or polycystic kidney

By visualizing the histology of each of these organs, one can broaden the list of possibilities. For example, the liver is made up of a capsule, parenchyma, fibrous tissue, ducts, arteries, and veins. Considering the capsule, one would think of hematoma or subdiaphragmatic abscess; considering the parenchyma brings to mind hepatoma; the fibrous tissue suggests alcoholic cirrhosis while the duct suggests biliary cirrhosis; the veins would prompt consideration of hepatic vein thrombosis or pyelophlebitis.

Applying the second step, as was done under the category of pain, one can develop a list of possibilities using a mnemonic. In this instance, it is helpful to use the mnemonic **MINT**. Here is how that works:

M—**Malformation** suggests hepatic or renal cysts.
I—**Inflammation** or intoxication suggests hepatitis, alcoholic cirrhosis, pancreatitis with a pseudocyst, cholecystitis, subdiaphragmatic abscess, liver abscess, perinephric abscess, or diverticular abscess.
N—**Neoplasm** suggests hematoma, metastatic neoplasm, cholangiocarcinoma, carcinoma of the pancreas, hypernephroma, or colon carcinoma.
T—**Trauma** would bring to mind laceration, contusion, or hematoma of any one of these organs.

Once again, by putting the anatomy and/or histology together with the etiologic classification, one can develop a very useful table (see page 19).

Now, the clinician has a list of possibilities that will help him or her ask the right questions in the interview with the patient. It will also help the clinician to determine which tests to order in the workup.

● Bloody Discharge

Any body orifice may be the site of a bloody discharge. It usually is the cause of great alarm, as it should be in most cases. That is because a bloody discharge often signifies malignancy. In most cases, a bloody discharge should be considered malignant until proven otherwise.

What basic science should be used to develop the differential diagnosis of a bloody discharge? The answer is anatomy, of course. For example, a 56-year-old woman complains of hematuria for several hours. The clinician knows the site of bleeding may be anywhere along the urinary tract. Starting from the bottom up, he or she can visualize the urethra, bladder, ureters, and kidneys. By simply applying one's knowledge of what is common, it is possible to develop a useful list of diagnoses as follows:

1. Urethra: Urethritis, stone
2. Bladder: Cystitis, stone, neoplasm
3. Ureter: Stone
4. Kidney: Stone, glomerulonephritis, neoplasm, polycystic kidney

The astute clinician will want a more exacting and extensive list of diagnostic possibilities. To obtain this, he or she can proceed to the second step: Recalling the etiologic possibilities by using a mnemonic such as **VANISH** as follows:

V—**Vascular** suggests embolism, thrombosis, or subacute bacterial endocarditis.
A—**Anomaly** suggests polycystic kidney, double ureter, horseshoe kidney, hereditary nephritis, and medullary sponge kidney.
N—**Neoplasm** suggests hypernephroma, Wilms tumor, or carcinoma of the bladder or prostate.
I—**Inflammation** suggests cystitis, pyelonephritis, glomerulonephritis, or tuberculosis.
S—**Stones** can be found in the kidney, ureter, bladder, or urethra and are a common cause of hematuria.
H—**Hemorrhage** should bring to mind trauma anywhere along the urinary tract as well as hematologic disorders such as Henoch–Schönlein purpura, disseminated intravascular coagulation (DIC), and hypoprothrombinemia.

Here again, one can combine steps one and two to make a very useful table of the diagnostic possibilities (see Table 35). Now having a list of possible causes of the patient's symptoms makes the interview and workup more meaningful.

● Nonbloody Discharge

The differential diagnosis of a nonbloody discharge, like that of a bloody discharge, begins with the basic science of *anatomy*. Visualizing where the discharge could come from means visualizing the anatomic "tree" or tract of the organ system involved. Unlike a bloody discharge, a nonbloody discharge is most likely due to inflammation. For example, a 48-year-old black man presents with a productive cough of 2 weeks duration. Visualizing the respiratory tree, we find the nasopharynx, larynx, trachea, bronchi, and alveoli. Now, translating each structure into common inflammatory diseases that may involve each of them, we can develop a useful list of diagnostic possibilities as follows:

1. Nasopharynx: Rhinitis, sinusitis
2. Larynx: Laryngitis
3. Trachea: Tracheobronchitis

4. Bronchi: Bronchitis, bronchiectasis, foreign body, bronchial asthma
5. Alveoli: Pneumonia, lung abscess, pneumoconiosis, congestive heart failure

Proceeding to the second step, we can develop a list of causes of productive sputum further by recalling the etiologic categories of respiratory diseases with the help of the mnemonic **MINT**. This would translate into a list of diagnoses as follows:

M—Malformations do not lead to a nonbloody discharge of themselves but predispose to infection. Bronchiectasis and lung cysts are examples of malformations in the lung that can cause productive sputum.

I—Inflammation would bring to mind rhinitis, sinusitis, pharyngitis, laryngitis, tracheobronchitis and abscess, or pneumonia. Hay fever and asthma should be included here.

N—Neoplasms predispose to infection. Thus a bronchogenic carcinoma or bronchial adenoma may cause pneumonia or bronchitis with productive sputum.

T—Toxins would be suggested by this category and should bring to mind pneumoconiosis, foreign body, and lipoid pneumonia as causes of a nonbloody discharge.

As with the other symptom categories, a differential diagnosis table can be constructed by combining the first and second steps in this process (see page 393, Table 53).

One can develop inflammation further by thinking of the smallest organism to the largest. Considering the alveoli or lung would prompt recall of viral pneumonia, mycoplasma, psittacosis, bacterial pneumonia or tuberculosis, fungal pneumonia such as histoplasmosis, and parasitic infestation such as *Pneumocystis carinii* or *Echinococcus*.

Now, with these diagnostic possibilities in mind, one can proceed with the interview asking meaningful questions that will help pinpoint the diagnosis.

● Functional Changes

Functional changes take place because of an alteration in the physiology or biochemistry of an organ system. Consequently, a differential diagnosis can be best developed by using physiology or biochemistry. For example, a 24-year-old black woman presents with a 2-day history of jaundice and anorexia. Jaundice results from an elevation in the bilirubin level in the blood. Using pathophysiology, one can appreciate that an increased serum bilirubin may result from increased *production* of bilirubin as occurs in hemolytic anemia or decreased *excretion* of bilirubin by a diseased liver or obstructed biliary tree. Now, one can translate these categories into a list of possibilities using common causes as follows:

1. Increased production: Sickle cell anemia, hereditary spherocytosis, acquired hemolytic anemia
2. Decreased excretion by a diseased liver: Viral hepatitis, toxic hepatitis, cirrhosis
3. Decreased excretion due to bile duct obstruction: Biliary cirrhosis, common duct stone, neoplasm

This list may be abbreviated, but it would provide the clinician with a basis for a meaningful interview of the patient and a logical laboratory workup. Thinking of increased production, one would ask about other symptoms of sickle cell anemia, such as joint pain, cramps, and the fever of sickle cell crisis. Thinking of bile duct obstruction, one would ask about previous attacks of right upper quadrant pain with fever and nausea or vomiting to substantiate a diagnosis of cholecystitis or common duct stone.

In the workup, one would not forget to order a serum haptoglobin level to exclude hemolytic anemia or sickle cell preparation. One would also consider a gallbladder sonogram if the hepatitis profile were normal.

Now, for a more extensive list of possibilities, a second step can be taken to develop functional changes like jaundice using etiologic categories. The mnemonic **MINT** can be applied as follows:

M—Malformation would help recall congenital bile duct atresia and hereditary hemolytic anemias.

I—Inflammation would bring to mind viral hepatitis, amebic abscess, lupoid hepatitis, and acquired hemolytic anemia.

N—Neoplasm would suggest hepatoma, carcinoma anywhere along the biliary tree, and metastatic carcinoma.

T—Toxins would remind one of chlorpromazine, carbon tetrachloride, alcoholic cirrhosis, and so on.

A third step can be taken to develop a table as has been done in the other categories of symptoms or signs previously discussed.

● Abnormal Laboratory Values

As with functional changes, the principal basic sciences used to develop the differential diagnosis of abnormal laboratory values will be physiology and biochemistry.

For example, the clinician has just received a complete blood cell count showing a reduction of hemoglobin and hematocrit. Using physiology, he or she can recall that anemia may develop from a decreased intake or absorption of iron, B_{12}, or folic acid, a decreased production of red cells in the bone marrow, or increased destruction of red cells in the spleen or blood circulation. Now, the clinician can prepare a simple list of possibilities using common etiologies as follows:

1. Decreased intake: Iron deficiency anemia, starvation, folic acid deficiency
2. Decreased absorption: Pernicious anemia, malabsorption syndrome
3. Decreased production: Aplastic anemia, myelophthisic anemia
4. Increased destruction: Hemolytic anemia, DIC, malaria, etc.

The list of possibilities can be expanded by taking this sign to the second and third steps, as demonstrated above.

A unique feature of this fourth edition is the case histories in each section. This allows the student to test his or her ability to apply what has been learned. The correct answers are in Appendix B.

The methods outlined in this introduction now will be applied to each symptom and sign in the rest of this book. It is the hope of the author that the reader will eventually be able to apply these methods smoothly and efficiently in his or her daily practice of medicine.

One other method that has assisted the author immensely in his quest for a diagnosis is prayer. The Bible says, "the Lord will give wisdom to anyone who asks for it" (James 1:5). It is highly recommended that this method be applied in the daily practice of medicine also.

A

A

ABDOMINAL MASS

● Abdominal Mass, Generalized

As the physician examines the abdomen, how can he or she recall all of the causes of a mass or swelling? The physician should consider the possibilities for the mass's composition. It may be **air**, in which case the physician would think of air in the peritoneum with rupture of a viscus, particularly a peptic ulcer, or it may be air in the intestinal tract from focal or generalized distention, in which case the physician would recall gastric dilatation, intestinal obstruction related to numerous causes (see page 18), or paralytic ileus. The mass may be **fluid**, in which case the physician would recall fluid in the abdominal wall (anasarca), the peritoneum (ascites, page 3) and its various causes, and fluid (urine) accumulation in the bladder or intestine or cysts of other abdominal organs. The lWatter brings to mind ovarian, pancreatic, and omental cysts. The mass may be **blood** in the peritoneal wall, the peritoneum, or any of the organ systems of the abdomen. The mass may be a solid **inorganic substance**, such as the fecal accumulation in celiac disease and Hirschsprung disease. Finally, the mass may be a **hypertrophy**, **swelling**, or **neoplasm** of any one of the organs or tissues in the abdomen.

This is where **anatomy** comes in. In the abdominal wall, there may be an accumulation of fat (obesity). The **liver** may be enlarged by neoplasm or obstruction of its vascular supply (e.g., Budd–Chiari syndrome or cardiac cirrhosis) or by obstruction of the biliary tree with neoplasms or biliary cirrhosis. The **spleen** may become massively enlarged by hypertrophy, hyperplasia in Gaucher disease, infiltration of cells in chronic myelogenous leukemia and myeloid metaplasia, or by inflammation in kala azar. The **kidney** rarely enlarges to the point at which it causes a generalized abdominal swelling in hydronephrosis, but a Wilms tumor or carcinoma may occasionally become extremely large.

The **bladder**, as mentioned above, may be enlarged sufficiently to present a generalized abdominal swelling when it becomes obstructed, but a neoplasm of the bladder will not present as a huge mass. The **uterus** presents as a generalized abdominal mass in late stages of pregnancy, but ovarian cysts should be first considered in huge masses arising from the female genital tract. Pancreatic cysts and pseudocysts are possible causes of a generalized abdominal swelling, although they are usually localized to the right upper quadrant (RUQ) or epigastrium. It would be unusual for an aortic aneurysm to grow to a size sufficient to cause a generalized abdominal mass, but it is frequently mentioned in differential diagnosis texts.

The above method is one method of developing a differential diagnosis of generalized abdominal swelling or mass. Relying solely on anatomy and cross-indexing the various structures with the mnemonic **MINT** is another. This mnemonic is suggested as an exercise for the reader. Take each organ system as a tract. Thus, the **gastrointestinal (GI) tract** presents most commonly with a diffuse swelling in intestinal obstruction and paralytic ileus; the **biliary tract** and pancreas with hepatitis, neoplasms, and pancreatic pseudocysts. The **urinary tract** presents with a diffuse "mass" in bladder neck obstruction. The female genital tract may be the cause of a huge abdominal mass in ovarian cysts, neoplasms, and pregnancy. Apply the same technique to the spleen and abdominal wall to complete the picture.

There are, in addition, certain conditions that cause abdominal swelling that is more apparent than real. Lumbar lordosis causes abdominal protuberance, as does visceroptosis. A huge ventral hernia or diastasis recti may mimic an abdominal swelling. Psychogenic protrusion of the belly by straining is another cause.

Approach to the Diagnosis
What can be done to work up a diffuse abdominal swelling? It is important to catheterize the bladder if there is any question that this may be the cause. A flat plate of the abdomen and lateral decubiti and upright films will help in diagnosing intestinal obstruction, a ruptured viscus, or peritoneal fluid. A pregnancy test must be done in women of childbearing age. If pregnancy or ovarian cysts can be definitively excluded by ultrasonography, then a computed tomography (CT) scan or diagnostic peritoneal tap may be helpful in the diagnosis.

Other Useful Tests
1. Complete blood count (CBC)
2. Amylase and lipase levels (pancreatic pseudocyst)
3. Liver profile (ascites)
4. Laparoscopy (ovarian cysts, metastatic carcinoma, tuberculous peritonitis)
5. Lymphangiogram (retroperitoneal sarcoma)
6. Surgery consult
7. Gynecology consult
8. Exploratory laparotomy
9. Alpha-fetoprotein (hepatoma)

● Right Upper Quadrant Mass

When the clinician lays his or her hand on the RUQ and feels a mass, he or she should visualize the anatomy and the differential diagnosis should become clear. Proceeding from the skin, the physician encounters the subcutaneous tissue, fascia, muscle, peritoneum, liver, hepatic flexure of the colon, gallbladder, duodenum, pancreas, kidney, and adrenal gland. The blood vessels and lymphatics to these organs and the bile and pancreatic ducts should be considered. Then, because masses are caused by a limited

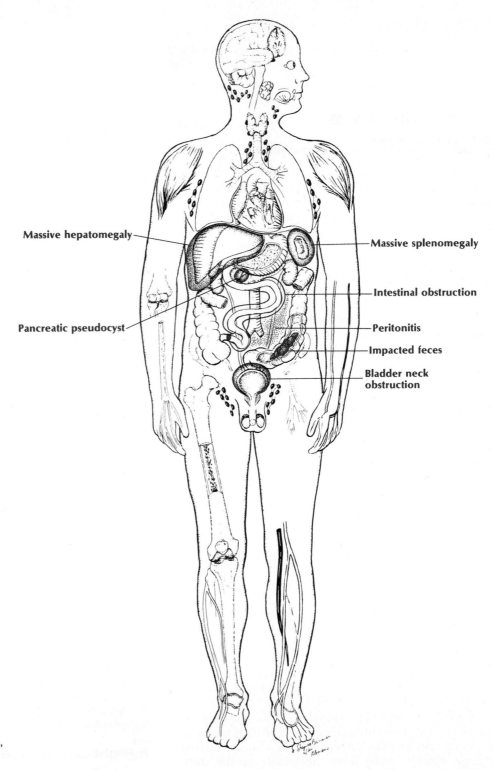

● **FIGURE 1** Abdominal mass, generalized.

number of etiologies, apply the mnemonic **MINT** to each organ. The differential using these methods is developed in Table 1.

Skin malformations do not usually cause a mass, but inflammation of the skin is manifested by cellulitis and carbuncles, and neoplasms are manifested as carcinomas, both primary and metastatic. Trauma of the skin is usually manifested by obvious contusions or lacerations. A mass of the **subcutaneous tissue** may be a lipoma, fibroma, metastatic carcinoma, cellulitis, or contusion. A mass disease of the **fascia** is usually the result of a hernia. The causes of hepatomegaly are reviewed on page 226, but if the mass is in the liver, it is usually hepatitis, amebic or septic abscess, carcinoma (primary or metastatic), contusion,

A

TABLE 1   Right Upper Quadrant Mass

	M Malformation	I Inflammation	N Neoplasm	T Trauma
Skin	Sebaceous cyst	Abscess	Carcinomas (primary or metastatic)	Contusion
Subcutaneous Tissue and Fascia	Hernia	Cellulitis	Metastatic carcinoma Lipoma	Contusion
Muscle		Myositis		Contusion
Liver	Cyst Riedel lobe	Abscess Hepatitis	Carcinoma (primary and metastatic)	Contusion Laceration
Hepatic Flexure of Colon	Diverticulum Malrotation	Diverticulitis Retrocecal appendix	Carcinoma of the colon	Contusion Perforation
Gallbladder and Ducts	Hydrops	Cholecystitis Cholelithiasis	Pancreatic carcinoma Cholangioma Choledochal carcinoma	Contusion
Duodenum		Perforation of ulcer with subphrenic abscess		
Pancreas	Pancreatic cyst	Acute and chronic pancreatitis	Carcinoma of the head of the pancreas	Traumatic pseudocyst
Kidney	Renal cyst Hydronephrosis Polycystic kidney	Hydronephrosis Pyonephrosis Perinephric abscess	Wilms tumor Hypernephroma	Contusion Laceration
Adrenal Gland			Neuroblastoma Pheochromocytoma Adrenal carcinoma	
Lymph Nodes			Hodgkin lymphoma Metastatic carcinoma	

or laceration. A Riedel lobe should not be mistaken for a large gallbladder. The **hepatic flexure of the colon** may be enlarged by diverticulitis, carcinoma, granulomatous colitis, contusion, or volvulus. Malrotation may cause a mass in infants. A retrocecal appendix should not be forgotten here either.

An enlarged gallbladder accounts for the mass in the RUQ in many cases. The enlargement may be caused by cholecystitis, obstruction of the neck of the cystic duct by a stone causing gallbladder hydrops, Courvoisier–Terrier syndrome caused by obstruction of the bile duct by carcinoma of the head of the pancreas, or cholangiocarcinoma.

The **pancreas** may be enlarged in M—**Malformations** by congenital or acquired pancreatic cysts, I—**Inflammation** of an acute or chronic pancreatitis, N—**Neoplasm**, and T—**Traumatic** pseudocysts.

A **duodenal** diverticulum is not usually felt as a mass, but a perforated duodenal ulcer may manifest itself by a palpable subphrenic abscess in the right anterior intraperitoneal pouch. Malformations of the **kidney** often cause

hydronephrosis, whereas inflammation may cause a perinephric abscess and thus an RUQ mass. Carcinoma or Wilms tumor of the kidney is frequently responsible for a large kidney.

Carcinoma of the **adrenal gland** is not usually palpable until late in the disease process, but a neuroblastoma is palpable early. Other lesions of the adrenal gland are not usually associated with a mass.

Aneurysms, emboli, and thromboses of the vessels supplying these organs usually do not produce a mass, but a thrombosis of the hepatic vein (the well-known Budd–Chiari syndrome) causes hepatomegaly, and emboli and thrombi of the mesenteric vessels of the colon may cause focal enlargement from obstruction and infarction. Visualizing the lymphatics should recall Hodgkin lymphoma in the portal area.

Approach to the Diagnosis
Acute onset of the RUQ mass with a history of trauma is no doubt a laceration or contusion of the liver or kidney: A surgeon should be consulted immediately. When an

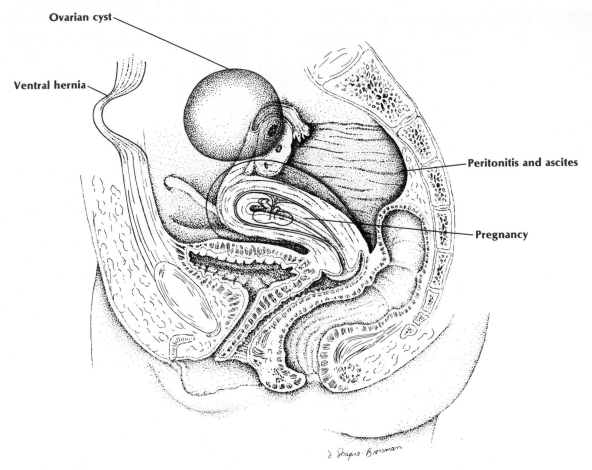

Ovarian cyst

Ventral hernia

Peritonitis and ascites

Pregnancy

J. Shapiro-Brennman

● **FIGURE 2** Abdominal mass, generalized.

RUQ mass is discovered unexpectedly or during a routine physical examination, one may proceed more deliberately. Ultrasonography will help determine if the mass is a gallbladder, liver, or pancreatic cyst. A CBC, chemistry profile, and liver panel will help determine if the mass is hepatic in origin. An intravenous pyelogram (IVP), urinalysis, or urine culture will help determine if it is renal in origin. However, a CT scan can resolve the dilemma quickly in most cases so it may be the most cost-effective approach. Then, one can determine which specialist to refer the patient to without hesitation. It is important to remember that whereas most masses will require referral to a specialist, fecal impactions and abdominal wall hematomas can be handled by the primary care physician.

Other Useful Tests
1. Amylase and lipase levels (pancreatic carcinoma, pancreatic cysts)
2. Barium enema (colon carcinoma)
3. Cholecystogram (gallstones)
4. Gallium scan (subphrenic abscess)
5. Aortogram (aortic aneurysm)
6. Small-bowel series (tumor)
7. Gastroenterology consult
8. Exploratory laparoscopy

Case Presentation #1

A 56-year-old white man who complained of mild weight loss and loss of appetite for 3 months is found to have an RUQ mass on examination.

Question #1. Utilizing the methods described above, what is your list of possibilities at this point?

Your physical examination also reveals icteric sclera, clay-colored stools, and slight hepatomegaly.

Question #2. What is your differential diagnosis now?

(See Appendix B for the answers.)

● Left Upper Quadrant Mass

The differential diagnosis for left upper quadrant (LUQ) masses is not a great deal different from that of the RUQ. The anatomy is similar: Just replace the liver with the spleen and the gallbladder with the stomach. The presence of the aorta on the side of the abdomen should not be forgotten. Again, **anatomy** is the key, as shown in Table 2. Cross-index the various organs and tissues with the etiologies using **MINT** as the mnemonic.

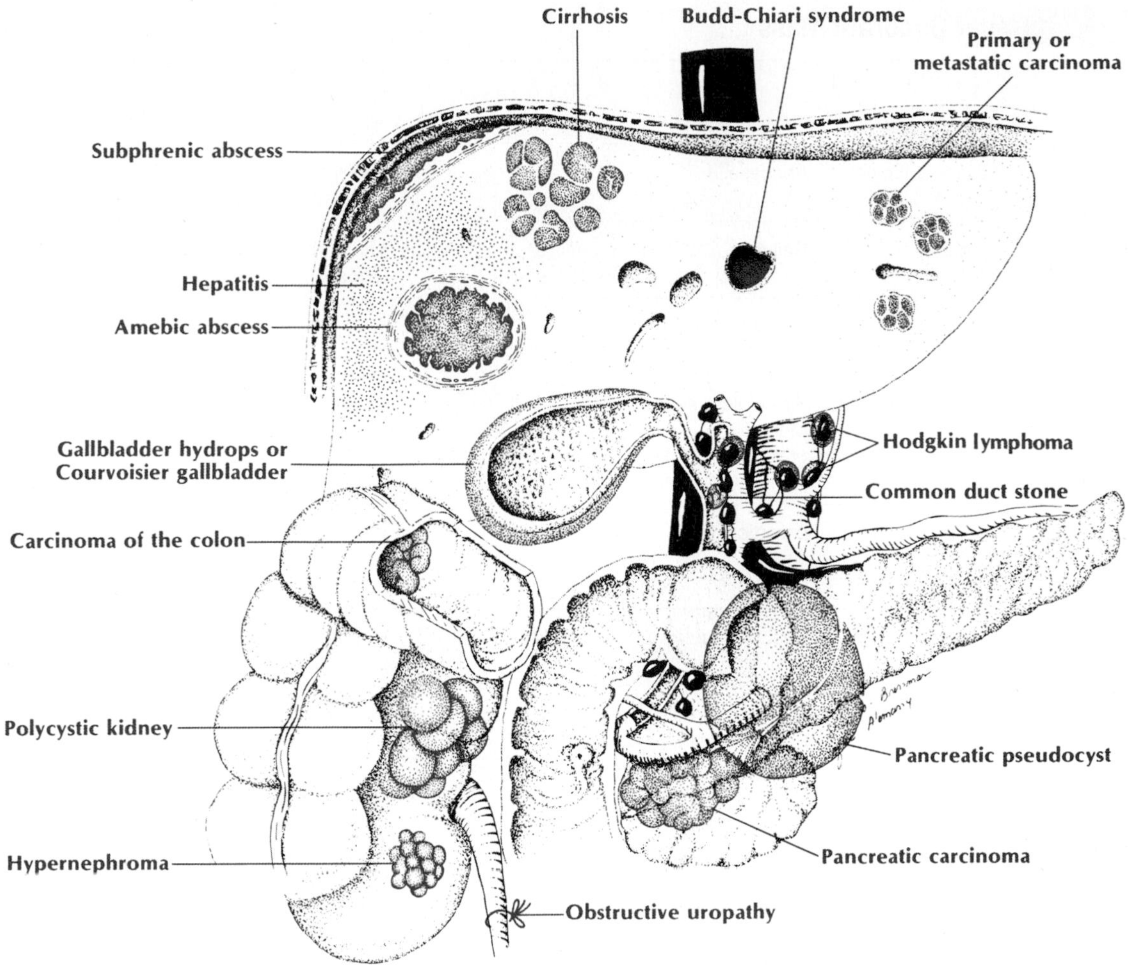

● **FIGURE 3** Abdominal mass, right upper quadrant.

M—**Malformations** of the skin, subcutaneous tissue, fascia, and muscle are usually hernias; for the spleen, they are **aneurysms**; for the splenic flexure of the colon, they are mainly volvulus, intussusceptions, and diverticula. Gastric dilatation of the stomach is caused by obstruction or pneumonia. Cysts are common for the pancreas, just as polycystic disease, single cysts, and hydronephrosis are common for the kidney. There is no common malformation for the adrenal gland.

I—**Inflammatory** conditions of the skin, subcutaneous tissue, muscle, and fascia are usually abscesses and cellulitis. In the spleen, a host of systemic inflammatory lesions can cause enlargement (see page 392), but primary infections of the spleen are unusual. The colon may be inflamed by diverticulitis, granulomatous colitis, and, occasionally, by tuberculosis. Inflammatory disease of the stomach does not usually produce a mass, but if an ulcer perforates or if a diverticulum ruptures, a subphrenic abscess may form in the left hypochondrium. Inflammatory pseudocysts may form in the tail of the pancreas. A palpable perinephric abscess and an enlarged kidney from acute pyelonephritis or tuberculosis may be felt, but inflammatory lesions of the adrenal gland are rarely palpable.

N—**Neoplasms** of the organs mentioned above account for most of the masses in the LUQ. Carcinoma of the stomach or colon, Hodgkin lymphoma, chronic leukemias involving the spleen, Wilms tumor, carcinoma of the kidney, and neuroblastoma must be considered. A retroperitoneal sarcoma is occasionally responsible for an LUQ mass.

T—**Trauma** to the spleen or kidney will produce a tender mass in the LUQ. Less common traumatic lesions here include contusion of the muscle and perforation of the stomach or colon. It should be noted that the left lobe of the liver may project into the LUQ; therefore, tumor and abscess of the liver must be considered.

Approach to the Diagnosis

The presence or absence of other symptoms and signs is the key to the clinical diagnosis of an LUQ mass. The presence of jaundice would suggest that the mass is a large spleen. The presence of blood in the stool would suggest carcinoma of the colon. The presence of hematuria would suggest that the mass is renal in origin. An enema should be done to exclude fecal impaction before an extensive workup is performed.

A conservative workup will include a CBC, sedimentation rate, urinalysis, chemistry panel, platelet count, stool

TABLE 2 **Left Upper Quadrant Mass**

	M Malformation	I Inflammation	N Neoplasm	T Trauma
Skin	Sebaceous cyst	Abscess	Carcinoma (primary or metastatic)	Contusion
Subcutaneous Tissue and Fascia	Hernia	Cellulitis	Metastatic tumor Lipoma	Contusion
Muscle		Myositis		Contusion
Spleen	Aneurysm Accessory spleen	Tuberculosis Systemic disease Malaria	Hodgkin lymphoma Chronic leukemia	Contusion Laceration
Stomach	Gastric dilatation	Perforated ulcer with subphrenic abscess	Carcinoma of the stomach	Perforation
Splenic Flexure of the Colon	Diverticulum Volvulus Intussusception	Diverticulitis	Carcinoma of the colon	Contusion Perforation
Pancreas	Pancreatic cyst	Pseudocyst from pancreatitis	Carcinoma of the pancreas	Traumatic pseudocyst
Kidney	Hydronephrosis Polycystic kidney Renal cyst	Hydronephrosis Pyonephrosis Perinephric abscess	Wilms tumor Hypernephroma	Contusion Laceration
Adrenal Gland			Neuroblastoma Pheochromocytoma Adrenal carcinoma	
Lymph Nodes			Hodgkin lymphoma Retroperitoneal lymphosarcoma	
Blood Vessels	Aortic aneurysm			

for occult blood, coagulation profile, and a flat plate of the abdomen. On the basis of these results, the clinician can determine whether to do an upper GI series, barium enema, IVP, or CT scan of the abdomen. Another approach would be to do the CT scan immediately. In the long run, the latter approach may be more cost-effective. It is usually prudent to get a surgical or gastroenterological consult to help decide between the two approaches.

Other Useful Tests
1. Amylase and lipase levels (pancreatic pseudocyst or tumor)
2. Bone marrow examination (splenomegaly)
3. Liver–spleen scan (splenomegaly)
4. Sonogram (renal cyst, pancreatic cyst)
5. Colonoscopy (colon carcinoma)
6. Laparoscopy
7. Biopsy of mass (neoplasm)
8. Gallium scan (abscess)

● Right Lower Quadrant Mass

Anatomy is once again the key to developing a differential diagnosis of a right lower quadrant (RLQ) mass.

Underneath the skin, subcutaneous tissue, fascia, and muscle lie the cecum, appendix, terminal ileum, iliac artery and vein, and ileum. In the female, the fallopian tube and ovary should be included. Occasionally a ptosed kidney also will be felt here. Now, apply the etiologic mnemonic **MINT** to each organ, and you should have a reliable differential diagnosis, like that in Table 3. The important lesions to remember here are the following:

M—**Malformations** such as inguinal and femoral hernias may be present.
I—**Inflammations** include acute appendicitis with abscess, tubo-ovarian abscesses, and regional ileitis.
N—**Neoplasms** to be considered in this area are carcinoma of the cecum and ovarian tumors.
T—**Traumatic** lesions include fracture or contusion of the ileum and perforation of the bowel from a stab wound.

The lymph nodes may be involved with tuberculosis or actinomycosis. The cecum may also be enlarged by accumulation of *Ascaris* or other parasites. The omentum can contribute to adhesions of the bowel to form a mass, or it may develop cysts.

A

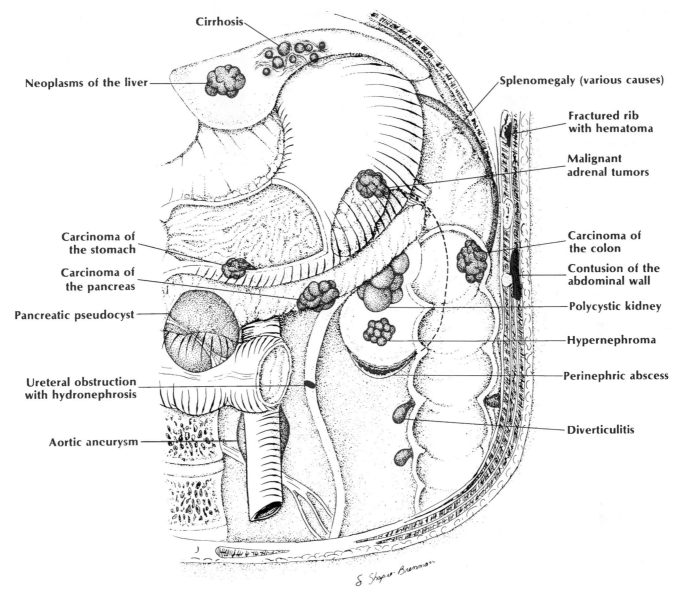

Cirrhosis

Neoplasms of the liver

Splenomegaly (various causes)

Fractured rib with hematoma

Malignant adrenal tumors

Carcinoma of the stomach

Carcinoma of the pancreas

Pancreatic pseudocyst

Carcinoma of the colon

Contusion of the abdominal wall

Polycystic kidney

Hypernephroma

Ureteral obstruction with hydronephrosis

Perinephric abscess

Aortic aneurysm

Diverticulitis

S. Shapiro-Brennan

● **FIGURE 4** Abdominal mass, left upper quadrant.

Approach to the Diagnosis

As with other abdominal masses, it is important to look for other symptoms and signs that will help determine the origin of the mass. If there are fever and chills, an appendiceal or diverticular abscess is possible. Blood in the stool suggests a diagnosis of colon carcinoma. If there is amenorrhea or vaginal bleeding in a woman of childbearing age, an ectopic pregnancy must be considered. A long history of chronic diarrhea with or without blood in the stools suggests Crohn disease.

The initial workup will include a CBC, sedimentation rate, chemistry panel, stool for occult blood, pregnancy test, and flat plate of the abdomen. If there is fever and an acute presentation, consultation with a general surgeon to consider an immediate exploratory laparotomy is indicated.

With a more insidious onset of the RLQ mass, the clinician has a choice of ordering a CT scan of the abdomen and pelvis after performing the initial diagnostic studies or proceeding systematically with a barium enema, IVP, or small-bowel series to determine the origin of the mass. A gastroenterology or gynecology consult may be the best way to resolve this dilemma.

Other Useful Tests

1. Sonogram (ectopic pregnancy)
2. Peritoneal tap (ruptured ectopic, peritoneal abscess)
3. Colonoscopy (colonic neoplasm)
4. Serum protein electrophoresis (plasmacytoma)
5. Indium scan (peritoneal abscess)
6. Aortogram (aortic aneurysm)
7. Lymphangiogram (retroperitoneal tumor)
8. Laparoscopy (neoplasm, ectopic pregnancy)

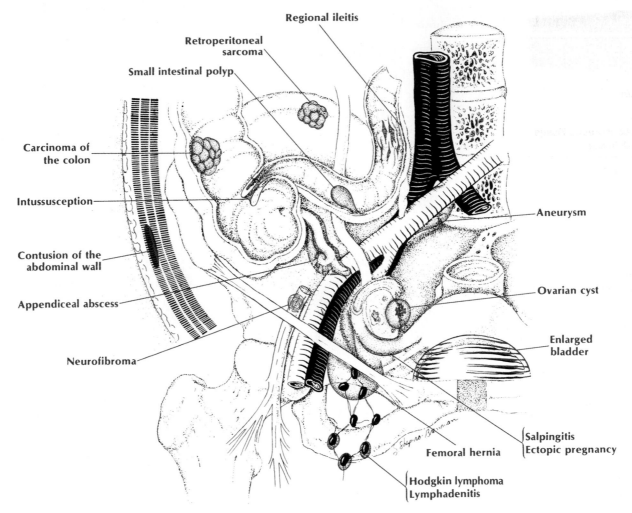

● **FIGURE 5** Abdominal mass, right lower quadrant.

Case Presentation #2

A 12-year-old white boy complained of sore throat, fever and chills, and nausea and vomiting for 3 days. On examination, he was found to have an RLQ mass.

Question #1. Utilizing the methods described above, what is your list of possible causes at this point?

There is marked tenderness and rebound over the mass. Laboratory evaluation showed a white blood cell (WBC) count of 18,500 with a shift to the left. A peritoneal tap revealed mucopurulent fluid.

Question #2. What are your diagnostic possibilities now?

(See Appendix B for the answers.)

● Left Lower Quadrant Mass

To quickly develop a list of etiologies of a left lower quadrant (LLQ) mass, visualize the **anatomy** of the area. Compared to the RUQ, the number of organs there is few. Beneath the skin, subcutaneous tissue, fascia, and muscle are the sigmoid

colon, the iliac artery and veins, the aorta, and the ileum. In the female, one must remember the fallopian tube and ovary. Occasionally, the kidney drops into this region (nephroptosis) and the omentum may cause adhesion. Now apply the mnemonic **MINT** to each organ and the list of possibilities in Table 4 is completed without any difficulty.

Lesions of the **skin** and **fascia** are similar to those in upper quadrants with one exception: Because of the inguinal and femoral canals, hernias (especially indirect inguinal hernias) are much more frequent. In the **sigmoid colon** the following conditions should be considered:

M—**Malformations** include diverticula and volvulus.
I—**Inflammatory** conditions include diverticulitis, abscesses, and granulomatous and ulcerative colitis.
N—**Neoplasms** such as polyps and carcinomas may be present.
T—**Trauma** to this area may involve perforations and contusions.

This list excludes an important consideration, that of fecal impaction. If the patient is given an enema, the mass will often disappear. Less common causes of masses in the sigmoid colon are tuberculosis and amebiasis and other parasites.

Table 3	Right Lower Quadrant Mass			
	M **Malformation**	**I** **Inflammation**	**N** **Neoplasm**	**T** **Trauma**
Skin	Sebaceous cyst	Abscess	Primary or metastatic carcinoma	Contusion
Subcutaneous Tissue and Fascia	Hernia	Cellulitis	Metastatic carcinoma Lipoma	Contusion
Cecum	Intussusception Diverticulum Intestinal obstruction	Diverticulitis Granulomatous colitis Parasites Amebiasis Ulcerative colitis	Carcinoma of the cecum	Perforation Contusion
Muscle		Psoas abscess Myositis		Contusion
Appendix	Fecalith	Appendicitis Appendiceal abscess	Carcinoid	Perforation
Terminal Ileum	Intussusception Meckel diverticulum Intestinal obstruction	Regional ileitis Typhoid Tuberculosis	Polyp Carcinoid Sarcoma	Perforation Contusion
Iliac Blood Vessels	Aneurysm	Thrombophlebitis		
Lymph Nodes		Tuberculous adenitis	Metastatic tumor	
Ilium		Osteomyelitis	Sarcoma	Fracture or contusion

There may be aneurysms of the **iliac artery** or **aorta** and thrombosis of the **iliac vein**, although the latter is not usually palpable. The **iliac lymph nodes** may enlarge from Hodgkin lymphoma, metastatic carcinoma, or tuberculosis. **Tubal** and **ovarian** lesions that should come to mind are malignant and benign ovarian cysts, tubo-ovarian abscesses, ectopic pregnancy, and endometriosis. A sarcoma or other tumor of the **ileum** may be palpable, but abscesses of the sacroiliac joint are rarely palpable.

Approach to the Diagnosis

The approach to this diagnosis includes a careful pelvic and rectal examination, a search for the presence of blood in the stool, a history of weight loss, tenderness of the mass, fever and other symptoms, and a laboratory workup. As mentioned above, an enema may diagnose and treat a fecal impaction. A surgical consult is wise at this point. Stool examination (for blood, ova, and parasites), sigmoidoscopy, and barium enemas are the most useful diagnostic procedures other than a colonoscopy. Arteriography and gallium scans (for diverticular and other abscesses) and the CT scan have become useful additions to the diagnostic armamentarium. Peritoneoscopy and exploratory laparotomy are still necessary in many cases.

Other Useful Tests

1. Sonogram (ovarian cyst, ectopic pregnancy)
2. Peritoneal tap (ruptured ectopic, peritoneal abscess)
3. IVP (pelvic kidney)
4. Pregnancy test (ectopic pregnancy)
5. CBC (infection, anemia)
6. Sedimentation rate (abscess, pelvic inflammatory disease [PID])
7. Gastroenterology consult

● Epigastric Mass

In developing the differential diagnosis of an epigastric mass, one merely needs to visualize the anatomy of the epigastrium from skin to spine. The conditions are presented in outline form in Table 5, but the important conditions are emphasized in the following discussion.

1. **Abdominal wall:** Here the physician must consider ventral hernias, contusions in the wall, the xiphoid cartilage (which occasionally fools the novice), and lipomas or sebaceous cysts.
2. **Diaphragm:** A subphrenic abscess may be felt here.
3. **Liver:** The liver extends into the epigastrium and occasionally into the LUQ; thus, any cause of hepatomegaly (see page 220) may present as an epigastric mass.
4. **Omentum:** This may be enlarged by a cyst, a mass of adhesions, tuberculoma, or metastatic carcinoma.
5. **Stomach:** The acute dilatation in pneumonia or pyloric stenosis needs to be recalled. However, one usually thinks of carcinoma of the stomach or a perforated ulcer when this organ is visualized.

TABLE 4   Left Lower Quadrant Mass

	M Malformation	I Inflammation	N Neoplasm	T Trauma
Skin	Sebaceous cyst	Abscess	Primary and metastatic carcinomas	Contusion
Subcutaneous Tissue and Fascia	Hernia	Cellulitis	Metastatic carcinoma Lipoma	Contusion
Muscle		Myositis		Contusion
Sigmoid Colon	Intestinal obstruction	Diverticulum Volvulus Diverticulitis and abscess Tuberculosis Granulomatous and ulcerative colitis	Carcinoma and polyp	Perforation Contusion Foreign body
Tube and Ovary	Hydatid cyst of Morgagni Ectopic pregnancy	Tubo-ovarian abscess	Ovarian cyst and carcinoma	
Iliac Artery and Veins and Aorta	Aneurysm	Thrombophlebitis		
Lymph Nodes		Tuberculous and acute infectious adenitis	Metastatic tumor	
Ilium		Osteomyelitis	Sarcoma	Fracture or contusion

6. **Colon:** Carcinoma, toxic megacolon, or diverticulitis may cause a mass in this organ, but a hard chunk of feces also may do so.
7. **Pancreas:** Important conditions that must be considered here are carcinoma of the pancreas and pancreatic cysts. Occasionally, chronic pancreatitis may present as a mass.
8. **Retroperitoneal lymph nodes:** Lymphoma, retroperitoneal sarcoma, and metastatic tumor may make these nodes palpable.
9. **Aorta:** An aortic aneurysm may be felt, but more often the examiner is fooled by a normal or slightly enlarged aorta.
10. **Spine:** Deformities of the spine (e.g., lordosis) may make it especially prominent, but a fracture, metastatic neoplasm, myeloma, or arthritis may do the same.

Approach to the Diagnosis
The association of other symptoms and signs are very helpful in determining the origin of an epigastric mass. If there is jaundice, the mass is probably an enlarged liver. Fever and chills suggests a subphrenic abscess displacing the liver downward or an abscessed gallbladder. A mass associated with a history of anorexia and wasting suggests pancreatic or gastric carcinoma. A history of alcoholism suggests that the mass is an enlarged liver or pancreatic pseudocyst. Blood in the stool suggests carcinoma of the stomach or colon. A history of constipation would warrant a cleansing enema to rule out a fecal impaction before ordering an expensive workup. If the mass pulsates, one would consider an aortic aneurysm in the differential diagnosis.

The initial workup should include a CBC, urinalysis, chemistry panel, amylase and lipase levels, stool for occult blood, and flat and upright x-rays of the abdomen. If a presentation is acute, a general surgeon should be consulted to consider immediate exploratory laparotomy. If the development was more insidious and the patient is in no acute distress, a more systematic workup can be done at this point. Based on the results of the initial workup, one can proceed with an upper GI series, a barium enema, or ultrasonography of the gallbladder and pancreas. However, a more expeditious route to the diagnosis would be to order a CT scan of the abdomen. It is wise to consult a surgeon or gastroenterologist to help decide what method would be the most cost-effective and prudent.

Other Useful Tests
1. Liver function tests (cirrhosis or carcinoma of the liver)
2. Hepatitis profile (hepatitis)
3. Gastroscopy (gastric carcinoma)
4. Colonoscopy (colon carcinoma)
5. Peritoneal tap (metastatic neoplasm, peritonitis)
6. Laparoscopy (metastatic neoplasm)
7. Aortogram (aortic aneurysm)
8. Gallium scan (subphrenic abscess)

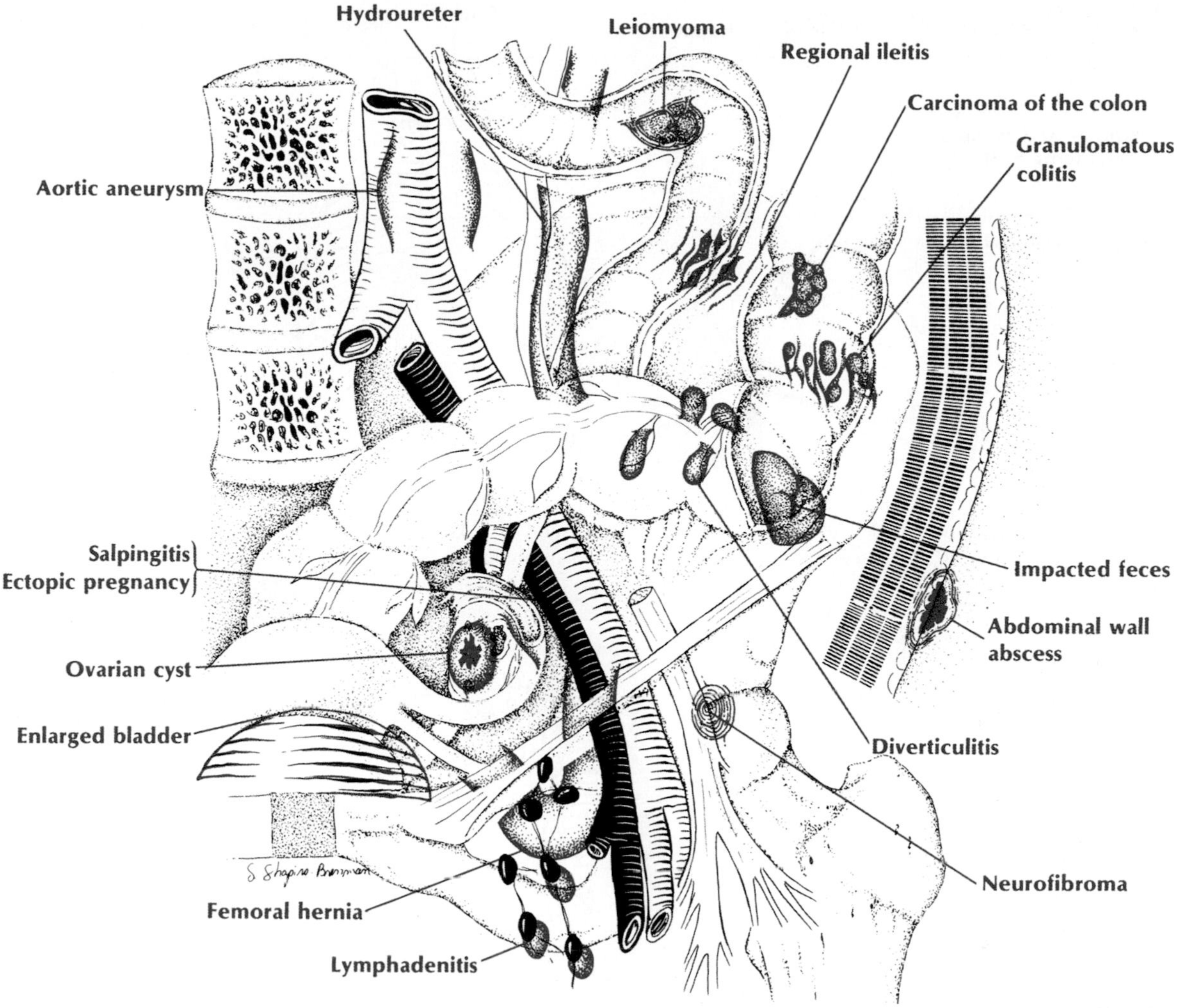

A

● FIGURE 6 Abdominal mass, left lower quadrant.

 9. Liver biopsy (cirrhosis, neoplasm)
10. Liver–spleen scan (hepatomegaly)
11. Exploratory laparotomy
12. Bentiromide excretion test (chronic pancreatitis)

Case Presentation #3

A 42-year-old alcoholic black man was found to have a midepigastric mass on examination.

Question #1. Utilizing the methods described above, what are the various diagnostic possibilities?

   Additional history reveals that he has been hospitalized for recurrent bouts of acute pancreatitis in the past. His serum amylase and lipase were mildly elevated. His stool is negative for occult blood.

Question #2. What are the diagnostic possibilities now?

(See Appendix B for the answers.)

● Hypogastric Mass

More physicians have been fooled by a hypogastric mass than by a mass in any other area. How many times can you recall the mass disappearing on the operating table after catheterization of the bladder? More often than not, the mass is more apparent than real because of a lumbar lordosis or a diastasis recti.

   Anatomy is the key to the differential diagnosis. There are not many organs here normally. Under the skin, subcutaneous tissue, fascia, and rectus abdominus muscles, the bladder, terminal aorta, and lumbosacral spine may be palpated in a thin male. In the female, the uterus may be palpated on bimanual pelvic examination. When there is visceroptosis, the transverse colon will be palpated.

   Under pathologic conditions, however, the lymph nodes, sigmoid colon, fallopian tube and ovary, and small intestines may be palpated as well as a pelvic kidney. Applying the mnemonic **MINT** to these organs results in the extensive differential diagnosis in Table 6. The discussion that follows mentions only the most significant causes of a hypogastric mass.

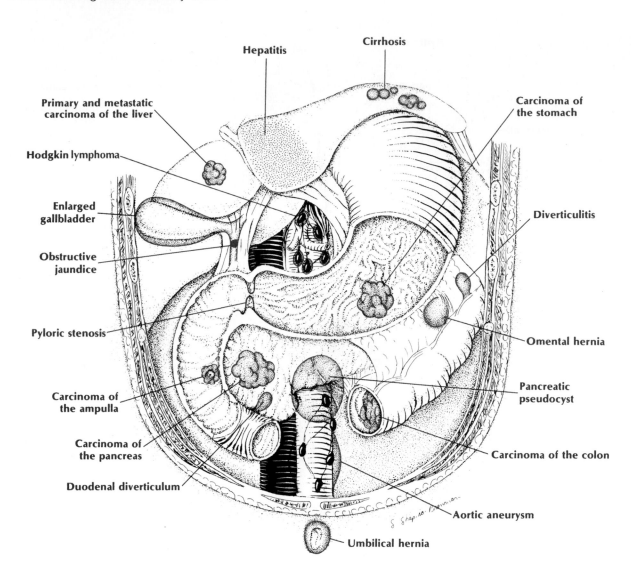

● **FIGURE 7** Abdominal mass, epigastric.

Lipomas of the skin, ventral hernias, and diastasis recti form the most frequently encountered disorders in the covering of the hypogastrium. The **bladder** may be obstructed by strictures and prostatism (see page 351), but bladder carcinoma and stones may also be palpable. Bladder rupture should be considered in trauma to the perineum. The **uterus** may be enlarged by pregnancy, endometritis, fibroid, choriocarcinoma, or endometrial carcinoma. An **ovarian** or **tubal mass** may be caused by a benign or malignant ovarian cyst, an ectopic pregnancy, or a tubo-ovarian abscess. The **aorta** may present as a mass in aneurysms or thrombosis and severe arteriosclerosis of the terminal aorta. Finally, the **lumbosacral spine** may present as a hypogastric mass in the severe lordosis of Pott disease, spondylolisthesis, metastatic carcinoma, and lumbar spondylosis. The **preaortic lymph nodes** may greatly enlarge in tuberculosis, Hodgkin lymphoma, and metastatic carcinoma. If the **transverse colon** drops to the hypogastrium, a carcinoma or inflamed and abscessed diverticulum may be felt. Volvulus may present a mass here.

Ascites from cirrhosis of the liver, ruptured abdominal viscus, or bacterial or tuberculous peritonitis is often encountered and is difficult to differentiate from an ovarian cyst and a distended bladder. Careful percussion or ultrasonic evaluation will be extremely helpful, but a peritoneoscopy or a peritoneal tap in the lateral quadrants may be necessary.

Approach to the Diagnosis
Before the clinician can evaluate a hypogastric mass, it is important to have the patient empty his or her bladder. If the mass is still present, catheterization for residual urine or ultrasonography can determine if the mass is a distended bladder due to a neurogenic bladder or bladder neck obstruction. If there are objective neurologic findings, there may be a neurogenic bladder and the patient should be referred to a neurologist. If the clinician suspects bladder neck obstruction, a referral to a urologist is in order.

After the possibility that the mass is a distended bladder has been excluded, one should consider ruling out pregnancy in women of childbearing age. A pregnancy test is done: If the test is positive, ultrasonography may be done, particularly if an ectopic pregnancy is suspected or the patient denies that she could be pregnant.

A

TABLE 5	**Epigastric Mass**			
	M **Malformation**	**I** **Inflammation**	**N** **Neoplasm**	**T** **Trauma**
Abdominal Wall	Hernia	Cellulitis Carbuncles	Lipoma Sebaceous cyst	Contusion
Diaphragm	Hiatal hernia	Subphrenic abscess		
Liver	Cyst Hemangioma	Abscess Hepatitis	Hepatoma Metastatic carcinoma	Contusion Laceration
Omentum	Adhesion Cyst	Peritonitis Tuberculoma	Metastatic carcinoma	Traumatic fat necrosis Hemorrhage
Stomach	Hypertrophic pyloric stenosis	Gastric ulcer Gastric dilatation Gastric syphilis	Gastric carcinoma	Hemorrhage Stab wound
Colon	Hirschsprung disease Intussusception Volvulus	Diverticulitis Toxic megacolon	Colon carcinoma Polyp	Contusion Laceration
Pancreas	Cyst Pseudocyst	Pancreatitis	Carcinoma of pancreas	Contusion
Retroperitoneal Lymph Nodes		Tuberculosis	Lymphoma Sarcoma Metastatic carcinoma	
Aorta	Aneurysm			
Spine	Lordosis Scoliosis	Tuberculosis Arthritis Osteomyelitis	Metastatic carcinoma Myeloma Hodgkin lymphoma	Fracture Herniated disc Hematoma

After a distended bladder and pregnancy have been removed from consideration, the next step would be a CT scan of the abdomen and pelvis. It is probably wise to consult a gynecologist, general surgeon, or urologist before ordering this expensive test. Their wisdom may make the test unnecessary.

Other Useful Tests
1. Stool for occult blood (rectal carcinoma)
2. CBC
3. Urinalysis (bladder neoplasm or stone)
4. Urine culture (cystitis, bladder diverticulum)
5. IVP (malformation neoplasm, pelvic kidney)
6. Barium enema (rectal or sigmoid carcinoma)
7. Colonoscopy (sigmoid or colon carcinoma)
8. Culdoscopy (ectopic pregnancy, ovarian cyst)
9. Laparoscopy (ovarian cyst, ectopic pregnancy, other pelvic mass)
10. Exploratory laparotomy
11. Aortogram (aortic aneurysm)
12. X-ray of the lumbosacral spine (deformities of the spine)
13. Lymphangiogram (retroperitoneal lymph nodes)

ABDOMINAL PAIN

● Abdominal Pain, Generalized

The **GI tract** is the only "organ" that really covers the abdomen from one end to the other. Anything that causes an irritation of all or a large portion of this "tube" may cause generalized abdominal pain. Thus, gastritis, viral and bacterial gastroenteritis, irritable bowel syndrome, ulcerative colitis, and amebic colitis fall into this category. The remainder of the causes of generalized abdominal pain can be developed by using the mnemonic **ROS** with the anatomy of the entire abdomen.

When faced with a patient with diffuse abdominal pain, think of **R** for **ruptured viscus**. Now take each organ and consider the possibility of its having ruptured. Thus, the stomach and duodenum suggest a ruptured peptic ulcer; the pancreas, an acute hemorrhagic pancreatitis; the gallbladder, a ruptured cholecystitis. The liver and spleen usually rupture from trauma, whereas the fallopian tube may rupture from an ectopic pregnancy. The colon ruptures from diverticulitis, ulcerative colitis, or carcinoma. What is the one thing that should make the

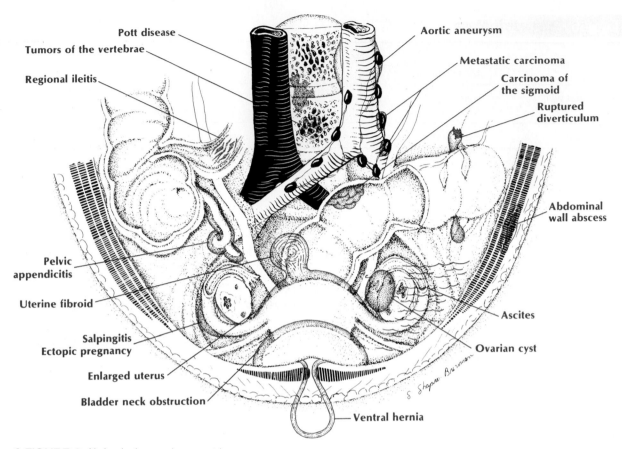

● **FIGURE 8** Abdominal mass, hypogastric.

physician suspect a ruptured viscus? Rebound tenderness is the answer. In addition, one or both testicles may be drawn up (Collins sign). If only the right testicle is drawn up, suspect a ruptured appendix or peptic ulcer. If only the left is drawn up, suspect a ruptured diverticulum. If both are drawn up, suspect pancreatitis or a generalized peritonitis.

Now take the letter **O**. This signifies intestinal **obstruction**. Think of adhesion hernia, volvulus, paralytic ileus, intussusception, fecal impaction, carcinoma, mesenteric infarction, regional ileitis, and malrotation. The best way to recall all these is with the mnemonic **VINDICATE**.

Next take the letter **S**. This signifies the **systemic** diseases that may irritate the intestines, the peritoneum, or both. Once again the mnemonic **VINDICATE** will remind one to recall the important offenders.

V—Vascular suggests the anemias, congestive heart failure (CHF), coagulation disorders, and mesenteric artery occlusion, embolism, or thrombosis.

I—Inflammatory includes tuberculous, gonococcal and pneumococcal peritonitis, and trichinosis.

N—Neoplasms should suggest leukemia and metastatic carcinoma.

D—Deficiency might suggest the gastroenteritis of pellagra.

I—Intoxication reminds one of lead colic, uremia, and the venom of a black widow spider bite.

C—Congenital suggests porphyria and sickle cell disease.

A—Autoimmune brings to mind periarteritis nodosa, rheumatic fever, Henoch–Schonlein purpura, and dermatomyositis.

T—Trauma would suggest the paralytic ileus of trauma anywhere, the crush syndrome, and hemoperitoneum.

E—Endocrine disease suggests diabetic ketoacidosis, addisonian crisis, and hypocalcemia.

Approach to the Diagnosis

If the onset is acute, a general surgeon should be consulted at the outset. Ominous signs include boardlike rigidity, rebound tenderness, and shock with nausea and vomiting. With a history of trauma and hypotension, peritoneal lavage may diagnose a ruptured spleen. Hyperactive bowel sounds of a high-pitched tinkling character with distention and obstipation suggest intestinal obstruction. In contrast, normal bowel sounds, little distention, good vital signs, and minimal tenderness suggest gastroenteritis or other diffuse irritation of the bowel.

It is wise to pass a nasogastric tube and attach to suction and proceed with a CBC, urinalysis, an immediate flat plate and upright films of the abdomen, chest x-ray, serum amylase and lipase levels, and chemistry panel. Sometimes, lateral decubitus films are necessary to reveal the stepladder pattern of intestinal obstruction. A pregnancy test should be ordered if age and gender dictates it.

If these tests fail to confirm the clinical diagnosis and the patient's condition is deteriorating, it is probably wise

TABLE 6 Mass in the Hypogastrium

	M Acquired or Congenital Malformation	I Inflammation	N Neoplasm	T Trauma
Skin	Sebaceous cyst	Abscess	Primary and metastatic tumors Lipoma	Contusion
Subcutaneous Tissue and Fascia	Ventral hernia	Cellulitis	Primary and metastatic tumors Lipoma Neurofibroma	Contusion
Muscle	Diastasis recti	Myositis		Contusion
Bladder	Diverticulum Obstruction Stone		Carcinoma of bladder or prostate Prostatic hypertrophy	Ruptured bladder
Transverse Colon	Diverticulum Volvulus Intussusception	Diverticular abscess Granulomatous colitis Toxic megacolon	Carcinoma of colon	Contusion Perforation
Uterus	Pregnancy Endometriosis	Endometritis Parametritis	Fibroids Endometrial carcinoma Cervical carcinoma Choriocarcinoma	Perforation Contusion
Tube and Ovary	Ectopic pregnancy	Tubo-ovarian abscess	Ovarian cyst (benign and malignant)	Perforation Rupture
Aorta	Aneurysm Leriche syndrome Arteriosclerosis			Perforation
Lumbosacral Spine	Spondylolisthesis Lordosis	Pott disease Osteomyelitis	Metastatic tumor	Herniated disc
Preaortic Lymph Nodes		Tuberculous adenitis	Metastatic carcinoma Hodgkin lymphoma	Herniated disc
Peritoneum	Obstruction of portal vein with ascites	Ascites from tuberculosis or gonorrhea	Metastatic carcinoma with ascites	Bloody ascites from perforation of viscus

to proceed immediately with an exploratory laparotomy. If the patient's condition is stable, one may order more diagnostic tests depending on the location of the pain and other symptoms and signs. For example, if the pain seems more localized to the RUQ, a gallbladder ultrasound or nuclear scan may be ordered. If it is still considered generalized, perhaps a CT scan of the abdomen and pelvis is indicated. Monitoring vital signs and doing repeated CBCs, serum amylase levels, and flat plates of the abdomen are useful in borderline cases.

Other Useful Tests
1. Quantitative urine amylase level
2. Four-quadrant peritoneal tap (peritonitis, pancreatitis, ruptured ectopic pregnancy)
3. Urine porphobilinogen (porphyria)
4. IVP (renal calculus)
5. Serial cardiac enzymes (myocardial infarct)
6. Serial electrocardiograms (ECGs)
7. Double enema (intestinal obstruction)
8. Esophagoscopy (reflux esophagitis)
9. Gastroscopy (peptic ulcer)
10. Colonoscopy (diverticulitis, carcinoma)
11. Laparoscopy (ruptured viscus, PID)
12. Culdocentesis (ruptured ectopic pregnancy)
13. Pelvic sonogram (ruptured ectopic pregnancy)
14. Angiogram (mesenteric thrombosis)
15. Breath test or stool tests for *Helicobacter pylori* (peptic ulcer)
16. Lipid profile (hypertriglyceridemia and chylomicronemia syndrome)

● Right Upper Quadrant Pain

The patient is complaining of RUQ pain and you cannot just give him or her a bag of pills and send him or her home.

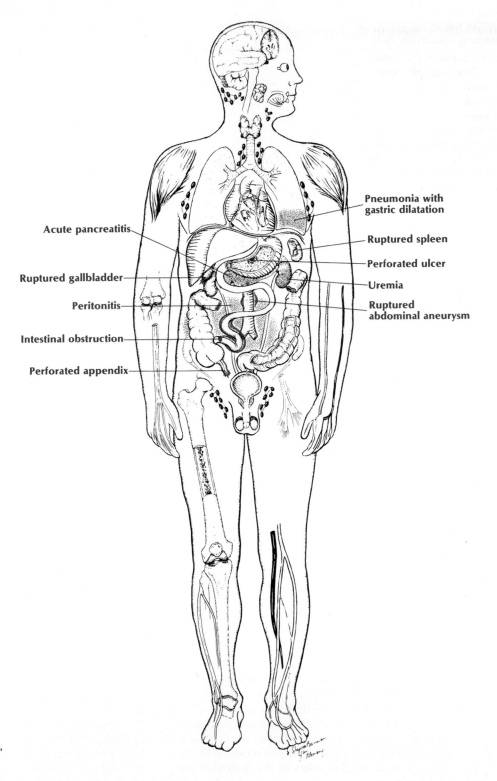

Acute pancreatitis

Ruptured gallbladder

Peritonitis

Intestinal obstruction

Perforated appendix

Pneumonia with gastric dilatation

Ruptured spleen

Perforated ulcer

Uremia

Ruptured abdominal aneurysm

● **FIGURE 9** Abdominal pain, generalized.

The patient's condition may be serious. However, you are in a hurry to get out of the office because you have another important appointment. What do you do? The key is to visualize the **anatomy**. Imagine the liver, gallbladder, bile ducts, hepatic flexure of the colon, duodenum, and head of the pancreas. Surrounding these are the skin, fascia, ribs, and thoracic and lumbar spine, with the intercostal nerves and arteries and abdominal muscle.

Pain is usually from **inflammation**, **trauma**, or **infarction**. The patient gives no history of trauma, but he or she could have a contusion of the muscle from coughing hard. That is not likely, however, unless the patient has other symptoms of the respiratory tract.

The possible sources of inflammation should be narrowed down first. The **liver** can be inflamed from hepatitis (most likely viral), the **gallbladder** from **cholecystitis** (most likely induced by stones and bacteria), or the **bile ducts** from cholangitis. The **colon** may be involved with diverticulitis, a segment of granulomatous colitis, or perhaps there is a retrocecal appendix. The **duodenum**, of course, would most likely have a peptic ulcer which could cause an obstruction or a perforation if the patient is vomiting, or pallor and shock if the patient is bleeding. The **pancreas** could be inflamed with pancreatitis, especially if the patient drinks alcohol.

These are the most important intra-abdominal considerations, but if the mnemonic **VINDICATE** in Table 7 were applied one might not forget the Budd–Chiari syndrome (thrombosis of the hepatic veins), portal vein thrombosis, or pyelophlebitis; these are rare. In addition, toxic hepatitis from isoniazid, thorazine, and erythromycin estolate (Ilosone), for example, can be painful. Collagen diseases affecting the liver are another possibility.

Now let us round out the differential diagnosis with extra-abdominal disorders. The **skin** may be involved with herpes zoster or cellulitis. A **fascial rent** may cause a hernia, particularly if there was previous upper abdominal surgery. Compression of the **nerve roots** by a herniated disc, thoracic spondylosis, or a spinal cord tumor is possible, but unlikely. Systemic conditions, such as lead colic and porphyria, and involvement of another organ, such as the kidney, must be considered (pyelonephritis or renal colic).

Approach to the Diagnosis

As in the case of generalized abdominal pain, an immediate CBC, urinalysis, chemistry profile, serum amylase and lipase levels, and flat plate and upright films of the abdomen are ordered. If cholecystitis is suspected, ultrasonography or nuclear scanning of the gallbladder (hepatoiminodiacetic acid [HIDA] scan) is ordered. If there is jaundice, a common duct stone can be ruled out by endoscopic retrograde cholangiopancreatography (ERCP).

Other Useful Tests

1. Surgery consult
2. CT scan of the abdomen
3. Quantitative urine amylase
4. Urine porphobilinogen (porphyria)
5. Gallium scan (subphrenic abscess)
6. IVP (renal stone)
7. Liver function studies (common duct stone)
8. Blood lead level
9. Pregnancy test (ruptured ectopic pregnancy)
10. X-ray of thoracolumbar spine (radiculopathy)
11. Laparoscopy (ruptured viscus)
12. Aortogram (dissecting aneurysm)
13. Lymphangiogram (Hodgkin lymphoma)
14. Exploratory laparotomy
15. MRI
16. Endoscopic ultrasonography

A

Case Presentation #4

A 38-year-old obese white woman complained of RUQ pain, nausea, and vomiting of 2 days duration.

Question #1. Utilizing the methods applied above, what is your list of possible causes at this point?

Further history reveals the pain is colicky; she is the mother of four children and had a few similar attacks in the past 5 years but never this severe. Examination reveals icteric sclera, tenderness, and rebound in the RUQ but no mass or hepatomegaly.

Question #2. What is your list of possibilities at this point?

(See Appendix B for the answers.)

● Left Upper Quadrant Pain

Anatomy is the key to recalling the many causes of abdominal pain in the LUQ by visualizing the structures layer by layer. In the first layer are the skin, abdominal wall, and ribs; in the second layer, the spleen, colon, and stomach; and in the third layer, the pancreas, adrenal gland, kidney, aorta, and spine. Now it is possible to cross-index the organs with the various etiologies contained in the mnemonic **VINDICATE** (Table 8). The following discussion emphasizes the most important of these.

1. **Abdominal wall and ribs:** Pain will occur most commonly from herpes zoster, contusion, hernia, rib fracture, or metastatic tumor.
2. **Spleen:** Painful splenic infarcts are not unusual in subacute bacterial endocarditis (SBE), polycythemia, sickle cell anemia, leukemia, periarteritis nodosa, and other autoimmune disorders. A ruptured spleen is an important consideration in abdominal injuries, particularly those in children and in patients with infectious mononucleosis.
3. **Stomach:** Acute gaseous distention of the stomach in gastritis, pneumonia, and pyloric obstruction is a common cause of LUQ pain. Gastric carcinoma that extends beyond the wall of the stomach may cause pain. Episodic obstruction of the stomach in the "cascade stomach" should be considered in the differential diagnosis. Herniation of the stomach through the diaphragm occasionally causes LUQ pain.
4. **Colon:** An inflamed diverticulum or an inflamed splenic flexure from granulomatous colitis may cause pain in the LUQ. Less commonly, the colon develops a perforating or constricting carcinoma in this area, which obstructs the bowel. A mesenteric infarct of the colon, as well as gas or impacted feces in the splenic flexure, may also cause LUQ pain.
5. **Pancreas:** Acute pancreatitis, pancreatic pseudocyst, and carcinoma of the pancreas may cause LUQ pain.
6. **Adrenal gland:** Adrenal infarction from emboli or Waterhouse–Friderichsen syndrome may cause pain, but neoplasms rarely do until they have become massive.

TABLE 7 Right Upper Quadrant Pain

	V Vascular	I Inflammatory	N Neoplasm	D Degenerative	I Intoxication or Idiopathic	C Congenital or Acquired Anomaly	A Autoimmune or Allergic	T Trauma	E Endocrine	Foreign Body
Skin		Herpes zoster Cellulitis								
Muscle and Fascia		Diaphragmatic abscess Trichinosis				Ventral hernia Incisional hernia		Contusion Cough Hemorrhage		
Liver	Infarct Pyelophlebitis	Hepatitis Hepatic abscess	Carcinoma		Alcoholic hepatitis			Contusion Laceration		
Gallbladder		Cholecystitis Cholangitis	Cholangioma					Traumatic rupture		Calculus
Duodenum	Mesenteric thrombosis	Ulcer Duodenitis			Ulcer·	Diverticulum Obstruction				
Colon		Diverticulitis Colitis				Diverticulum Obstruction				
Pancreas		Pancreatitis	Pancreatic carcinoma			Cyst				Calculus
Lymph Nodes		Mesenteric adenitis	Hodgkin lymphoma Lymphosarcoma							
Adrenal Gland	Adrenal infarct	Waterhouse–Friderichsen syndrome Tuberculosis	Neuroblastoma Adrenal carcinoma							
Kidney	Occlusion Embolism Renal vein thrombosis	Pyelonephritis			Gout	Hydronephrosis		Contusion Laceration	Hyperparathyroidism	Calculus
Thoracic Spine		Tuberculosis Osteomyelitis	Primary, metastatic, multiple myeloma	Osteoarthritis			Rheumatoid spondylitis	Herniated disc Fracture		
Referred	See Table 11									

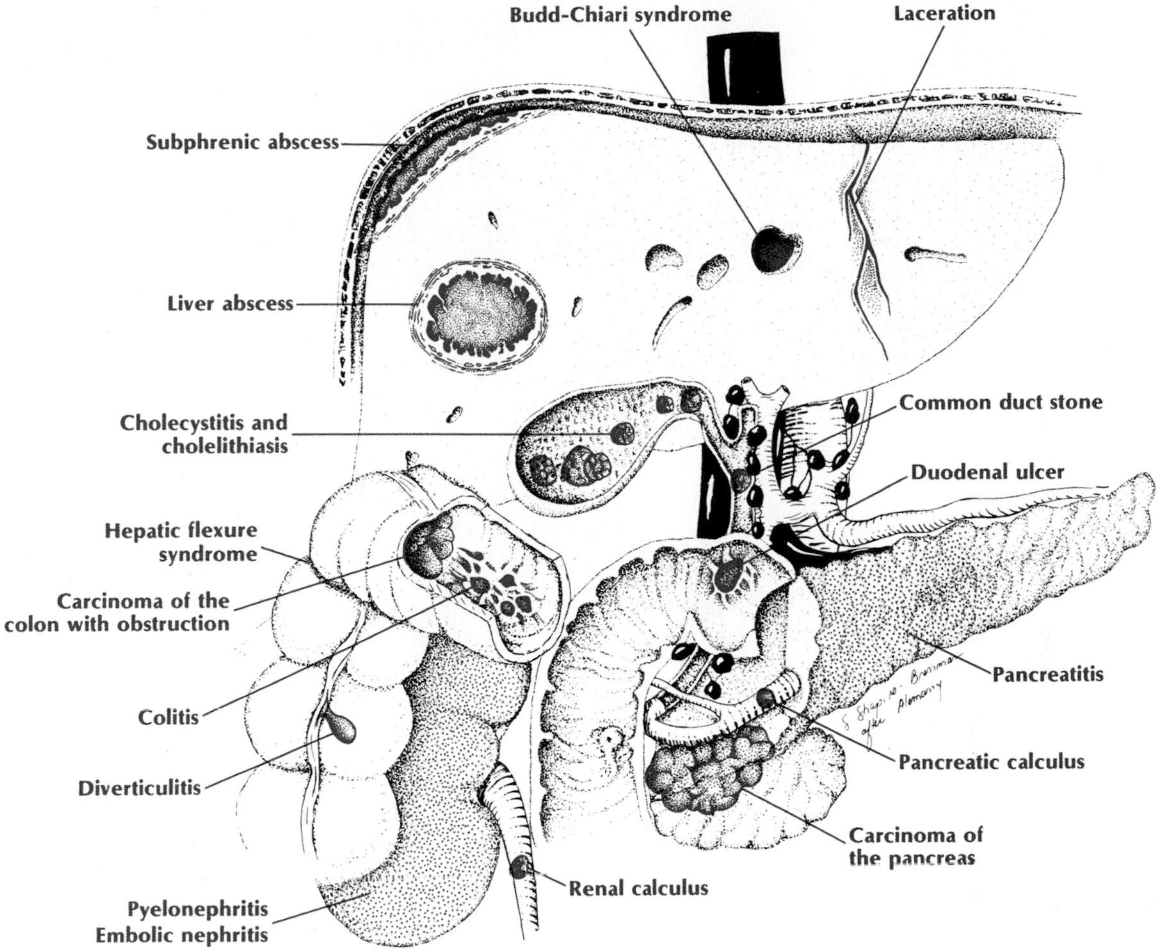

● **FIGURE 10** Abdominal pain, right upper quadrant.

7. **Kidney:** Renal infarct, renal calculus, acute pyelonephritis, and nephroptosis with a Dietl crisis may cause LUQ pain. Perinephric abscess must also be considered.
8. **Aorta:** Dissecting or atherosclerotic aneurysms of the aorta may cause LUQ pain, especially when they occlude a feeding artery to one of the structures there.
9. **Spine:** Herniated disc, tuberculosis, multiple myeloma, osteoarthritis, tabes dorsalis, spinal cord tumor, and anything else that may compress or irritate the intercostal nerve roots can cause LUQ pain.

Approach to the Diagnosis
The presence or absence of other symptoms and signs will be most helpful in the diagnosis. In acute cases, a surgeon is consulted and a flat plate of the abdomen, CBC, urinalysis, and perhaps a serum amylase level should be done. If necessary, a CT scan of the abdomen is also done. Gastroscopy and colonoscopy may be desirable before other x-rays are done. In chronic cases, however, an upper GI series, barium enema, and stool examination for blood, ova, and parasites are indicated.

Other Useful Tests
1. Four-quadrant peritoneal tap (ruptured spleen)
2. Quantitative urine amylase

3. IVP (renal calculus)
4. Stool for occult blood (carcinoma, diverticulitis)
5. Gallium scan (diverticulitis, etc.)
6. X-ray of thoracolumbar spine (radiculopathy)
7. Small-bowel series (Meckel diverticulum)
8. Laparoscopy (ruptured viscus or peritonitis)
9. Aortogram (dissecting aneurysm)
10. Lymphangiogram (retroperitoneal sarcoma)
11. Exploratory laparotomy

● Right Lower Quadrant Pain

Most cases of acute RLQ pain are considered appendicitis until proven otherwise, but every physician has been fooled by this axiom more times than he or she would like to remember. For this reason, the astute clinician will want to have a good list of possibilities in mind. Anatomy is the key to recalling an inclusive list of causes of all RLQ pain. Visualizing the structures, layer by layer, one finds the skin and abdominal wall in the first layer; the terminal ileum, cecum, appendix, and Meckel diverticulum in the second layer; the ureters, tubes, and ovaries (in women) in the third layer; and the muscles, spine, and terminal aorta in the fourth layer. Now the organs can be cross-indexed with the various etiologies that may be encountered by using

TABLE 8 Left Upper Quadrant Pain

	V Vascular	I Inflammatory	N Neoplasm	D Degenerative and Deficiency	I Intoxication	C Congenital	A Autoimmune or Allergic	T Trauma	E Endocrine
Abdominal Wall	Ruptured vein	Cellulitis	Metastatic carcinoma of ribs					Contusion Hernia	
Spleen	Infarct Aneurysm	Infectious mononucleosis Subacute bacterial endocarditis	Leukemia Hodgkin lymphoma				Periarteritis nodosa	Ruptured spleen	
Stomach		Gastritis Gastric ulcer	Gastric carcinoma		Gastric dilatation in pneumonia	Cascade stomach Hiatal hernia		Ruptured stomach	
Colon	Mesenteric thrombosis	Diverticulitis Mucous colitis Parasites	Colon carcinoma			Diverticulum	Granulomatous colitis	Ruptured colon	
Pancreas		Pancreatitis	Pancreatic carcinoma Pancreatic cyst						
Adrenal Gland	Infarct		Malignancy with infarction						Waterhouse–Friderichsen syndrome
Kidney	Embolism Infarction	Pyelonephritis Perinephric abscess	Hypernephroma			Nephroptosis			Renal calculus
Aorta	Atherosclerotic aneurysm			Medionecrosis with dissecting aneurysm					
Spine		Tuberculosis of the spine Tabes dorsalis	Myeloma Metastatic carcinoma Spinal cord tumor	Osteoarthritis				Fracture Ruptured disc	Osteoporosis

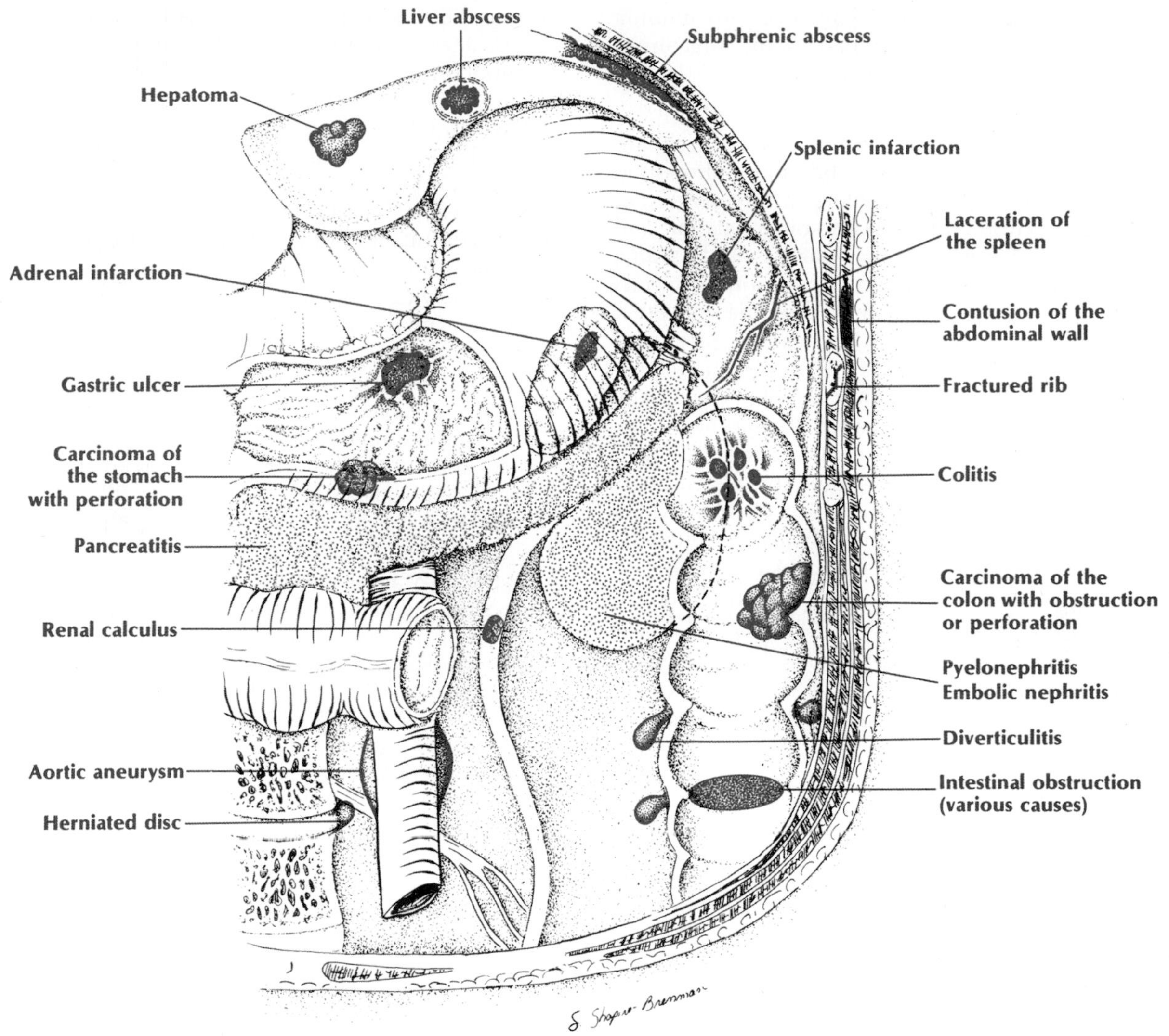

● **FIGURE 11** Abdominal pain, left upper quadrant.

the mnemonic **VINDICATE** (Table 9). The following discussion emphasizes the most important diseases in the differential diagnosis.

1. **Skin and abdominal wall:** Herpes zoster, cellulitis, contusion, and especially inguinal or femoral hernias are significant causes of RLQ pain.
2. **Appendix:** Appendicitis is a major cause of RLQ pain.
3. **Terminal ileum:** Regional ileitis, tuberculosis, or typhoid and intussusceptions may involve the ileum and cause severe pain. Mesenteric adenitis and infarcts may also affect the ileum.
4. **Cecum:** Diverticulitis, colitis (e.g., granulomatous or amebic), and colon carcinoma are culprits that may cause RLQ pain originating in the cecum. Impacted feces are also a possible cause.
5. **Meckel diverticulum:** This congenital anomaly may become obstructed and inflamed, develop a pancreatitis or a perforated peptic ulcer, or communicate with a periumbilical cellulitis. All of these may cause RLQ pain.

6. **Ureters:** Renal calculi and hydronephrosis may cause RLQ pain.
7. **Ovary and fallopian tubes:** A mumps oophoritis may cause pain in the RLQ. Ovarian cysts may twist on their pedicles or rupture, causing pain, as may the rupture of a small graafian follicle in the normal cycle (mittelschmerz). Three significant lesions may involve the tube: salpingitis, endometriosis, and ectopic pregnancy. All three are painful.
8. **Aorta:** Dissecting aneurysms or emboli of the terminal aorta and its branches may seize the patient with acute pain.
9. **Pelvis and spine:** Osteoarthritis, ruptured disc, metastatic carcinoma, Pott disease, and rheumatoid spondylitis should be considered here.
10. **Miscellaneous structures:** A ruptured peptic ulcer or inflamed gallbladder may leak fluid into the right colic gutter and cause RLQ pain. Any of the numerous causes of intestinal obstruction (e.g., adhesions or volvulus) may cause pain. Omental infarcts are another

miscellaneous cause. Referred pain from pneumonia or pulmonary infarct has encouraged some surgeons to insist on a chest x-ray prior to surgery.

Approach to the Diagnosis

Obviously, acute RLQ pain is suspected to be acute appendicitis until proven otherwise. Now abdominal ultrasound or CT scan can establish the diagnosis before surgery in over 90% of cases. However, it is wise to order flat plate and upright films of the abdomen, CBC, urinalysis, and an amylase level before surgery to dodge a curveball. Some surgeons want a chest x-ray as well, because pneumonia and other chest conditions can present with RLQ pain. A pregnancy test should be ordered for women of childbearing age to help rule out a ruptured ectopic pregnancy, but ultrasonography is even better. Surprisingly, many patients get to the operating room without a rectal or vaginal examination. RLQ pain in a child less than 2 years old should be considered intussusceptions until proven otherwise. In cases of chronic RLQ pain, contrast studies such as a barium enema, IVP, upper GI series, and cholecystogram may be indicated. If these are not diagnostic, further investigation with colonoscopy, cystoscopy, culdoscopy, or laparoscopy may be needed. A CT scan of the abdomen and pelvis can often reveal the diagnosis.

Other Useful Tests

1. Stool for occult blood (mesenteric thrombosis, neoplasm)
2. Stool for ova and parasites
3. Gallium or indium scan (diverticulitis, abscess)
4. Angiogram (mesenteric thrombosis)
5. X-ray of lumbar spine (herniated disc, etc.)
6. Urine culture, sensitivity, and colony count
7. Chemistry panel
8. Sedimentation rate (inflammation)
9. Lymphangiogram (Hodgkin lymphoma)
10. Urine porphobilinogen (porphyria)
11. Small-bowel series (Meckel diverticulum)
12. Blood lead level

● Left Lower Quadrant Pain

The anatomy of the LLQ, like that of the RLQ, provides a basis for recalling the causes of pain. There are fewer structures to deal with; thus, the differential diagnosis is not difficult. Visualizing the structures layer by layer, there are the skin and abdominal wall in the first layer; the sigmoid colon, omentum, and portions of small intestine in the second layer; the ureter, fallopian tubes, and ovaries (in women) in the third layer; and the aorta, pelvis, and spine beneath all these structures. Now, by using the mnemonic **VINDICATE**, the organs can be cross-indexed with the various etiologies that may cause pain in this area (Table 10). The following discussion emphasizes the most important diseases that must be considered in the differential diagnosis.

1. **Skin and abdominal wall:** Herpes zoster, cellulitis, contusion, and, especially, inguinal or femoral hernias are significant causes of LLQ pain.
2. **Small intestine:** Regional ileitis, intussusception, adhesion, volvulus, and other conditions that cause intestinal obstruction should be considered here.

3. **Sigmoid colon:** Diverticulitis, ischemic colitis, mesenteric adenitis and infarct, and granulomatous colitis are important causes. Carcinoma of the sigmoid may induce pain by perforating or obstructing the colon.
4. **Ureters:** Ureteral colic must be considered in the differential diagnosis of LLQ pain.
5. **Ovary and fallopian tubes:** A mumps oophoritis, ovarian cysts that twist on their pedicles or rupture, and small graafian follicles of the normal cycle that rupture are all included in the differential diagnosis of LLQ pain. The tubes may cause pain if there is an ectopic pregnancy, if they are inflamed by a salpingitis, or if they are infiltrated by endometriosis.
6. **Aorta:** Dissecting aneurysms and emboli of the terminal aorta may cause acute lower quadrant pain.
7. **Pelvis and spine:** Osteoarthritis, a ruptured disc, metastatic carcinoma, Pott disease, and rheumatoid spondylitis should be considered here.
8. **Miscellaneous:** Occasionally, pain in the bladder, prostate, or uterus is referred to the LLQ. A fibroid of the uterus may twist and cause pain. Impacted feces may cause severe pain. Referred pain from pneumonia, pleurisy, and myocardial infarction is uncommon but must be considered. Metabolic conditions that cause generalized abdominal pain and that should be remembered are listed on page 16.

Approach to the Diagnosis

There is no doubt about the value of a good history and physical examination, including both the rectal and pelvic areas. After this, the signs and symptoms should be summarized and grouped together; in many cases, this technique will pinpoint the diagnosis.

The laboratory workup can now proceed. In acute cases, the physician should order a flat plate of the abdomen, CBC, urinalysis (and examine it himself or herself), and serum amylase level before exploratory surgery. A pregnancy test is ordered in women of childbearing age. In chronic cases, sigmoidoscopy, barium enema, upper GI series, small-bowel follow-through, and stool examination for blood, ova, and parasites should be done before culdoscopy, peritoneoscopy, or colonoscopy is contemplated. An exploratory laparotomy remains a useful diagnostic tool even in chronic cases of LLQ pain.

Other Useful Tests

1. CT scan of the abdomen and pelvis
2. Gallium or indium scan (diverticular abscess, tubo-ovarian abscess)
3. Sonogram (ruptured ectopic pregnancy)
4. IVP
5. Examination of all urine for stones
6. Vaginal culture
7. Stool culture
8. Urine culture, sensitivity, and colony count
9. X-ray of lumbar spine (herniated disc, radiculopathy)
10. Peritoneal tap (ruptured ectopic pregnancy)
11. Aortogram (dissecting aneurysms)
12. Angiogram (mesenteric infarction)
13. Exploratory laparotomy

TABLE 9 Right Lower Quadrant Pain

	V Vascular	I Inflammatory	N Neoplasm	D Degenerative and Deficiency	I Intoxication	C Congenital	A Autoimmune Allergic	T Trauma	E Endocrine
Skin and Abdominal Wall		Herpes zoster Cellulitis				Inguinal hernia Femoral hernia		Contusion Incisional hernia	
Terminal Ileum	Mesenteric infarct	Tuberculosis Typhoid Mesenteric adenitis				Intussusception	Regional ileitis Whipple disease		
Cecum		Diverticulitis Amebic colitis Shigella Ascaris	Colon carcinoma		Toxic megacolon	Diverticulum	Granulomatous colitis	Impacted feces Ruptured bowel	
Appendix		Appendicitis Enterobiasis	Carcinoid					Fecalith	
Meckel Diverticulum		Meckel diverticulitis Cellulitis				Ectopic gastric and pancreatic tissue			
Ureter		Ureteritis				Aberrant blood vessel or congenital band			Ureteral calculus
Ovary and Tubes		Mumps Oophoritis Salpingitis	Ovarian cyst Neoplasm Endometriosis			Ectopic pregnancy			Ruptured graafian follicle (mittelschmerz)
Aorta	Dissecting aneurysm Embolism								
Spine and Pelvis	Pott disease	Metastatic carcinoma Myeloma Hodgkin lymphoma	Osteoarthritis				Rheumatoid spondylitis Ileitis	Fracture Ruptured disc	

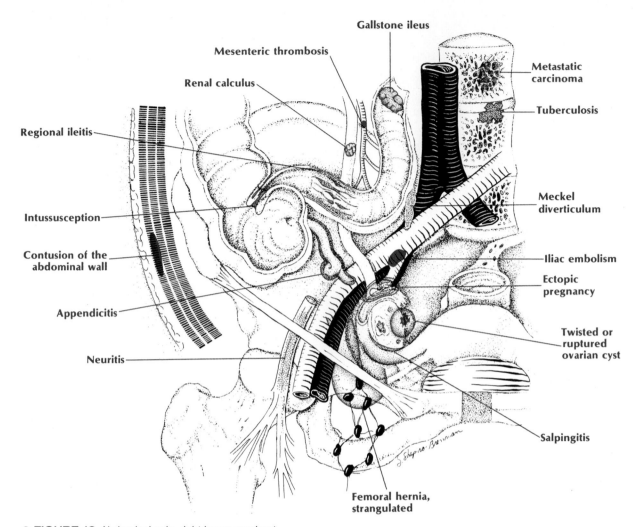

● **FIGURE 12** Abdominal pain, right lower quadrant.

Case Presentation #5

A 25-year-old white woman complained of a sudden onset of LLQ pain and occasional nausea and vomiting on the day of admission.

Question #1. Utilizing the methods described above, what are the possible causes of this patient's condition at this point?

Further history reveals she had intermittent vaginal bleeding for 2 weeks and she was treated for a vaginal discharge several months ago. Vaginal examination revealed a tender adnexal mass.

Question #2. What are the diagnostic possibilities now?

(See Appendix B for the answers.)

● Epigastric Pain

By mental dissection of the epigastrium layer by layer from the skin to the thoracolumbar spine, one encounters all the important organs that are the sites of origin of epigastric pain (Table 11). **Anatomy**, therefore, is the basic science used to develop this differential diagnosis.

The **skin** may be the site of the pain in herpes zoster, as it is in other types of pain, although it is less likely to be midline. Cellulitis and other lesions of the skin will be readily apparent. However, muscle and fascial conditions may be missed if one does not specifically think of this layer. Thus, epigastric hernia, hiatal hernia, or contusion of the muscle will be missed, as will diaphragmatic abscesses and trichinosis of the diaphragm.

The **stomach** and **duodenum** are the next organs encountered; both are prominent causes of epigastric pain. Ulcers, especially perforated ulcers, cause severe pain. Gastritis (syphilitic, toxic, or atrophic) causes a milder form of pain. Pyloric stenosis (from whatever cause), cascade stomach, diverticula, and carcinoma or sarcoma round out the differential diagnosis here. Good collateral circulation makes vascular occlusion a less likely cause.

The **colon** and **small intestines** lie just below the stomach, so one must not forget ileitis, colitis (ulcerative or granulomatous), appendicitis, diverticulitis, Meckel diverticulum,

TABLE 10 Left Lower Quadrant Pain

	V Vascular	I Inflammatory	N Neoplasm	D Degenerative and Deficiency	I Intoxication	C Congenital	A Autoimmune Allergic	T Trauma	E Endocrine
Skin and Abdominal Wall		Herpes zoster Cellulitis				Inguinal and femoral hernias		Contusion Hernia	
Small Intestine	Mesenteric thrombosis	Parasite	Polyp with intussusception Carcinoma Leiomyoma		Uremia Lead colic	Intussusception Porphyria Congenital polyposis	Regional ileitis	Rupture Hematoma Adhesion	Diabetic ketosis
Sigmoid Colon	Ischemic colitis Mesenteric infarct	Diverticulitis Mesenteric adenitis	Carcinoma of the sigmoid				Granulomatous colitis	Contusion Perforation Adhesion	
Ureters		Ureteritis	Papilloma			Congenital band ureterocele			Ureteral calculus
Ovary and Tubes		Mumps Oophoritis Salpingitis	Benign and malignant ovarian tumors Endometriosis			Ovarian cyst Ectopic pregnancy		Contusion Rupture	Ruptured graafian follicle (mittelschmerz)
Aorta	Dissecting aneurysm Emboli								
Spine and Pelvis		Pott disease	Metastatic carcinoma Myeloma	Osteoarthritis		Spondylolisthesis	Rheumatoid spondylitis	Fracture Ruptured disc	

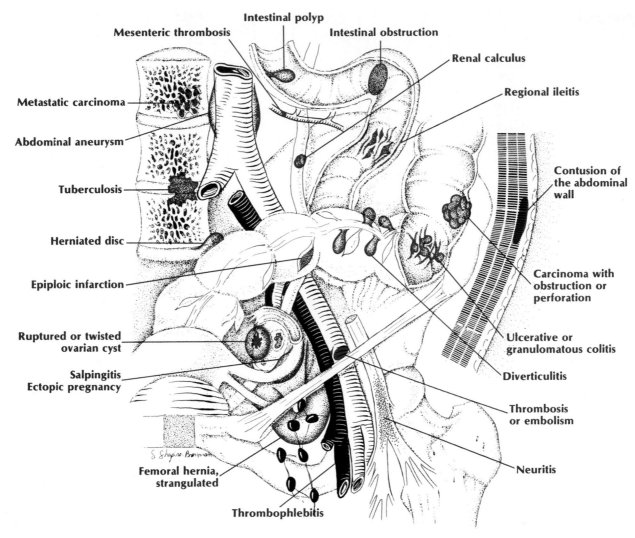

● **FIGURE 13** Abdominal pain, left lower quadrant.

and transverse colon carcinoma that ulcerates through the wall. Intestinal parasites and mesenteric thrombosis are additional causes that originate here. The various forms of intestinal obstruction are more important than parasites and mesenteric thrombosis.

The **pancreas** sits at the next layer, and acute pancreatitis is a particularly severe form of epigastric pain. Chronic pancreatitis, carcinoma, cysts of the pancreas, and mucoviscidosis cause less severe forms of epigastric pain. The **lymph nodes** may be involved by Hodgkin lymphoma and lymphosarcoma, leading to intestinal obstruction, but mesenteric adenitis is a much more likely cause. When the retroperitoneal nodes are involved by neoplasms (e.g., sarcoma), the pain is usually referred to the back.

The **blood vessels** are contained in the next layer, and one is reminded of aortic aneurysm, abdominal angina, periarteritis nodosa, and other forms of vasculitis. The sympathetic and parasympathetic nerves are involved by lead colic, porphyria, and black widow spider venom. Conditions of the **thoracic spine** are present in the final layer. Cord tumor, tuberculosis, herniated disc,

osteoarthritis, and rheumatoid spondylitis can all lead to midepigastric pain.

Omission of the systemic diseases and diseases of other abdominal organs that sometimes cause epigastric pain is inexcusable. Pneumonia, myocardial infarction (inferior wall, particularly), rheumatic fever, epilepsy, and migraine are just a few systemic conditions that are associated with epigastric or generalized abdominal pain.

Cholecystitis, hepatitis, and pyelonephritis are some local diseases that also produce midepigastric or generalized abdominal pain, which is why the target system has a useful application here. The center circle of the target is the stomach, the pancreas, and other organs in Table 11. The next circle covers the liver, kidney, gallbladder, heart, and ovaries. A further circle covers the brain and the testicles.

Approach to the Diagnosis

The approach to the diagnosis of midepigastric pain is identical to that for generalized abdominal pain (see page 29).

TABLE 11 Epigastric Pain

	V Vascular	I Inflammatory	N Neoplasm	D Degenerative and Deficiency	I Intoxication Idiopathic	C Congenital Acquired Anomaly	A Autoimmune Allergic	T Trauma	E Endocrine
Skin		Herpes zoster Cellulitis							
Muscle and Fascia		Diaphragmatic abscess Trichinosis				Epigastric hernia Hiatal hernia		Contusion Cough hemorrhage	
Stomach		Gastritis Ulcer Syphilis	Carcinoma Sarcoma	Atrophic gastritis	Gastritis Ulcer	Cascade stomach Pyloric stenosis			Zollinger–Ellison syndrome
Duodenum		Ulcer			Ulcer	Diverticulitis			Zollinger–Ellison syndrome
Intestines	Mesenteric thrombosis	Appendicitis Ileitis Colitis Parasites	Polyp Carcinoma Sarcoma		Dumping syndrome	Meckel or colonic diverticulum Intestinal obstruction			Adrenal insufficiency
Pancreas		Pancreatitis	Pancreatic carcinomas		Pancreatitis				
Lymph Nodes		Mesenteric adenitis	Hodgkin lymphoma Lymphosarcoma			Mucoviscoidosis Pancreatic cyst			
Blood Vessels	Aortic aneurysm Abdominal angina						Periarteritis nodosa		
Nerves		Herpes zoster			Lead colic Porphyria Arachnidism				
Thoracic Spine		Tuberculosis Osteomyelitis	Primary tumor or metastasis	Osteoporosis Arthritis			Rheumatoid spondylitis	Fracture Herniated disc	
Local Referred	Coronary insufficiency Myocardial infarction Congestive heart failure	Hepatitis Cholecystitis Pyelonephritis	Hepatic carcinoma						
Systemic Referred	Pulmonary embolism	Pneumonia Epididymitis	Endometriosis Peritoneal carcinomatosis	Epilepsy Migraine Electrolyte imbalance			Rheumatic fever	Fractured ribs	Diabetes mellitus

A

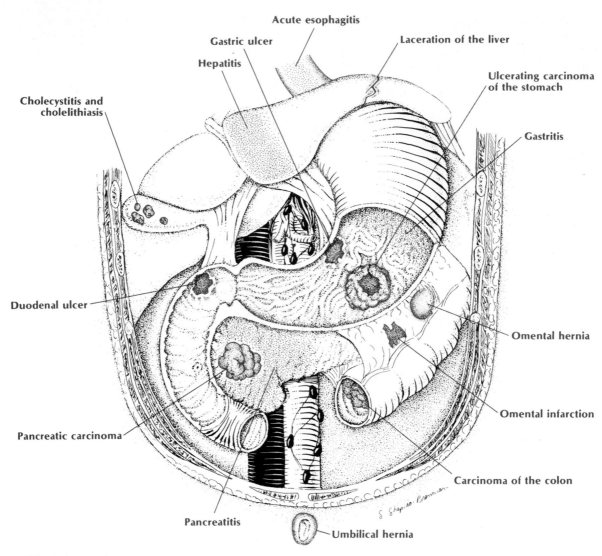

Acute esophagitis

Gastric ulcer

Hepatitis

Laceration of the liver

Ulcerating carcinoma of the stomach

Cholecystitis and cholelithiasis

Gastritis

Duodenal ulcer

Omental hernia

Omental infarction

Pancreatic carcinoma

Carcinoma of the colon

Pancreatitis

Umbilical hernia

● **FIGURE 14** Abdominal pain, epigastric.

● Hypogastric Pain

Anatomy is the basic science that will open the door to this differential diagnosis. Visualizing the structures in the hypogastrium, one sees the abdominal wall, the bladder and urinary tract, the female genital tract, the sigmoid colon and rectum, the iliac vessels, the aorta and vena cava, and the lumbosacral spine. Occasionally, other organs fall into the hypogastrium; thus, they must be considered too. A pelvic kidney, visceroptosis of the transverse colon, and a pelvic appendix all may occur. Now that one has the organs in mind it is necessary only to apply the mnemonic **MINT** to recall the causes of hypogastric pain.

In the **abdominal wall**,

M—Malformations bring to mind ventral hernias and urachal cysts or sinuses with associated cellulitis.
I—Inflammation includes cellulitis, carbuncle, and other skin infections.
N—Neoplasms of the abdominal wall do not usually present with pain.

T—Trauma suggests contusion of the rectus abdominus muscles or stab wound.

In the **urinary tract**,

M—Malformations recall diverticulum, cystocele, ureterocele, bladder neck obstruction from stricture and calculus, and phimosis and paraphimosis.
I—Inflammation suggests cystitis, prostatitis and urethritis, and Hunner ulcers.
N—Neoplasms suggest transitional cell papilloma and carcinoma and prostate carcinoma.
T—Trauma recalls ruptured bladder.

In the **female genital tract**,

M—Malformations that may cause pain include a retroverted uterus, an ectopic pregnancy, and various congenital cysts (e.g., hydatid cyst of Morgagni) that may twist on their pedicles.
I—Inflammation of the vagina and cervix is not usually painful except on intercourse, but endometritis and tubo-ovarian abscesses are associated with pain and fever.

N—**Neoplasms** such as carcinoma of the cervix and uterus do not cause pain unless they extend beyond the uterus or obstruct the menstrual flow. However, fibroids often cause dysmenorrhea and severe pain if they twist on their pedicles, and endometriosis may spread throughout the pelvis and cause chronic or acute pain. **T—Trauma** such as perforation of the uterus during a dilatation and curettage (D & C), delivery, or by the introduction of a foreign body during sexual relations may cause abdominal pain.

The **sigmoid colon** and **rectum** may be the site of pain in

M—**Malformations** such as diverticulitis.
I—**Inflammations** such as ulcerative colitis with perforation, granulomatous colitis with perforation, amebic colitis, and ischemic colitis.
N—**Neoplasms** that spread beyond the lumen of the bowel or cause obstruction.
T—**Trauma** from introduction of instruments or foreign bodies.

Pain in the hypogastrium may also be caused by a dissecting aneurysm of the **aorta** or phlebitis of the **iliac veins** or the inferior **vena cava**. The **lumbosacral spine** may be the site of pain in

M—**Malformations** such as spondylolisthesis and scoliosis, but these are usually associated with back pain.

I—**Inflammatory** conditions of the spine such as tuberculosis and rheumatoid spondylitis are much more likely to cause hypogastric pain.
N—**Neoplasms**, particularly metastatic carcinoma, multiple myeloma, and Hodgkin lymphoma may cause hypogastric pain.
T—**Trauma** of the spine may cause a herniated disc fracture or hematoma of the spine and surrounding muscles, producing hypogastric pain from a distended bladder or paralytic ileus, among other things.

The appendix and small intestine may occasionally end up in the pelvis; therefore, appendicitis and regional ileitis should not be forgotten as possible causes of hypogastric pain.

Approach to the Diagnosis

In cases of hypogastric pain, it is most important to do a good pelvic and rectal examination. Because the most common cause of hypogastric pain is cystitis or other urinary tract infection, it is essential to examine the urine (personally) and to do a culture sensitivity and colony count regardless of the findings on routine urinalysis. A vaginal culture should also be done in women on special media for *Chlamydia* and gonococcus to help rule out PID. Urethral smear and culture is done if there is a urethral discharge. Acute hypogastric pain may require a flat plate of the abdomen, CBC, chemistry panel, and amylase

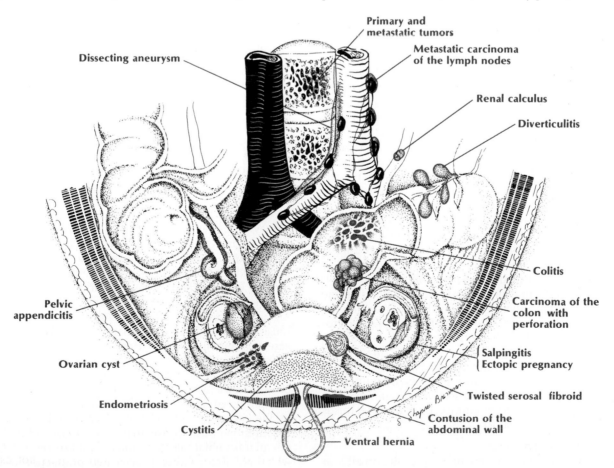

● **FIGURE 15** Abdominal pain, hypogastric.

level depending on the seriousness of the patient's condition. A general surgeon may need to be consulted. Ultrasonography may be ordered to further evaluate any suspicious pelvic mass. A pregnancy test should be ordered in women of childbearing age. Three conditions that must be ruled out in the female patient are ruptured ectopic pregnancy, PID, and endometriosis. That is why a gynecologist should be consulted early if these conditions are suspected in acute cases. Chronic cases may need an IVP and cystoscopy if a urinary tract infection, stone, or neoplasm is suspected. If a problem in the lower bowel is suspected, colonoscopy or barium enema may be necessary. If there is any question about a perforated bowel or mesenteric infarction, a CT scan of the abdomen and pelvis should be done first.

Other Useful Tests
1. Stool for occult blood (mesenteric infarct, diverticulitis, neoplasm)
2. Stool for ova and parasites
3. Stool culture
4. Urine porphobilinogen (porphyria)
5. Sedimentation rate (PID)
6. Tuberculin test
7. Culdoscopy (ectopic pregnancy)
8. Laparoscopy (PID, endometriosis)
9. Exploratory laparotomy
10. Angiogram (mesenteric infarct)

ABSENT OR DIMINISHED PULSE

Anatomy is once again the simplest way to recall the many causes of an absent or diminished pulse. By visualizing the arterial tree, we can recall the various causes. Beginning at the top of the tree, we have the **heart**, which should prompt the recall of shock and CHF. Proceeding down the tree to the **aorta** we have dissecting aneurysm, Takayasu disease, and coarctation of the aorta as prominent causes of absent or diminished pulses. A large saddle embolism at the terminal aorta may cause absent or diminished pulses in the lower extremities. Arteriosclerosis of the terminal aorta as seen in Leriche syndrome may produce a similar picture. Proceeding further down the tree to the **larger arteries**, we are reminded of the subclavian steal syndrome in the upper extremities and femoral artery thrombosis, embolism, or arteriosclerosis affecting the lower extremities.

Extrinsic pressure from a thoracic outlet syndrome may also affect the subclavian artery. Finally reaching the **peripheral arteries**, we encounter peripheral arteriosclerosis, embolism, and thrombosis. These arteries also may be affected by external compression in fractures, tumors, and other masses of the extremities. An arteriovenous fistula of the extremity arteries may produce an absent or diminished pulse also. Significant anemia or dehydration may produce a diminished pulse in all extremities, but of course, this is usually associated with shock.

Approach to the Diagnosis
Clinically it is useful to take the blood pressure on all four extremities and do a thorough examination of the optic fundus and heart. Ultrasonography of the vessels involved is an excellent noninvasive technique for further evaluation. If a dissecting aneurysm is suspected, aortography and surgery must be planned immediately. Laboratory evaluation includes a CBC, blood cultures to rule out bacterial endocarditis, serial ECGs, and serial cardiac enzymes. Arteriography of the vessel or vessels involved will ultimately be necessary in most cases. Magnetic resonance angiography is an expensive but adequate alternative in some cases when contrast arteriography is considered hazardous.

Other Useful Tests
1. Chest x-ray (dissecting aneurysm)
2. Sedimentation rate (mediastinitis, collagen disease)
3. Urinalysis (dissecting aneurysm)
4. Chemistry panel (myocardial infarction with embolism)
5. Venereal disease research laboratory (VDRL) test (syphilitic aneurysm)
6. Echocardiography (CHF)
7. 24-hour Holter monitor (cardiac arrhythmia)
8. Cardiology consult
9. Four-vessel cerebral angiography (subclavian steal syndrome)
10. Plain films of the extremities (fracture, mass)
11. Protein electrophoresis (collagen disease, multiple myeloma)

ACIDOSIS (DECREASED PH)

Developing a list of possible causes of acidosis is also best approached by using the physiologic model of production, transport, excretion, or degradation.

Production: Acids are produced as the end products of metabolism; thus, sugar is broken down to water and carbon dioxide (CO_2) (carbolic acid), fats are broken down to keto acids, and protein is broken down to sulfur-containing amino acids. In pathophysiologic states, there may be increased production of these acids. This should call to mind **diabetic acidosis**, **lactic acidosis**, and **starvation** as diagnostic possibilities when one is faced with a patient within acidosis.

Transport: If there is inadequate transport of acid to the kidney for excretion (as occurs in various forms of **shock** [prerenal azotemia]), acidosis may develop.

Excretion: Finally, these acids must be excreted by the lungs and the kidney. Thus, CO_2 retention occurs in pulmonary emphysema leading to pulmonary acidosis, while retention of sulfates and phosphates occurs in uremia causing uremic acidosis. Primary diseases of the kidney that may cause uremia acidosis are glomerulonephritis, collagen disease, toxic nephritis from various drugs, and end-stage renal disease from a host of causes. Chronic obstructive uropathy from renal stones, bladder neck obstruction, and congenital anomalies may also lead to uremic acidosis. Acidosis is also produced by a decrease in **production** of bicarbonate by the kidney or an increased excretion of bicarbonate in the intestinal tract. Consequently, one must add to the differential list renal tubular acidosis and Fanconi syndrome, which are associated with decreased production of bicarbonate while not producing uremia at the same time. In

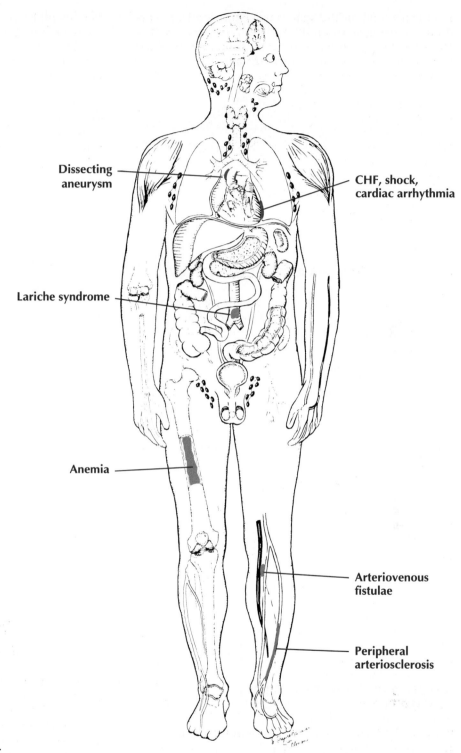

● FIGURE 16 Absent or diminished pulse.

addition, diarrhea of many causes must be added to the list because it is associated with increased excretion of bicarbonate. Finally, the mechanism of **regulation** of bicarbonate production should bring to mind conditions with acidosis related to decreased production of bicarbonate. In Addison disease, there is little or no aldosterone hormone to induce the kidneys to produce bicarbonate; lack of this hormone leads to acidosis. Drugs such as acetazolamide diuretic also interfere with the kidney's ability to produce bicarbonate, causing acidosis.

Approach to the Diagnosis
The laboratory will be of greatest assistance in determining the cause of acidosis. An elevated blood sugar and serum

acetone level will help diagnose diabetic acidosis. An elevated blood urea nitrogen (BUN) level would point to uremia acidosis. Arterial blood gases may show an increased CO_2, isolating pulmonary emphysema as the cause.

Other Useful Tests

1. CBC (shock, septicemia, lactic acidosis)
2. Urinalysis (renal tubular acidosis, uremia)
3. Chemistry panel (diabetes, uremia, Addison disease)
4. Serial electrolytes (diabetic acidosis, renal disease, Addison disease)
5. Lactic acid (shock, lactic acidosis)
6. Pulmonary function tests (pulmonary emphysema)
7. ECG (CHF)
8. Pulmonology consult
9. Nephrology consult

ACID PHOSPHATASE ELEVATION

An elevated acid phosphatase level usually points to metastatic carcinoma of the prostate. However, because other tissues can **produce** acid phosphatase, the clinician should consider liver disease, hematologic disorders, Gaucher disease, and Niemann–Pick disease in the differential diagnosis. In addition, diseases of the bone such as osteogenic sarcoma and Paget disease may cause an elevation in acid phosphatase level.

Approach to the Diagnosis

Clinically the prostate should be examined and a prostate-specific antigen (PSA) test ordered. If either one or both of these are positive, a urologist should be consulted for prostate biopsy. A skeletal survey is ordered. If the survey results are unremarkable, a bone scan should be done.

Other Useful Tests

1. CBC
2. Sedimentation rate
3. Chemistry profile (metastatic carcinoma, Paget disease)
4. Protein electrophoresis (malignancy)
5. Liver profile (Gaucher disease, other liver disease)
6. Sonogram of the prostate (prostate carcinoma)
7. CT scan of the abdomen and pelvis (metastatic malignancy)

ALKALINE PHOSPHATASE ELEVATION

Developing a list of diagnostic possibilities for an elevated alkaline phosphatase level involves the use of biochemistry and physiology. As with other laboratory values, we need to know where alkaline phosphatase is produced, how it is transported, and how it is degraded or excreted. Alkaline phosphatase is **produced** in many tissues but in terms of pathophysiology, only the osteoblasts of the bone need be recalled. Thus, disorders that increase osteoblastic activity such as metastatic tumors of the bone, osteogenic sarcoma, Paget disease, and primary and secondary hyperparathyroidism may cause the

alkaline phosphatase level to increase and must be considered in the differential. **Transport** of blood alkaline phosphatase does not seem to be affected by disease. However, the **excretion** of alkaline phosphatase seems to take place in the liver by an undetermined pathway, but anything that blocks the cholangioles or biliary tree will usually cause an elevation of alkaline phosphatase. Consequently, carcinoma of the head of the pancreas, common duct stones, carcinoma of the ampulla of Vater, and drugs that produce cholestasis (such as chlorpromazine) may cause an elevated alkaline phosphatase. Metastatic carcinoma of the liver probably produces an elevated alkaline phosphatase by blocking individual cholangioles. In addition to the above diagnostic possibilities, there are disorders that cause an elevated alkaline phosphatase level by an unknown mechanism such as pregnancy, sepsis, and gynecologic malignancies that must be included in the differential.

Approach to the Diagnosis

If the elevated alkaline phosphatase level is related to liver disease, the clinical examination will often show jaundice or hepatomegaly. If it is related to bone disease, the clinical examination will show bone pain, pathologic fracture, or bone mass. A liver profile will also help diagnose a liver disorder, but a CT scan of the abdomen may be necessary. A skeletal survey will usually reveal bony metastasis and other disorders of the bone, but a bone scan may be necessary to show early metastasis to the bone. A serum parathyroid hormone (PTH) level will help diagnose primary hyperparathyroidism, whereas secondary hyperparathyroidism (rickets, etc.) will require the specialized tests listed below.

Other Useful Tests

1. CBC
2. Chemistry profile (liver disease)
3. Sedimentation rate (hepatitis)
4. Urinalysis (renal tubular acidosis)
5. 24-hour urine calcium (hyperparathyroidism, malignancy)
6. Gallbladder ultrasound (common duct stone)
7. ERCP (obstructive jaundice)
8. Transhepatic cholangiogram (obstructive jaundice)
9. Liver biopsy (cirrhosis, hepatitis)
10. Bone biopsy (metastatic malignancy)
11. D-xylose absorption test (malabsorption syndrome)
12. Acid phosphatase (metastatic cancer of the prostate)
13. PSA (metastatic cancer of the prostate)
14. Vitamin D metabolites (25-hydroxycholecalciferol) (rickets, osteomalacia)
15. Exploratory laparotomy

ALKALOSIS (INCREASED PH)

The differential diagnosis of alkalosis, like acidosis, begins with using the physiologic model of **production, excretion**, or **degradation**.

Production: Bicarbonate is produced in the kidneys. Excessive production of bicarbonate occurs in primary

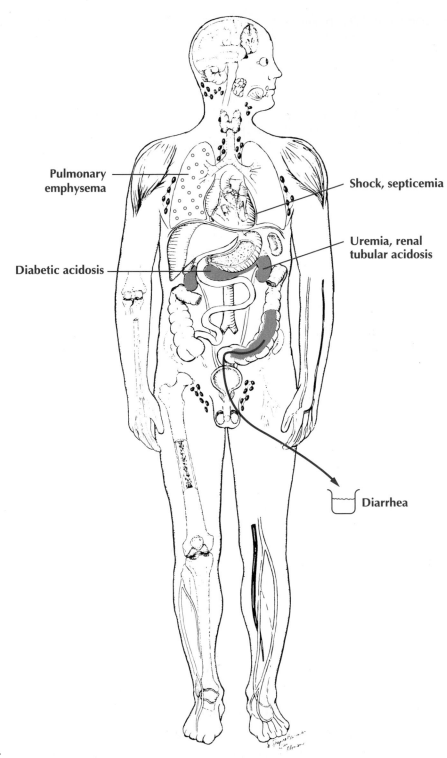

● **FIGURE 17** Acidosis (decreased pH).

or secondary aldosteronism where the hormone aldosterone induces increased bicarbonate production and excessive excretion of the hydrogen (H^+) ion in exchange for sodium (Na^+) reabsorption. The same mechanism occurs in exogenous steroid administration and Bartter syndrome.

Excretion: This mechanism should help recall salicylate toxicity and hyperventilation as causes of alkalosis. In these conditions, the pH is raised because of excessive excretion of CO_2 through the lungs.

Excessive **excretion** of acid also occurs in pyloric stenosis, intestinal obstruction, and other causes of excessive vomiting leading to alkalosis. Prolonged nasogastric suctioning may lead to alkalosis by the same mechanism. Chronic antacid use, various diuretics, and Cushing disease may also induce alkalosis.

Approach to the Diagnosis

Taking a drug history and noting hyperventilation or vomiting during the clinical evaluation will assist in the diagnosis. Serial electrolytes, arterial blood gases, and drug screen are first-line laboratory tests to assist in the diagnosis.

Other Useful Tests

1. CBC (intestinal obstruction)
2. Urinalysis (renal calculi, salicylates)
3. Chemistry profile (aldosteronism, diuretic use)
4. Serum amylase and lipase levels (acute pancreatitis with vomiting)
5. Flat plate of the abdomen (intestinal obstruction)
6. Chest x-ray (pneumonia, pulmonary infarction)
7. Gastroscopy (pyloric stenosis)
8. Plasma renin and aldosterone levels (aldosteronism)
9. Urine aldosterone (primary aldosteronism)
10. Endocrinology consult
11. CT scan of the abdomen (adrenal hyperplasia or adenoma)
12. Surgery consult

AMNESIA

The most common causes of this disorder are head injury, epilepsy, migraine, drug use, and hysteria. However, it is wise to have a systematic method of remembering the many etiologies to avoid mistakes in diagnosis. The mnemonic **VINDICATE** provides an excellent method.

V—Vascular disorders include cerebral arteriosclerosis, hemorrhage, thrombosis, embolism, and migraine. Transient cerebral ischemia (TIA) may cause amnesia.

I—Inflammatory disorders include meningitis, encephalitis, cerebral abscess, malaria and other cerebral parasites, and neurosyphilis. Amnesia and delirium may be caused by high fever regardless of the cause of the fever.

N—Neoplasm of the brain including primary and metastatic lesions may cause a sudden loss of memory.

D—Deficiency of thiamine brings to mind Wernicke encephalopathy as a cause of sudden memory loss, but pellagra and pernicious anemia are also associated with memory loss even though it is not usually acute. Degenerative disorders such as Alzheimer disease are associated with gradual onset of memory loss so are not likely to be confused with amnesia.

I—Intoxication with lysergic acid diethylamide (LSD), alcohol, bromides, opiates, and a host of other drugs can produce acute amnesia. Uremia, hypoxemia, and liver failure can do the same.

C—Convulsive states, especially temporal lobe epilepsy, can be associated with transient amnesia. However, this amnesia rarely lasts more than 1 to 2 hours as it is likely to be confused with the amnesia of hysteria.

A—Autoimmune disorders include the acute cerebritis of lupus erythematosus that may be associated with a transient amnesia. Other collagen disorders may do the same.

T—Trauma should help recall concussion and epidural and subdural hematomas.

E—Endocrine disorders include hypoglycemia and diabetic acidosis. Hypoparathyroidism and other hypocalcemic states may cause seizures and temporary memory loss. Emotional causes of amnesia include hysteria, depressive psychosis, and schizophrenia. Malingering could be recalled under this category.

Approach to the Diagnosis

The workup of amnesia must include a drug screen, CT scan, or magnetic resonance imaging (MRI) and often an electroencephalogram (EEG) to rule out epilepsy. Migraine may be ruled out by a careful history. A neurologist or psychiatrist will need to be consulted in most cases. If there is fever, a CBC, chemistry panel, antinuclear antibody (ANA), urinalysis, and blood cultures should be ordered. A spinal tap may be necessary as well.

Other Useful Tests

1. Carotid sonogram (TIA)
2. Psychometric testing (hysteria)
3. Four-vessel cerebral angiography (TIA)
4. Histamine test (migraine)
5. Glucose tolerance test (insulinoma)
6. VDRL test (neurosyphilis)
7. Blood smear for malarial parasites (malaria)
8. Response to intravenous thiamine (Wernicke encephalopathy)
9. Magnetic resonance angiography (basilar insufficiency)
10. Serum B_{12} and folate levels (pernicious anemia)

ANAL MASS

Aside from the common external hemorrhoids (which will not be seen in many cases unless the patient is asked to bear down), anal masses may include any of the following:

1. **Skin tag** from previous ruptured or incised hemorrhoids
2. **Sentinel piles** from rectal fissure
3. **Perirectal abscess**
4. **Condyloma latum** (syphilitic wart)
5. **Condyloma acuminatum** or **viral warts**
6. **Rectal prolapse**

It is important to keep all of them in mind when the anus is being examined because often you will not see them unless you remember to look for them. A surgical consult is wise before ordering diagnostic tests.

ANEMIA

In developing a list of diagnostic possibilities in cases of anemia, **physiology** is the key. Anemia may be caused by a decrease in red cell production, a break in the transport system (blood loss), or excessive red cell destruction.

Decreased production: This should bring to mind iron deficiency anemia, folate deficiency, and pernicious anemia. Production also is decreased when the bone marrow is infiltrated with leukemia or metastatic neoplasms.

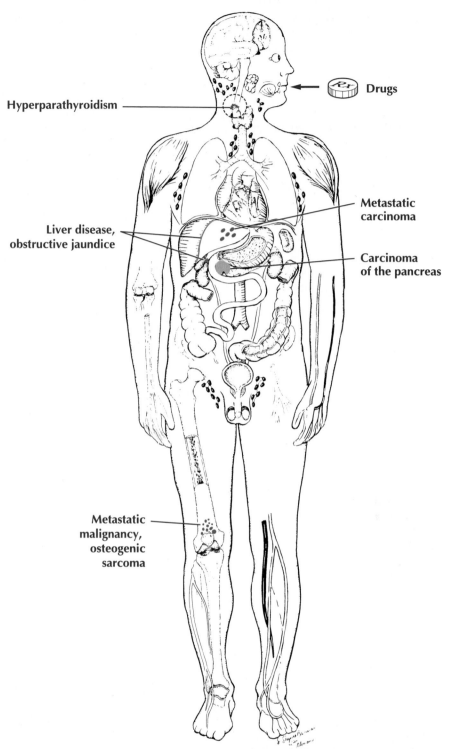

Hyperparathyroidism

Drugs

Liver disease,
obstructive jaundice

Metastatic
carcinoma

Carcinoma
of the pancreas

Metastatic
malignancy,
osteogenic
sarcoma

● **FIGURE 18** Alkaline phosphatase elevation.

Replacement of the marrow by fibrous tissue (as occurs in myelofibrosis) also decreases production. Cirrhosis of the liver may be associated with anemia due to lack of ability to store B_{12}, folic acid, and iron, thus reducing production. Decreased production should also bring to mind aplastic anemia, toxic or idiopathic.

Break in the transport system (blood loss): Trauma to any part of the body may cause significant blood loss. Massive hematemesis associated with esophageal varices or gastric ulcers is also obvious. However, chronic GI blood loss from bleeding ulcers, neoplasms, and diverticulitis is not. Also, insidious is the anemia associated with excessive menses or metrorrhagia. This can be dysfunctional or associated with fibroids or endometrial carcinoma and other tumors.

Increased destruction: This should prompt recall of the hemolytic anemias—hereditary or acquired. Sickle cell

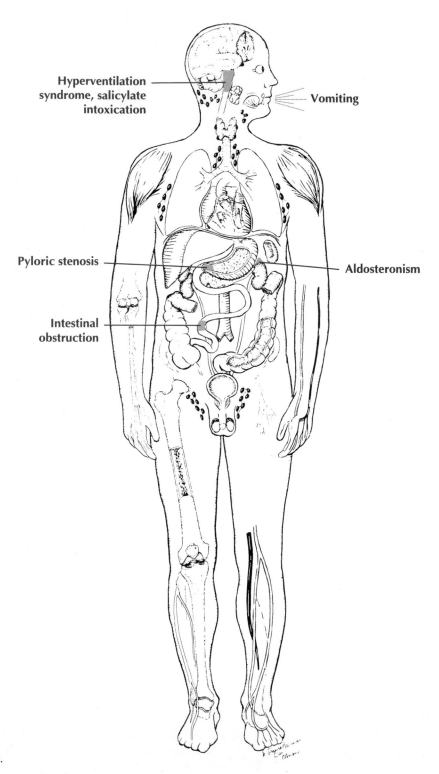

● **FIGURE 19** Alkalosis (increased pH).

anemia, thalassemia (major and minor), and hereditary spherocytosis are the major genetic anemias. Acquired hemolytic anemias include hemolytic anemias associated with lymphoma, leukemia, collagen disease, and idiopathic type. Hemolytic anemia may also be associated with infectious diseases such as malaria, Oroya fever, babesiosis, and septicemia. The hemolytic anemia associated with transfusion should not pose a diagnostic dilemma. Finally,

toxins and drugs such as phenacetin, primaquine, and lead may induce a hemolytic anemia.

Miscellaneous conditions: A large spleen from whatever cause may induce anemia based on both excessive red cell destruction and decreased red cell production. Hypothyroidism is also associated with an anemia that may be due to multiple causes. Simple chronic anemia associated with chronic inflammatory conditions, neoplasms,

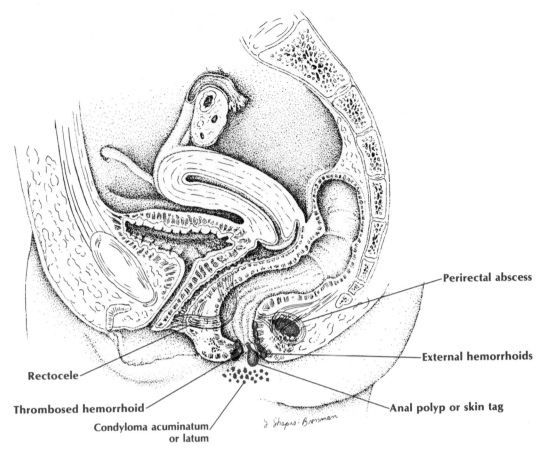

Perirectal abscess

External hemorrhoids

Anal polyp or skin tag

Rectocele

Thrombosed hemorrhoid

Condyloma acuminatum
or latum

● **FIGURE 20** Anal mass.

and renal disease is also caused by both decreased production and increased destruction of red cells.

Approach to the Diagnosis
Clinical evaluation should involve looking for occult blood in the stool, noting jaundice and splenomegaly, and taking a careful history to exclude drugs, toxins, blood loss, or nutrition as possible factors. The history should focus on possible causes of chronic blood loss such as tarry stools, hematemesis, or excessive menstruation. On physical examination, one may also note a smooth tongue (pernicious anemia), spoon nails (iron deficiency anemia), and myxedema. The initial laboratory workup includes a CBC and differential, serum iron and iron-binding capacity or ferritin levels, serum B_{12} and folic acid levels, chemistry profile, and serum haptoglobin level. The clinician should look at a blood smear. If these studies are not revealing, a hematologist should be consulted for a bone marrow examination.

Other Useful Tests
1. Sedimentation rate (infectious disease)
2. Red cell indices (pernicious anemia, iron deficiency anemia)
3. Reticulocyte count (hemolytic anemia)
4. Gastric analysis (pernicious anemia)
5. Schilling test (pernicious anemia)
6. Liver spleen scan (hemolytic anemia)
7. CT scan (liver or spleen size, malignancy)
8. Bone marrow biopsy (aplastic anemia)
9. Therapeutic trials (pernicious anemia, iron deficiency anemia)
10. Platelet count (aplastic anemia)
11. GI series (bleeding gastric ulcer, malignancy)
12. Barium enema (malignancy, colitis)
13. Endoscopy (malignancy, ulcer, diverticulitis)
14. Red blood cell survival (hemolytic anemia)
15. Serum erythropoietin (chronic renal disease)
16. Urinary, methylmalonic acid (pernicious anemia)
17. Peripheral bloodsmear (malaria, babesiosis)

ANKLE CLONUS AND HYPERACTIVE AND PATHOLOGIC REFLEXES

As with most neurologic signs, the differential diagnosis of ankle clonus and hyperactive and pathologic reflexes can be developed by using anatomy. The most commonly used pathologic reflexes are the Babinski and Hoffman signs. The reader is referred to physical diagnosis texts for a more extensive list. Ankle clonus and hyperactive and pathologic reflexes are usually caused by a pyramidal tract lesion. If we follow this tract from its origin in the cerebrum to its termination in the spinal cord, we

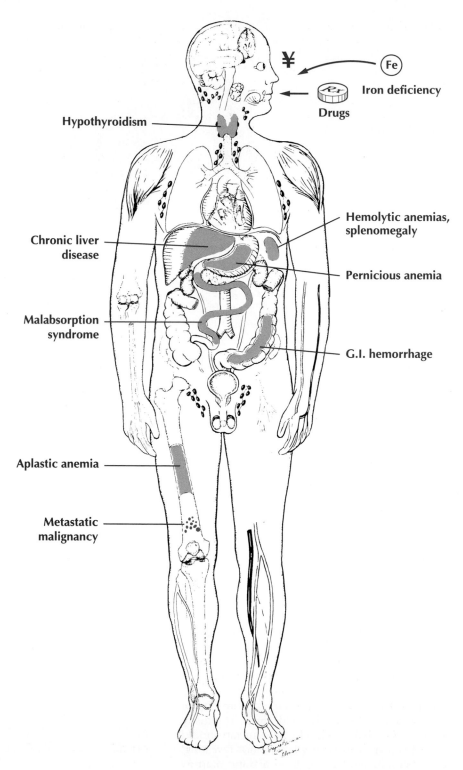

Hypothyroidism

Iron deficiency

Drugs

Chronic liver disease

Hemolytic anemias, splenomegaly

Pernicious anemia

Malabsorption syndrome

G.I. hemorrhage

Aplastic anemia

Metastatic malignancy

● **FIGURE 21** Anemia.

will be able to recall the many disorders that may cause them. It is helpful to cross-index these with the mnemonic **VINDICATE** at each level.

● **Cerebrum**

V—Vascular disorders include cerebral hemorrhage, thrombosis, aneurysms, and embolism.

I—Inflammation will help recall viral encephalitis, encephalomyelitis, cerebral abscess, venous sinus thrombosis, and central nervous system (CNS) syphilis.

N—Neoplasms include gliomas, meningiomas, and metastasis.

D—Degenerative disorders will help recall Alzheimer disease and the other degenerative diseases.

I—**Intoxication** reminds one of lead encephalopathy, alcoholism, and other toxins that affect the brain.

C—**Congenital** disorders include the reticuloendothelioses, Schilder disease, and cerebral palsy.

A—**Autoimmune** disorders include multiple sclerosis and the various collagen diseases that may affect the brain.

T—**Traumatic** disorders include epidural and subdural hematomas, intracerebral hematomas, and depressed skull fractures.

E—**Endocrine** disorders rarely cause pyramidal tract lesions.

● Brainstem

Applying the mnemonic **VINDICATE** to the brainstem, we can recall the following possibilities:

V—**Vascular** disorders include basilar and vertebral aneurysms, thrombosis, and insufficiency.

I—**Inflammatory** disorders associated with pyramidal tract signs include encephalomyelitis, abscess, and basilar meningitis.

N—**Neoplasms** in the brainstem are similar to those in the cerebrum but also include the acoustic neuroma, colloid cyst of the third ventricle, and chordomas.

D—**Degenerative** disorders include syringobulbia, lateral sclerosis, and Friedreich ataxia. **Deficiency diseases** include Wernicke encephalopathy and pernicious anemia.

I—**Intoxication** includes lead, alcohol, bromide, and drug reactions.

C—**Congenital** disorders with pyramidal tract involvement in the brainstem include platybasia and Arnold–Chiari malformation.

A—**Autoimmune** disorders bring to mind multiple sclerosis and other demyelinating diseases.

T—**Traumatic** disorders include basilar skull fracture and posterior fossa subdural hematoma.

E—**Endocrine** disorders of the brainstem prompt recall of an advanced chromophobe adenoma or craniopharyngioma.

● Spinal Cord

V—**Vascular** lesions of the spinal cord are anterior spinal artery occlusion and dissecting aneurysm of the aorta.

I—**Inflammatory** lesions of the spinal cord include epidural abscess, transverse myelitis, and meningovascular lues.

N—**Neoplasms** of the spinal cord include neurofibromas, meningiomas, and metastatic tumors. These frequently compress the pyramidal tracts.

D—There are a large number of **degenerative diseases** that affect the pyramidal tracts. These include amyotrophic lateral sclerosis, syringomyelia, subacute combined degeneration, and Friedreich ataxia.

I—**Intoxication** will help recall radiation myelitis and the side effects of spinal anesthesia.

C—**Congenital** disorders of the spinal cord include arteriovenous malformations and diastematomyelia. Cervical spondylosis associated with a progressive myelopathy is often associated with a congenital narrowing of the cervical spinal canal.

A—**Autoimmune** helps recall multiple sclerosis as a common cause of pyramidal tract lesions in the spinal cord.

T—**Trauma** will help recall fractures, epidural hematomas, and ruptured discs that compress the spinal cord.

E—**Endocrine** disorders do not usually affect the spinal cord and pyramidal tracts unless there is metastasis from an endocrine tumor to the spine.

Approach to the Diagnosis

A neurologist should be consulted at the outset. The neurologist will be able to determine whether a CT scan or MRI should be ordered and whether it should be of the brain, brainstem, or spinal cord. If there are obvious cranial nerve signs, the imaging study will include the brain and brainstem. Spinal cord lesions usually require x-ray of the spine and possibly myelography and spinal fluid analysis. In suspected intracranial pathology, a spinal tap should not be done until a CT scan or MRI has ruled out a space-occupying lesion.

Other Useful Tests

1. Carotid sonogram (carotid thrombosis)
2. ECG (cardiac arrhythmia)
3. Blood cultures (SBE)
4. VDRL test (neurosyphilis)
5. Four-vessel cerebral angiogram (carotid embolism, thrombosis)
6. Chemistry panel (myocardial infarct with embolism)
7. Urine drug screen (drug abuse)
8. ANA test (collagen disease)
9. Blood lead level (lead encephalopathy)
10. Serum B_{12} and folate levels (pernicious anemia)
11. Tuberculin test
12. Fluorescent treponemal antibody absorption (FTA-ABS) test (neurosyphilis)

ANOREXIA

Physiology is the most appropriate basic science to use in developing a list of the causes of anorexia. A good appetite depends on a psychic desire for food; a happy GI tract that is secreting hydrochloric acid, pancreatic and intestinal enzymes, and bile in the proper amounts; a smooth absorption of food; a smooth transport of food and oxygen to the cell; and an adequate uptake of food and oxygen by the cells. Examining each of these physiologic mechanisms provides a useful recall of the differential diagnosis of anorexia.

1. **Psychic desire for food:** This may be impaired in functional depression, psychosis, anorexia nervosa, and organic brain syndromes (e.g., cerebral arteriosclerosis, senile dementia, and tumors).
2. **GI disease:** Esophagitis, esophageal carcinoma, gastritis, gastric and duodenal ulcers, gastric carcinoma, intestinal parasites, regional enteritis, intestinal obstruction, ulcerative colitis, diverticulitis, chronic appendicitis, and colonic neoplasm are the most important diseases to consider here. Many drugs increase acid production (e.g., caffeine) and cause gastritis (e.g., aspirin, corticosteroids,

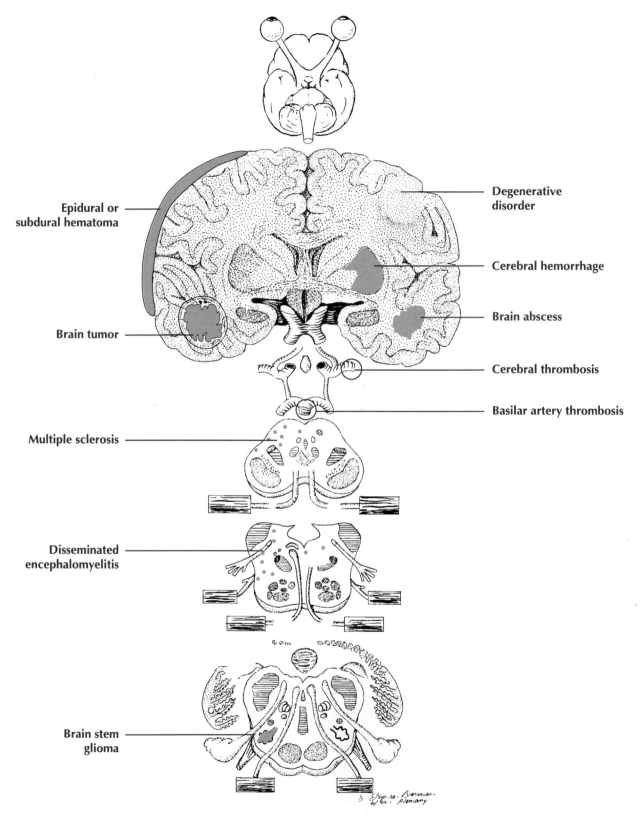

● FIGURE 22 Ankle clonus and hyperactive and pathologic reflexes.

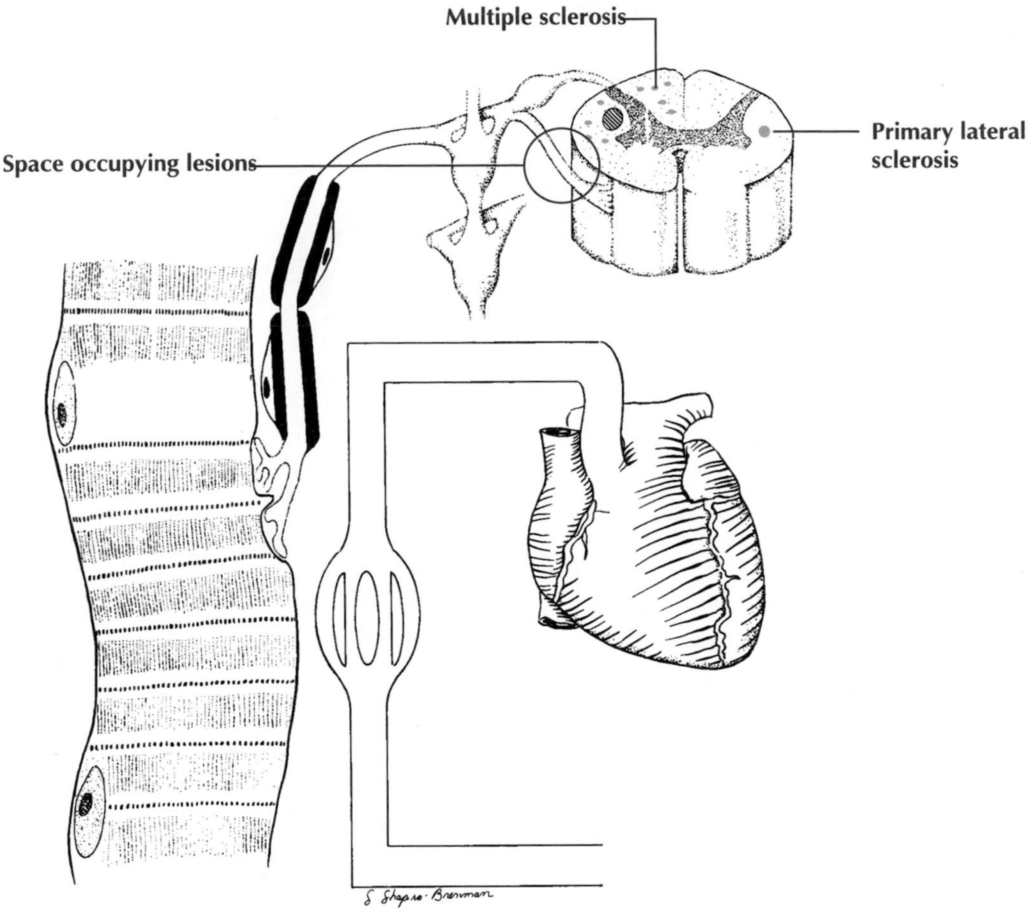

● **FIGURE 23** Ankle clonus and hyperactive and pathologic reflexes.

and reserpine) or interfere with intestinal motility and cause anorexia.

3. **Decreased pancreatic enzymes:** Pancreatitis, fibrocystic disease, pancreatic carcinomas, and ampullary carcinomas are considered here.

4. **Proper bile secretion:** Gallstones, cholecystitis, cholangitis, liver disease, and carcinoma of the pancreas and bile ducts must be considered here.

5. **Smooth absorption of food:** Celiac disease and the many other causes of malabsorption are brought to mind in this category.

6. **Smooth transport of food and oxygen:** Anything that interferes with oxygen and food reaching the cell may be considered here. Pulmonary diseases that interfere with the intake of oxygen or release of CO_2 are recalled here, as are anemia and CHF.

7. **Uptake of food and oxygen by the cell:** This will be decreased in diabetes mellitus (when there is no insulin to provide the transfer of glucose across the cell membrane); in hypothyroidism (when the cell metabolism is slow, uptake of oxygen and food is also slow); in adrenal insufficiency, where the proper relation of sodium (Na^+), chloride (Cl^-), and potassium (K^+) is interfered with; in uremia, hepatic failure, and other toxic states from drugs that interfere with cell metabolism; and in histotoxic anoxia, where the uptake of oxygen by the

cell is impaired (e.g., cyanide poisoning). Chronic infections such as pulmonary tuberculosis may also produce anorexia by this mechanism.

Approach to the Diagnosis

Loss of appetite usually is related to one of four things: (i) a psychiatric disorder, (ii) an endocrine disorder, (iii) a malignancy, or (iv) a chronic disease. If the general physical examination is normal, it is wise to get a psychiatric consult at the onset. Alternatively, one may order a psychometric test such as the Minnesota Multiphasic Personality Inventory (MMPI).

The organic causes of anorexia are usually associated with significant weight loss. The combination with anorexia of other symptoms and signs will help make the diagnosis. Anorexia with jaundice points to hepatitis or liver neoplasm as the cause. Anorexia with nonpitting edema would suggest hypothyroidism. Anorexia with dysphagia would suggest an esophageal neoplasm. Anorexia with tanning of the skin would suggest adrenal insufficiency.

The initial workup of anorexia includes a CBC; sedimentation rate; urinalysis; chemistry panel; stool for occult blood, ovum, and parasites; chest x-ray; and flat plate of the abdomen. If hypothyroidism is suspected, a free thyroxine index (FT_4) and thyroid-stimulating hormonesensitive (S-TSH) assay is ordered. If liver disease is suspected, a liver

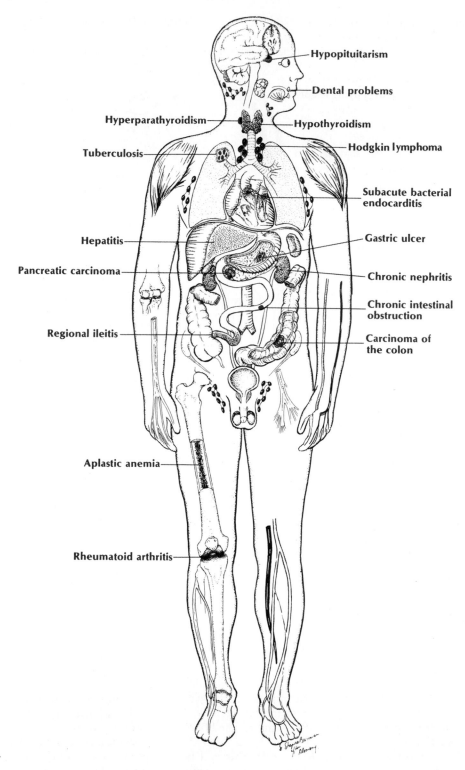

Hypopituitarism

Dental problems

Hyperparathyroidism

Hypothyroidism

Tuberculosis

Hodgkin lymphoma

Subacute bacterial endocarditis

Hepatitis

Gastric ulcer

Pancreatic carcinoma

Chronic nephritis

Chronic intestinal obstruction

Regional ileitis

Carcinoma of the colon

Aplastic anemia

Rheumatoid arthritis

● **FIGURE 24** Anorexia.

profile or hepatitis profile may be ordered. If malabsorption syndrome is suspected, one can order a D-xylose absorption test or quantitative stool fat analysis. If CHF is suspected, a circulation time is a good screening test. If pancreatic carcinoma or other GI malignancy is suspected, a CT scan of the abdomen may be ordered. It is best to consult a gastroenterologist before ordering these expensive tests. He or she can decide if endoscopic procedures or other studies would be more useful before ordering a CT scan.

Other Useful Tests
1. Fever chart (chronic infectious disease)
2. Serum amylase and lipase (pancreatic carcinoma)
3. Carcinoembryonic antigen (CEA) (GI neoplasm)

4. Schilling test (pernicious anemia)
5. Barium enema (colon neoplasm)
6. Upper GI series and esophagram (GI malignancy, cardiospasm)
7. Small-bowel series (regional enteritis, neoplasm)
8. Sonogram (hepatic cyst, pancreatic cyst)
9. Esophagoscopy (carcinoma)
10. Gastroscopy (gastric ulcer or malignancy)
11. Colonoscopy (colonic neoplasm)
12. Follicle-stimulating hormone (FSH) and luteinizing hormone (LH) assays (anorexia nervosa, hypopituitarism)

ANOSMIA OR UNUSUAL ODOR

Anatomy is an excellent method of recalling the possible causes of anosmia and unusual odors.

1. **Nasal passages:** Focusing on the nasal passages, one can recall upper respiratory infections, allergic rhinitis, chronic rhinitis of smoking and/or overdose of decongestants, polyps, sinusitis, and nasopharyngeal carcinomas.
2. **Olfactory nerves** may be affected by fracture of the cribriform plate or neoplasms.
3. The **olfactory groove** may be affected by trauma, neoplasm (particularly a meningioma), or cerebral abscess.
4. **Cerebrum:** Considering the cerebrum will prompt the recall of general paresis, encephalitis, basilar meningitis, multiple sclerosis, and tumor of the frontal lobe. It should also help recall epilepsy, cerebral aneurysms, and migraine. Unfortunately, this method will not help recall the various drugs such as captopril and penicillamine that may cause anosmia. It will also not prompt the recall of hysteria and various systemic diseases (hypothyroidism, diabetes, renal failure, hepatic failure, and pernicious anemia). By using the mnemonic **VINDICATE** these will not be missed.

Approach to the Diagnosis
If the disorder is the result of an acute infectious process, nothing needs be done. If it is associated with trauma or there has been a gradual onset, it is important to get a CT scan to rule out skull fracture or neoplasm. It is essential to rule out drug and alcohol use at the outset by a careful history and urine screen.

A good nasopharyngeal examination and nasopharyngoscopy must be done if local disease is suspected. These may need to be complemented by x-rays or CT scan of the sinuses. Systemic disease can be ruled out by a CBC, chemistry panel, thyroid profile, serum B_{12} test, glucose tolerance test, and liver profile. If epilepsy is suspected, a wake-and-sleep EEG needs to be done.

Other Useful Tests
1. Neurology consult
2. Otolaryngology consult
3. MRI of the brain (brain tumor)
4. Nasal smear for eosinophils (allergic rhinitis)
5. ANA titer (collagen disease)
6. Spinal tap (multiple sclerosis)

ANURIA AND OLIGURIA

Diminished output of urine (oliguria with less than 500 mL of output in 24 hours) and no output of urine (anuria) are best understood using **pathophysiology**. The causes may be divided into prerenal (where less fluid is delivered to the kidney for filtration), renal (where the kidney is unable to produce urine because of intrinsic disease), and postrenal (where the kidney is obstructed and the urine cannot be excreted).

1. **Prerenal causes:** Anything that reduces the blood flow to the kidney may cause anuria. Thus, shock from hemorrhage, myocardial infarction, dehydration, drugs, or septicemia may be the cause. CHF in which the effective renal plasma flow is reduced is also a possibility. Intestinal obstruction or intense diarrhea may cause the loss of enormous amounts of fluid through vomiting or diarrhea, and the accompanying shock results in anuria. Embolic glomerulonephritis, bilateral renal artery thrombosis, and dissecting aneurysms may cause renal shutdown.
2. **Renal causes:** These may be analyzed with the mnemonic **VINDICATE** so that none are missed.

   V—**Vascular** lesions include embolic glomerulonephritis and dissecting aneurysm; transfusion reactions are considered as well as intravascular hemolysis of any cause.

   I—**Inflammatory** lesions include pyelonephritis, necrotizing papillitis, and renal tuberculosis.

   N—**Neoplasms** of the kidney rarely cause anuria because only one kidney is affected at a time.

   D—**Degenerative** conditions are unlikely to cause anuria.

   I—**Intoxication** from numerous antibiotics (e.g., gentamicin, sulfa, streptomycin) and from gold, arsenic, chloroform, carbon tetrachloride, or phenol, for example, is a common cause of anuria. Renal calculi and nephrocalcinosis should be considered here.

   C—**Congenital** disorders include polycystic kidneys and medullary sponge kidneys.

   A—**Autoimmune** disorders form the largest group of renal causes of anuria. Lupus erythematosus, polyarteritis nodosa, acute glomerulonephritis, amyloidosis, Wegener granulomatosis, and scleroderma are included here.

   T—**Trauma** includes contusions and lacerations of the kidney for completeness; however, lower nephron nephrosis from crush injury or burns is not unusual.

   E—**Endocrine** disorders include diabetic glomerulosclerosis, necrotizing papillitis from diabetes, and nephrocalcinosis from hyperparathyroidism and related disorders.
3. **Postrenal causes:** The mnemonic **MINT** will help recall this group of disorders that obstruct the kidneys and bladder.

   M—**Malformations** may cause anuria; they include congenital bands, aberrant vessels over the ureters, horseshoe kidney, and ureteroceles.

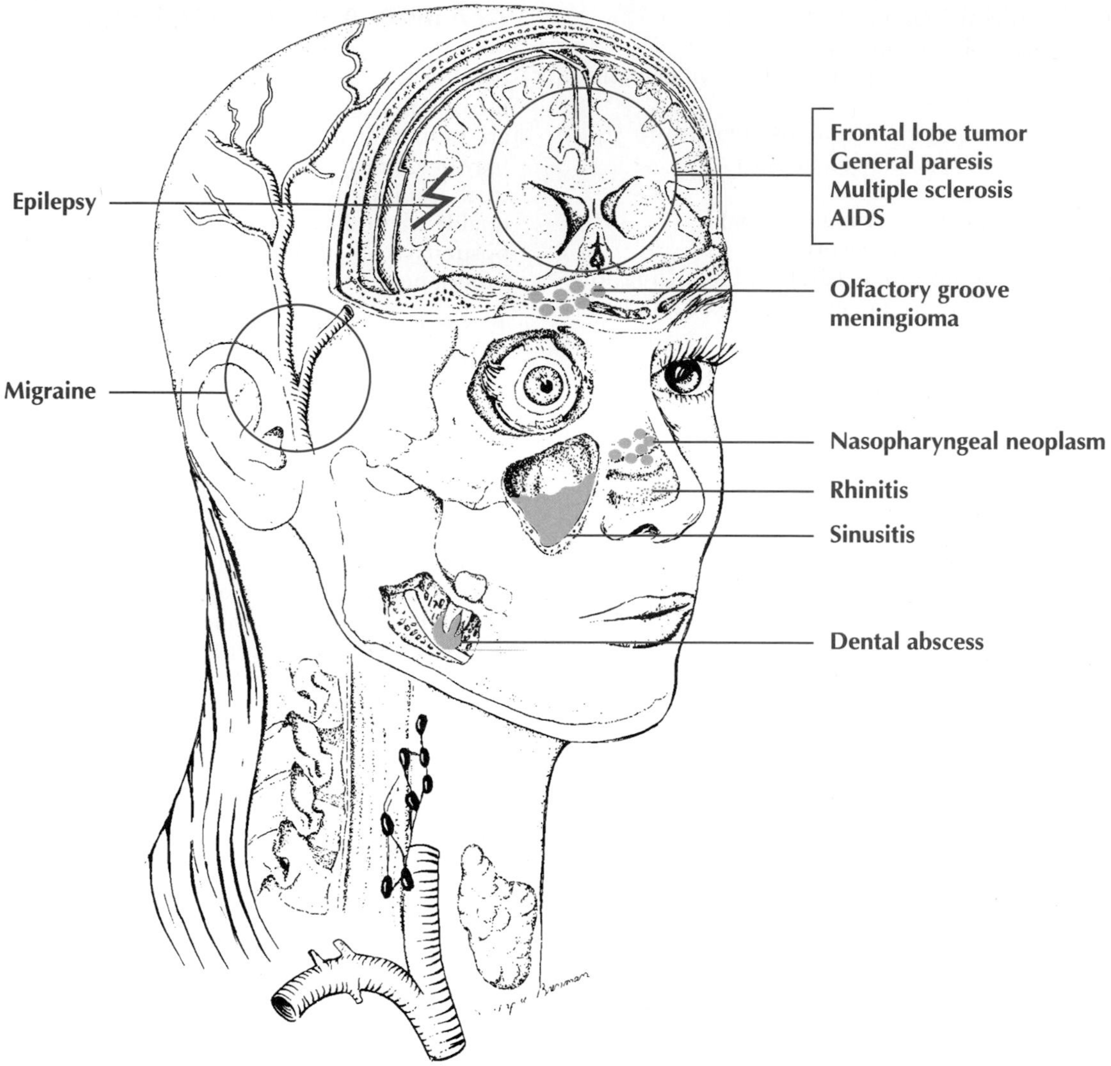

● FIGURE 25 Anosmia or unusual odor.

I—**Inflammation** includes cystitis, urethritis, and prostatitis.

N—**Neoplasms** include carcinomas of the bladder obstructing both ureters, prostatic hypertrophy, and carcinomas of the uterus or cervix involving both ureters. **N** also signifies neurologic disorders such as polio, multiple sclerosis, and acute trauma to the spinal cord that may cause anuria.

T—**Trauma** signifies surgical ligation of the ureters, ruptured bladder, and instrumentation of the urinary tract.

Approach to the Diagnosis

The clinical picture will be helpful in determining the cause of anuria. In cases of prerenal azotemia, there will be decreased skin turgor and orthostatic hypotension if the cause is volume depletion. If the cause is CHF, there will be jugular vein distention, hepatomegaly, and pedal edema. Patients with postrenal azotemia may have an enlarged prostate, a distended bladder, and other signs of obstructive uropathy. Patients with renal azotemia may have bilateral flank masses (polycystic kidney), hypertension, peripheral emboli (embolic glomerulonephritis), or a rash (collagen disease, interstitial nephritis).

The initial workup includes a CBC; urinalysis; urine culture and sensitivity; personal examination of the urine for casts, and so forth; chemistry panel; spot urine sodium; serum and urine osmolality; flat plate of the abdomen for kidney size; chest x-ray; and ECG. The bladder is catheterized for residual urine; if this is significant, postrenal azotemia is likely and a urologist is consulted. He or she will most likely do a cystoscopy and retrograde pyelography after the patient's condition is stabilized. Ultrasonography can be used to determine if there is significant residual urine also.

The laboratory studies will determine whether there is prerenal or renal azotemia. If the sodium concentration in the spot urine is <10 mEq/L, prerenal azotemia is likely. Also, in prerenal azotemia, the BUN/creatinine ratio is 20:1 or greater and the urine osmolality is 450 mOsm per kilogram of water or greater. The urine sediment will show granular and red cell casts in most cases of renal azotemia, and the BUN/creatinine ratio will be 10:1 or less.

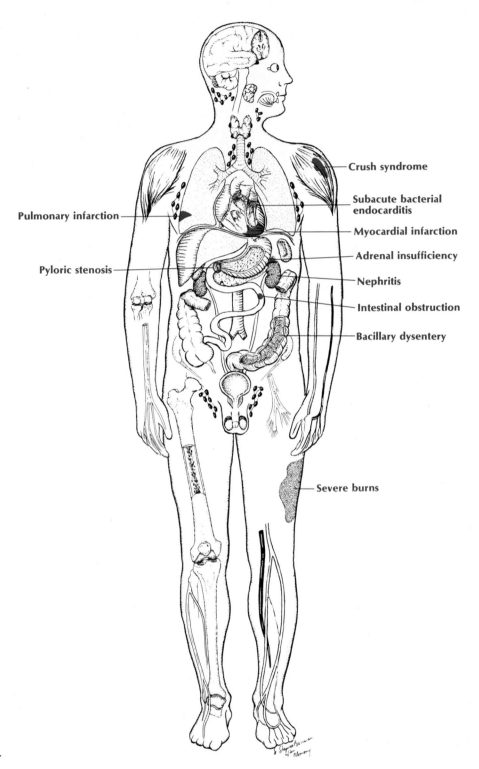

Crush syndrome

Subacute bacterial endocarditis

Pulmonary infarction

Myocardial infarction

Adrenal insufficiency

Pyloric stenosis

Nephritis

Intestinal obstruction

Bacillary dysentery

Severe burns

● **FIGURE 26** Anuria and oliguria.

Further workup will depend on what the presumptive diagnosis is. If volume depletion is the cause, intravenous saline and plasma volume expanders are given while carefully monitoring the urine output. If this is ineffective, furosemide and a mannitol drip can be utilized to reestablish urine output. If these measures are ineffective, the patient obviously has a renal cause for his or her anuria, and a urologist should be consulted.

Renal causes can be differentiated by further workup. If intravascular hemolysis is suspected, a serum haptoglobin test should be ordered. If dissecting aneurysm or bilateral renal artery stenosis is suspected, aortography and angiography would be done. If polycystic kidney disease is suspected, ultrasonography or CT scan of the abdomen may be done. Eosinophilia of the blood or urine will be found in drug-induced nephritis. If a collagen disease is suspected, one

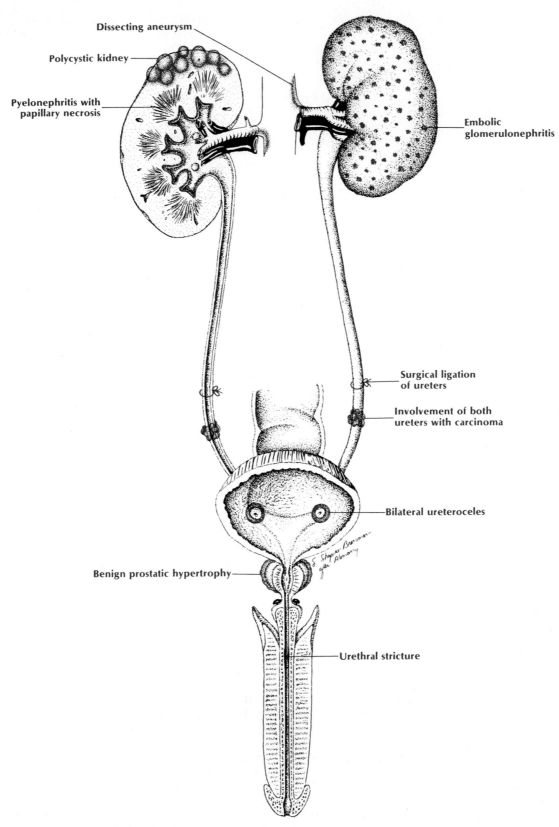

● **FIGURE 27** Anuria and oliguria.

should order an ANA, double-stranded DNA (dsDNA) antibody titer, or lupus erythematosus cell prep. A renal biopsy may also be necessary in these and many other disorders.

Other Useful Tests
1. Serum protein electrophoresis (multiple myeloma)
2. Anti-streptolysin O (ASO) titer (acute glomerulonephritis)
3. Blood cultures (bacterial endocarditis)
4. Serum complement (acute glomerulonephritis, collagen disease)

APHASIA, APRAXIA, AND AGNOSIA

These disorders signify a dysfunction of the cerebrum. Aphasia must be distinguished from dysarthria, which could also be due to involvement of the brain stem or cerebellum. Patients with dysarthria have no difficulty recognizing or interpreting words or phrases, but speech is garbled and difficult to understand by the clinician. The mnemonic **VINDICATE** would be useful in developing the differential diagnosis of these symptoms and signs.

V—Vascular should bring to mind TIA, cerebral thrombosis, embolism, hemorrhage. Cerebral or arteriosclerosis should also be considered.
I—Inflammation conditions include viral encephalitis, brain abscess, and human immunodeficiency virus (HIV) infections.
N—Neoplasm brings to mind primary and metastatic tumors.
D—Degenerative disorders include Alzheimer disease, Pick disease, Huntington chorea, and dementia with Lewy bodies. There is also a condition known as progressive aphasia without dementia.
I—Intoxication should suggest the possibility of alcohol or drug intoxication and Korsakoff psychosis.
C—Congenital disorders include cerebral palsy, the leukodystrophies, and congenital abnormalities of the brain such as hydrocephalus and microcephaly. Cerebral aneurysm and atrioventricular (A-V) anomalies might also be brought to mind in this category.
A—Autoimmune disorders include multiple sclerosis, lupus erythematosus, thrombotic thrombocytopenic purpura, and other collagen disorders.
T—Trauma should bring to mind epidural, subdural, and intracerebral hematomas related to trauma.
E—Endocrine disorders are not particularly suggestive of cerebral pathology, but an amniotic fluid embolism may rarely be responsible for aphasia, apraxia, or agnosia. Hypoparathyroidism may bring about seizures which could cause transient aphasia in the postictal phase.

Approach to the Diagnosis
A thorough neurologic examination may disclose hemiparesis suggesting a cerebrovascular accident or papilledema suggesting a space-occupying lesion. The history would be very important in ruling out alcohol or drug intoxication, trauma, or autoimmune disorders. A CT scan would be useful in acute cases, whereas an MRI would be best for cases with a gradual onset. These studies would be most definitive for an infarct, space-occupying lesion, or degenerative disorders. A VDRL test, ANA, CBC, and sedimentation rate would be helpful to rule out systemic causes. A urine drug screen may be necessary. For cases of intermittent symptoms, an EEG should be done to rule out epilepsy, and a carotid scan should be done to rule out carotid stenosis or plaque formation. A neurologist should be consulted if four-vessel angiography is contemplated.

ARM PAIN

An **anatomic** breakdown of the arm into its components is the key to a sound differential diagnosis in arm pain. Pain may be referred from more proximal portions of the extremity such as the shoulder (e.g., bursitis) or brachial plexus (e.g., cervical rib), so these areas must also be examined.

Beginning with the **skin** and **subcutaneous tissue**, one recalls herpes zoster, cellulitis, contusions, and a variety of dermatologic conditions that should be obvious. Weber–Christian disease, which usually affects the thighs, is more obscure. Rheumatoid and rheumatic nodules may occur on the skin and are, of course, painful. Beneath the skin the **muscles**, **fascia**, and **bursae** are frequent sites of inflammation and trauma. Contusions, rupture of the ligaments, and bursitis (particularly tennis elbow) are common acute traumatic conditions (bursitis, however, is more likely the result of chronic strain). Inflammatory lesions of the muscles include epidemic myalgia, trichinosis, nonarticular rheumatism, and dermatomyositis. Muscle cramping from hypocalcemia or other electrolyte disturbances must be considered in the differential diagnosis of arm pain.

The superficial and deep veins are the site of thrombophlebitis and hemorrhage, both prominent causes of arm pain. The **arteries** may be involved by emboli (from auricular fibrillation, myocardial infarction, and SBE), thrombosis (especially in Buerger disease and blood dyscrasias such as sickle cell anemia), and vasculitis (periarteritis nodosa is one example). Acute trauma to the artery may cause pain. When one moves centrally along the arterial pathways, additional causes of pain come to mind. For example, dissecting aneurysms or acute subclavian steal syndrome may cause severe pain down the arm, but pain is referred to the arm from a myocardial infarct as well. When superficial or deep infections of the arm spread to the lymphatics, lymphangitis may develop and cause arm pain.

The nerves may be a source of pain, both centrally and locally. Buerger disease, cellulitis, and osteomyelitis may involve the nerve locally. Neuromas may cause focal pain in the distribution of the involved peripheral nerve. Carpal tunnel syndrome, which may be caused by rheumatoid arthritis, amyloidosis, acromegaly, hypothyroidism, or multiple myeloma, may compress the median nerve (and occasionally the ulnar nerve) to cause pain in the hand and even up the arm. Moving up the nerve pathways, another frequent spot for nerve compression is the brachial plexus. Pancoast tumors, cervical ribs, and the scalenus anticus syndrome may be the cause of arm pain originating from the plexus.

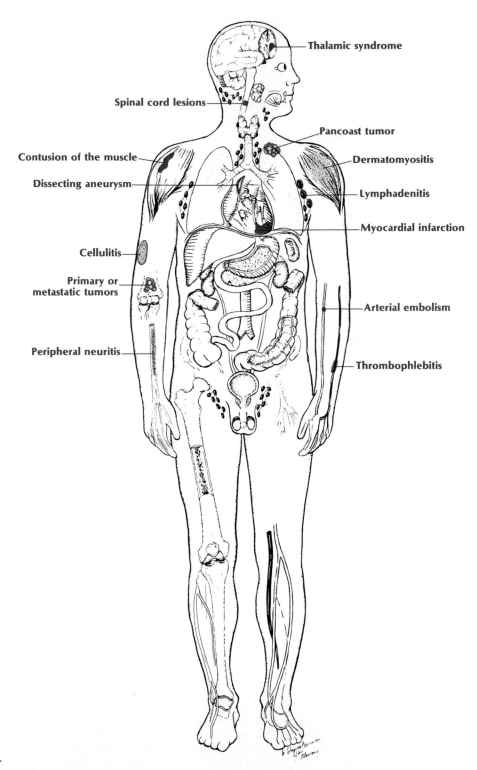

Thalamic syndrome

Spinal cord lesions

Pancoast tumor

Contusion of the muscle

Dermatomyositis

Dissecting aneurysm

Lymphadenitis

Myocardial infarction

Cellulitis

Primary or metastatic tumors

Arterial embolism

Peripheral neuritis

Thrombophlebitis

● **FIGURE 28** Arm pain.

The **cervical nerve roots** may be compressed by diseases of the spine and spinal cord. A herniated disc, cervical spondylosis, metastatic carcinoma, tuberculosis of the spine, multiple myeloma, and cord tumors (e.g., meningiomas, neurofibromas, and ependymomas) are the most notable. Syringomyelia and tabes dorsalis are other sources of arm pain that originate in the spinal cord. As one moves up the cord to the **brainstem**, one recalls the thalamic syndrome (usually caused by occlusion of the thalamogeniculate artery) as a cause of pain in the arm.

The **bone** and **joints** are deeper in the arm. They prompt the diagnosis of osteomyelitis, primary and metastatic bone tumors, and diseases of the joints such as osteoarthritis, rheumatoid arthritis, gout, gonococcal arthritis, and Reiter syndrome. In adolescents with elbow pain, look for

A

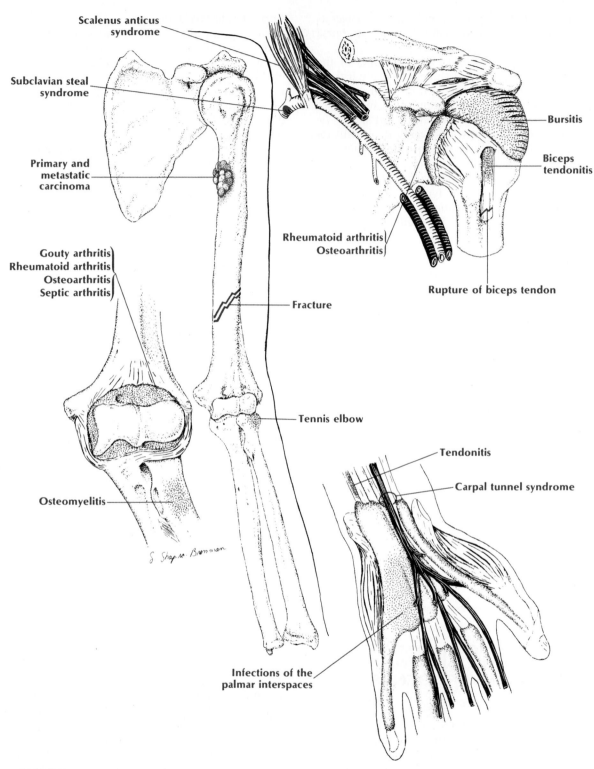

Scalenus anticus
syndrome

Subclavian steal
syndrome

Primary and
metastatic
carcinoma

Gouty arthritis
Rheumatoid arthritis
Osteoarthritis
Septic arthritis

Osteomyelitis

Bursitis

Biceps
tendonitis

Rheumatoid arthritis
Osteoarthritis

Rupture of biceps tendon

Fracture

Tennis elbow

Tendonitis

Carpal tunnel syndrome

Infections of the
palmar interspaces

● **FIGURE 29** Arm pain, local causes.

osteochondritis dissecans. A more extensive discussion of joint disorders can be found on page 274. Systemic diseases that cause arm pain from peripheral nerve involvement include diabetes mellitus (with ischemic neuropathy), periarteritis nodosa, and macroglobulinemia. Sickle cell anemia may also cause an ischemic neuropathy.

Approach to the Diagnosis

The association of other symptoms and signs found on a good history and physical examination is most important in pinpointing the diagnosis. Thus, arm pain with tenderness and limitation of motion at the elbow suggests tennis elbow, gout, or rheumatoid arthritis. Arm pain with loss of sensation in the distribution of the median nerve suggests carpal tunnel syndrome. Injection of lidocaine into bursa or trigger points may be diagnostic.

The laboratory workup should include x-rays of the involved area and of the cervical spine, especially if there is a radicular distribution of the pain. It is important to do anteroposterior (AP), lateral, and oblique films in all cases. If there are focal neurologic signs, a neurologist should be consulted before ordering an MRI: A cervical rib will not be missed in this way. An ECG and myocardial enzymes may be necessary to exclude a myocardial infarct, and an exercise tolerance test will help to exclude coronary insufficiency. Arteriogram, phlebogram, lymphangiogram, electromyogram with nerve conduction studies, myelogram, and nerve blocks will be necessary in specific cases.

Other Useful Tests

1. Stellate ganglion block (reflex sympathetic dystrophy)
2. Dermatomal somatosensory evoked potentials (DSEPs) (neuropathy, radiculopathy, demyelinating disease)
3. Arthritis panel
4. Chest x-ray (Pancoast tumor)
5. MRI of shoulder (torn rotator cuff)

Case Presentation #6

A 44-year-old white male executive complained of recurrent pain radiating down his left arm into his fingers for 3 months.

Question #1. Utilizing the methods described above, what are the possible diagnoses that you would entertain at this point?

Further history reveals that the patient was involved in an auto accident 1 year ago. He complained of neck pain at that time but was treated in the emergency room and released. Neurologic examination at this time reveals a diminished biceps reflex and hypesthesia and hypalgesia in the left thumb and index finger. Adson tests are negative.

Question #2. What are the most likely possibilities now?

(See Appendix B for the answers.)

ASPARTATE AMINOTRANSFERASE, ALANINE AMINOTRANSFERASE, AND LACTIC DEHYDROGENASE ELEVATION

When the chemistry profile shows an elevation of these enzymes, recall the tissues that produce a large amount of these enzymes: the liver, heart, and skeletal muscles. This translates into hepatitis, myocardial infarction, and dermatomyositis as the principal conditions to consider in the differential diagnosis. When only the aspartate aminotransferase (AST) level is elevated, liver disease is the primary consideration. When only the lactate dehydrogenase (LDH) level is elevated, pulmonary infarction should be high on the list of possibilities and a lung scan should be ordered. CHF may also produce a significant elevation of the AST with little or no elevation of the LDH.

Approach to the Diagnosis

Obviously, the first condition to rule out is myocardial infarction. This is done by ordering serial MB isoenzyme of creatine phosphokinase (MB-CPKs) and ECGs. Serum cardiac troponin levels may also be helpful. Next, determine if the patient is on heparin, because this may elevate the alanine aminotransferase (ALT) level. Various muscle diseases (dermatomyositis, muscular dystrophy, muscle trauma, etc.) may be excluded by ordering CPK enzymes also, particularly the MM (MM isoenzyme of CPK) fraction. Patients using statins (HMGCoA reductase inhibitors) may have elevated transaminases and CPK. Liver disease can be revealed by a liver profile, CT scan of the abdomen, and gallbladder ultrasonography.

Other Useful Tests

1. CBC
2. Urinalysis
3. Sedimentation rate (neoplasm, dermatomyositis)
4. Repeated chemistry profile (myocardial infarct, muscle disease)
5. Serum amylase level (pancreatitis)
6. Lung scan (pulmonary infarct)
7. Electromyogram (dermatomyositis, muscle disease)
8. ANA analysis (dermatomyositis)
9. Muscle biopsy (collagen disease, muscular dystrophy)
10. Liver biopsy

AURAL DISCHARGE (OTORRHEA)

The differential diagnosis of a nonbloody discharge of the ear can best be done by using **anatomy**. Visualize the components of the ear apparatus. A discharge may arise from the external canal, the middle ear, the mastoids and petrous bone, the inner ear, or the cerebrospinal fluid. As elsewhere in the body, nonbloody discharge signifies inflammation and infectious or allergic conditions, but foreign bodies and malignancies can trigger an infection by causing an obstruction or lowering resistance.

The **external canal** may be involved by bacterial infection as in furunculosis, diffuse otitis externa, and Eaton agent pneumonia and by **viral infection** in herpes zoster (Ramsay Hunt syndrome). Fungi may infest the external canal, particularly when wax or a foreign body accumulates. Atopic, contact, or seborrheic dermatitis may also involve the external canal.

In the **middle ear**, bacterial infections may produce an acute or chronic purulent otitis media with or without rupture of the drum, but a serous otitis media from allergy, viral infections, or obstruction of the eustachian tube does not usually cause otorrhea. In addition to perforation, otitis media may lead to mastoiditis, petrositis, and ultimately to a chronic granuloma called a cholesteatoma. All of these are usually associated with a chronic continuous or intermittent nonbloody discharge.

Conditions arising in the **inner ear** (e.g., labyrinthitis) are rarely associated with otorrhea, but a basilar skull fracture may lead to cerebrospinal otorrhea. This is usually bloody at onset, but if it goes unrecognized it may become clear or, when infected, purulent.

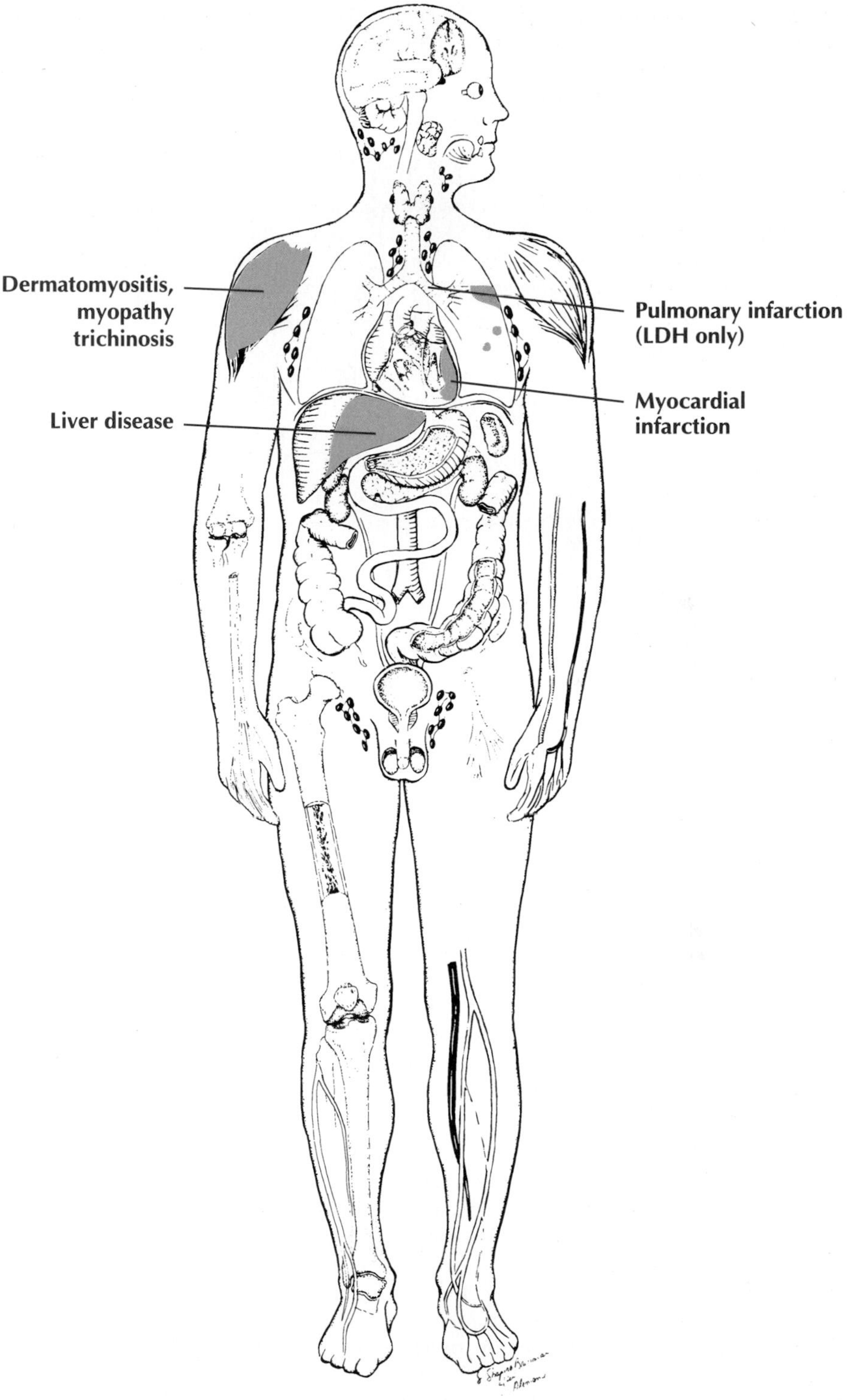

● **FIGURE 30** Aspartate aminotransferase (AST, SGOT), alanine aminotransferase (ALT), and lactic dehydrogenase (LDH) elevation.

Approach to the Diagnosis

The approach to the diagnosis of an aural discharge is similar to the approach for discharges from any body orifice. After careful examination for a foreign body or obstruction, the discharge is cultured and appropriate therapy begun. A Gram stain of the material often aids in the determination of the most appropriate antibiotic. If the discharge is chronic, x-rays of the mastoids and petrous bones may be necessary, as well as tomography. Obviously, referral to an otolaryngologist is wise at this point.

Other Useful Tests

1. CBC (infection)
2. Sedimentation rate (inflammation)
3. Acid-fast bacillus (AFB) and fungal smear and culture
4. Tuberculin test

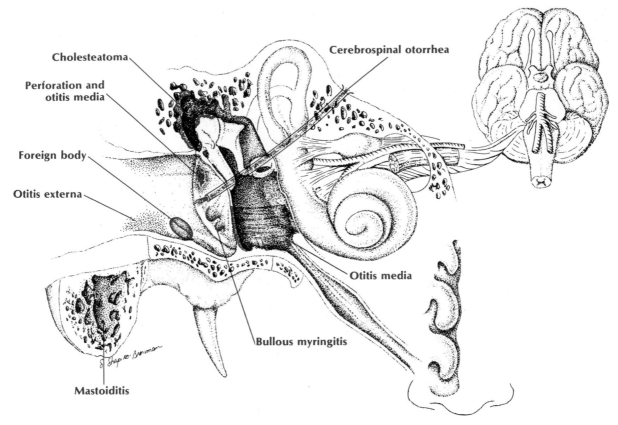

Cholesteatoma

Perforation and otitis media

Foreign body

Otitis externa

Cerebrospinal otorrhea

Otitis media

Bullous myringitis

Mastoiditis

● **FIGURE 31** Aural discharge.

5. VDRL test (syphilis)
6. CT scan of the brain, mastoids, petrous bones (neoplasm, mastoiditis, cholesteatoma)
7. Biopsy
8. Tympanogram (otitis media)
9. Radioactive iodine serum albumin (RISA) study (CSF otorrhea)

AUSCULTATORY SIGNS OF PULMONARY DISEASE

It is questionable whether this topic should be included in a differential diagnosis book, but because it is important for the clinician to be able to recall a fairly complete list of possible causes for these signs while he or she is still examining the patient, a discussion is included here. Regardless of what the sign is, it almost invariably may be considered the result of local disease of the lung or heart. Infrequently, a disease of another organ might have spread to the lung. Cross-indexing these topics with the mnemonic of etiologies, **VINDICATE**, will provide a useful list of possibilities.

● Lung

V—**Vascular** diseases include pulmonary embolism, infarction, and Goodpasture disease.
I—**Inflammatory** disease suggests viral, bacterial tuberculosis, parasitic and fungal pneumonia, and lung abscess. Pleurisy must also be considered.

N—**Neoplasms** remind one of carcinoma of the lungs (primary or metastatic) and bronchial adenomas.
D—**Degenerative** disease suggests emphysema and pulmonary fibrosis.
I—**Intoxication** brings to mind the pneumoconioses and changes from drugs such as nitrofurantoin.
C—**Congenital** disorders include cystic fibrosis, α_1-antitrypsin deficiency, bronchiectasis, alveolar proteinosis, atelectasis, and lung cysts.
A—**Autoimmune** diseases include rheumatoid arthritis, lupus, Wegener granulomatosis, periarteritis nodosa, and scleroderma. The **A** also stands for **allergic** diseases, including asthma and Löffler syndrome.
T—**Trauma** should suggest pneumothorax and hemopneumothorax.
E—**Endocrine** disease suggests the bronchoconstriction of the carcinoid syndrome.

● Heart

V—**Vascular** diseases of the heart that cause auscultatory signs include myocardial infarction and hypertension with CHF and the various arrhythmias associated with them.
I—**Inflammatory** diseases of the heart also affect the lungs. Subacute and acute bacterial endocarditis may shed emboli in the lung if the right side of the heart is affected. Myocarditis may cause failure, and pericarditis may cause pleural effusion.
N—**Neoplasms** of the heart rarely affect the lung.

D—**Degenerative** diseases include muscular dystrophy and other cardiomyopathies.

I—**Intoxication** reminds one of alcoholic myocardiopathy with CHF and arrhythmias that may lead to emboli. Digitalis and other cardiac drugs may do the same. Electrolyte disturbances must also be considered here.

C—**Congenital** heart diseases bring to mind a host of diseases that may cause failure.

A—**Autoimmune** diseases, especially lupus erythematosus, scleroderma, and amyloidosis, affect the heart and lung.

T—**Traumatic** hemopericardium or aneurysm of the heart may cause auscultatory changes of the lung.

E—**Endocrine** diseases such as hyperthyroidism, hypothyroidism, acromegaly, and diabetes mellitus affect the heart and may ultimately lead to CHF and edema in the lungs. Endocrine causes of hypertension (aldosteronism and Cushing syndrome) may lead to hypertensive cardiovascular disease (HCVD) and CHF.

● Diseases of Other Organs

V—**Vascular** suggests pulmonary embolism from systemic phlebitis.

I—**Inflammation** includes embolic abscesses or pneumonitis of the lungs and pulmonary tuberculosis, tularemia, plague, *Echinococcus*, *Paragonimus westermani*, histoplasmosis, and so forth. Shock lung from septicemia is a possible cause.

N—**Neoplasms** suggest metastatic carcinoma from other organs. Meigs syndrome is also suggested here.

D—**Degenerative** suggests nothing here, although pleural effusion may result from nephrosis and cirrhosis.

I—**Intoxication** may result from ingested turpentine or other products that subsequently affect the lung. Aspiration pneumonitis must be considered in this category.

C—**Congenital** disorders, especially neurologic diseases and esophageal atresia, may lead to recurrent pneumonia.

A—**Autoimmune** diseases have been reviewed above.

T—**Trauma** and burns anywhere may result in pulmonary edema from shock lung.

E—**Endocrine** diseases have been discussed above.

Approach to the Diagnosis
Clinically, the grouping together of signs provides the best way of narrowing the differential diagnosis.

Rales
1. Bilateral crepitant rales, lack of dullness, and normal breath sounds suggest pulmonary edema or pneumonitis.
2. Focal crepitant rales, reduced alveolar breathing, dullness to percussion, and increased tactile and vocal fremitus suggest lobar pneumonia or pulmonary infarction.
3. Bilateral sibilant and sonorous rales without dullness and with increased bronchial breathing suggest asthma, chronic bronchitis and emphysema, acute bronchitis or bronchiolitis, and cardiac asthma.
4. Focal crepitant rales and amphoric breathing with dullness below and hyperresonance above suggest a lung abscess or cavitation.

Hyperresonance
1. Hyperresonance bilaterally with diminished breath sounds bilaterally and sibilant rales suggests pulmonary emphysema or asthma.
2. Focal hyperresonance with diminished or absent breath sounds and no rales suggests pneumothorax.
3. Focal hyperresonance with normal or only diminished breath sounds suggests a large bulla.

Dullness or Flatness
1. Dullness with diminished breath sounds and no rales suggests atelectasis or pleural effusion from empyema, CHF, or pulmonary infarct. In atelectasis, there is no hyperresonance or egophony above the dullness.
2. Dullness with diminished breath sounds and crepitant rales suggests pneumonia or pulmonary infarct. If there is bronchophony as well, there is probably no associated effusion. If there is no bronchophony but hyperresonance and egophony above the dullness, then an associated pleural effusion should be considered.

Laboratory Workup
Crepitant rales should prompt a sputum examination, smear and culture, possibly a tuberculin test, venous pressure and circulation time, chest roentgenogram, and ECG to secure the diagnosis. If the chest x-ray film shows no consolidation and the individual is in no acute distress, a pulmonary function study may help. If it shows a reduced vital capacity with a normal timed vital capacity, CHF is the most likely diagnosis. In acute cases, shock lung or adult respiratory distress syndrome must be considered.

Other Useful Tests
1. CBC (pneumonia)
2. Sedimentation rate (pneumonia)
3. Tuberculin test
4. Sputum smear and culture (pneumonia)
5. Sputum smear and culture for fungi (histoplasmosis, etc.)
6. Sputum cytology (carcinoma of the lung)
7. ANA test (collagen disease)
8. Coccidioidin skin test
9. Histoplasmin skin test
10. Blastomycin skin test
11. Rheumatoid arthritis test (rheumatoid arthritis involving the lung)
12. Kveim test (sarcoidosis)
13. X-ray of the hands (sarcoidosis)
14. Lymph node biopsy (neoplasm, sarcoidosis)
15. Bronchoscopy (neoplasm)
16. CT scan of the lung (neoplasm, bronchiectasis)
17. Echocardiogram (CHF, valvular heart disease)
18. Lung biopsy (neoplasm)
19. HIV antibody titer (acquired immunodeficiency syndrome [AIDS])

AXILLARY MASS

When the physician palpates a mass in the right axilla, his or her first thought is that it is a lymph node. Although in most cases this is probably right, it is a good idea to first

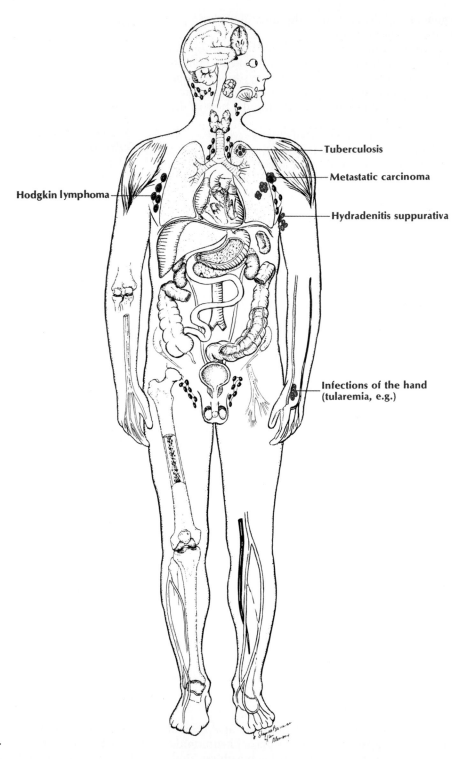

Hodgkin lymphoma

Tuberculosis

Metastatic carcinoma

Hydradenitis suppurativa

Infections of the hand
(tularemia, e.g.)

● **FIGURE 32** Axillary mass.

think of the **anatomy**: the skin and its glands, the lymph nodes, the axillary artery, subcutaneous tissue, muscles, and ribs. Thus, in addition to an enlarged lymph node, one must consider skin conditions such as sebaceous cysts and hidradenitis suppurativa; lesions of the subcutaneous tissue such as cellulitis, lipomas, and accessory breast tissue; and axillary aneurysms and primary and metastatic tumors of the ribs.

The lymph nodes are involved primarily by infection or malignancy. If other groups of lymph nodes are involved (e.g., anterior cervical or groin), then consider the differential under generalized lymphadenopathy (see page 301). For focal lymphadenopathy, look for infection in the areas that feed the gland. There may be a minor wound of the arm or hand that has become infected or there may be an infection in the lung, breast, or back. Tularemia often causes axillary adenopathy even though the wound in the hand is insignificant. The node may be involved with tuberculosis or a fungal infection such as actinomycosis, but there is also usually a site of infection in the lung.

If infection has been excluded, then malignancy must be considered. Hodgkin lymphoma, carcinoma of the breast, and carcinoma of the lung are the chief offenders, but lymphosarcoma and metastasis from other sites must be considered.

Approach to the Diagnosis

A unilateral tender axillary mass with an exudate is usually a sebaceous cyst or hidradenitis suppurativa. All that is required is incision and drainage, culture of the exudate, and antibiotics. After the infection has cleared, it can be excised. A unilateral, nontender mass is most likely a lymph node harboring metastasis or Hodgkin lymphoma. Lymph node biopsy is indicated. If the lymph node is associated with an infection of the breast or the arm, the swelling should subside after the infection is treated. Bilateral axillary lymphadenopathy would be an indication for a more extensive workup (see page 292).

Other Useful Tests

1. Needle aspiration and culture and sensitivity of the material retrieved (infection)
2. CBC
3. Sedimentation rate (inflammatory)
4. Chemistry panel (metastatic neoplasm, systemic infection)
5. Tuberculin test
6. Kveim test (sarcoidosis)
7. Coccidioidin skin test (coccidiomycosis)
8. Chest x-ray (tuberculosis, neoplasm)
9. Mammogram (neoplasm)
10. Lymphangiogram (Hodgkin lymphoma)
11. Angiogram (axillary aneurysm)
12. Exploratory surgery

B

BACK MASS

It is not uncommon for a patient to complain of a lump on his or her back. Most of the time, the lesion is a sebaceous cyst or lipoma. However, there are other types of back masses, and a simple method of recall is needed. **Anatomy** is the key. If the mnemonic **MINT** is applied to most of these structures, all of the important lesions can be recalled.

SKIN

M—**Malformations** include pilonidal cysts and sebaceous cysts.
I—**Inflammation** suggests carbuncles and furuncles.
N—**Neoplasms** include hemangiomas, neurofibromas, lipomas, and metastatic tumors.
T—**Trauma,** of course, suggests contusions.

SUBCUTANEOUS TISSUE AND FASCIA

M—**Malformations** include hernias of Petit triangle.
I—**Inflammation** suggests lesions such as rheumatoid nodules and abscesses.
N—**Neoplasms** encompass those mentioned above.
T—**Trauma** includes contusions and lacerations. Anasarca may produce edema of the back.

MUSCLE

Muscle is frequently nodular in fibromyositis, and a bursa may occasionally swell significantly. Rupture of a muscle or ligament and contusions are traumatic lesions that may present a mass. Muscle spasm from back injuries is often significant enough to cause a "mass."

BONE

Lesions of the bone are usually responsible for the deeper masses in the back.
M—**Malformations** include spina bifida, which may be occult or manifest as a swelling such as meningocele or meningomyelocele.
I—**Inflammation** suggests the gibbus of Pott disease (tuberculosis of the spine).
N—**Neoplasm** suggests metastatic neoplasm and multiple myeloma of the spine which may protrude from beneath the skin.
T—**Trauma** suggests the obvious mass of a fracture dislocation or hematoma of the periosteum of the spine.

RETROPERITONEAL STRUCTURE

Wilms tumors of the kidney and perinephric abscesses may present as a mass in the back.

● Approach to the Diagnosis

With skin lesions, excision or biopsy is frequently the best approach. Masses of the deeper structures cannot be approached as aggressively until certain conditions have been ruled out by computed tomography (CT) scans and bone scans. If a meningocele or similar congenital lesion is suspected, a neurosurgeon must be consulted.

● Other Useful Tests

1. X-ray of the thoracic or lumbosacral spine (malformations, neoplasm)
2. Magnetic resonance imaging (MRI) of the thoracic or lumbar spine (malformation, neoplasm)
3. Intravenous pyelogram (IVP) (Wilms tumor, perinephric abscess)
4. Tuberculin test
5. Serum protein electrophoresis (multiple myeloma)
6. Myelogram
7. Exploratory surgery

BALDNESS

A clever mnemonic to apply here is **HAIR**. The **H** stands for **hereditary** baldness and **hormonal** baldness, such as that caused by hypothyroidism and hyperthyroidism. The **A** stands for **alopecia areata** and **autoimmune** disease, such as lupus erythematosus. The **I** stands for **inflammatory** conditions, most notably tinea capitis, impetigo, or any condition associated with prolonged fever. The **I** also stands for **intoxication**, with arsenic and gold therapy most important here. Finally, the **R** stands for **radiation**. This is particularly significant today with so many victims of neoplasms being treated with this modality.

● Approach to the Diagnosis

The Wood lamp and scrapings of any scaly material are useful in distinguishing tinea capitis from lupus and other disorders, but taking a skin biopsy of any unusual lesion is wise. Referral to a dermatologist is best if fungus or other infections are ruled out and the findings from thyroid function studies are normal. When there is diffuse hair loss, hypogonadism may be ruled out by ordering serum luteinizing hormone (LH), follicle-stimulating hormone (FSH), testosterone and estrogen.

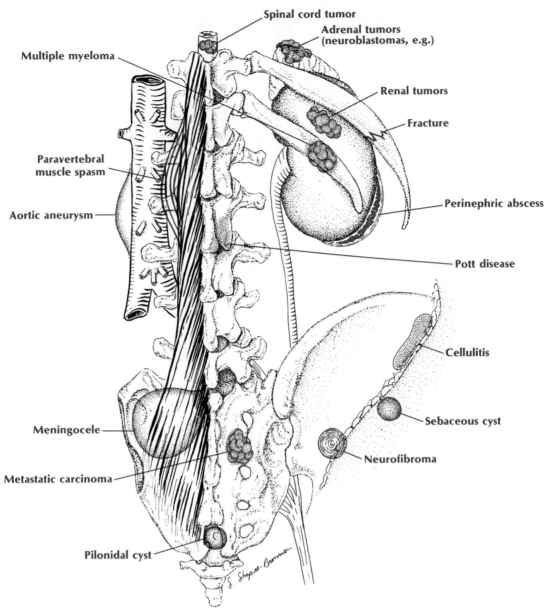

● FIGURE 1 Back mass.

BLEEDING UNDER THE SKIN

Conditions of the skin, subcutaneous tissue, vascular wall, and blood may all be associated with bleeding under the skin or purpura, thus both **anatomy** and **physiology** must be used to develop this differential (Table 12). The **skin** may hemorrhage from infections such as smallpox, scabies, chickenpox, and measles, especially when the patient traumatizes the area to relieve the itching. A bug bite also may cause hemorrhage by this means. Focal and metastatic neoplasms may cause hemorrhage in the skin, whereas degeneration of the skin may lead to senile purpura. Trauma is by far the most common cause of hemorrhage of the skin.

The **subcutaneous tissue** is distinguished separately, so that one will recall the Ehlers–Danlos syndrome and pseudoxanthoma elasticum. The **vascular wall** may be

damaged by numerous etiologies. The most important infectious etiologies are subacute bacterial endocarditis and meningococcemia, but typhoid fever, Weil disease, and Rocky Mountain spotted fever should not be forgotten. Systemic neoplasms that infiltrate the vascular wall (such as leukemia) are significant causes, but these usually cause purpura by inducing thrombocytopenia. Vascular degeneration and deficiency diseases (such as scurvy) are uncommon causes of purpura. Toxic conditions are more likely to be related to bone marrow suppression of platelets. Congenital lesions such as hereditary telangiectasias are important to remember.

Most important of all are the allergic and autoimmune disorders, because something can be done to alleviate the condition (e.g., steroids or immunosuppressants). Henoch–Schönlein purpura is a significant form of allergic

TABLE 12   Bleeding Under the Skin (Purpura)

	V Vascular	I Inflammatory	N Neoplasm	D Degenerative	I Intoxication	C Congenital	A Allergic and Autoimmune	T Trauma	E Endocrine
Skin		Smallpox Scabies Chickenpox Measles	Focal and metastatic neoplasms	Senile purpura				Bug bite Scratching (most common cause)	
Subcutaneous Tissue						Ehlers–Danlos syndrome Pseudoxanthoma elasticum			
Vascular Wall		Subacute bacterial endocarditis Meningococcemia Typhoid fever Weil disease Rocky Mountain spotted fever	Leukemia (systemic neoplasm)	Scurvy	Telangiectasis (hereditary) Von Willebrand disease	Henoch–Schönlein purpura Periarteritis nodosa		Ruptured varicose vein Crush injury Whooping cough Contusion	Cushing syndrome Waterhouse–Friderichson syndrome
Blood			Leukemia Overgrowth Myelophthisic anemia	Aplastic anemia	Gold injection Salicylate ingestion Potassium iodide Quinidine Ergot, heparin, and dicoumarol therapy Salicylate toxicity	Hemophilia von Willebrand disease Hereditary thrombasthenia	Idiopathic thrombocytopenia Lupus erythematosus		

B

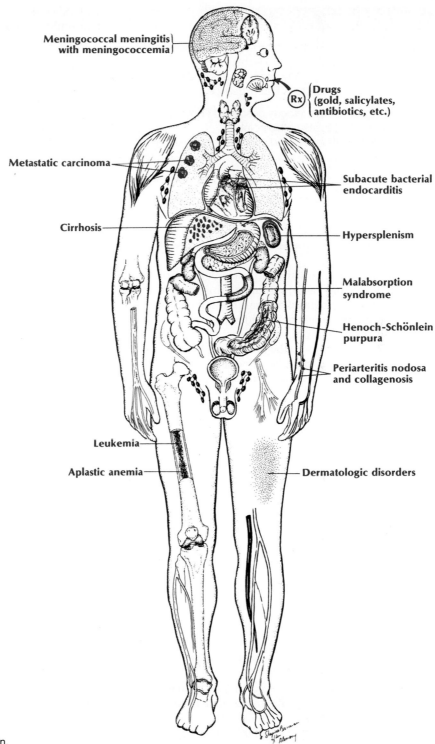

● **FIGURE 2** Bleeding under the skin.

vasculitis, but periarteritis nodosa is important as well. Trauma is just as important here as in the skin. Thus, a ruptured varicose vein, crush injury, whooping cough, or contusions are important causes of purpura. Endocrine disorders also cause vascular purpura (as in Cushing syndrome).

Disorders of the **blood** figure prominently in purpura. Significant among these are the numerous disorders that cause suppression or increased destruction of platelets. Toxic disorders such as gold injections, salicylate ingestion, potassium iodide, quinidine, ergot, and chloral hydrate are just a few of these. It is best to assume that any drug may cause purpura until proven otherwise. Leukemic overgrowth of the bone marrow may cause purpura because of thrombocytopenia, but any neoplasm that infiltrates the marrow (myelophthisic anemia) must be considered. Autoimmune disease suggests the purpura of idiopathic thrombocytopenic purpura (ITP) and lupus erythematosus.

Degenerative disorders bring to mind aplastic anemia, although this is often caused by drug suppression of the bone marrow. Congenital disorders are more often the cause of coagulation disorders such as hemophilia, but coagulation disorders are often associated with heparin and dicoumarol therapy as well. Trauma and endocrine disorders do not figure as prominently here. There may still be a platelet disorder even though the platelet count is normal. Thus, one should investigate for hereditary thrombasthenia and salicylate toxicity, among other things, by doing a clot retraction test as a screen.

● Approach to the Diagnosis

The clinical approach to purpura involves taking a drug history and a good family history, and ordering appropriate coagulation studies, tourniquet testing, and other tests. Referral to a hematologist is wise in obscure cases.

● Other Useful Tests

1. Complete blood count (CBC) (aplastic anemia, leukemia, collagen disease)
2. Sedimentation rate (systemic infection, inflammation)
3. Coagulation time (hemophilia, disseminated intravascular coagulation [DIC])
4. Partial thromboplastin time (hemophilia, DIC)
5. Bleeding time (vasculitis, vascular purpura)
6. Prothrombin time (liver disease, drug toxicity, etc.)
7. Platelet count (aplastic anemia, leukemia, collagen disease, ITP)
8. Rumpel–Leede test (vascular purpura, ITP, collagen disease)
9. Thromboplastin generation test (DIC, hemophilia)
10. Bone marrow examination (leukemia, aplastic anemia, myelophthisic anemia)
11. Antinuclear antibody (ANA) analysis (collagen disease)
12. Blood cultures (septicemia, DIC)
13. Coombs test (autoimmune disorders)
14. Monospot test (infectious mononucleosis)
15. CT scan of abdomen (neoplasm, splenomegaly)
16. Skin biopsy (Ehlers–Danlos syndrome etc.)
17. Muscle biopsy (collagen disease)
18. Liver–spleen scan (metastasis, splenomegaly)
19. Bone scan (metastatic neoplasm)
20. Test for fibrin split product (DIC)

BLURRED VISION, BLINDNESS, AND SCOTOMATA

The causes of blurred vision and blindness can best be recalled with the use of **anatomy**. If the path of light is followed through the eye to the nervous system, the various components of the eye and nervous system that may be involved may be considered in terms of the common diseases that may affect them.

Conjunctiva: Chemical, allergic, and infectious conjunctivitis may cause blurred vision, but it rarely causes blindness. A pterygium may grow across the cornea and impair vision. Trachoma may cause blindness if left untreated.

Cornea: Foreign bodies, keratitis, herpes ulcers, and keratoconus may cause blurred vision and blindness. Congenital syphilis forms an extensive progressive interstitial keratitis. Trachoma may cause corneal ulcers and blurred vision.

Canal of Schlemm: At the angle of the iris and cornea, the canal of Schlemm prompts the recall of glaucoma because obstruction of this area figures so prominently in the pathophysiology.

Iris: Iritis from sarcoid, tuberculosis, histoplasmosis, and other causes is considered here. **Iridocyclitis** occurs when both the lens and iris are involved.

Lens: The two most common causes of blurred vision, cataracts and refractive errors, are considered here. Cataracts may result from diabetes, myotonic dystrophy, galactosemia, and many systemic diseases. They are also congenital and senile, posttraumatic, and associated with various mental deficiency states. Refractive errors include myopia, hyperopia, and astigmatism. These are usually correctable. The lens may be dislocated in Marfan syndrome (page Appendix A).

Vitreous humor: Hemorrhages of the vitreous humor and precipitation of triglycerides (lipemia retinalis) may cause blurred vision.

Retina: Chorioretinitis causes blurred vision and blindness and may result from syphilis, tuberculosis, toxoplasmosis, retinitis pigmentosa, and proliferative retinitis in diabetes mellitus. Retinal detachment may result from all the above. Retinal hemorrhages, exudates of hypertension, diabetes, lupus erythematosus, aplastic anemia, and subacute bacterial endocarditis are all possible causes of blurred vision and blindness.

Retinal artery: Occlusion of the retinal artery is a prominent cause of blurred vision or blindness in older people. Emboli, thrombi, and vasculitis secondary to temporal arteritis are all possible causes of the occlusion. Migraine and birth control pills should be considered, and migraine, in particular, should be a prominent consideration in scintillating scotomata.

Retinal vein: Retinal vein thrombosis is a possibility here. Following the course of the vein, however, one encounters the cavernous sinus, and a thrombosis here may lead to bilateral blurred vision and blindness.

Optic nerve: Papilledema, optic neuritis, and optic atrophy are the most important conditions to consider. The papilledema is usually due to an intracranial space-occupying lesion, but hypertension and benign intracranial hypertension need attention in the differential. Optic neuritis requires the consideration of multiple sclerosis, neurosyphilis, tuberculosis, diabetes mellitus, sinusitis, and lead poisoning. Optic atrophy should suggest syphilis, methyl alcohol poisoning, hereditary optic atrophy, Foster Kennedy syndrome (frontal lobe tumors), and various congenital anomalies. It may be secondary to diseases of the retina. The optic nerve may be severed by an orbital fracture.

Optic chiasma: Pituitary tumors, sphenoid ridge meningiomas, colloid cysts of the third ventricle, aneurysms, and cavernous sinus thrombosis are possible causes. Syphilitic or tuberculosis meningitis may also involve the chiasma, as may the spread of a Schmincke tumor from the nasopharynx. Basilar skull fractures infrequently involve the chiasma.

Optic tract, optic radiations, and occipital cortex: Intracranial hematomas, cerebral thrombi or emboli, transient ischemic attacks (TIAs), aneurysms, cerebral tumors, and abscesses may involve these structures. Certain forms of acute and chronic encephalitis may also involve these areas, causing blurred vision and blindness. Cortical blindness may result from an occlusion of both posterior cerebral arteries at their origin from the basilar artery. Head trauma may cause transient cortical blindness in children. The neurologic workup is usually negative.

● Approach to the Diagnosis

A careful eye examination with magnification and fluorescence to rule out a foreign body and ulcers is essential in the acute case of blurred vision. Ophthalmoscopic examination may reveal optic neuritis or a retinal vein thrombosis. Visual field examination by confrontation may reveal a field defect. If these test results are negative, ocular tension should be checked to rule out glaucoma. A history of migraine, the use of birth control pills, and alcohol intake must be investigated. If there is headache on the side of the lesion, a sedimentation rate is done, steroids should probably be started immediately, and referral to a neurologist

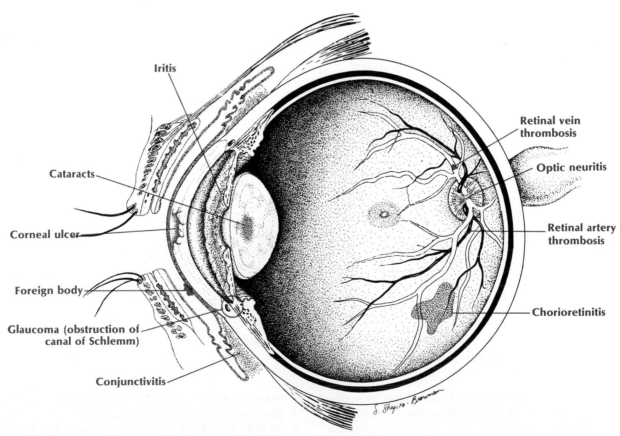

● **FIGURE 3** Blurred vision, blindness, and scotomata.

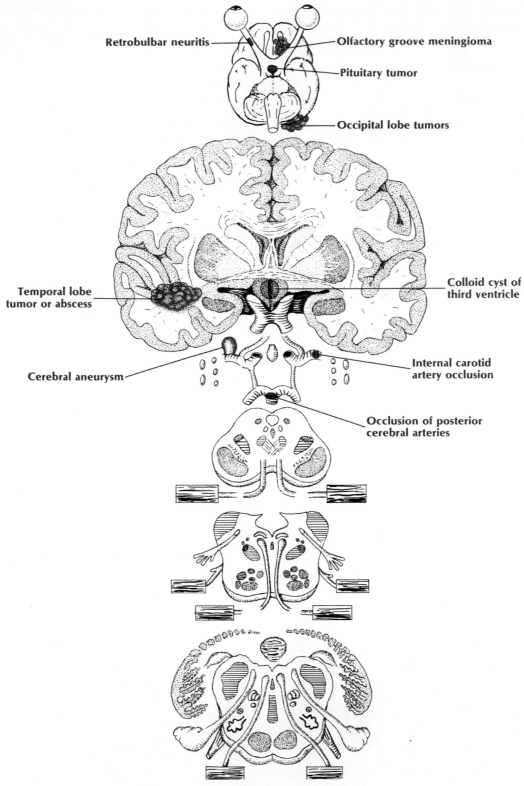

● **FIGURE 4** Blurred vision, blindness, and scotomata.

made promptly in case temporal arteritis is possible, especially in an aged individual. Otherwise, referral to an ophthalmologist is necessary. The ophthalmologist will perform visual field examinations with perimetry and a slit lamp examination, and will look for refractive errors. If other neurologic findings are present, a CT scan, skull x-ray film, and spinal tap may be indicated. A neurologic consultant can determine this.

Case Presentation #8

A 66-year-old white female diabetic was brought to the emergency room because of sudden onset of blurred vision in the right eye.

Question #1. Applying the methods discussed above, what are the possible diagnoses at this point?

Neurologic examination revealed constriction of the right visual field, a left central facial palsy, weakness of the left upper and lower extremities, and a positive Babinski sign on the left.

Question #2. What is your diagnosis?

_____

(See Appendix B for the answer.)

● Other Useful Tests

1. Venereal disease research laboratory (VDRL) test (syphilis)
2. Toxicology screen (drug abuse)
3. Tuberculin test
4. Histoplasmosis skin test
5. Serology for histoplasmosis
6. Serology for toxoplasmosis
7. Kveim test (sarcoidosis)
8. MRI (brain tumor)
9. Visual evoked potentials (multiple sclerosis)
10. ANA (collagen disease)
11. Pituitary function studies
12. Four-vessel cerebral angiography
13. Relative afferent pupillary defect (RAPD) (glaucoma, retinal detachment)

BRADYCARDIA

Bradycardia (a heart rate below 60 beats per minute) is not infrequently found during a routine physical examination. Visualizing the conduction system of the heart recalls the sick sinus syndrome, atrioventricular (A-V) nodal rhythm, or A-V block but, unfortunately, it does not help recall the many causes of these disorders. The mnemonic **VINDICATE** is the most useful aid in my experience.

V—Vascular diseases suggest myocardial infarction, especially inferior wall and anteroseptal infarctions. Arteriosclerosis may also cause focal ischemia of the conducting system.

I—Inflammatory disease suggests viral myocarditis, diphtheria, and Chagas disease.

N—Neurologic disorders may be considered, because neoplasms of the heart are infrequent. Neurologic **disorders** include vasovagal syncope (common faint), cerebral concussion, and anything else that might cause an increased intracranial pressure (e.g., subarachnoid hemorrhage and cerebral tumor).

D—Degenerative and **deficiency** diseases suggest beriberi and myocardial fibroelastosis.

I—Intoxication suggests alcoholic myocardiopathy, digitalis, propranolol (Inderal), procainamide, and quinidine toxicity or effects, as well as other cardiac drugs. The hypokalemia of chlorothiazide diuretics and the hyperkalemia of uremia, triamterene (Dyrenium), and spironolactone also are suggested.

C—Congenital disorders that might cause bradycardia include many congenital heart diseases, sickle cell anemia, glycogen storage disease, and muscular dystrophy.

A—Autoimmune disorders constitute a large group of diseases that may cause bradycardia or heart block. Sarcoidosis, amyloidosis, lupus erythematosus, and rheumatic fever are some of the most important ones.

T—Trauma is not a significant cause; however, a stab wound could sever the conduction system.

E—Endocrine disorders include myxedema and endocrine diseases that cause electrolyte disturbance such as Addison disease (hyperkalemia), aldosteronism (hypokalemia), and hyperparathyroidism (hypercalcemia).

● Approach to the Diagnosis

The finding of bradycardia in an otherwise healthy adult is probably normal. Nevertheless, other symptoms and signs should be looked for. Fever suggests meningitis, yellow fever, or a cerebral abscess. A history of syncope requires that sinus arrest or complete heart block be ruled out. If a heart murmur is present, aortic stenosis must be considered. If there is nonpitting edema and brittle hair and nails, myxedema should be ruled out. If there is a history of chest pain, perhaps the patient has had a recent myocardial infarction. It is important to find out what medications the patient is taking. β-blockers, digitalis, quinidine, and various cholinergic drugs may induce bradycardia.

The initial workup should include a CBC, urinalysis, thyroid profile, sedimentation rate, chemistry panel, electrocardiogram (ECG), and chest x-ray. If there is fever, febrile agglutinins and a laboratory survey for other infections should be made. If there is nuchal rigidity, a spinal tap should be done, preferably after a CT scan. If a myocardial infarction is suspected, serial cardiac enzymes and ECGs should be done. If valvular heart disease is suspected, echocardiography should be done. If there is a history of syncope, the patient needs 24- to 48-hour Holter monitoring. When this is unrevealing, a continuous-loop event recording may be conducted over a 1- to 2-week period.

● Other Useful Tests

1. Exercise stress testing (heart block, coronary insufficiency)
2. His bundle study (heart block)
3. Serum digitalis level
4. VDRL test (cardiac syphilis)
5. ANA analysis (collagen disease)
6. Coronary angiogram (myocardial infarction, coronary insufficiency)
7. Angiocardiogram (valvular heart disease)

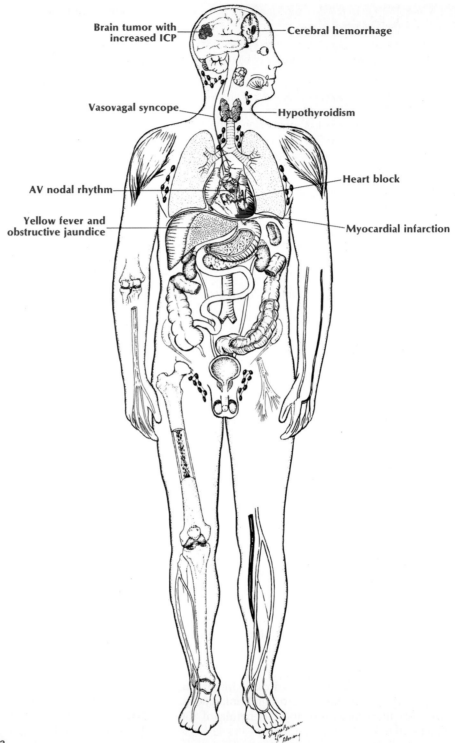

Brain tumor with
increased ICP

Cerebral hemorrhage

Vasovagal syncope

Hypothyroidism

AV nodal rhythm

Heart block

Yellow fever and
obstructive jaundice

Myocardial infarction

● **FIGURE 5** Bradycardia.

BREAST DISCHARGE

A purulent discharge from the breast, just like a purulent discharge from any other body orifice, should signify inflammation (mastitis or breast abscess), yet this is not the most common cause of a nonbloody discharge from the breast. Obviously, the most common cause is lactation.

This is, of course, physiologic in the postpartum period, but what about other periods of a woman's life? The cause in these cases is usually a pituitary, hypothalamic, or ovarian disturbance causing excessive production of prolactin. Among these disturbances are pituitary tumors, Chiari–Frommel syndrome, empty sella syndrome, and ovarian atrophy or tumors. Hyperthyroidism may occasionally

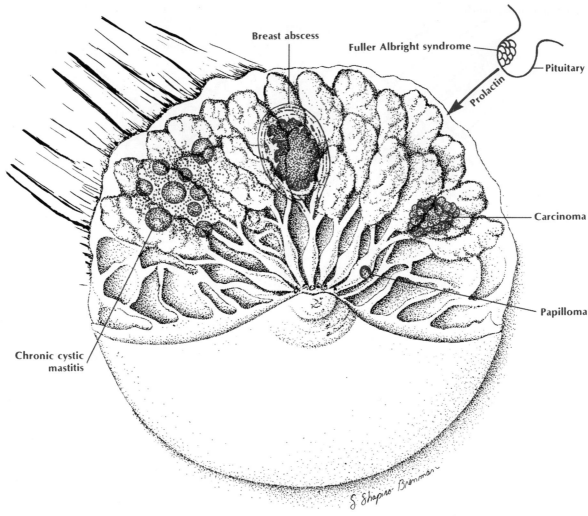

Breast abscess

Fuller Albright syndrome

Pituitary

Prolactin

Carcinoma

Papilloma

Chronic cystic mastitis

● **FIGURE 6** Breast discharge.

be responsible. Certain drugs such as chlorpromazine hydrochloride (Thorazine) and methyldopa (Aldomet) may also cause galactorrhea. Certainly malignancy, particularly papillomas or carcinomas of the ducts, should be considered, but they usually produce a bloody discharge.

● Approach to the Diagnosis

The workup of purulent breast discharge is usually simply a smear and culture and occasionally a white blood cell count and differential. A trial of antibiotics may be initiated regardless of the results. When these are fruitless, an acid-fast smear and culture may be indicated; however, this rarely occurs. It concerns me that tuberculosis is almost invariably given too much space in other differential diagnosis textbooks. Mammography is ordered next. For an endocrine workup, skull x-ray films, a CT scan or MRI of the brain, and determination of serum prolactin levels may be done, but it is wise to refer the patient to an endocrinologist for further evaluation and diagnostic assessment.

● Other Useful Tests

1. Cytology study of exudate (neoplasm)
2. Fine-needle aspiration (cysts)
3. Biopsy (neoplasm)
4. Lymph node biopsy (neoplasm)
5. Sonogram (distinguish cyst from neoplasm)
6. Thyroid profile (hypothyroidism)

BREAST MASS OR SWELLING

Developing a differential of this condition can be done either histologically or with the mnemonic **MINT**. After all, once each structure or tissue is identified, the significant lesions are either inflammatory or neoplastic. Let us apply the histologic method.

A **skin** or **subcutaneous mass** is most commonly an abscess, sebaceous cyst, lipoma, or neurofibroma. (For a more detailed discussion of masses of the skin, see page 381.) The **supporting tissue** of the breast may be involved

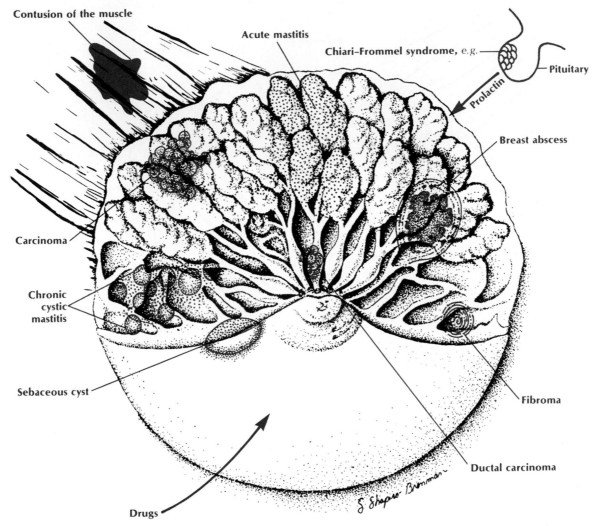

● **FIGURE 7** Breast mass.

by cellulitis, fatty necrosis, fibromas, or sarcomas. The **breast tissue** can be inflamed by bacteria in **acute mastitis**, obstructed and inflamed on a chronic basis in cystic mastitis, or diffusely and painfully swollen bilaterally by drugs (e.g., chlorpromazine and α-methyldopa) or endocrine disturbances (e.g., pregnancy or Chiari–Frommel syndrome). Carcinoma of the breast usually forms a nontender, firm swelling in one breast. Ductal carcinoma presents with a mass and often with a bloody discharge. Trauma may involve any of the histologic components of the breast, but the history and physical examination usually make the diagnosis clear.

● **Approach to the Diagnosis**

When faced with a mass in the breast, the physician's first step should be a careful examination of the breasts and the surrounding area. If the mass is tender, it is likely to be inflammatory or traumatic. If it is not tender, one should suspect a tumor. If it transilluminates, it is probably a cyst. Obviously, the primary concern of both physician and patient is whether the mass is a neoplasm. A careful search for enlarged lymph nodes in the axilla and the neck or a

mass in the other breast is important. Mammography and ultrasonography are the next most important steps, but a breast biopsy is still necessary in most cases. A truly cystic mass may be punctured for fluid analysis and Papanicolaou tests. A biopsy should be taken of a suspicious mass even if mammography findings are negative.

● **Other Useful Tests**

1. CBC (infection)
2. Culture of discharge (breast abscess)
3. Serum prolactin level (pituitary adenoma)
4. CT scan of the brain (pituitary adenoma)
5. MRI
6. Single photon emission computed tomography scan
7. Positron emission tomography scan

BREAST PAIN

Division of the breast anatomically into various components is interesting but not worthwhile in the differential diagnosis of breast pain. It is rather more instructive and

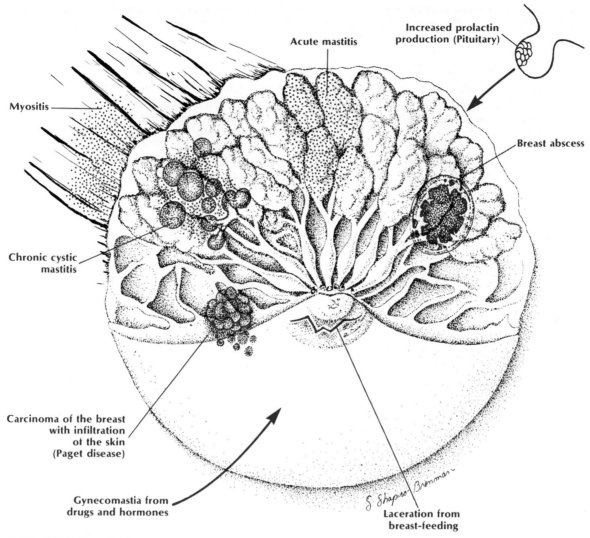

● **FIGURE 8** Breast pain.

practical to use **VINDICATE** in developing a list of causes of this symptom.

V—Vascular infarction in this area is rare, although a pulmonary or myocardial infarction may refer pain to the breast, and congestive heart failure may distend the veins of the breast sufficiently to cause mastitis.

I—Inflammation in the form of acute bacterial mastitis occurs in breastfeeding mothers, but it is infrequent. Under other circumstances, chronic cystic mastitis is a common cause of unilateral or bilateral breast pain. A breast abscess may develop during lactation. Herpes zoster may affect the skin and nerve roots supplying the breast.

N—Neoplasms of the breast, like neoplasms elsewhere, are an unlikely cause of **breast** pain, but if they infiltrate the skin (i.e., in Paget disease) or axillary nerves or obstruct the ducts they may cause pain.

D—Degenerative conditions are rarely a cause of breast pain.

I—Intoxication: A number of drugs (e.g., chlorpromazine and α-methyldopa) may cause gynecomastia and pain.

Alcoholism, estrogen, and birth control pills are probably more frequent causes.

C—Congenital anomalies are not a significant cause of breast pain.

A—Allergic-autoimmune conditions are also unlikely causes of breast pain.

T—Trauma from a bite on the breast by a feeding infant is a common cause of acute mastitis and pain. Frequent sexual relations and masturbation of the breasts may induce pain, although some women are reluctant to admit that their breasts have been traumatized this way.

E—Endocrine causes of breast pain are numerous. Menstruation, menarche, pregnancy, and menopause are associated with bilateral swollen and painful breasts. Hyperestrogenemia from endogenous or exogenous sources is also a frequent cause. Estrogen from birth control pills, estrogen therapy for menopause, and the increase of blood **estrogen** in chronic liver disease and ovarian tumors are a few of the etiologies in this group. Any pituitary condition associated with an increased output of prolactin may cause swollen, painful, and, of course, lactating breasts. The Chiari–Frommel syndrome is one of these conditions.

● Approach to the Diagnosis

The diagnosis of a painful breast is usually made by taking a careful history. What drugs is the patient taking? Associated symptoms and signs (see sections on bloody discharge, page 297 and swelling, page 81) are also important. A culture of the discharge, mammography, and determination of serum, estrogen, and prolactin levels may be important, but referral to an endocrinologist is wise when the history does not provide a simple solution, especially when the pain is bilateral. Biopsy (frozen section) is necessary when tumor is suspected and mammography is equivocal, because faith in mammography has declined somewhat in recent years.

● Other Useful Tests

1. CBC (infection)
2. Sedimentation rate (infection)
3. Chest x-ray (metastasis)
4. CT scan of the brain (pituitary adenoma)
5. Sonogram (cyst)
6. Aspiration (cyst)
7. Discontinuation of suspicious drugs
8. Pregnancy test
9. Surgery consult

C

CARDIAC ARRHYTHMIAS

With few exceptions, the etiologies of cardiac arrhythmias like those of bradycardia can best be recalled using the mnemonic **VINDICATE**. The exceptions are from one pathophysiologic cause: **obstruction** and consequent dilatation of one or more of the chambers of the heart. Thus, mitral stenosis with obstruction and dilatation of the left atrium is a prominent cause of atrial arrhythmias, especially of auricular fibrillation. Hypertension and aortic stenosis may cause a number of atrial and ventricular arrhythmias. Pulmonary hypertension resulting from pulmonary emphysema, fibrosis, or pneumonia with consequent right ventricular and atrial obstruction and dilatation cause arrhythmias, especially atrial arrhythmias. Getting back to **VINDICATE** completes the recall of the causes of arrhythmias.

V—**Vascular** diseases include myocardial infarction, coronary insufficiency, and coronary artery emboli.

I—**Inflammatory** diseases include viral myocarditis, diphtheria, syphilis, tuberculosis, and Chagas disease.

N—**Neoplasms** include atrial myxomas, but the N also stands for neuropsychiatric causes. Paroxysmal atrial tachycardia is especially likely to result from emotional causes.

D—**Degenerative** diseases include Friedreich ataxia, myotonic dystrophy, myocardial fibroelastosis, and other myocardiopathies.

I—**Intoxication** suggests the largest number of causes of arrhythmia: Alcohol, caffeine, tobacco, digitalis, quinidine, propranolol, and procainamide are just a few. Diuretics cause electrolyte disturbances that may cause or contribute to cardiac arrhythmias.

C—**Congenital** disorders recall congenital heart diseases, many of which cause recurrent arrhythmias. The Wolff–Parkinson–White syndrome predisposes to atrial tachycardia. Muscular dystrophy may cause myocardiopathy and arrhythmias. Von Gierke disease and gargoylism also need to be remembered.

A—**Autoimmune** disorders suggest the arrhythmias of amyloidosis, sarcoidosis, scleroderma, periarteritis nodosa, and rheumatic fever.

T—**Trauma** suggests the arrhythmias in shock, burns, stab wounds to the heart, and head injuries. Electric shock is a cause of ventricular fibrillation.

E—**Endocrinopathies** should remind one of hyperthyroidism, a prominent cause of atrial fibrillation, Addison disease, and aldosteronism, which disturb the electrolytes sufficiently to cause arrhythmias. Pheochromocytomas may cause atrial tachycardia from the tremendous output of epinephrine.

● Approach to the Diagnosis

The diagnosis depends a lot on the type of arrhythmia. Atrial premature contractions are usually benign, and an extensive workup is unnecessary unless other physical signs indicate the need for it. Infrequent ventricular premature contractions (VPCs) in otherwise healthy individuals probably can be handled the same way. When VPCs are frequent or multifocal, an exercise tolerance test, echocardiogram, and perhaps coronary angiography are indicated. Runs of ventricular tachycardia require an extensive workup, including coronary angiography, but usually there will be other signs to indicate the need for this.

Atrial tachycardia and fibrillation require a workup of hyperthyroidism and pulmonary disease, systemic hypertension, and congestive heart failure (CHF). Atrial obstruction and dilatation should be excluded by echocardiography. Carotid sinus massage will distinguish rapid atrial arrhythmias from sinus tachycardia.

Any arrhythmia warrants an electrocardiogram (ECG) and possibly repeated ECGs. The Holter monitor should be used if there is doubt about the type of arrhythmia.

● Other Useful Tests

1. Complete blood count (CBC) (anemia)
2. Thyroid profile (hyperthyroidism, hypothyroidism)
3. Urinalysis (renal disease)
4. Chemistry panel (uremia, electrolyte imbalance)
5. Sedimentation rate (infection)
6. Serial cardiac enzymes (myocardial infarction)
7. Serum and urine osmolality (CHF)
8. Exercise tolerance test (coronary insufficiency)
9. Serial ECGs (myocardial infarction)
10. Signal-averaging ECG and electrophysiologic testing (localize site of irritable focus)
11. Pulmonary function tests (CHF, emphysema)
12. Echocardiogram (CHF, valvular heart disease)
13. Coronary angiogram (coronary insufficiency)
14. Drug screen (chronic drug abuse)
15. Hold all drugs (drug intoxication)
16. B-type natriuretic peptide (BNP) (CHF)

CARDIOMEGALY

If an x-ray film demonstrates cardiomegaly, the physician must find out what is causing this condition (Table 13). You have already listened to the patient and he or she does not have a murmur. This seems to exclude the common groups of causes—congenital and rheumatic heart disease. (It really does not.) The patient does not have hypertension and denies symptoms of heart failure. The ECG is normal. Now what do you do?

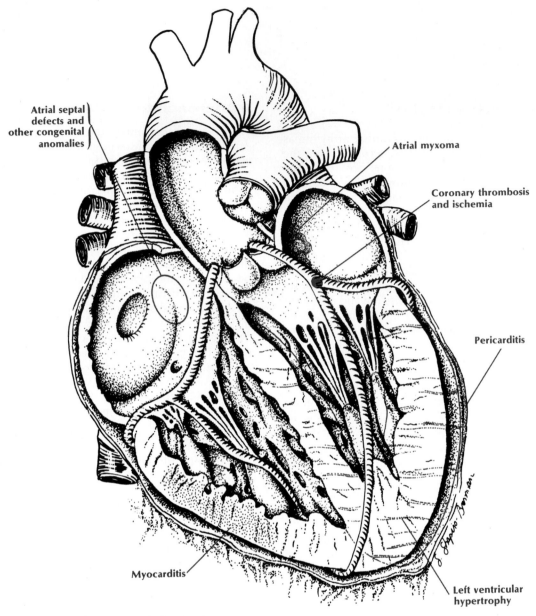

Atrial septal defects and other congenital anomalies

Atrial myxoma

Coronary thrombosis and ischemia

Pericarditis

Left ventricular hypertrophy

Myocarditis

● **FIGURE 1** Cardiac arrhythmias, local causes.

This situation is all too common, and I hope this chapter will remedy that situation. The basic sciences of **histology** and **physiology** are, of course, the key to an immediate differential diagnosis. Remember that the heart is divided into three basic layers: endocardium, myocardium, and pericardium; each of these can be cross-indexed with the etiologic classification using the mnemonic **VINDICATE**. The pathophysiologic mechanism, **obstruction**, provides the remaining disorders in the differential diagnosis. This is applied to the pulmonary and systemic circulations and cross-indexed with the various etiologic groups. Let us begin with the **endocardium**.

V—Vascular lesions include the ball–valve thrombosis.
I—Inflammatory lesions bring to mind acute and subacute bacterial endocarditis and syphilitic valvular disease.

N—Neoplasms suggest an atrial myxoma.
D—Degenerative disease signals atherosclerotic valvular disease.
I—Intoxication does not suggest any particular condition, because most toxins involve the myocardium.
C—Congenital suggests a host of valvular and septal defects and transposition of the blood vessels of the heart.
A—Autoimmune suggests the important rheumatic carditis and also Libman–Sack endocarditis of lupus erythematosus.
T—Trauma suggests all the valvular or septal defects that can occur from surgery.
E—Endocrine suggests the pulmonic and tricuspid valvular defects that result from carcinoid syndrome.

TABLE 13 Cardiomegaly

	V Vascular	I Inflammatory	N Neoplasm	D Degenerative and Deficiency	I Intoxication Idiopathic	C Congenital	A Autoimmune Allergic	T Trauma	E Endocrine
Endocardium	Ball valve thrombus	Bacterial endocarditis Subacute bacterial endocarditis Syphilis	Myxoma	Atherosclerotic valvular disease		Congenital valvular and septal defects	Lupus endocarditis Rheumatic fever	Valvular perforation or lacerating surgery	Carcinoid syndrome
Myocardium	Coronary insufficiency Myocardial infarction Congestive heart failure	Diphtheria Trypanosomiasis Syphilis Viral myocarditis	Rhabdomyosarcoma	Beriberi Muscular dystrophy	Hemochromatosis Alcoholism Amyloidosis Gout	Hurler disease von Gierke disease Myocardial fibroelastosis Subaortic stenosis	Rheumatic fever Rheumatic arthritis scleroderma	Traumatic aneurysm Postpericardiotomy syndrome	Hyperthyroidism Diabetic arteriolar sclerosis Hypothyroidism
Pericardium	Hemopericardium	Tuberculosis Viral pericarditis	Metastatic carcinoma		Idiopathic pericarditis		Rheumatic fever	Hemopericardium	
Systemic Circulation	Renal artery stenosis		Polycythemia vera Hypernephroma	Anemia Paget disease	Essential hypertension Dissecting aneurysm	Coarctation of aorta Patent ductus	Periarteritis nodosa Glomerulonephritis	Arteriovenous fistula	Adrenal tumor
Pulmonary Circulation	Pulmonary embolism and infarction	Chronic bronchitis and emphysema Tuberculosis Fungi	Carcinomatosis		Pulmonary fibrosis Primary pulmonary hypertension				

C

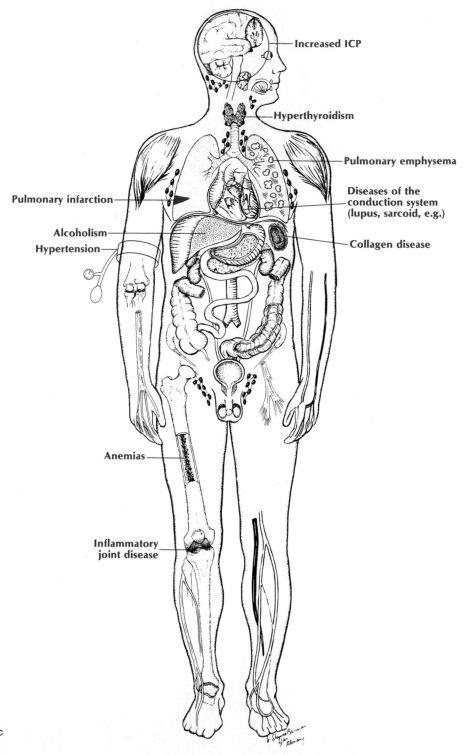

● FIGURE 2 Cardiac arrhythmias, systemic causes.

In the **myocardium**, one encounters a large number of diseases; therefore, only the most common ones will be mentioned here.

V—Vascular should immediately suggest coronary insufficiency and myocardial infarction.

I—Inflammation could indicate viral myocarditis, but it would hardly be expected to remind one of diphtheria and syphilitic myocarditis because these rarely are seen.

N—Neoplasms of the myocardium are rare, thus rhabdomyosarcoma needs to be mentioned here for completeness only.

D—Degenerative and **deficiency** diseases should signal beriberi and muscular dystrophy, but these are also infrequently encountered.

I—Intoxicating and **idiopathic** disorders of the myocardium, especially alcoholism, are much more common. Others include hemochromatosis, amyloidosis, and gout.

C

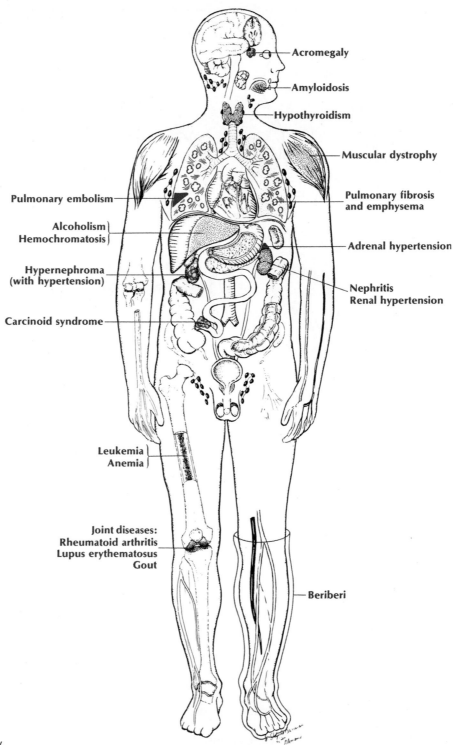

Acromegaly

Amyloidosis

Hypothyroidism

Muscular dystrophy

Pulmonary embolism

Pulmonary fibrosis
and emphysema

Alcoholism
Hemochromatosis

Adrenal hypertension

Hypernephroma
(with hypertension)

Nephritis
Renal hypertension

Carcinoid syndrome

Leukemia
Anemia

Joint diseases:
Rheumatoid arthritis
Lupus erythematosus
Gout

Beriberi

● **FIGURE 3** Cardiomegaly.

C—**Congenital** disorders include Von Gierke disease and myocardial fibroelastosis.

A—**Autoimmune** again suggests rheumatic fever and the collagen diseases.

T—**Trauma** suggests posttraumatic aneurysms.

E—**Endocrine** disorders include two treatable disorders: hyperthyroidism and hypothyroidism.

The **pericardium** is not frequently the cause of "cardiomegaly," but tuberculosis and idiopathic pericarditis should be considered, as should hemopericardium, especially in the course of a myocardial infarction. **Obstruction** in the pulmonary circulation can result from the following:

V—**Vascular** from pulmonary infarction.

I—**Inflammatory** from chronic bronchitis and emphysema or from chronic infections such as tuberculosis and various fungi.

N—**Neoplastic** from primary or metastatic carcinoma.

D—**Degenerative**

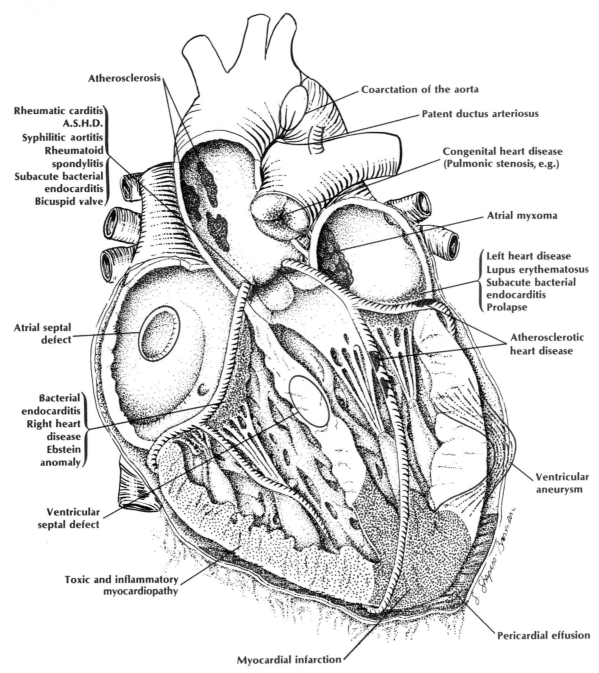

● **FIGURE 4** Cardiomegaly, local causes.

I—Idiopathic or **Intoxication** in pulmonary fibrosis and primary pulmonary hypertension.

C—Congenital disorders include pulmonic stenosis and hemangiomas.

A—Autoimmune diseases include collagen diseases.

T—Trauma may cause an arteriovenous aneurysm or pneumothorax obstructing the pulmonary circulation.

E—Endocrine disorders do not obstruct the pulmonary vasculature.

Under **systemic circulation** comes essential or secondary hypertension caused by coarctation of the aorta, periarteritis nodosa, or the many renal and adrenal diseases. Dissecting aneurysms of the aorta may rupture into the pericardium causing cardiomegaly.

● **Approach to the Diagnosis**

The diagnosis of cardiomegaly can be further developed by a good history and the association of other symptoms and signs. Is there a history of hypertension, alcoholism, rheumatic fever, or other systemic disease? Has the patient experienced shortness of breath, angina, fever, joint pains, and so forth? Are there findings of pedal edema, hepatomegaly, or jugular venous distention (CHF)? Are there hypertension and proteinuria (renal disease or essential hypertension)? Is there a significant heart murmur (congenital heart disease, rheumatic heart disease)?

The diagnostic workup will include a CBC, urinalysis, chemistry panel, sedimentation rate, chest x-ray, and ECG. At this point, it is wise to consult a cardiologist. Echocardiography will be helpful in diagnosing valvular heart disease, myocardiopathy, and pericardial effusion. If CHF is suspected, a venous pressure and circulation time as well as spirometry will support the diagnosis. Echocardiography can diagnose CHF by determining the left ventricular ejection fraction (LVEF). If there is unexplained fever, an antistreptolysin O (ASO) titer or streptozyme test should be ordered to rule out rheumatic fever, and perhaps serial blood cultures should be done to exclude subacute bacterial endocarditis. If there is hypertension, the patient may need a hypertensive workup (see page 238).

● Other Useful Tests

1. Exercise tolerance test (coronary insufficiency)
2. Thallium scan (coronary insufficiency)
3. Phonocardiogram (valvular heart disease)
4. Antinuclear antibody (ANA) analysis (collagen disease)
5. Cardiac catheterization studies (congenital heart disease, rheumatic heart disease)
6. Angiocardiogram (valvular heart disease)
7. Coronary arteriogram (coronary insufficiency)
8. Thyroid profile (myxedema)
9. 24-hour urine catecholamine (pheochromocytoma)
10. Urine thiamine afterload (beriberi)
11. Muscle biopsy (collagen disease, trichinosis)
12. Computed tomography (CT) scan (mediastinal mass)
13. Magnetic resonance imaging (MRI) (dissecting aneurysm)

C

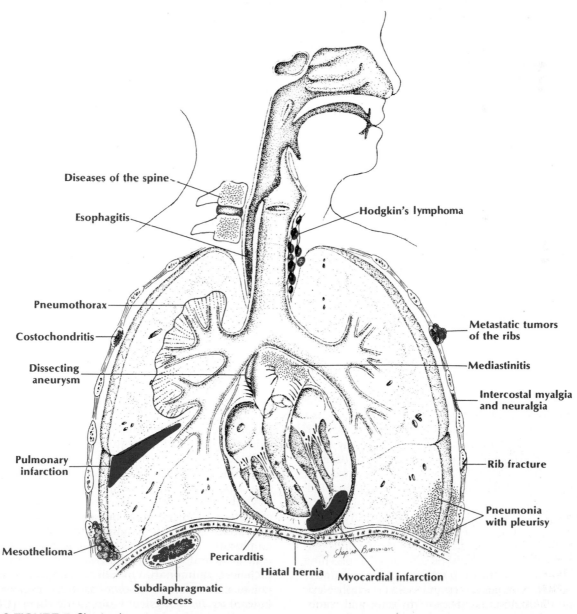

● **FIGURE 5** Chest pain.

CERVICAL BRUIT

Anatomy is the key to the differential diagnosis of a cervical bruit. Visualizing the neck, we have the carotid, innominate, and subclavian arteries; the jugular, innominate, and subclavian veins; the thyroid, scalenus anticus muscle, and cervical ribs, all of which may be involved in this sign.

Arteries: This should prompt the recall of a carotid or subclavian artery stenosis (subclavian steal syndrome) or an aneurysm. It should also remind us of aortic murmurs that may be transmitted to the neck from a stenosed aortic valve, calcific aortitis, or an aortic aneurysm.

Veins: A venous hum may be heard in the neck as a result of a circuitous route that blood must take in the veins. This is of course usually benign.

Thyroid: This prompts the recall of the bruit heard over the thyroid in Grave disease.

Muscles: Occasionally a bruit is heard in the neck in patients with scalenus anticus syndrome or other forms of thoracic outlet syndrome.

Cervical rib: The subclavian artery may also be compressed by a cervical rib producing a cervical bruit.

● Approach to the Diagnosis

A history of diaphoresis, weight loss, or heat intolerance would arouse suspicion of hyperthyroidism. A history of transient hemiplegia, amaurosis fugax, or other intermittent neurologic symptomatology should point to a carotid stenosis or subclavian steal syndrome. Physical findings of pallor or spoon nails would point to anemia. An enlarged thyroid prompts the suspicion of hyperthyroidism. If there's a diminished pulse on the side of the bruit, look for thoracic outlet syndrome or subclavian steal syndrome. The diagnostic workup may need to include a CBC, thyroid panel, and carotid duplex scan.

Consult a neurologist if there are objective neurologic signs. Four-vessel angiography needs to be considered if a carotid stenosis or subclavian steal syndrome is suspected. If the bruit seems to be transmitted from the chest, echocardiography may be needed.

CHEST PAIN

Hardly a day goes by in a busy practitioner's office that he or she is not confronted with a patient complaining of chest pain. The main concern, of course, is to exclude an acute myocardial infarction, which is not an easy task in many cases. The practitioner frequently admits the patient for observation, which is the safe thing to do when there is any doubt. With a list of virtually all the diagnostic possibilities in mind, however, fewer patients will require admission for observation. **Anatomy** forms the basis for formulating such a list.

Visualizing the organs of the chest and cross-indexing them with the various etiologies (Table 14), one finds that at least 30 or 40 conditions must be considered. Proceeding from the superficial to the deep structures, one encounters the **skin**, considers herpes zoster, and looks for a rash. Next, there is **muscle**; trichinosis, dermatomyositis, and contusion of the muscle must be considered. Cough-induced contusions should not be forgotten. In the same layer, the **ribs** and **cartilage** remind one of rib fractures, Tietze syndrome, metastatic carcinoma, and multiple myeloma. Other rarer conditions of the rib are shown in Table 14.

Many causes of chest pain arise from the pleura. Pneumonia with pleurisy, empyema, pulmonary infarction, and neoplasms of the **pleura** must be considered. Tuberculous pleurisy and other infectious agents are not uncommon. In contrast, conditions of the lung are less likely to cause chest pain unless they involve the pleura: This is certainly true of pneumonia and neoplasms. A pneumothorax, however, is a very common cause of chest pain, especially in young adults.

Visualize the **heart**, and the **pericardium** comes to mind. This is a source of chest pain in acute idiopathic pericarditis, rheumatic carditis, and tuberculous and neoplastic pericarditis. The **myocardium** is the source of the most serious form of chest pain, myocardial infarction, but here again the pain is more severe if the pericardium is involved. Angina pectoris and chronic coronary insufficiency are common causes of chest pain arising from the myocardium. Myocarditis (e.g., viral) causes less severe pain, but inflammation of the myocardium from postinfarction syndrome or postpericardiotomy syndrome can be extremely painful. The endocardium is the source of mild chest pain in mitral valve prolapse.

Now visualize the other central structures: The **esophagus** reminds one of reflux esophagitis and hiatal hernia, the **mediastinum** suggests mediastinitis and substernal thyroiditis or Hodgkin lymphoma (usually not too painful), the **aorta** suggests dissecting aneurysms, and the **thoracic spine** suggests spinal cord tumors, osteoarthritis, Pott disease, fractures, herniated discs, as well as the other conditions listed in Table 14.

This chapter would not be complete unless referred pain to the chest was considered. Thus, abdominal conditions such as cholecystitis, pancreatitis, and splenic flexure syndrome may present with chest pain. Conditions of the neck that press the cervical nerves may also cause chest pain, particularly scalenus anticus syndrome, cervical ribs, and herniated discs of the cervical spine: Neurocirculatory asthenia is associated with atypical chest pain; a psychiatric evaluation will assist in this diagnosis.

● Approach to the Diagnosis

A possible myocardial infarction must be the first consideration in all adults with acute chest pain, especially if there are significant alterations of the vital signs. Consequently, serial ECGs, serial cardiac enzymes including troponins, and hospitalization will often be necessary. After this condition has been excluded, we can turn our attention to the other possibilities. A tablespoon of xylocaine viscus may be administered to rule out reflux esophagitis. Arterial blood gases, chest x-ray, and a lung scan or helical CT scan of the chest may be ordered to exclude a pulmonary embolism. Pulmonary angiography may be necessary in some cases. A chest x-ray may be ordered to rule out pneumonia. Acute chest pain related to esophagitis is often relieved by swallowing lidocaine

TABLE 14 Chest Pain

	V Vascular	I Inflammatory	N Neoplasm	D Degenerative and Deficiency	I Intoxication Idiopathic	C Congenital	A Autoimmune Allergic	T Trauma	E Endocrine
Skin		Herpes zoster							
Muscles		Epidemic pleurodynia Trichinosis Diaphragmatic abscess			Intercostal neuralgia		Dermatomyositis	Contusion Cough-induced hemorrhage into muscle	
Ribs and Cartilages		Osteomyelitis Tietze syndrome	Metastatic carcinoma Multiple myeloma sarcoma	Osteitis deformans				Fracture contusion	Osteitis fibrosa cystica
Pleura	Pulmonary infarction	Pleurisy Tuberculosis Fungus Empyema	Metastatic carcinoma Mesenthelioma						
Lung		Pneumonia	Carcinoma (primary and metastatic)		Pneumothorax		Pneumothorax		
Pericardium		Viral pericarditis Rheumatic fever Tuberculosis	Metastatic carcinoma		Uremia				
Myocardium	Myocardial infarct Coronary insufficiency	Myocarditis					Postinfarction syndrome	Postcommissurotomy syndrome Contusion	
Aorta	Aneurysm	Aortitis		Medionecrosis				Ruptured aorta	
Esophagus		Ulcer Esophagitis	Esophageal carcinoma		E.g., lye erosion	Diverticulum Hiatal hernia		Ruptured esophagus	
Mediastinum		Mediastinitis	Dermoid cyst Hodgkin lymphoma						Substernal thyroiditis
Thoracic Vertebrae		Osteomyelitis Pott disease	Metastatic carcinoma	Osteoporosis Osteoarthritis			Rheumatoid spondylitis	Fracture Herniated disc	Osteoporosis Osteomalacia
Spinal Cord		Syphilis Tuberculosis Neuralgia	Tumor				Transverse myelitis	Hematomyelia	

viscus, an extremely useful tool in the differential diagnosis. Relief of the pain with nitroglycerin under the tongue or by spray will support the diagnosis of coronary insufficiency. Tenderness of the costochondral junctions with relief on lidocaine injection into the point of maximum tenderness suggests Tietze syndrome (costochondritis). In cases of chronic chest pain, an exercise tolerance test with thallium scan should be done to rule out coronary insufficiency or myocardial infarction. It may be wise to do immediate coronary angiography if the condition deteriorates so that balloon angiography, bypass surgery, or reperfusion therapy may be initiated. Dissecting aneurysm is revealed by CT scan or MRI of the chest.

● Other Useful Tests

1. CBC
2. Sedimentation rate (pneumonia, infarction)
3. Sputum smear and culture (pneumonia)
4. Bernstein test (reflux esophagitis)
5. Serum cardiac troponin levels (myocardial infarction)
6. D-dimer testing (pulmonary embolism)
7. Esophagoscopy (reflux esophagitis)
8. X-ray of the spine (radiculopathy)
9. Echocardiogram (pericarditis)
10. 24-hour Holter monitoring (coronary insufficiency)
11. Gallbladder sonogram
12. Ambulatory pH monitoring (esophagitis)
13. Helical CT scan (pulmonary embolism)
14. Single photon emission computed tomography (SPECT) scan (coronary insufficiency)
15. Therapeutic trial of antacids or proton pump inhibitors (reflux esophagitis)

Case Presentation #9

A 58-year-old white male executive was brought to the emergency room at midnight complaining of severe substernal chest pain of 2 hours duration.

Question #1. Utilizing the methods outlined above, what is your list of possible diagnoses at this point?

Additional history reveals that the patient has had several previous attacks of a similar nature over the past 10 years, but never lasting this long. The pain does not radiate to the neck or down the arm, and is not accompanied by diaphoresis. The pain is often relieved by antacids but is increased by deep breathing. There is no history of alcohol intake. Physical examination, ECG, and laboratory studies are unremarkable.

Question #2. What are the possible diagnoses to consider at this point?

(See Appendix B for the answers.)

CHEST WALL MASS

The differential diagnosis of this symptom and sign is similar to that of chest pain: **Anatomy** is the key to both. After visualizing all the organs of the chest and cross-indexing them with the mnemonic **MINT**, a convenient and extensive differential list can be constructed as in Table 15. The discussion that follows will also concentrate on the most significant of these.

TABLE 15 Mass in the Chest Wall

	M Malformation	I Inflammation	N Neoplasm	T Trauma
Skin and Subcutaneous Tissue	Neurofibroma Venous engorgement Sebaceous cyst	Cellulitis Abscess	Lipoma	Contusion
Muscle		Myositis	(Rare)	Contusion
Ribs	Pigeon breast Xiphoid prominence	Osteomyelitis Tuberculosis Tietze syndrome	Osteoma Mtiple myeloma Metastatic carcinoma	Fracture Contusion
Lungs and Pleura		Tuberculosis Emphysema Lung abscess	Carcinoma or mesenthelioma with direct extension	Hemorrhage Pneumothorax Subcutaneous emphysema
Heart and Pericardium	Cardiomegaly Aneurysm	Tuberculous or idiopathic pericarditis	Metastatic carcinoma to pericardium	Traumatic aneurysm
Aorta	Aneurysm			Traumatic aneurysm
Mediastinum	Superior vena cava obstruction	Mediastinitis	Hodgkin lymphoma Dermoid cyst	

The significant lesions of the **skin** and **subcutaneous tissues** include sebaceous cysts, cellulitis, neurofibromas, lipomas, and contusions. Unlike the abdomen, the chest seldom is the source of a hernia. In the **ribs**, look for fractures, contusions, multiple myeloma, and primary and metastatic tumors. In the **cartilage**, there may be a protruding xiphoid process or a lump at the costochondral junctions in Tietze syndrome. Years ago it was common for empyema, lung abscesses, pleural and monary tuberculosis, and fungi (actinomycosis especially) to work their way out to the skin and form a mass or fistula: This is now unusual. Carcinoma of the lung and mesenthelioma, however, may form a mass on the chest wall by direct extension. In the **mediastinal structures**, aortic aneurysms used to be a common cause of a pulsating chest wall mass, but they are now rarely seen. Cardiomegaly and pericardial effusions occasionally cause a noticeable protuberance of the precardium but not as frequently as in the past. Tumors of the mediastinum may also cause chest wall masses or protuberances.

● Approach to the Diagnosis

The approach to this diagnosis is again a good clinical history and physical examination along with correlation of signs and symptoms. Chest x-ray films with special views and tomography will diagnose most cases, but a biopsy, arteriography, CT scans, and exploratory surgery may be necessary, especially if the lesion turns out to be noninfectious. It is important not to be fooled by a congenital anomaly (e.g., pigeon breast).

● Other Useful Tests

1. CBC
2. Radioactive iodine (RAI) uptake and scan (goiter, thyroid neoplasm)

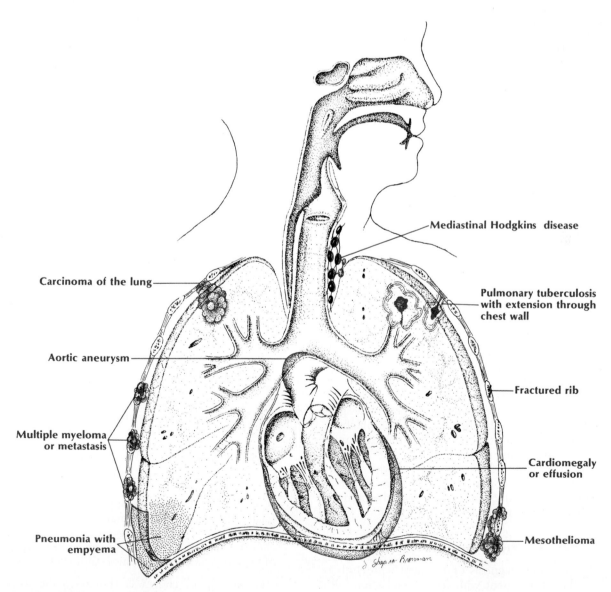

● **FIGURE 6** Chest wall mass.

3. Sedimentation rate (inflammation, abscess)
4. Incision and drainage (I & D) and culture
5. Bone scan (metastatic carcinoma)
6. Barium swallow (diverticulum, cardiac size)
7. Mammogram
8. Sonogram (cystic mass)
9. Aortogram (aortic aneurysm)
10. Mediastinoscopy (neoplasm of mediastinum)
11. CT scan of mediastinum or chest (neoplasm, aneurysm, abscess)

CHILLS

A chill with chattering of the teeth and shaking followed by a fever is almost invariably due to an infectious process. Furthermore, the infection is usually bacterial, and the chill indicates that the bacteria have invaded the bloodstream. The exceptions to the above are discussed later in this chapter.

Anatomy is the key to a differential diagnosis. To start with, each organ in the body can be infected by an "itis" of the parenchyma, an "itis" of the capsule, or an abscess.

1. **"Itis" of the parenchyma:** Here one should recall encephalitis, otitis media, mastoiditis, pharyngitis, pneumonitis, endocarditis, pyelonephritis, hepatitis, cholecystitis, cholangitis, gastroenteritis, appendicitis, diverticulitis, prostatitis, orchitis, endometritis, salpingitis, cellulitis, osteomyelitis, and arthritis. Because some of these infections are frequently viral (e.g., hepatitis, gastroenteritis, and encephalitis), a chill would be unusual. Myositis is usually viral but in trichinosis, a chill is not rare.
2. **"Itis" of the capsule:** In this group are meningitis, pleuritis or pleurisy, pericarditis, and peritonitis.
3. **Abscess:** This should prompt the recall of cerebral abscess, epidural or subdural abscess, dental abscess, retropharyngeal abscess, lung abscess or empyema, liver abscess, subdiaphragmatic abscess, perinephric abscess, abscessed diverticulum, appendiceal abscess, tubo-ovarian abscess, pelvic abscess, prostatic abscess, and furuncles or carbuncles. Abscesses are especially prone to cause chills.
4. **Systemic infection:** Some systemic infections are particularly likely to be associated with a chill. Malaria, relapsing fever, Weil disease, rat-bite fever, yellow fever, smallpox, Rocky Mountain spotted fever, acute poliomyelitis, and pulmonary tuberculosis belong in this group.
5. **Venous thrombosis:** Phlebitis in various portions of the body is often associated with chills. Cavernous sinus thrombosis, lateral sinus thrombosis, pyelophlebitis, and, less frequently, thrombophlebitis of the extremities may be associated with a chill.
6. **Miscellaneous:** Chills are often associated with intravenous injection of drugs or antibiotics, transfusion, hemolytic anemia, and introduction of contaminated equipment into the body. Chills are rare in rheumatic fever.

● Approach to the Diagnosis

The approach to the diagnosis of a patient with chills is similar to that of a patient with fever. Association with other signs (e.g., jaundice or dysuria) will often point to the organ involved. However, when fever and chills are the only symptoms, a workup similar to that found below may be necessary. Careful charting of the temperature while the patient remains off aspirin or other antipyretics will be rewarding, especially in the diagnosis of malaria.

● Other Useful Tests

1. CBC (infection)
2. Sedimentation rate (inflammation, neoplasm)
3. Urinalysis (pyelonephritis)
4. Urine culture and sensitivity (urinary tract infection [UTI])
5. Culture discharge from any body orifice
6. Blood cultures (bacterial endocarditis, septicemia)
7. Bone marrow smear and culture (bacterial endocarditis, metastasis)
8. Blood smear for parasites (malaria)
9. Febrile agglutinins
10. Monospot test (infectious mononucleosis)
11. ASO titer (rheumatic fever)
12. Sickle cell prep (sickle cell anemia)
13. Cerebrospinal fluid (CSF) smear and culture (meningitis, encephalitis)
14. Tuberculin test
15. Other skin test as indicated
16. Chest x-ray
17. Flat plate of abdomen
18. Gallbladder sonogram (cholecystitis)
19. ANA (collagen disease)
20. CT scan of abdomen and pelvis (abscess)
21. Indium scan (occult abscess)

CHOREA

The causes of this symptom lend themselves easily to recall. Simply remember the word **VINDICATE**. There are usually just one or two diseases for each letter.

V—Vascular suggests an infarction of the subthalamic nucleus, which produces hemiballism.
I—Inflammatory lesions suggest the various forms of viral encephalitis.
N—Neoplasms of the brainstem include gliomas and metastatic carcinoma.
D—Degenerative disease suggests Huntington chorea.
I—Intoxication suggests Wilson disease, phenothiazine, lead or manganese toxicity, and carbon monoxide poisoning.
C—Congenital chorea suggests the chorea of cerebral palsy.
A—Autoimmune disease suggests the Sydenham chorea of rheumatic fever.
T—Trauma suggests chorea from concussion, basilar skull fracture, or intracerebral hematoma.
E—Endocrine and **epilepsy** suggest the possibility that the chorea is related to an epileptic focus. The hyperkinesis of hyperthyroidism sometimes stimulates chorea.

The workup of chorea is similar to the workup of tremor (see page 420).

C

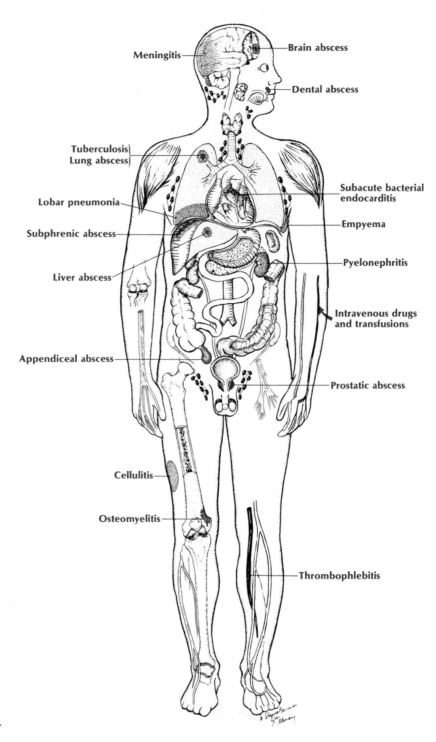

Meningitis

Brain abscess

Dental abscess

Tuberculosis
Lung abscess

Subacute bacterial
endocarditis

Lobar pneumonia

Empyema

Subphrenic abscess

Pyelonephritis

Liver abscess

Intravenous drugs
and transfusions

Appendiceal abscess

Prostatic abscess

Cellulitis

Osteomyelitis

Thrombophlebitis

● **FIGURE 7** Chills.

CLUBBING AND PULMONARY OSTEOARTHROPATHY

Although there have been arguments in the past over whether clubbing and pulmonary osteoarthropathy are just two clinical manifestations of the same thing, I take the position that they are; their differential diagnosis, therefore, will be considered together.

When presented with a case of clubbing, one might simply use **anatomy** and think of all the major internal organs (except the kidney); one would then be closer to an accurate and reliable differential diagnosis. To be more scientific, apply basic physiology to provide an extensive and organized differential diagnosis. The important basic science, then, is **physiology**; according to Mauer,[1] the principle common denominator is **anoxia**. Table 16 is developed on this basis. Anoxic anoxia or poor intake of oxygen would suggest the first category of disease, pulmonary;

[1] Mauer EF. Etiology of clubbed fingers. *Am Heart J*. 34:852–853; 1947.

TABLE 16 Clubbing and Pulmonary Osteoarthropathy

	V Vascular	I Inflammatory	N Neoplasm	D Degenerative and Deficiency	I Intoxication Idiopathic	C Congenital	A Autoimmune	T Trauma	E Endocrine
Anoxic Anoxia (Pulmonary Disease)		Tuberculosis Lung abscess Emphysema Chronic bronchitis	Carcinoma of the lung		Pulmonary fibrosis Emphysema	Cystic fibrosis Bronchiectasis	Sarcoidosis		
Shunt Anoxia (Cardiovascular Disease)	Pulmonary embolus		Pulmonary hemangioma		Adhesive pericarditis	Congenital heart disease Tetralogy of Fallot Pulmonic stenosis			
Anemic Anoxia		Amebiasis Ascaris Chronic osteomyelitis	Carcinoma of the GI tract Hodgkin lymphoma		Cirrhosis of the liver		Regional Ileitis Ulcerative colitis		
Histotoxic Anoxia		Subacute bacterial endocarditis	Carcinoma of the GI tract		Biliary cirrhosis				Myxedema
Miscellaneous	Aortic and brachial artery aneurysm		Polycythemia vera Nasopharyngeal tumor	Syringomyelia	Idiopathic clubbing				

GI, gastrointestinal.

most significant among these are chronic diseases of the lung, including chronic bronchitis and emphysema, empyema, pulmonary tuberculosis, carcinoma of the lung, pneumoconiosis, bronchiectasis, and pulmonary fibrosis. Acute pneumonia, pneumothorax, and bronchial asthma (where there may be many short episodes of anoxia) do not usually lead to clubbing.

In the next group of disorders, the lungs may be normal but a significant amount of blood never reaches the alveoli; I call this **shunt anoxia**. Here are classified the tetralogy of Fallot and other congenital anomalies of the heart, recurrent pulmonary emboli, cirrhosis of the liver (associated with small pulmonary arteriovenous shunts), and pulmonary hemangiomas. Many conditions associated with anemia may present with clubbing. Thus,

anemic anoxia may be a factor in portal cirrhosis, biliary cirrhosis, Banti disease, chronic malaria, and subacute bacterial endocarditis. It may also be a factor in disorders of the gastrointestinal tract, such as regional ileitis, ulcerative colitis, and carcinoma of the colon. Stagnant anoxia is not usually associated with clubbing, but this may be because severe anoxia in CHF and shock are usually transient.

Histotoxic anoxia is Mauer's other explanation for clubbing in patients without low arterial oxygen saturation. The theory is hindered by chronic inflammatory diseases. This group includes subacute bacterial endocarditis, myxedema, ulcerative colitis, intestinal tuberculosis, and amebic dysentery. Of course, this is a regular occurrence in chronic methemoglobinemia or sulfhemoglobinemia.

C

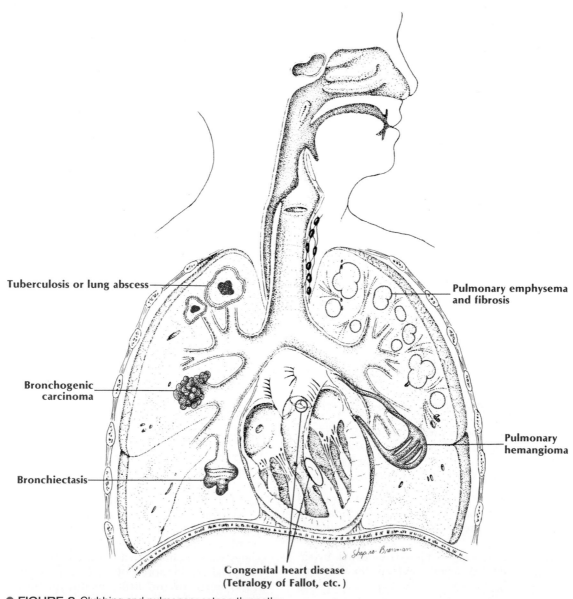

Tuberculosis or lung abscess

Bronchogenic carcinoma

Bronchiectasis

Pulmonary emphysema and fibrosis

Pulmonary hemangioma

Congenital heart disease (Tetralogy of Fallot, etc.)

● **FIGURE 8** Clubbing and pulmonary osteoarthropathy.

● Approach to the Diagnosis

The clinical approach to clubbing involves being certain that clubbing is present. A curved fingernail is not good evidence, and the "drumstick" appearance (which makes the finger look like a true club) does not occur until late. Early clubbing is determined by the angle between the nail-covered portion and the skin-covered portion of the dorsal surface of the terminal phalanx. Normally this angle is 160 degrees. When the angle becomes 180 degrees and disappears, that is, when the terminal phalanx becomes flat, clubbing exists.

Careful examination for cyanosis and a thorough evaluation of the heart and lungs will determine the cause in most cases. Pulmonary function studies, and arterial blood gases before and after exercise and before and after 100% oxygen, will help confirm the diagnosis in many cases. Of course, lung scans and angiocardiography are frequently necessary. Blood cultures, stool culture and examination, and thorough radiologic studies of the gastrointestinal tract will be necessary in obscure cases.

● Other Useful Tests

1. CBC (anemia)
2. Chemistry panel (liver disease)
3. Tuberculin test
4. Chest x-ray (neoplasm, bronchiectasis)
5. Sputum culture and sensitivity (lung abscess)
6. Sputum cytology (carcinoma of the lung)
7. Sputum for acid-fast bacillus (AFB) smear and culture (tuberculosis)
8. Histoplasmin skin test
9. Coccidioidin skin test
10. Blastomycin skin test
11. Bronchoscopy (neoplasm, bronchiectasis)
12. Lung biopsy (neoplasm, silicosis)
13. Exploratory surgery

COMA AND SOMNOLENCE

Somnolence is a deep sleep from which the patient can be aroused. Coma is an unconscious state from which the patient cannot be aroused. Because somnolence may be simply an early stage of coma, its etiologies are almost all identical to the etiologies of coma. The few exceptions are mentioned at the close of this discussion.

While in medical school, I discovered a little text, *Aids to Medical Diagnosis* by G. E. F. Sutton.[2] I have never forgotten the unique little mnemonic provided in the text for remembering the causes of coma, A-E-I-O-U, the vowels.

A—Accidents suggest cerebral concussion and epidural and subdural hematomas. The **A** also stands for arterial occlusions, arteriosclerosis, aneurysms, and autoimmune disorders.

E—Endocrine disorders such as myxedema coma, hyperparathyroidism, diabetic coma, and insulin shock are

included in this category. The **E** also stands for the coma following an epileptic seizure.

I—Inflammatory and **intoxication** disorders such as encephalitis, cerebral abscess, meningitis, alcoholism, and opiates or barbiturates are included in this category.

O—Organ failure should suggest hepatic coma, respiratory failure, and uremia.

U—Uremia was used by Sutton, but because it is included above in organ failure, I prefer to use the **U** to designate the "undefined" disorders such as narcolepsy and conversion hysteria.

Therefore, with the vowels **A, E, I, O,** and **U**, one has a useful system for recalling the causes of coma and somnolence. **VINDICATE** can be used in a similar manner, but I prefer to let the reader develop the etiologies using this mnemonic as an exercise. There are two other approaches to the differential diagnosis of coma that may be more instructive. These are the **anatomic** and **physiologic** approaches.

If one visualizes the **anatomy** of the head from the skull on into the ventricles and cross-indexes the various layers with the mnemonic **MINT**, one will have an excellent means of recalling the causes of coma and somnolence demonstrated in Table 17. The important conditions resulting from disease of each anatomic structure are reviewed here.

Thinking of the **skull** reminds one of depressed skull fractures and epidural and subdural hematomas. In visualizing the **meninges**, meningitis and subarachnoid hemorrhages are recalled. Moving deeper into the **brain** itself will suggest encephalitis, encephalopathies (e.g., alcoholic), and brain tumors. Considering the **arteries** at the base of the brain, one should recall arterial occlusions, hemorrhages, and emboli. The **blood supply** prompts the recall of anoxia and other metabolic disorders that may be responsible for coma. The **veins** suggest venous sinus thrombosis as the cause of coma. Finally, the **pituitary** should help recall not only the coma of hypopituitarism but all the other endocrinopathies. This, then, is the anatomic approach to the differential diagnosis of coma and somnolence.

For the physiologic approach, simply ask the question, "What does the brain cell need to 'keep awake' or to continue functioning?" It needs a good supply of oxygen, glucose, and vitamins; the proper amount of insulin; an appropriate electrolyte and acid–base medium; and a proper amount of fluid in that medium. In addition, the brain cell cannot afford to have any toxic substance in that medium that might block the use or action of these metabolic substances. Now one is in a position to take each category and discuss the diseases that may result in a disturbance of brain cell function.

1. **Decreased supply of oxygen:** Focal anoxia from an arterial thrombosis, embolism, or hemorrhage falls into this category. Generalized anoxia from severe anemia and pulmonary or heart disease can also be recalled here.
2. **Decreased or increased supply of glucose:** Any hypoglycemic state (e.g., malabsorption syndrome, severe cirrhosis, glycogen storage disease, and hypopituitarism) may cause coma. In contrast, coma may be caused by hyperglycemia (nonketotic hyperosmolar diabetic coma).
3. **Too much or too little insulin:** In this category one should recall excessive exogenous insulin, insulinomas,

[2] Sutton GEF. *Aids to Medical Diagnosis*, Blackwell Publishing Co.

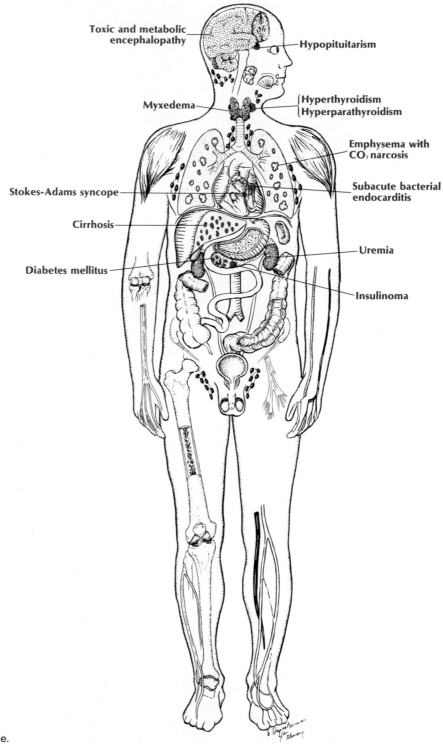

Toxic and metabolic
encephalopathy

Hypopituitarism

Myxedema

Hyperthyroidism
Hyperparathyroidism

Emphysema with
CO₂ narcosis

Stokes-Adams syncope

Subacute bacterial
endocarditis

Cirrhosis

Diabetes mellitus

Uremia

Insulinoma

● **FIGURE 9** Coma and somnolence.

and functional hypoglycemia, as well as diabetic acidosis (too little insulin).

4. **Avitaminosis:** Wernicke encephalopathy from thiamine deficiency, the hypocalcemia and possible tetany of rickets, and the dementia with somnolence of pellagra might be recalled here.

5. **Disturbances of electrolyte and acid–base equilibrium:** Here one should recall the coma of hyponatremia, hypokalemia, hyperkalemia (e.g., Addison disease, uremia, and diuretics), hypocalcemia (hypoparathyroidism, rickets, uremia, and malabsorption syndrome), hypercalcemia (e.g., hyperparathyroidism and metastatic tumors of the bone), and hypomagnesemia. The coma of diabetic acidosis, lactic acidosis, carbon dioxide (CO_2) narcosis, and alkalosis (hyperventilation syndrome) will also be recalled here.

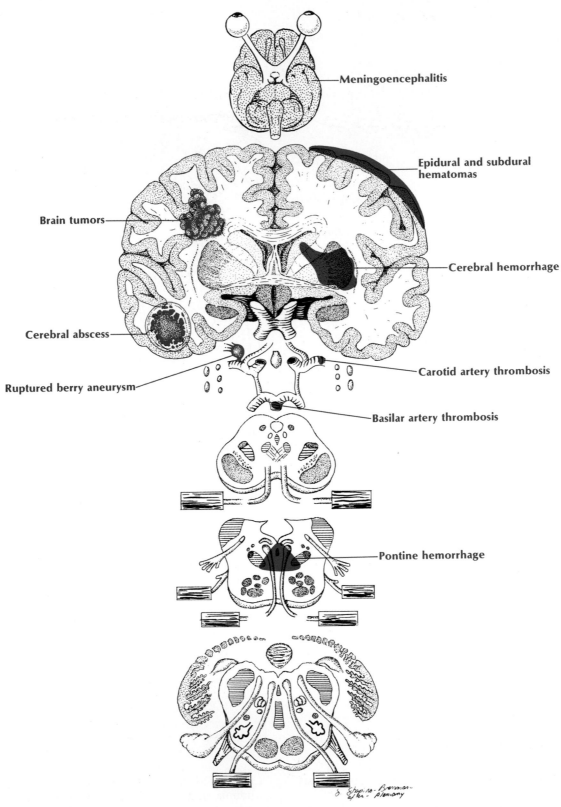

● **FIGURE 10** Coma and somnolence.

C

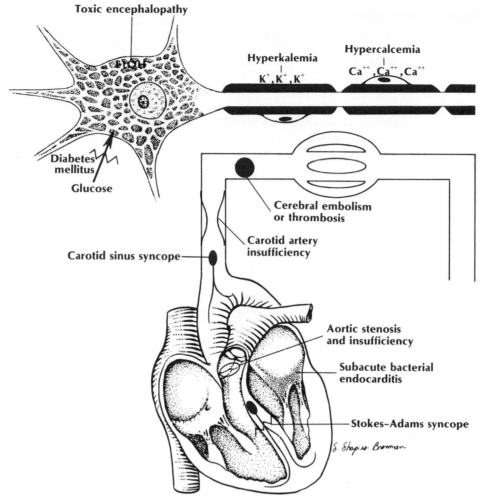

Toxic encephalopathy

Hyperkalemia
K^+,K^+,K^+

Hypercalcemia
Ca^{++},Ca^{++},Ca^{++}

Diabetes mellitus

Glucose

Cerebral embolism or thrombosis

Carotid artery insufficiency

Carotid sinus syncope

Aortic stenosis and insufficiency

Subacute bacterial endocarditis

Stokes–Adams syncope

● **FIGURE 11** Coma and somnolence.

6. **Increased fluid in the cell medium:** This should suggest cerebral edema from brain tumors, hemorrhages, hydrocephalus, encephalitis and meningitis, and cerebral concussions.
7. **Toxic substances that block the utilization or action of metabolic substances:** In this category are extrinsic substances like lead, alcohol, lysergic acid diethylamide (LSD), opiates, and a list of other drugs. It should also include intrinsic toxins from hepatic coma, uremia, and CO_2 narcosis.

Somnolence, as suggested in the introduction, is an indication of a few conditions that are not as likely to present with frank coma: These are endogenous depression, narcolepsy, cerebral arteriosclerosis, and encephalitis lethargica. The physiologic approach should also suggest myxedema coma, but it is difficult to fit it into any of the aforementioned categories.

● Approach to the Diagnosis

Obviously, a neurologic examination and a good history from a family member or friend are invaluable in the diagnosis of coma. However, one should not delay ordering laboratory work until the examination and history are accomplished. A CBC, blood urea nitrogen (BUN), fasting blood sugar (FBS), serum osmolality, electrolytes, blood gases, urinalysis, and drug screen are ordered immediately. If there is little or no history available and insulin shock is suspected, glucose or glucagon is administered before the laboratory reports are back, although this is done with more caution today for fear of aggravating a case of nonketotic, hyperosmolar diabetic coma.

It has been my experience that the neurologic examination is best performed simultaneously with the taking of a history from a relative or friend. In this way, various telltale neurologic signs can be found with alacrity. A unilateral dilated pupil (suggesting a subdural hematoma or aneurysm), acetone breath (suggesting diabetic acidosis), contusion of the skull (suggesting cerebral concussion or hematoma), and nuchal rigidity (suggesting a subarachnoid hemorrhage in meningitis) are just a few of the signs that can help to rapidly identify the cause of the coma.

Coma without focal neurologic findings should suggest a metabolic or toxic cause. In that case, an intensive laboratory workup as listed below would be indicated. A spinal tap may be indicated if there is fever as well. In contrast,

TABLE 17	**Coma and Somnolence**			
	M Malformation	**I** Inflammation	**N** Neoplasm	**T** Trauma
Skull				Depressed skull fracture Epidural or subdural hematoma
Meninges	Subarachnoid hemorrhage (from aneurysms)	Meningitis		Subarachnoid hemorrhage
Brain and Parenchyma	Porencephalic cyst Birth trauma or anoxia Kernicterus	Encephalitis Toxic and metabolic encephalopathies Alcoholism	Brain tumor	Cerebral concussion or contusion
Arteries	Arterial occlusion Hemorrhage Embolism	Subacute bacterial endocarditis Embolism Anoxia	Hemangioma	Fat embolus Arterial embolus
Veins	Arteriovenous malformation	Venous sinus thrombosis		
Pituitary	Hypopituitarism and other endocrinopathies		Pituitary adenoma	Postpartum hemorrhage

coma with focal neurologic signs suggests tumor, abscess, hematoma or cerebral embolism, thrombosis, or hemorrhage. The clinician should proceed with a skull x-ray film and CT scan immediately. When these are not available, immediate referral to a large medical center is necessary. Electroencephalography (EEG) and a spinal tap may identify the cause. A spinal tap should be considered with extreme caution even if there is no papilledema. Of course, a spinal tap is never done in the presence of papilledema unless a neurologist is consulted and CT findings are negative. One indication for a spinal tap under these circumstances might be meningitis. Another might be "benign intracranial hypertension."

● Other Useful Tests

1. CBC (septicemia, meningitis)
2. Sedimentation rate (inflammation)
3. Chemistry panel (diabetic acidosis, hypoglycemia, uremia, electrolyte imbalance)
4. Drug screen (drug intoxication)
5. Arterial blood gas (hypoxia, hypercarbia)
6. Blood lead level (lead encephalopathy)
7. Urine porphobilinogens (porphyria)
8. Blood cultures (septicemia)
9. Thyroid profile (myxedema coma)
10. Blood ammonia level (hepatic coma)
11. ECG (CHF, cardiac arrhythmia)
12. CT scan of the brain (encephalitis, hematoma, abscess)
13. Electroencephalogram (EEG) (level of coma assessment, epilepsy)
14. Spinal tap (meningitis, encephalitis, subarachnoid hemorrhage)
15. Serum and urine osmolality, syndrome of inappropriate antidiuretic hormone secretion (SIADH)

Case Presentation #10

A 34-year-old white man was admitted to the hospital ward in a comatosed state. History reveals he had been suffering with fever and chills for 1 week prior to admission. Neurologic examination revealed only diminished reflexes in the right extremities and a right Babinski sign. There was no nuchal rigidity.

Question #1. Given the method described above, what would be your list of possible causes of this man's condition at this point?

Physical examination revealed an apical systolic murmur and a few small petechiae of the trunk and extremities.

Question #2. What is your list of possibilities now?

(See Appendix B for the answers.)

CONSTIPATION

The causes of constipation can be recalled on a physiologic basis. Normal defecation requires feces that are of proper consistency, good muscular contraction of the walls of the large intestine, and unobstructed passage of the stool. It follows that constipation will result from insufficient intake of food and water, inhibition of muscular contraction of the bowels, or obstruction to the passage of stools. The obstruction can be high or low and intrinsic or extrinsic.

1. **Insufficient intake 1of food and water:** Starvation or anything that interferes with the appetite will cause constipation. Senility, anorexia nervosa, chronic tonsillitis,

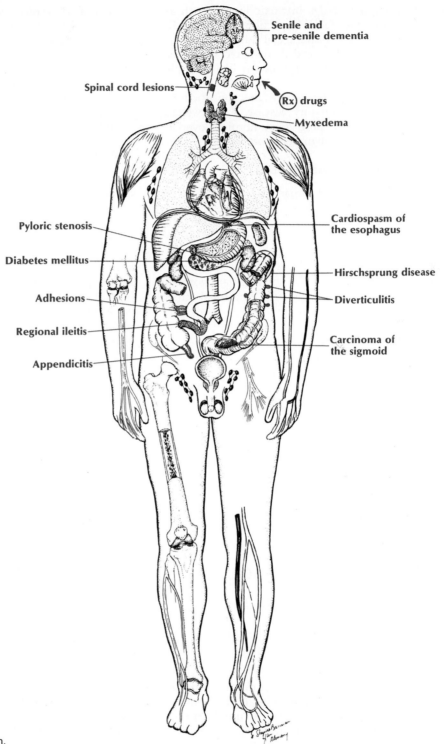

Senile and
pre-senile dementia

Spinal cord lesions

(Rx) drugs

Myxedema

Pyloric stenosis

Cardiospasm of
the esophagus

Diabetes mellitus

Hirschsprung disease

Adhesions

Diverticulitis

Regional ileitis

Carcinoma of
the sigmoid

Appendicitis

● **FIGURE 12** Constipation.

and cardiospasm of the esophagus are examples. Lack of fluid intake will cause a hard stool and constipation.

2. **Poor bowel motility and contractability:** Neurologic conditions such as poliomyelitis and tabes dorsalis may be considered in this group. In Hirschsprung disease, there is lack of the myenteric plexus, causing poor contraction of the bowel wall. Anxiety and depression may interfere with bowel motility and lead to constipation.

Certain drugs (such as atropine derivatives, tranquilizers, opiates, and barbiturates) interfere with bowel motility and cause constipation. Uremia and diabetic acidosis may cause a paralytic ileus.

3. **Obstruction:**
    A. **High obstruction** includes pyloric stenosis, volvulus, intussusception, regional ileitis, adhesions, and incarcerated hernias.

B. **Low obstruction** includes **intrinsic** lesions such as polyps, carcinomas, fecal impactions, and conditions that cause spasm of the rectal sphincter, such as proctitis, hemorrhoids, rectal fissures, rectal fistulas, and abscesses and spinal cord lesions like multiple sclerosis.

C. **Extrinsic** conditions that cause low obstructions include pelvic inflammatory disease, a retroverted uterus, endometriosis, pregnancy, fibroids, ovarian cysts, and a large prostate or pelvic abscess.

● Approach to the Diagnosis

Rectal examination for a fecal impaction and subsequent enemas are the first steps if no contraindication exists. This may disclose a fissure, inflamed hemorrhoid, or abscess. Pelvic examination must be done in all female patients. If nothing is found here a proctoscopic examination and barium enema would be indicated, provided the neurologic examination and a flat plate of the abdomen are normal. Careful inquiry about diet, drugs, and emotional stress should be made.

● Other Useful Tests

1. Glucose tolerance test (diabetic neuropathy)
2. Stool for occult blood (rectal or colon carcinoma)
3. Serum electrolytes (motility disorder)
4. Thyroid function tests (hypothyroidism)
5. Urine porphobilinogen (porphyria)
6. Urine drug screen (drug abuse)
7. Colonoscopy (colon carcinoma)
8. Defecography (motility disorder)
9. Anorectal manometry (neuropathy)
10. Gastroenterology consult
11. Psychometric testing
12. Therapeutic trial of stool softeners or psyllium fibers

CONSTRICTED PUPILS (MIOSIS)

The best method to develop a list of the causes of a constricted pupil is to use **neuroanatomy**. One simply follows the nerve pathways from the end organ (iris) through the peripheral portion of the nerves to the central nervous system (brainstem) (Table 18).

1. **End organ:** Iritis, keratitis, or cholinergic drugs may be the cause of the constricted pupil in this location. Poisoning with organophosphates allows the accumulation of acetylcholine at the synaptic junctions causing miosis. Hyperopia and presbyopia are also possible causes.
2. **Peripheral nerves:** Constriction of the pupil may occur from lesions anywhere along the sympathetic pathway as it branches around the internal carotid artery (aneurysms, thrombosis, and migraine), enters the stellate ganglion in the neck (scalenus anticus syndrome, tumors or adenopathy in the neck), and follows the preganglionic pathway into the spinal cord (aneurysm of the aorta, mediastinal tumors, spinal cord tumors, or other space-occupying lesions).

3. **Central nervous system:** Lesions involving the sympathetic pathways of the brainstem (posterior inferior cerebellar tumors, occlusion, brainstem tumors, hemorrhages, encephalitis, or toxic encephalopathy) will cause miosis. Both pupils are constricted in the Argyll Robertson pupil of neurosyphilis in which the damage is located in the pretectal nucleus of the midbrain. Morphine characteristically causes bilateral constriction of the pupils, probably based on its central nervous system effects.

● Approach to the Diagnosis

In unilateral miosis, the clinician must look for local conditions such as iritis and keratitis. If there is an associated ptosis and enophthalmos, Horner syndrome is present. The lesion is undoubtedly located somewhere along the sympathetic pathway. Miosis alone, however, may be due to a sympathetic lesion. Bilateral miosis and coma should suggest narcotic intoxication or a brain stem lesion (possibly a pontine hemorrhage). Bilateral miosis in an alert individual with pupils that fail to react to light but react to accommodation is clear evidence of an Argyll Robertson pupil. Partial Argyll Robertson pupils do occur. Bilateral miosis in older individuals without loss of the light reflexes suggests hyperopia or arteriosclerosis.

The laboratory workup may include an x-ray film of the cervical spine, chest and skull roentgenogram, a CT scan or MRI of the brain, and a spinal tap or arteriograms, depending on the association of other symptoms and signs. A starch test to determine if sweating function is lost on the side of the lesion will help locate the level of the sympathetic nerve lesion.

● Other Useful Tests

1. Venereal disease research laboratory (VDRL) test (neurosyphilis)
2. Histoplasmin skin test (iriditis)
3. Toxoplasma serology (iridocyclitis)
4. Epinephrine test (Horner syndrome)
5. Slit lamp examination (iriditis, keratitis)
6. Tonometry (glaucoma)
7. Mecholyl test (Argyll Robertson pupil)

Case Presentation #11

A 24-year-old white male medical student was found to have miosis, partial ptosis, and enopthalmos of the left eye on a routine life insurance examination. On further questioning, he admitted he had intermittent weakness of his left arm and hand.

Question #1. Applying the methods from the above discussion, what are your diagnostic possibilities at this point?

Complete neurologic examination was normal except for a weak left radial pulse.

Question #2. What are your diagnoses now?

(See Appendix B for the answers.)

C

Table 18   Constricted Pupils (Miosis)

	V Vascular	I Inflammatory	N Neoplasm	D Degenerative	I Intoxication	C Congenital	A Allergic and Autoimmune	T Trauma	E Endocrine
End Organ		Iritis Keratitis		Hyperopia Presbyopia	Cholinergic drug	Hyperopia Congenital myosis Arachnodactyly	Amyloidosis		Hypoparathyroidism
Peripheral Sympathetic Pathways	Carotid aneurysm and thrombosis Migraine Aortic aneurysm	Cervical adenitis Mediastinitis	Hodgkin lymphoma Mediastinal tumor Pancoast tumor			Cervical rib Klumpke paralysis		Brachial plexus trauma	
Brainstem	Posterior inferior cerebellar artery occlusion Pontine hemorrhage	Encephalitis Neurosyphilis (Argyll Robertson pupil)	Brainstem tumor		Toxic encephalopathy (e.g., morphine)				
Spinal Cord		Poliomyelitis Tuberculosis Epidural abscess Transverse myelitis	Spinal cord tumor Metastatic tumor to the spine	Syringomyelia			Multiple sclerosis	Fracture Herniated disc	

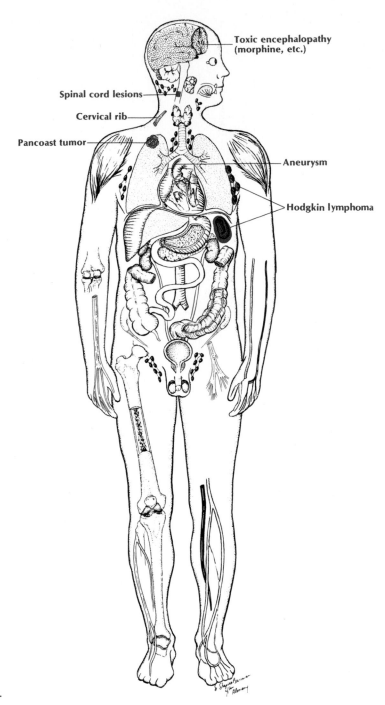

● FIGURE 13 Constricted pupils (miosis).

CONVULSIONS

To formulate a differential diagnosis of convulsions, one must use both **physiology** and **anatomy**. The anatomic causes are charted in Table 19.

Irritability of the nerve cell is caused by the same physiologic factors that lead to irritability of a muscle cell: anoxia, hypoglycemia, and electrolyte imbalances. Any condition causing anoxia may cause a seizure; thus, focal arterial spasm (e.g., transient ischemic attack [TIA]) may lead to seizures. Obstruction of the artery by emboli, thrombi, or

atheromatous plaques may cause focal anoxia and seizures, whereas diffuse cerebral anoxia is more likely to cause syncope and coma. Acute blood loss (anemic anoxia) and acute reduction in cardiac output (as in Stokes–Adams disease and various arrhythmias) are infrequent causes of seizures. Aortic stenosis and insufficiency may occasionally cause seizures by relative reduction in cardiac output compared to demand (as during exercise).

Hypoglycemia is more likely to cause a coma than a seizure. Anything that severely reduces the blood sugar (<40 mg/dL), such as exogenous insulin overdose, islet

C

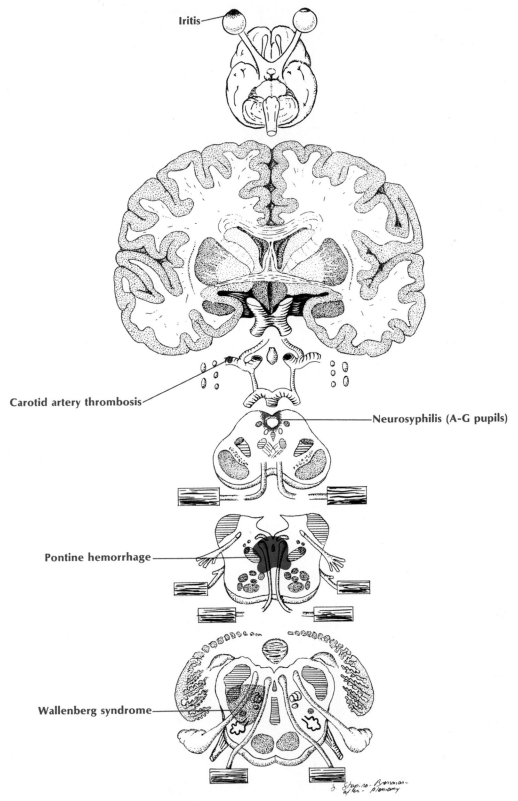

Iritis

Carotid artery thrombosis

Neurosyphilis (A-G pupils)

Pontine hemorrhage

Wallenberg syndrome

● **FIGURE 14** Constricted pupils (miosis).

TABLE 19 Convulsions

	V Vascular	I Inflammatory	N Neoplasm	D Degenerative and Deficiency	I Intoxication and Idiopathic	C Congenital	A Autoimmune Allergic	T Trauma	E Endocrine and Metabolic
Brain Cell and Axon	Hypertensive hemorrhage	Viral encephalitis Syphilis Tetanus Rabies		Pyridoxine deficiency Cortical atrophy	Lead Wilson disease Bromide Alcohol Kernicterus Uremia Eclampsia	Schilder disease Porencephaly Birth trauma Anoxia	Multiple sclerosis	Concussion Intracerebral hematoma	Hypoglycemia Hypocalcemia (see physiology)
Supporting Tissue		Tuberculoma Cysticercosis Other parasites	Glioma Neurofibroma Metastasis	Tay–Sachs disease Histiocytosis X		von Gierke disease	Cerebral urticaria		Addison disease
Meninges	Subarachnoid hemorrhage	Meningitis Epidural abscess	Meningioma Hodgkin lymphoma		Phenylketonuria			Subdural hematoma	
Skull								Depressed fracture Epidural hematoma	
Arteries	Infarct Embolism		Hemangioma Angioma			Aneurysm A-V anomaly	Periarteritis nodosa Lupus	A-V aneurysm	
Veins		Venous sinus thrombosis				A-V anomaly Sturge–Weber syndrome			
Blood		Septicemia	Leukemia Polycythemia vera	Aplastic anemia	Coumadin and heparin therapy		ITP		
Heart	Arrhythmia Heart block Myocardial infarction	Subacute bacterial endocarditis	Atrial myxoma with embolism		Drug-induced arrhythmia Heart block	Aortic stenosis	Rheumatic heart disease with aortic stenosis		Hyperthyroidism with auricular fibrillation and embolism

cell adenoma, Addison disease, and hypopituitarism, may cause a seizure.

Irritability of the nerve cell is more often caused by electrolyte alterations. The same equation that applied to muscle applies here:

$$\text{Neuronal irritability} \times \frac{Na^+, K^+, pH}{Ca^{++}, Mg^{++}, H^+}$$

Hypocalcemia may at first lead to tetany, simulating a convulsion. The causes of hypocalcemia include hypoparathyroidism, vitamin D deficiency, malabsorption syndrome, calcium-losing nephropathy, and chronic nephritis. Ionizable calcium is decreased by alkalosis, respiratory or metabolic. Hypomagnesemia must be ruled out, especially in chronic alcoholics and in malabsorption syndromes. Water intoxication should be considered in inappropriate antidiuretic hormone (ADH) syndrome (relative dilution of both calcium and magnesium).

Moving from the physiologic causes of seizures to the anatomic analysis, the physician's main consideration is that something mechanical is irritating the nerve cell. The nerve cell may be irritated by a tumor of the supporting tissue, an abscess, or a hematoma. Pressure from inflammatory lesions in the meninges (i.e., meningitis or epidural abscess) or hemorrhage into this layer (subdural or epidural hematoma and subarachnoid hemorrhages) may be the mechanical irritant. Focal accumulation of fluid in the brain substance as in encephalitis, concussions, and increased intracranial pressure from whatever causes may lead to a seizure. A depressed skull fracture is occasionally the mechanical irritant, as is a scar from an old skull injury. Infiltration of the brain by metals such as lead and copper (i.e., Wilson disease) are worth considering in children, particularly infiltration of the brain by a foreign cell (i.e., leukemia). Reticuloendotheliosis and mucopolysaccharidosis should be considered. Turning to exogenous factors, one must consider a host of chemicals and drugs that may cause seizures, most commonly alcohol, paint thinners, lidocaine (Xylocaine), phenothiazine drugs, and bromides. A bolus of almost any substance may occasionally cause seizures if it is large enough.

Occasionally, degenerative and demyelinating disease may present with seizures. In contrast, lupus erythematosus and other collagen diseases may frequently present with seizures. Finally, one should not forget idiopathic epilepsy.

● Approach to the Diagnosis

The first thing to do is ascertain whether the motor disturbance or episode of loss of consciousness was really a seizure. Hysterical seizures are not associated with incontinence or tongue biting. There is often an aura with real seizures but not so with hysterical seizures.

Next, a careful history from the immediate family or friend is important. Be sure to ask about previous head trauma (including birth trauma), anoxia, meningitis, or encephalitis. Inquiry into drug or alcohol abuse is essential.

A thorough neurologic examination is a must. If the clinician is too busy or not equipped to do this, referral to a neurologist is done at this point. If there are focal neurologic signs or papilledema, there is a strong chance that the patient has a space-occupying lesion such as tumor, subdural hematoma, or abscess and will need a neurologist anyway.

The clinical picture will help determine the cause of the seizures. If there is alcohol or drug use, toxic encephalopathy is suspected. If there is fever, meningitis or encephalitis must be considered in the differential diagnosis. If there is a heart murmur or irregular heart beat, cerebral embolism should be suspected. A history of trauma suggests posttraumatic epilepsy. A history of optic neuritis makes one suspicious of multiple sclerosis. A history of high-risk sexual behavior suggests that acquired immunodeficiency syndrome (AIDS) may be the cause. A history of cancer makes it important to rule out cerebral metastasis.

The initial workup should include a CBC, urinalysis, sedimentation rate, ANA, VDRL test, chemistry panel, drug screen, wake-and-sleep EEG, and skull x-ray. Patients with suspected grand mal epilepsy or focal motor seizures need either a CT scan or MRI to rule out a space-occupying lesion. This is true of all patients with complex partial seizures as well.

Patients suspected of having meningitis or encephalitis need a spinal tap. Patients with possible cerebral embolism need an ECG, echocardiogram, blood cultures, and a cardiology consult. If AIDS is suspected, a human immunodeficiency virus (HIV) antibody titer is ordered. Patients with possible multiple sclerosis need a spinal fluid analysis, and visual, somatosensory, or brainstem-evoked potential studies. Elderly patients should have a chest x-ray done to exclude a primary tumor of the lung.

● Other Useful Tests

1. Holter monitoring (heart block)
2. Ambulatory EEG monitoring (epilepsy with infrequent seizures)
3. 72-hour fast (hypoglycemia)
4. 24-hour urine calcium (hypoparathyroidism)
5. Stool for ova and parasites (cysticercosis)
6. Urine porphobilinogen (porphyria)
7. Blood lead level (lead encephalopathy)
8. Therapeutic trial of anticonvulsants

Case Presentation #12

A 56-year-old black male mechanic gave a 1-month history of daily generalized headaches (occasionally associated with nausea and vomiting) on awakening in the morning. On the day of admission, he had a generalized grand mal seizure.

Question #1. Based on the method described above, what would be your list of possible causes at this point?

Neurologic examination revealed hyperactive reflexes in the right lower extremity and a positive Babinski sign. His blood pressure is 110/76. The patient gives a history of chronic cough with occasional hemoptysis. He has smoked 1½ packs of cigarettes a day for 30 years.

Question #2. What is your list of possibilities now?

(See Appendix B for the answers.)

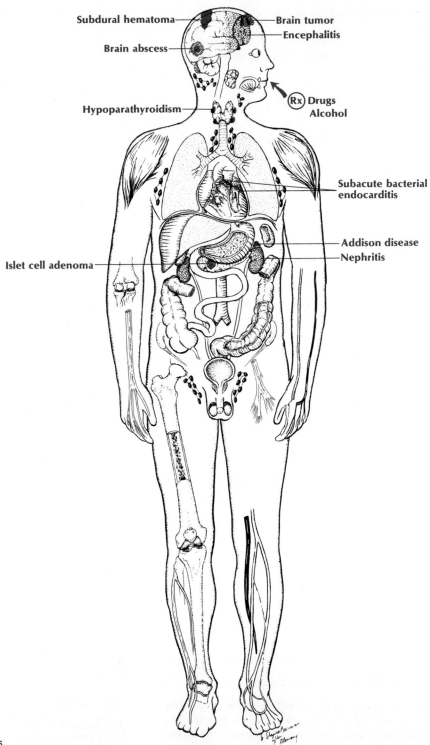

Subdural hematoma

Brain tumor
Encephalitis

Brain abscess

Rx Drugs
Alcohol

Hypoparathyroidism

Subacute bacterial
endocarditis

Addison disease
Nephritis

Islet cell adenoma

● **FIGURE 15** Convulsions.

COUGH

The differential diagnosis of cough is best developed with the use of **anatomy**. Cough may arise from an irritative focus anywhere along the respiratory tract. The irritation may be **intrinsic**, in which case it is usually inflammatory, neoplastic, or toxic, or it may be **extrinsic**, in which case it is often neoplastic or vascular (Table 20).

Intrinsic irritation: Pharyngitis, whether due to virus, *Streptococcus*, or diphtheria, is a common cause of cough. Hypertrophied tonsils or adenoids may also initiate the cough reflex. Other pharyngeal causes are angioneurotic edema, leukemia, and agranulocytosis. The **esophagus** is an extrinsic cause of cough in most cases, but a tracheo-esophageal fistula from esophageal carcinoma or reflux esophagitis with repeated aspiration of hydrochloric acid

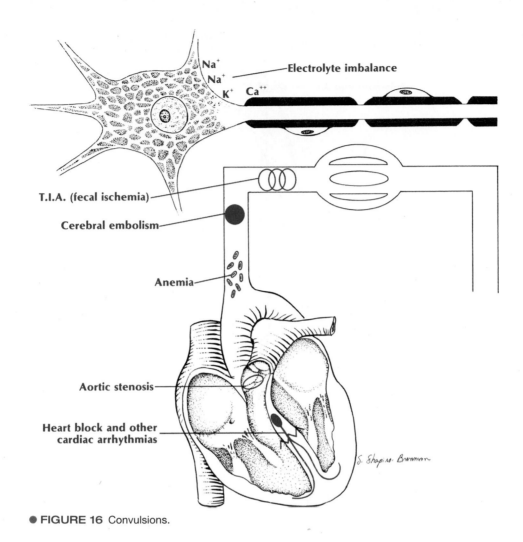

Na⁺
Na⁺
K⁺ Ca⁺⁺
—Electrolyte imbalance

T.I.A. (fecal ischemia)—

Cerebral embolism—

Anemia—

Aortic stenosis—

Heart block and other
cardiac arrhythmias—

S. Shapiro-Brennan

● **FIGURE 16** Convulsions.

(HCL) may cause a chronic cough. **Diverticula** of the esophagus may press on the trachea and cause a cough.

In the **larynx**, the numerous infections of the pharynx discussed above may irritate the cough centers but, in addition, laryngeal polyps, tuberculosis, and trauma from overuse are important causes. The more common causes of cough, especially a nonproductive cough, are in the **tracheobronchial** area. Numerous viruses cause tracheobronchitis, especially influenza, but bacterial causes such as whooping cough should always be considered. Tuberculosis and carcinoma are important here, as are toxic gases such as chlorine and cigarette smoke. Bronchiectasis, whether congenital or acquired, and the associated postnasal drip from chronic sinusitis must not be forgotten. A search for asthma is important in areas with high pollen counts.

In the **alveoli**, in addition to pneumonia, tuberculosis, and carcinoma (particularly metastatic), several new etiologies are added. Thus, pulmonary embolism, parasites, fungi (such as actinomycosis), pneumoconiosis, reticuloendothelioses, and autoimmune diseases (i.e., Wegener granuloma) should be included. Advanced AIDS may manifest itself with a productive cough due to pneumocystis carani.

Extrinsic irritation: The extrinsic causes are mainly from the structures of the mediastinum, especially the heart. A large heart from CHF or a single chamber enlargement (as in mitral stenosis) may compress the bronchus and recurrent laryngeal nerve and cause a cough. Pericarditis, aortic aneurysms, and rings are other cardiovascular causes. Finally, other structures in the mediastinum such as a substernal thyroid, a large lymph node from Hodgkin lymphoma, and occasionally a dermatoid cyst must be considered. Trauma can lead to a cough whether it hits the lung, mediastinum, or pericardium. Angiotensin-converting enzyme (ACE) inhibitors may cause cough, and other drugs are occasionally responsible.

● Approach to the Diagnosis

There is no problem diagnosing a patient with an acute cough. The association of fever and running nose make the common cold or influenza likely. A rapid lab test for influenza is now available. Clinically, exposure to dust, smoke, and various gases should be looked for in the patient presenting with a cough. Postnasal drip from chronic sinusitis should be ruled out. An allergic history (e.g., hay fever) is important. Cardiovascular disease should be carefully

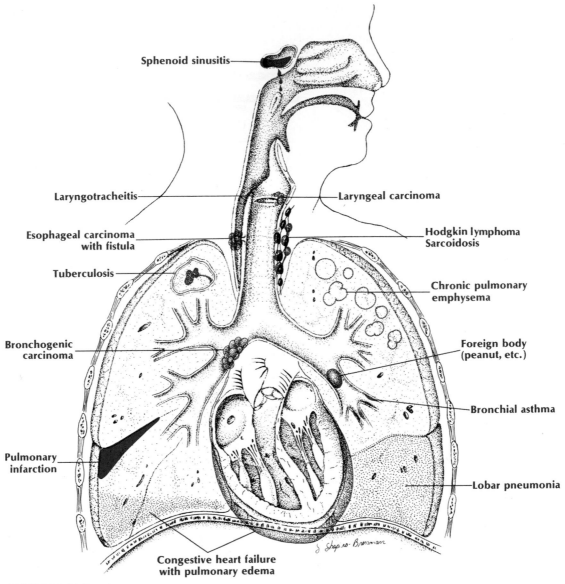

● **FIGURE 17** Cough.

excluded, especially when sputum is negative for routine cultures, tuberculosis, fungi, and Papanicolaou smears, and chest x-rays, bronchoscopy, and bronchography are normal. Hysterical cough should be considered, however, as well as reflux esophagitis and hiatal hernia. A sputum and nasal smear for eosinophils should be done to rule out asthma. A trial of therapy may be indicated. A CT scan of the chest is indicated if the above studies are negative.

● **Other Useful Tests**

1. CBC and C-reactive protein (CRP) (pneumonia)
2. Sedimentation rate (infection)
3. Sputum smear and culture (pneumonia)
4. Sputum volume study (bronchiectasis)
5. Sputum for eosinophils (asthma)
6. Arterial blood gases (chronic pulmonary disease)
7. Sputum cytology (neoplasm)
8. Sputum for AFB smear and culture (tuberculosis)
9. Sputum for fungal smear and culture
10. Tuberculin test
11. Histoplasmin skin test
12. Coccidioidin skin test
13. Blastomycin skin test
14. Sweat test (fibrocystic disease)
15. α_1-Antitrypsin assay (pulmonary disease due to α_1-antitrypsin deficiency)
16. Pulmonary function testing (CHF, chronic pulmonary disease)
17. Barium swallow (hiatal hernia with reflux esophagitis)
18. Cold agglutinins (mycoplasma pneumonia)
19. Serologic tests (Legionnaires disease, mycoplasma pneumonia)
20. X-ray of sinuses (sinusitis)
21. HIV antibody titer (AIDS)
22. Therapeutic trial of diuretics (CHF)
23. Special cultures for pertussis immigrants

TABLE 20 Cough

	V Vascular	I Inflammatory	N Neoplasm	D Degenerative and Deficiency	I Intoxication	C Congenital	A Autoimmune Allergic	T Trauma	E Endocrine
Pharynx		Bacterial or viral pharyngitis (diphtheria), tonsillitis	Leukemia Hypertrophied tonsils and adenoids		Agranulocytosis with pharyngitis		Angioneurotic edema		
Esophagus		Reflux esophagitis	Carcinoma			Diverticulum Tracheoesophageal fistula		Traumatic rupture or fistula	
Larynx		Laryngitis Singers nodes Tuberculosis	Carcinoma					Laryngitis from overuse	
Trachea		Tracheitis Tuberculosis Influenza Measles	Adenoma, carcinoma, or polyp		Chlorine or smoke				
Bronchi		Whooping cough Acute or chronic bronchitis Sinusitis	Bronchogenic carcinoma or adenoma	Bronchiectasis	Gas, smoking, paint	Bronchiectasis Cystic fibrosis	Asthmatic bronchitis	Foreign body	
Alveoli	Pulmonary embolism	Pneumonia Tuberculosis Parasites Fungi	Metastatic carcinoma or oat cell carcinoma	Emphysema bulla Pulmonary fibrosis	Pneumoconiosis Lipoid pneumonia	Reticuloendotheliosis Congenital cyst	Lupus Wegener granulomatosis	Pneumothorax Contusion Hemorrhage Laceration	
Pleura	Pulmonary embolism or congestive heart failure	Tuberculosis or other empyema	Mesenthelioma					Rib fracture	
Mediastinum	Aortic aneurysm	Mediastinitis	Hodgkin lymphoma Metastatic carcinoma			Dermoid cyst		Stab wound Gunshot wound	Substernal thyroid
Heart	Congestive heart failure	Syphilitic aneurysm Acute pericarditis		Dissecting aneurysm		Aortic ring Patent drug	Mitral stenosis with large atrium		

CREPITUS

In deciding what the cause of crepitus is, first think of what substances may be involved. There are three: gas, fluid, and bone. Next, visualize the anatomy of the area. If the crepitus is over a joint, it is most likely fluid in the joint or bursa, but it may also be loose bone or cartilage fragments. If the crepitus is over one of the long bones of the extremities, it may be due to a fracture, gas gangrene, or a bone tumor that has eroded the bony cortex. If the crepitus is over the lung, one has to consider the possibility of subcutaneous emphysema due to pneumothorax in addition to a fractured rib. Subcutaneous emphysema may also occur over an orbital fracture that has penetrated the maxillary or frontal sinus and around a tracheotomy site. Crepitus in the neck may also result from a ruptured esophagus, trachea, or major bronchus.

● Approach to the Diagnosis

Plain films of the area involved will identify subcutaneous emphysema, gas gangrene, fractures, and arthritic causes. Bone scans or CT scans help to identify bone tumors, fractures, and joint pathology in elusive cases. Arthroscopy is extremely valuable in diagnosing joint pathology. An orthopedic consultant should be consulted.

CYANOSIS

The causes of cyanosis may be quickly recalled by applying the basic science of **physiology**. Cyanosis is due to **decreased oxygenation of the blood**. The decrease, however, cannot be mild; there must be at least 5 g of reduced hemoglobin per 100 mL of blood if cyanosis is to appear.

It should be understood from the above that cyanosis will appear with less severe anoxia in polycythemia than it will in anemia. For example, a patient with 20 g of hemoglobin needs only one fourth of his or her blood unsaturated to show cyanosis, whereas a patient with 10 g of hemoglobin needs one half of his or her blood unsaturated to do the same.

Decreased oxygenation of the blood may result **from obstruction to the intake of oxygen** (e.g., acute laryngotracheitis, chronic bronchial asthma, chronic bronchitis, and emphysema or foreign body); **from the decreased absorption of oxygen**, as in conditions with alveolar–capillary block (sarcoidosis, pulmonary fibrosis, pneumonia, pulmonary edema, and alveolar proteinosis); or from a ventilation–perfusion defect (e.g., emphysema, pneumoconiosis, or sarcoidosis). Decreased oxygenation of the blood may also result **from decreased perfusion of the lung** with blood in shock, acute respiratory distress syndrome (ARDS), pulmonary embolism, pulmonary vascular shunts, or bypasses such as occur in pulmonary hemangiomas and congenital heart disease. Another cause of reduced intake of oxygen is an atmosphere with reduced concentration of oxygen. The hemoglobin may be unable to latch onto the oxygen in carbon monoxide poisoning and methemoglobinemia, but the cyanosis is associated with a cherry-red color to the lips and tongue in the former and a brownish hue in the latter; polycythemia vera may be associated with a cyanotic hue to the face in cold weather, but the arterial oxygen saturation is not necessarily decreased (Table 21).

Another approach to developing a differential diagnosis of cyanosis is to apply the mnemonic **VINDICATE** to the heart and lungs. This is suggested as an exercise for the reader.

TABLE 21 Cyanosis

	M Malformation	I Inflammatory Idiopathic	N Neoplasm	T Traumatic Toxication
Decreased Intake of Oxygen	Foreign body	Acute laryngotracheitis Chronic bronchitis and emphysema Asthma Whooping cough		Pneumoconiosis Lipoid pneumonia Drowning Pneumothorax Suffocation
Decreased Absorption of Oxygen		Sarcoidosis Pulmonary fibrosis Alveolar proteinosis Emphysema	Oat cell carcinoma Metastatic carcinoma	
Decreased Perfusion of the Lungs	Congenital heart disease (Tetralogy of Fallot)		Hemangioma	
Decreased Oxygen Combining Power of Blood				Carbon monoxide Sulfhemoglobinemia Methemoglobinemia

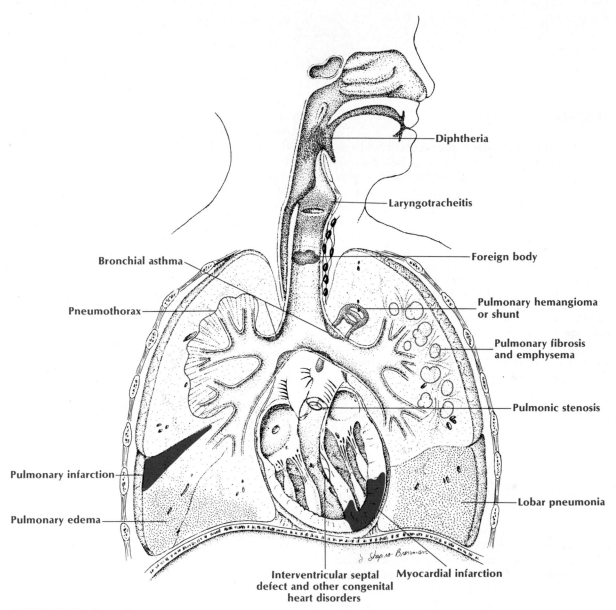

Diphtheria

Laryngotracheitis

Bronchial asthma

Foreign body

Pneumothorax

Pulmonary hemangioma
or shunt

Pulmonary fibrosis
and emphysema

Pulmonic stenosis

Pulmonary infarction

Lobar pneumonia

Pulmonary edema

Interventricular septal
defect and other congenital
heart disorders

Myocardial infarction

● **FIGURE 18** Cyanosis.

● Approach to the Diagnosis

The workup of cyanosis includes pulmonary function studies before and after bronchodilators, arterial blood gases, routine and before-and-after breathing 100% oxygen, venous pressure and circulation times, chest x-rays, ECGs, and ventilation–perfusion scans. It is unusual not to be able to pinpoint the cause.

● Other Useful Tests

1. CBC (pneumonia)
2. Tuberculin test (tuberculosis)
3. Lung scan (pulmonary embolism)
4. Echocardiogram (CHF, valvular heart disease)
5. Test for methemoglobinemia
6. Serial cardiac enzymes and ECGs (myocardial infarction)
7. Cardiac catheterization and angiocardiography (arteriovenous [A-V] shunts, valvular heart disease)
8. Pulmonary angiography (pulmonary embolism)
9. Hemoglobin electrophoresis (HbM disease)

D

DANDRUFF

The causes of dandruff are similar to the causes of baldness (see page 82), but a brief review will be made here because certain skin conditions should be added. Pityriasis simplex capitis is probably the most common cause, although no definite etiology has been established. Autoimmune disorders such as lupus erythematosus should be considered. Inflammatory disorders include ringworm (tinea capitis), impetigo, and seborrheic dermatitis. Idiopathic skin disorders such as psoriasis and lichen planus cause dandruff. These disorders can all be recalled by the same mnemonic that was applied in baldness, that is, **HAIR.**

H—Hereditary lesions include eczema and psoriasis.
A—Autoimmune disorders include lupus.
I—Inflammatory diseases include ringworm, impetigo, and seborrheic dermatitis. **I** also stands for idiopathic and thus includes pityriasis simplex capitis.
R—Radiation dermatitis.

The workup of dandruff is similar to that of baldness (see page 65).

DECREASED RESPIRATIONS, APNEA, AND CHEYNE-STOKES BREATHING

Nurses frequently become distressed and summon the intern during the night about these signs. Cheyne–Stokes respirations are a frequent source of bewilderment because they may occur at times with no direct evidence of damage to the nervous system. It would be interesting to discuss the physiology of respiration at length in this section, but it will be of little help in the differential diagnosis of apnea and in slow or Cheyne–Stokes respirations except in a few instances. In all cases, these are a result of an insult to the respiratory centers in the brain by some etiologic agent. The causes of these signs can best be remembered by the mnemonic **VINDICATE.**

V—Vascular includes cerebral thrombosis, embolism, and especially hemorrhage of the brainstem, which may cause depressed respirations or periodic apnea. Diffuse cerebral arteriosclerosis is another cause in this category.
I—Inflammatory disorders signify encephalitis, poliomyelitis, meningitis, and brain abscesses, particularly with increased intracranial pressure.
N—Neoplasms of the brainstem (primary or metastatic) and neoplasms of the cerebrum are associated with increased intracranial pressure and may cause depression of respirations and Cheyne–Stokes breathing.

D—Degenerative diseases of the brain, including senile and presenile dementia and Schilder disease, may cause these signs in the terminal stages.
I—Intoxication is an important category of etiologies of depressed or irregular respirations because the toxic substance may not be obvious at first. Failure of any organ system to function may lead to respiratory depression. When there is respiratory failure from emphysema or other causes, carbon dioxide (CO_2) builds up in the blood and CO_2 narcosis develops. In this state the important stimulus of high blood CO_2 on the respiratory centers is gradually lost and anoxia is the only stimulus left. Periodic or Cheyne–Stokes breathing frequently develops in the following manner: During respiration the blood oxygen builds up to a level at which the respiratory stimulus to anoxia is lost. Respirations cease. During apnea the blood oxygen falls to a point where there is sufficient anoxia to kick the respiratory center over again. The electrolyte disturbances and buildup of toxins in uremia, the high blood ammonia and other toxins that result from hepatic failure, and the anoxia of congestive heart failure (CHF) may all lead to apnea or depressed respirations.

Exogenous toxins are more commonly the cause in young people. Alcoholism, morphine, barbiturates, and a host of tranquilizers will cause respiratory depression in sufficient quantities.

C—Congenital disorders that cause these respiratory disturbances include Tay–Sachs disease, cerebral palsy, glycogen storage disease, reticuloendothelioses, epilepsy, and cerebral aneurysms with subarachnoid hemorrhage.
A—Autoimmune disorders such as lupus erythematosus and multiple sclerosis (MS) must be considered in this category.
T—Trauma is another frequent cause of apnea or Cheyne–Stokes respiration. Cerebral concussion, subdural, epidural, and intracerebral hematomas all may cause depressed respirations, especially when associated with increased intracranial pressure.
E—Endocrine disease reminds the reader that whereas diabetic coma may begin with Kussmaul breathing, in the advanced stages bradypnea and Cheyne–Stokes respirations develop from the severe acidosis. Pituitary and suprasellar tumors may grow sufficiently to compress the brainstem and cause apnea.

● Approach to the Diagnosis

Obviously, the association of other signs and symptoms will determine the workup in most cases. The most important things to do are to order a blood urea nitrogen (BUN) level, electrolytes, fasting blood sugar (FBS), arterial blood

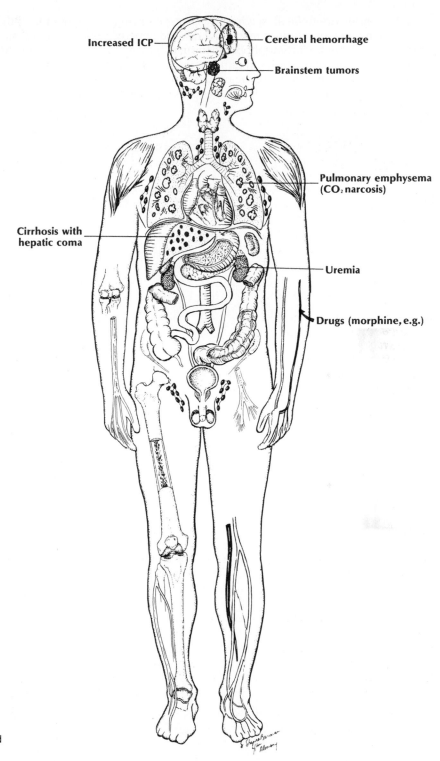

Increased ICP — Cerebral hemorrhage

Brainstem tumors

Pulmonary emphysema (CO₂ narcosis)

Cirrhosis with hepatic coma

Uremia

Drugs (morphine, e.g.)

D

● **FIGURE 1** Decreased respirations, apnea, and Cheyne–Stokes breathing.

gases, and a drug screen and to check for increased intracranial pressure by examining the eye grounds. If the history or physical findings suggest increased intracranial pressure, and other metabolic studies (e.g., BUN) are normal, a mannitol or urea drip is begun while awaiting the results of other investigations such as computed tomography (CT) scan, electroencephalogram (EEG), and echoencephalogram. A neurosurgeon should be consulted immediately.

DELAYED PUBERTY

Because most of the causes of delayed puberty are hormonal in origin, the key to recalling them will be visualizing the anatomy, particularly the endocrine glands.

Hypothalamus and pituitary: Lack of gonadotropin-releasing hormone from hypothalamic disorders such as Lawrence–Moon–Biedl syndrome, space-occupying lesions, trauma, or infection may cause delayed puberty in girls and boys. Chromophobe adenomas, prolactinomas, craniopharyngiomas, trauma, granulomas, and vascular lesions may decrease the production of growth hormone and other pituitary hormones causing delayed puberty.

Thyroid: Both hypothyroidism and hyperthyroidism in children may cause delayed puberty.

Adrenal gland: Visualizing this organ will prompt the recall of congenital adrenocortical hyperplasia and Cushing syndrome.

Ovaries: Ovarian dysgenesis (Turner syndrome etc.), autoimmune oophoritis, and Noonan syndrome are

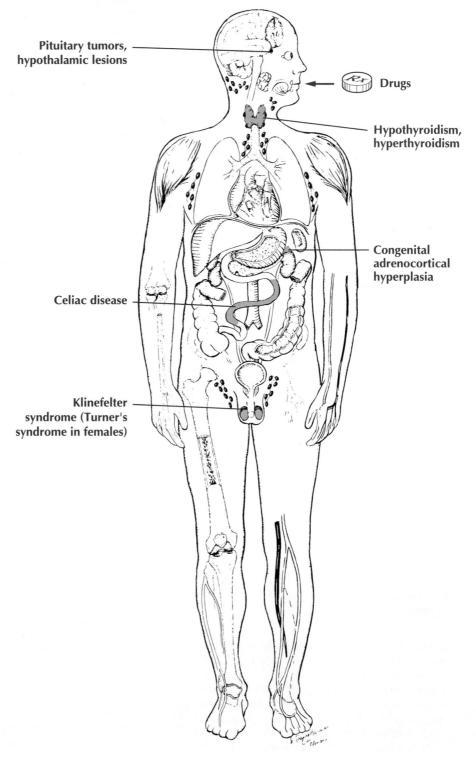

Pituitary tumors, hypothalamic lesions

Drugs

Hypothyroidism, hyperthyroidism

Congenital adrenocortical hyperplasia

Celiac disease

Klinefelter syndrome (Turner's syndrome in females)

● **FIGURE 2** Delayed puberty.

associated with delayed puberty in girls. A masculinizing tumor of the ovary will present with delayed puberty on occasion.

Testicles: Irradiation, Klinefelter syndrome, Noonan syndrome, castration, and anorchism may cause delayed puberty in boys. Mumps rarely is the cause.

The above method of recall will omit the chronic illnesses such as anorexia nervosa, malnutrition, renal failure, tuberculosis, celiac disease, collagen disease, and cyanotic heart disease that may cause delayed puberty. It also will not prompt the recall of drugs that cause delayed puberty such as thyroid hormone, anabolic steroids, and androgens in girls and thyroid hormones in boys. It is important to remember that over half the cases of delayed puberty in boys and 16% of cases in girls are due to constitutional delayed puberty.

● Approach to the Diagnosis

The physician is frequently consulted early about this problem by an overprotective parent, so it is important to remember that there is little cause for alarm until age 15 in boys and age 14 in girls. Nevertheless, a workup may be started early if other telltale signs of pathology such as short stature, web neck, or small or absent testicles are found. The workup will probably include a thyroid profile, serum testosterone (boys), estradiol (girls), and follicle-stimulating hormone (FSH) and luteinizing hormone (LH) assay. Urine gonadotropins are less expensive screening tests. Pelvic ultrasound and CT scans of the abdomen and pelvis will help to identify ovarian and adrenal causes. A CT scan or magnetic resonance imaging (MRI) of the brain will identify most pituitary causes.

● Other Useful Tests

1. Testicular biopsy (Klinefelter syndrome)
2. Buccal smear for Barr bodies (Klinefelter syndrome)
3. Complete blood count (CBC) and chemistry panel (renal failure)
4. Gynecology consult
5. Psychiatric consult
6. Visual field examination (pituitary tumor)
7. Serum growth hormone assay (pituitary tumor)
8. Urine drug screen (drug abuse)
9. Serum free cortisol (Cushing syndrome)
10. Full karyotyping (Klinefelter syndrome, Turner syndrome)
11. Laparoscopy (ovarian dysgenesis)
12. Serum prolactin (pituitary tumor)
13. Endocrine consult

DELIRIUM

The differential diagnosis of delirium is very similar to that for coma, and one finds the mnemonic **VINDICATE** useful in this regard.

V—Vascular disorders of the brain including hemorrhage, embolism, thrombosis, and arteriosclerosis may cause delirium.

I—Inflammatory disorders of the nervous system that may cause delirium include viral encephalitis, meningitis, syphilis, malaria and other parasites, rabies, and cerebral abscess. Generalized infections, usually when associated with fever, may be responsible.

N—Neoplasms of the brain are not usually associated with delirium until the end stages at which time the cause will be obvious.

D—Deficiency disorders that may be associated with delirium include Wernicke encephalopathy, pellagra, and pernicious anemia. Delirium may be associated with degenerative disorders such as Alzheimer disease.

I—Intoxication by an enormous number of exogenous and endogenous substances may cause delirium. Alcohol, cocaine, heroin, phencyclidine (PCP), marijuana, lead, arsenic, and manganese are just a few of the exogenous substances. Endogenous substances include uremia, ammonia from hepatic failure, hyperinsulinemia, diabetic ketosis, and porphyria. Delirium may be associated with the withdrawal of a patient from alcohol and/or any drug including morphine, cocaine, or tobacco.

C—Convulsive disorders may be associated with delirium either during or after the seizure.

A—Autoimmune disorders such as lupus erythematosus are associated with inflammation of vasculitis in the brain causing delirium.

T—Trauma may cause a concussion, cerebral hemorrhage, or subdural or epidural hematoma leading to delirium.

E—Endocrine disorders associated with delirium include insulinoma and diabetes.

● Approach to the Diagnosis

It is essential to get a history of drug or alcohol use from the patient or family, and a drug screen may be done in most cases. Infection is another common cause. The workup should also include a CBC, sedimentation rate, urinalysis, antinuclear antibody (ANA) analysis, chemistry panel, and electrolytes. A CT scan or MRI of the brain will be necessary in most cases. It may be wise to administer intravenous thiamine and glucose while awaiting the results of blood work. If there is a fever, blood cultures and possibly a spinal tap (after a CT scan or MRI has ruled out a space-occupying lesion) may be indicated. Arterial blood gas analysis and carboxyhemoglobin should be determined. A neurologist or neurosurgeon needs to be consulted early in the workup.

● Other Useful Tests

1. EEG (seizure disorder)
2. Venereal disease research laboratory (VDRL) test (neurosyphilis)
3. Carotid sonogram (carotid thrombosis)
4. Four-vessel angiography (transient ischemic attack [TIA])
5. Glucose tolerance test (diabetes, insulinoma)
6. Blood smear for malarial parasites (malaria)
7. Psychiatric consult
8. Urine porphobilinogen (porphyria)

Case Presentation #13

A 13-year-old boy is brought to the emergency room in a delirious state mumbling incomprehensible sentences and rolling his head back and forth. He is occasionally combative. His parents claim he has been this way since he came home 2 hours ago. His pupils are dilated but there are no other focal neurologic signs.

Question #1. Utilizing the techniques described above, what is your list of diagnostic possibilities at this point?

On questioning the parent's of the friends he was with before he came home this evening, it is discovered that he had taken two tablets of an illegal substance.

Question #2. What is your diagnosis now?

(See Appendix B for the answers.)

DELUSIONS

A delusion is a persistent false belief. The feeling that one is being followed or watched, that one has a bad odor even after frequent and careful bathing, that one is superior to others—all are examples of delusions. Although most patients presenting with a delusion have a functional disorder, the astute clinician knows the organic disorders of the brain that may be associated with a delusion. The mnemonic **VINDICATE** forms a simple method for ready recall of these disorders.

V—Vascular disorders suggest cerebral arteriosclerosis with lacunar infarcts or cerebral emboli.

I—Inflammatory disorders suggest cerebral abscess, tuberculomas, viral encephalitis (e.g., herpes simplex), and general paresis.

N—Neoplasms, both primary and metastatic, should always be considered, as these are potentially treatable.

D—Degenerative diseases include senile and presenile dementia, Huntington chorea, diffuse sclerosis, and many other conditions.

I—Intoxication brings to mind alcoholism, bromism, chronic use of both "uppers" and "downers," lysergic acid diethylamide (LSD), and cannabis. Uremia, CO_2 narcosis, chronic anoxia, electrolyte disorders, and early hepatic coma should also be considered.

C—Congenital diseases suggest Schilder disease, mongolism, Wilson disease, and many other conditions associated with mental retardation.

A—Autoimmune diseases focus on lupus erythematosus, allergic angiitis, and multiple sclerosis.

T—Trauma facilitates the recall of concussion and chronic subdural hematomas.

E—Endocrine disorders include suprasellar tumors that invade the hypothalamus, acromegaly, hypopituitarism, hyperthyroidism, Cushing syndrome, and adrenal insufficiency. Parathyroid dysfunction can also cause delusions.

● Approach to the Diagnosis

The important thing to do before referring these patients to a psychiatrist is to perform an evaluation of the mental status and a neurologic examination. Memory of recent events, orientation in time and place, ability to perform serial sevens, and interpretation of proverbial phrases should all be tested for. Psychologic testing may be warranted in borderline cases as well as an EEG, CT scan, skull roentgenogram, and spinal tap. A drug screen may also be indicated. Additional tests are listed below.

DEPRESSION, ANXIETY, AND OTHER ABNORMAL PSYCHIC STATES

It is simple enough to administer a sedative and refer the emotionally distressed patient to a psychiatrist, but the astute diagnostician will want to rule out an organic disease first. Almost every endocrine disease is associated with emotional disturbances, all of which are potentially curable. In addition, electrolyte and other metabolic disturbances, chronic anoxia, or failure of any organ system may lead to anxiety, depression, or a psychotic state. The mnemonic **VINDICATE** will help to recall this important group of disorders.

V—Vascular diseases include myocardial infarction, CHF, cerebral arteriosclerosis, and thrombosis.

I—Inflammatory diseases recall syphilis, encephalitis, tuberculosis, brain abscess, influenza, pneumonia, and any prolonged infectious state, particularly that of the hospitalized patient with tubes in every orifice.

N—Neoplasms include cerebral tumors, tumors of the endocrine glands, and any neoplasm which is metastatic or which affects the metabolism of the body by a hormone or enzyme which it secretes. Pancreatic carcinoma is frequently associated with depression.

D—Degenerative diseases and **deficiency** diseases suggest presenile and senile dementia, pellagra, Wilson disease, and atrophy of the various endocrine glands.

I—Intoxication suggests lead poisoning, alcoholism, bromism, hypercalcemia, hypocalcemia, manganese toxicity, hypokalemia, hypovolemia, uremia, anoxia from pulmonary disease, anemia, heart disease, and corticosteroid therapy, as well as many other drugs. Porphyria may cause depression or a psychotic state.

C—Congenital suggests the depression associated with many congenital neurologic diseases: epilepsy, muscular dystrophy, Friedreich ataxia, myotonic dystrophy, and the depression associated with congenital heart disease and congenital defects of many organ systems.

A—Autoimmune diseases include MS and lupus erythematosus.

T—Traumatic disorders include the now well-recognized posttraumatic neurosis or depression, neurocirculatory asthenia, and postconcussion syndrome. Compensation neurosis should be mentioned here. Sexual abuse is a common cause in children.

E—Endocrine diseases include hypopituitarism, acromegaly, hypothyroidism, apathetic hyperthyroidism,

D

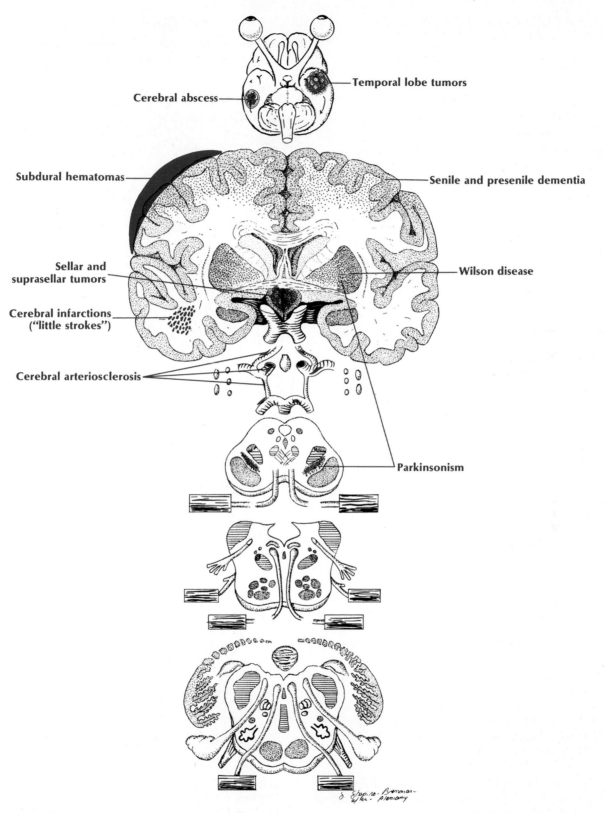

Cerebral abscess ——— **Temporal lobe tumors**

Subdural hematomas——— **Senile and presenile dementia**

Sellar and suprasellar tumors ——— **Wilson disease**

Cerebral infarctions ("little strokes")

Cerebral arteriosclerosis ———

Parkinsonism

● **FIGURE 3** Delusions.

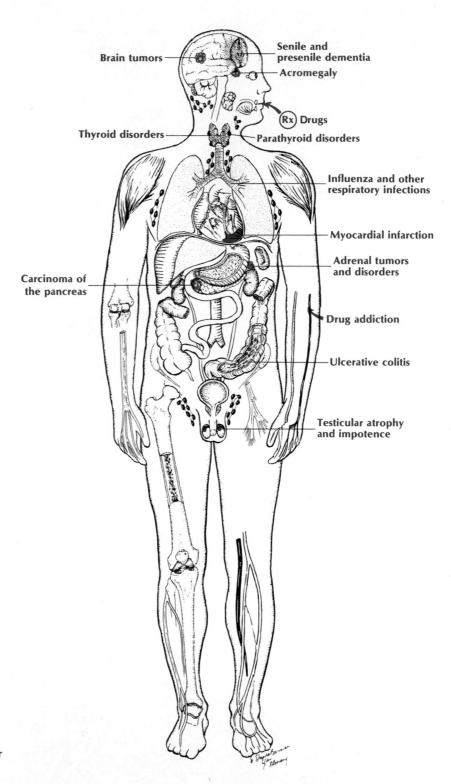

Brain tumors

Senile and
presenile dementia

Acromegaly

(Rx) Drugs

Thyroid disorders

Parathyroid disorders

Influenza and other
respiratory infections

Myocardial infarction

Adrenal tumors
and disorders

Carcinoma of
the pancreas

Drug addiction

Ulcerative colitis

Testicular atrophy
and impotence

● **FIGURE 4** Depression, anxiety, and other
abnormal psychic states.

hypoparathyroidism, hyperparathyroidism, diabetes mellitus, insuloma, hypogonadism, menopause, Cushing syndrome, and adrenal insufficiency.

● Approach to the Diagnosis

The association of other symptoms and signs is all important. For example, anxiety, tremor, tachycardia and diaphoresis may suggest alcohol withdrawal or hyperthyroidism. A triiodothyronine (T_3) level, total thyroxine (T_4) level, and free thyroxine index (FT_4), urine for porphobilinogen, serum electrolytes, toxicology screen, lead level, 24-hour urine, 17-ketosteroid level, and 17-hydroxycorticosteroid level should be done on anyone suspected of having endogenous depression. (Possibly all depressed patients should get this screen.) Skull x-ray film, EEG, CT scan, and even a spinal tap (to rule out MS and lues) may be worthwhile when other neurologic signs are present.

Case Presentation #14

A 62-year-old white woman is brought to your office because the family has noticed that she is depressed. The patient has insomnia, frequent nightmares, and weight loss over the past 6 months despite the fact that she has a good appetite.

Question #1. Utilizing the system provided above, what is your list of possibilities at this point?

Your examination reveals tachycardia, some lid retraction, and slight diffuse thyroid enlargement.

Question #2. What is your diagnosis now?

_____

(See Appendix B for the answers.)

DIARRHEA, ACUTE

Acute diarrhea is most likely infectious. Beginning with the smallest organism and working up to the largest will help recall the most common types of infectious diarrhea. The smallest organism prompts the recall of viral gastroenteritis. A midsized organism would suggest *Staphylococcus*, *Salmonella*, cholera, botulism, *Campylobacter*, *Escherichia coli*, *Clostridium difficile*, and bacillary dysentery. Moving up to the next largest organism, one would recall amebic dysentery and giardiasis. Both of these conditions move on to become a chronic diarrhea if left untreated. Patients with acquired immunodeficiency syndrome (AIDS) may have acute diarrhea from cryptosporidiosis. This organism is responsible for worldwide epidemics of diarrhea. Finally, larger organism such as *Trichinella spiralis* may also be associated with acute diarrhea.

Acute diarrhea is also caused by many drugs such as antibiotics, colchicine, ethacrynic acid, digitalis, and quinidine. Pseudomembranous enterocolitis is a severe diarrhea that follows antibiotic administration. Another form of noninfectious acute diarrhea is associated with ulcerative colitis and Crohn disease. This is often characterized by grossly bloody stools.

● Approach to the Diagnosis

The history may help differentiate many causes of acute diarrhea. Fever would help to distinguish *Salmonella*, *Shigella*, and *Campylobacter jejuni*. Blood in the stool also suggests *Salmonella*, *Shigella*, and *Campylobacter*, but may also be due to ulcerative colitis, amebic dysentery, or pseudomembranous colitis. If there is no blood in the stool, the patient most likely has viral gastroenteritis, staphylococcal toxin diarrhea, or traveler's diarrhea. If other members of the family are experiencing the same symptoms, the clinician should look for staphylococcal toxin diarrhea or botulism. Vomiting is associated with toxic staphylococcal

gastroenteritis and viral gastroenteritis, but is unlikely with giardiasis and pseudomembranous colitis.

All patients need to provide a stool sample for occult blood, culture, and smear for ovum parasites, and Giardia antigens. If there is a history of antibiotic use, the stool should be tested for *C. difficile* toxin B.

● Other Useful Tests

1. Stool smear for leukocytes
2. Culture for *Campylobacter* or *Yersinia*
3. Sigmoidoscopy
4. Colonoscopy
5. Stool for *Giardia* antigen
6. Swallowed string test (Giardiasis)

DIARRHEA, CHRONIC

The differential diagnosis of diarrhea may be approached from either an anatomic or a physiologic basis. The **anatomic** approach is used in Table 22. In the **stomach** and **duodenum**, pernicious anemia and Zollinger–Ellison syndrome are prominent causes. A carcinoma may form a fistula with the transverse colon and cause diarrhea. Viral gastroenteritis and *Giardia* infection may also be prominent causes.

Liver and biliary tract diseases of all types may cause diarrhea (steatorrhea) by decreasing the secretion of bile. Ampullary carcinoma and cirrhosis are illustrated here, but one should not forget the diarrhea of chronic cholecystitis. The **pancreas** is the source of important digestive enzymes; as a result, chronic pancreatitis and pancreatic carcinomas may be associated with diarrhea (steatorrhea) in adults, whereas cystic fibrosis should be considered in children. The pancreatic islet cell tumors may secrete gastrin or vasoactive intestinal peptide, causing diarrhea.

Most of the lesions causing diarrhea are in the **small intestine**. Thus, cholera, *Salmonella*, *Staphylococci*, typhoid, and tuberculosis attack here. The carcinoid syndrome, various polyps (especially Peutz–Jeghers), and regional ileitis are also important causes. Toxins and drugs (see Table 22) are common causes acting here, as are pellagra and other vitamin deficiencies and food allergies. Systemic autoimmune diseases such as scleroderma and Whipple disease are also important. Mesenteric artery insufficiency or obstruction should be considered both here and in the colon.

A wide variety of etiologic agents cause diarrhea by their action on the **colon**.

V—Vascular diseases include ischemic colitis.

I—Infectious agents such as bacillary dysentery (*Shigella*), *Escherichia coli*, *Campylobacter*, *Yersinia*, and amebiasis may ulcerate or inflame the colon.

N—Neoplasms such as carcinomas and polyps cause chronic irritation and exudates from the colon with hypermotility and diarrhea.

D—Degenerative lesions of the muscularis that cause diverticulosis and allow overgrowth of bacteria and

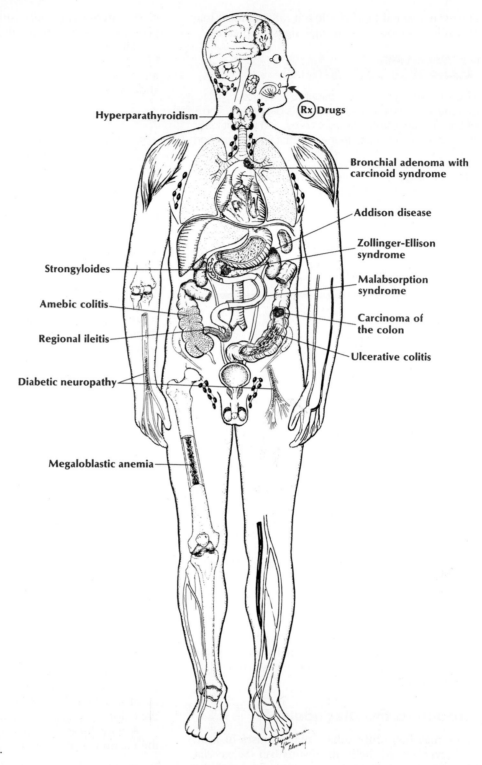

Hyperparathyroidism

Rx Drugs

Bronchial adenoma with carcinoid syndrome

Addison disease

Zollinger-Ellison syndrome

Malabsorption syndrome

Strongyloides

Amebic colitis

Regional ileitis

Carcinoma of the colon

Ulcerative colitis

Diabetic neuropathy

Megaloblastic anemia

● **FIGURE 5** Diarrhea.

chronic inflammation may lead to diarrhea, but this may be classified under the idiopathic category as well.

I—**Intoxicating** substances, osmotic cathartics, and antibiotics (by allowing overgrowth of bacteria and fungi) may involve the colon (e.g., pseudomembranous colitis). Mucous colitis or irritable bowel syndrome may best be classified as idiopathic.

C—**Congenital** lesions of the colon include the solitary diverticulum of the cecum, malrotation (more frequently associated with intestinal obstruction), and familial polyposis.

A—**Autoimmune** disease of the colon is common and includes both ulcerative colitis and granulomatous colitis.

TABLE 22   Diarrhea—Anatomic Classification

	V Vascular	I Inflammatory	N Neoplasm	D Degenerative and Deficiency	I Intoxication or Idiopathic	C Congenital	A Autoimmune or Allergic	T Trauma	E Endocrine
Stomach and Duodenum		Viral gastroenteritis Parasite	Carcinoma with fistula into intestines	Pernicious anemia Iron deficiency	Uremia Antacid			Surgery (e.g., blind loop)	Zollinger–Ellison syndrome
Liver and Biliary Tract		Chronic cholecystitis and lithiasis	Neoplasm obstructing bile ducts	Cirrhosis	Cirrhosis				
Pancreas		Chronic pancreatitis	Pancreatic carcinoma Islet cell adenoma		Radiation	Cystic fibrosis			Pancreatic cholera
Small Intestine	Mesenteric artery insufficiency	Cholera Botulism *Staphylococcus* *Salmonella* *Escherichia coli* Parasites Tuberculosis	Carcinoid Polyp Sarcoma Lymphoma	Pellagra Pyridoxine deficiency	Sprue Cathartic Mercurial Reserpine Antibiotic Alcohol Other drugs	Peutz–Jehgers diverticulum (Meckel)	Regional ileitis Whipple disease Scleroderma	Fistula	Hypoparathyroidism Hyperthyroidism Addison disease
Large Intestine	Mesenteric artery insufficiency	*Shigella* Amebiasis Other parasites	Polyp Carcinoma and other neoplasms		Mucus colitis Diverticulosis Antibiotic Hypervitaminosis Uremia	Familial polyposis	Ulcerative colitis Granulomatous colitis Food allergy		

T—**Trauma** is not a common cause of diarrhea anywhere in the intestinal tract, but certainly surgically induced fistulas may occur in the colon or anywhere else.

E—**Endocrine** disorders do not usually affect the colon directly.

Having considered the local causes of diarrhea, do not forget reflex diarrhea from diseases of other organs, such as pyelonephritis, salpingo-oophoritis, and central nervous system diseases.

Using Table 23, the reader can develop the differential diagnosis of diarrhea with **physiology**. Diarrhea may result from **increased intake** of fluids or bulk foods; **hyposecretion** of enzymes necessary for digestion of food; **hypersecretion** of gastrointestinal (GI) fluids and enzymes; **malabsorption** of various substances, particularly protein and fat; **exudations** of pus induced by granulomatous or ulcerative colitis and *Salmonella* or *Shigella* infections; **hypermobility** from stimulation by cathartics, various hormones (e.g., vasoactive intestinal peptides and gastrin), and **hypomobility** from autonomic dysfunction as occurs in diabetic neuropathy.

● Approach to the Diagnosis

Whichever method is applied (anatomic or physiologic), most causes of diarrhea can be recalled before interviewing the patient. Then one can proceed to ask the right questions to eliminate each suspected cause. Are other members of the family affected? Is there a history of recent travel abroad? Combinations of symptoms and signs will assist greatly in narrowing the differential diagnosis. For example, chronic diarrhea and copious mucus without blood suggests irritable bowel syndrome. Chronic diarrhea with mucus and blood suggests ulcerative colitis.

Physical examination is often unrewarding but it may disclose a hepatic, rectal, or pelvic source for the diarrhea; it may also indicate that the diarrhea is a sign of a systemic disease (e.g., scleroderma or hyperthyroidism). Rectal examination may reveal a fecal impaction. A warm stool examination for pus, pH (acid stool suggests lactase deficiency), fat and meat fibers, blood, ova, and parasites is most essential. Stool for immunoassay for lactoferrin may indicate bacterial infection. A stool culture is done. Proctoscopy (immediately if there is blood) followed by colonoscopy, barium enema, and upper GI series is usually necessary in all cases. A CT scan of the abdomen is occasionally necessary.

● Other Useful Tests

1. CBC (malabsorption syndrome)
2. Cathartic stool examination (intestinal parasites)
3. Small-bowel series (malabsorption syndrome)
4. Duodenal aspiration (giardiasis, *Strongyloides*)
5. Lactose tolerance test (lactase deficiency)
6. D-xylose absorption test (malabsorption syndrome)
7. Serum gastrin (gastrinoma)
8. Urine 5-hydroxyindoleacetic acid (5-HIAA) (malabsorption syndrome, carcinoid tumor)
9. Mucosal biopsy (malabsorption syndrome)
10. Colonoscopy and biopsy (ulcerative colitis, amebic colitis, granulomatous colitis)

11. Stool for *Giardia* antigen (giardiasis)
12. Human immunodeficiency virus (HIV) antibody titer (AIDS)
13. Angiogram (ischemic colitis)
14. Culture for *C. difficile* (pseudomembranous colitis)
15. Glucose tolerance test (diabetic enteropathy)
16. Stool for *C. difficile* toxin B
17. Psychometric testing (irritable bowel syndrome)
18. Hydrogen breath test (lactose intolerance)
19. Therapeutic trial of metronidazole (Giardiasis, *C. difficile*)

Case Presentation #15

A 54-year-old white man complained of chronic diarrhea for the past year. He had also noted frequent indigestion and heartburn and occasional midepigastric pain.

Question #1. Utilizing the methods provided above, what is your list of possibilities at this point?

Further history reveals that he has had occasional black stools and does not abuse alcohol or drugs. His physical examination is unremarkable, but stools test positive for occult blood. Fasting failed to eliminate the diarrhea.

Question #2. What is your diagnosis now?

(See Appendix B for the answers.)

DIFFICULTY SWALLOWING (DYSPHAGIA)

Swallowing is the function of the pharynx, larynx, and esophagus. This function may be impaired by two mechanisms: mechanical obstruction (e.g., carcinoma of the esophagus) and physiologic obstruction (e.g., pseudobulbar palsy).

Mechanical obstruction may result from intrinsic disease of the pharynx, larynx, and esophagus or extrinsic disease of the organs around the esophagus.

The mnemonic **VINDICATE** is useful in recalling the causes of mechanical obstruction as follows:

V—**Vascular** indicates aortic aneurysms and cardiomegaly.

I—**Inflammatory** should suggest pharyngitis, tonsillitis, esophagitis, and mediastinitis.

N—**Neoplasm** should bring to mind esophageal and bronchogenic carcinoma, and dermoid cysts of the mediastinum.

D—**Degenerative** and **deficiency** disease should suggest Plummer–Vinson syndrome or iron deficiency anemia.

I—**Intoxication** immediately indicates lye strictures.

C—**Congenital** and **acquired** anomalies should suggest esophageal atresia and diverticula.

A—**Autoimmune** disease suggests scleroderma.

T—**Trauma** would prompt the recall of ruptured esophagus, pulsion diverticulum, and foreign bodies that obstruct or injure the wall of the esophagus.

TABLE 23   Diarrhea—Physiologic Classification

	Hyposecretion	Hypersecretion	Hypermobility	Hypomobility	Primary Malabsorption	Exudative
Gastric	Pernicious anemia Iron deficiency Gastric resection	Zollinger–Ellison syndrome		Dumping syndrome		
Duodenal	Lactase deficiency Sucrase deficiency		Blind loop syndrome	Secretion-induced		
Biliary	Liver disease Obstructive jaundice			Cholecystokinin-induced	Cholecystokinin-induced Regional ileitis	
Pancreatic	Cystic fibrosis Chronic pancreatitis	"Pancreatic cholera" (islet cell adenoma with vasoactive intestinal peptide)		Gastrin Vasoactive intestinal peptide		
Small Intestine		Cholera (e.g., *Escherichia coli*)	Diabetic diarrhea Drugs	Coffee Serotonin-induced Cathartic Parasympathomimetic	Celiac sprue Tropical sprue Whipple disease Intestinal lymphoma Extensive resection	Regional ileitis Salmonellosis
Large Intestine		Protein-losing enteropathy (e.g., villous adenoma)				*Shigella* Ulcerative colitis Amebiasis

E—Endocrine disorders suggest the enlarged thyroid of endemic goiter and Graves disease.

Physiologic obstruction results from neuromuscular disorders at the end organ, myoneural junction, and lower and upper motor neurons.

1. **End organ:** This should suggest myotonic dystrophy, dermatomyositis, achalasia, and diffuse esophageal spasm.
2. **Myoneural junction:** This brings to mind myasthenia gravis.
3. **Lower motor neuron:** In this category one would recall poliomyelitis, diphtheritic polyneuritis, and brainstem tumors or infarctions.
4. **Upper motor neuron:** This structure prompts the recall of pseudobulbar palsy from cerebral thrombosis, embolism, or hemorrhage, multiple sclerosis, presenile dementia, and diffuse cerebral arteriosclerosis. It should also bring to mind Parkinson disease and other extrapyramidal disorders.

● Approach to the Diagnosis

The age of onset is significant because carcinoma of the esophagus is rare before age 50, whereas achalasia and reflux esophagitis are more common in young and middle-aged adults. In newborns, one must consider esophageal atresia. The onset is gradual in carcinoma and aortic aneurysms but more acute in reflux esophagitis and foreign bodies. Patients with achalasia have trouble swallowing both food and water, but those with carcinoma suffer the most, and often the only difficulty is swallowing food.

Association of other symptoms and signs is important. Neurologic findings will focus on the diagnosis of bulbar and pseudobulbar palsy whereas hematemesis and heartburn will suggest esophageal carcinoma or reflux esophagitis.

The barium swallow is still the most useful initial study to order. However, esophagoscopy and biopsy will lead to a definitive diagnosis in most cases of mechanical obstruction. If esophagoscopy is negative, one may resort to a mecholyl test to diagnose achalasia, a Tensilon test to exclude myasthenia gravis, and esophageal manometry to diagnose reflux esophagitis, scleroderma, and diffuse esophageal spasm.

● Other Useful Tests

1. CBC (Plummer–Vinson syndrome)
2. ANA analysis (collagen disease)
3. Sonogram (laryngeal obstruction)
4. Videofluoroscopy (oropharyngeal obstruction)
5. Ambulatory pH monitoring (reflux esophagitis)
6. CT scan of the mediastinum (mediastinal mass, aortic aneurysm)
7. Gastroenterology consult
8. Therapeutic trial of proton pump inhibitor (reflux esophagitis)
9. Solid food scintigraphy (achalasia)
10. Therapeutic trial of proton pump inhibitors (reflux esophagitis)

DIFFICULTY URINATING

This condition is characterized by a weak or interrupted urinary stream. Initiation of urination is difficult or slow, and the finish is just the same. Difficulty urinating must be distinguished from dysuria (page 144), which is painful urination, and anuria or oliguria (page 51), which is absent or reduced volume of urine. The pathophysiological cause of difficulty urinating is obstruction. If we then visualize the urinary tree from the prepuce on up to the bladder, we can visualize the causes of obstruction at each level. These are illustrated in the figure given for dysuria.

Prepuce—Phimosis and paraphimosis
Meatus—Meatal stricture
Urethral—Urethral stricture, urethral calculus
Prostate—Prostatitis, prostatic hypertrophy, prostatic carcinoma, prostatic calculus
Bladder—Bladder neck obstruction due to stricture, median bar hypertrophy, calculus or neoplasm
Extrinsic lesions of the bladder or urethra—Uterine fibroids, pregnant retroverted uterus, or carcinoma of the vagina
Lesions of the innervation of the bladder wall—This may be due to lower motor neuron disorders such as poliomyelitis, cauda equina tumors, or disks; tabes dorsalis; or diabetic neuropathy. It may also be due to upper motor neuron lesions such as MS, transverse myelitis, or spinal cord tumor.

● Approach to the Diagnosis

The first thing to do is to establish that there is an obstruction to the flow of urine. This may now be done with ultrasonography, but catheterization may still be done in the acute situation. The history will be helpful in many cases. Difficulty voiding in a young person will most likely point to a urethral stricture or prostatitis from previous gonorrhea or urethral injury, whereas difficulty voiding in an older man would suggest prostatic hypertrophy. A history of hematuria would suggest the possibility of a vesicle or urethral calculus. Ask if the patient is on any drugs or has a history of diabetes. A complete physical including a rectal and pelvic exam (in women) is done next. An abnormal neurological examination might point to diabetic neuropathy, MS, or spinal cord tumor.

The laboratory workup should include the CBC, urinalysis, chemistry panel, VDRL, and a urine culture and sensitivity. If these tests are negative, a urologist needs to be consulted for cystoscopy and cystometric testing.

● Other Useful Tests

1. Anaerobic cultures
2. Prostate-specific antigen (PSA) titer
3. Intravenous pyelogram (IVP) and voiding cystogram
4. Gynecology consult
5. Neurology consult
6. Electromyography (EMG) and nerve conduction velocity testing
7. Plain films of the thoracolumbar spine

8. MRI of the thoracic or lumbar spine
9. Laparoscopy
10. CT scan of the abdomen and pelvis
11. Therapeutic trial of tamsulosin (benign prostatic hyperplasia [BPH])

DILATED PUPILS (MYDRIASIS)

Like that of myosis, the differential diagnosis of dilated pupils or mydriasis can best be developed by applying **neuroanatomy** (Table 24). "Knowing where the lesion is, tells us what the lesion is." One simply follows the nerve pathway from the end organ up the oculomotor nerve to the termination in the brainstem. A dilated pupil, however, may also signify a lesion of the optic nerve and its pathways.

1. Lesions of the oculomotor nerve and pathways
   End organ: Lesions of the eye that cause dilated pupils include glaucoma, high myopia, anticholinergic drugs (e.g., atropine), and sympathomimetic drugs (such as neosynephrine).
   Peripheral portion of the oculomotor nerve: Important lesions here include aneurysms of the internal carotid artery and its branches, herniation of the brain in brain tumors, subdural hematomas and other space-occupying lesions, cavernous sinus thrombosis, sellar and suprasellar tumors, tuberculosis and syphilitic meningitis, and sphenoid ridge meningiomas. Diabetic neuropathy of the third cranial nerve does not usually cause mydriasis. Most of these lesions are associated with ptosis and paralysis of the other extraocular muscles supplied by the oculomotor nerve.
   Brainstem: Lesions here include MS, syphilis, encephalitis, Wernicke encephalopathy, brainstem gliomas, and Weber syndrome. Barbiturates and other drugs may cause dilated pupils by their central nervous system effects.
2. Optic nerve and pathways
   End organ: Keratitis, cataracts, retinitis, and occlusion of the ophthalmic artery are included here.
   Peripheral portion of the optic nerve: Aneurysms; optic neuritis; sellar and suprasellar tumors; optic nerve gliomas; primary optic atrophy from lues and other conditions; orbital fractures; exophthalmos; and cavernous sinus thrombosis are recalled in this category.
   Brainstem: The lesions involving the optic tract here are similar to those that involve the oculomotor nerve discussed above. Optic cortex (calcerine fissure) lesions may cause blindness, but there is no mydriasis.

● Approach to the Diagnosis

The clinical picture will often help to pinpoint the diagnosis. A history of drug use (narcotics, amphetamines, etc.) will suggest drug intoxication. Unilateral dilated pupil with ptosis would suggest oculomotor palsy, which may be due to a cerebral aneurysm or tumor or other space-occupying lesion. Early compression of the oculomotor nerve by a subdural hematoma or other mass may be indicated by a dilated pupil. Diabetic neuropathy may cause ptosis and

extraocular muscle palsy without a dilated pupil. Unilateral or bilateral dilated pupils with blurred vision may be due to glaucoma or iritis. Dilated pupils may also be associated with blindness (see page 167).

A dilated pupil with other neurologic findings is a clear indication for referral to a neurologist or neurosurgeon. He or she can best decide whether a CT scan or MRI is indicated.

Without focal neurologic signs the patient should have a drug screen. If that is negative, a referral to an ophthalmologist may be indicated. He or she may be able to do tonometry to rule out glaucoma and a slit lamp examination to evaluate for iritis and other conditions.

● Other Useful Tests

1. Spinal tap (MS)
2. Visual evoked potentials (MS)
3. Arteriogram (cerebral aneurysm)
4. Visual field examination (MS, glaucoma)
5. Mecholyl test (Adie pupil)

Case Presentation #16

A 26-year-old Hispanic man came to the emergency room complaining of drooping of the right eyelid and double vision. His wife had noted that his right pupil was dilated.

Question #1. Applying the method discussed above, what is your list of possibilities?

Further history reveals that he has had frequent headaches for the past week, and neurologic examination revealed nuchal rigidity in addition to the right oculomotor palsy.

Question #2. What is your diagnosis now?

(See Appendix B for the answers.)

DIZZINESS

Dizziness may mean true vertigo, which is a hallucination of movement of the patient or his environment, or lightheadedness, which is a feeling that one is going to faint (and sometimes does). The causes of lightheadedness are developed under the section on syncope (see page 418).

The diagnostic approach to dizziness or true vertigo uses **anatomy**, beginning with the external ear and working inwards toward the middle ear, labyrinth, auditory artery and nerve, and vesticular nuclei in the brainstem. Impacted wax or other foreign bodies in the **external ear** may cause vertigo. Otitis media, especially when it invades the mastoid or petrous bone, is the most important cause of vertigo in the middle ear. One should not forget serous otitis media from allergies or upper respiratory infections (URIs). If the **drum** is perforated, however, or if there is a perforation into the perilymph system, vertigo will occur, especially when water enters the ear.

TABLE 24 Dilated Pupils (Mydriasis)

	V Vascular	I Inflammatory	N Neoplasm	D Degenerative and Deficiency	I Intoxication	C Congenital	A Allergic and Autoimmune	T Trauma	E Endocrine
Oculomotor Nerve									
End organ	Aneurysm	Orbital cellulitis Tuberculosis Syphilis Cerebral abscess	Pituitary and brain tumors	Wernicke encephalopathy	Anticholinergic drug	Glaucoma	Multiple sclerosis	Trauma to the globe	Pheochromocytoma
Peripheral portion of the oculomotor nerve	Sinus thrombosis	Syphilis	Brainstem glioma		Neosynephrine	Myopia		Hematomas	Pituitary tumor (advanced)
Brainstem	Weber syndrome	Encephalitis			Barbiturate			Orbital fracture	
Optic Nerve									
End organ	Occlusion of ophthalmic artery Occlusion of internal carotid Cerebral aneurysm	Keratitis Retinitis Optic neuritis Basilar arachnoiditis	Retinoblastoma Pituitary and brain tumors	Cataract	Methyl alcohol	Cataract	Temporal arteritis	Orbital fracture	Cataract
Peripheral portion	Aneurysm	Tuberculosis	Optic nerve glioma Pituitary and brain tumors	Retinitis pigmentosa Weber optic atrophy	Tobacco		Multiple sclerosis	Hematoma	Exophthalmos
Brainstem	Sinus thrombosis	Syphilis							Cranial concussion

D

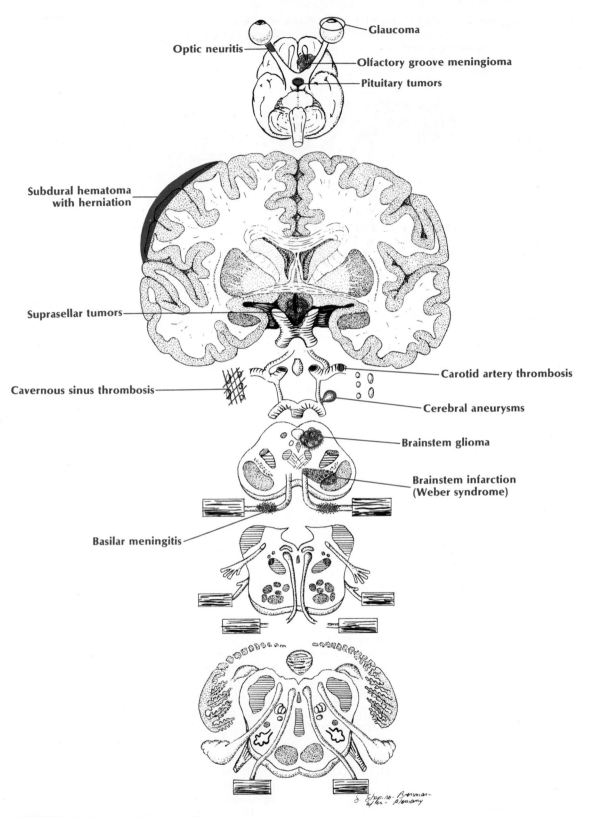

● **FIGURE 6** Dilated pupils (mydriasis).

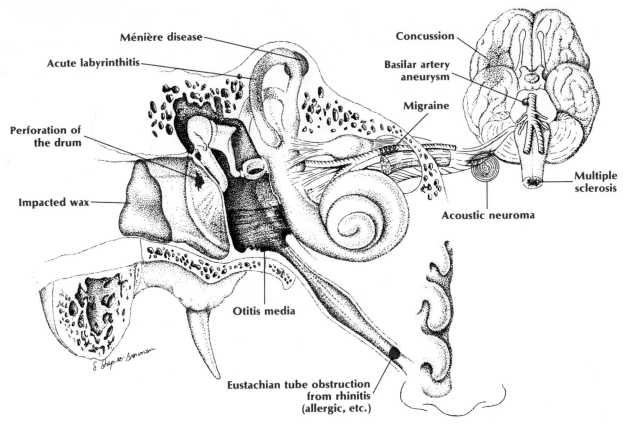

● **FIGURE 7** Dizziness.

The **inner ear** is the site of two important causes of vertigo, acute labyrinthitis and Ménière disease. Acute labyrinthitis is more often toxic than infectious (viral) in nature. Drugs such as streptomycin and gentomycin are common causes, but aspirin and quinidine should be considered with a host of other drugs. This can be determined by a good history without looking up the long list of drugs. Perhaps more common and more important from a legal standpoint is traumatic labyrinthitis from head injuries. The cause of Ménière disease is not known, but swelling of the endolymphatic ducts is probably the major pathophysiologic mechanism. If the **internal auditory artery** is obstructed by spasm (as occurs in migraine), basilar artery insufficiency, or thrombosis, vertigo will result. Rarely, an aneurysm of this artery or the basilar artery at its branching may compress or hemorrhage into the vestibular nerve and cause vertigo.

Additional neurologic causes of vertigo are acoustic neuromas and other brainstem tumors, petrositis, and vestibular neuronitis, which may involve the vestibular nerve or nucleus. Finally, central vertigo may result from MS, concussion, epilepsy, and cerebral tumors.

● **Approach to the Diagnosis**

The first step is to determine if the patient has true vertigo. True vertigo is the experience of subjective or objective rotation with respect to the environment. In other words, either the patient or his or her environment is turning. One other form of true vertigo is lateral pulsion. This is

the feeling that one is moving sideways when that is not the case.

The patient who does not experience true vertigo should have a syncope workup (see page 418). Narrowing the differential diagnosis of true vertigo depends on the presence or absence of other symptoms and signs. If there are other cranial nerve or long tract signs on neurologic examination, the patient may have a space-occupying lesion of the brain or brainstem or a hemorrhage, thrombosis, or embolism in the vertebral–basilar artery distribution. A neurology consult should be obtained.

If there is true vertigo, tinnitis, and deafness, one would consider inner ear pathology such as Ménière disease, syphilis, petrositis, mastoiditis, and acoustic neuroma. If there is vertigo without tinnitis, deafness, or focal neurologic signs, the clinician should suspect acute labyrinthitis, vestibular neuronitis, benign positional vertigo, and drug toxicity. The Dix–Hallpike maneuvers will pin down benign positional vertigo. If there are rapid respirations during the attack of vertigo, one would consider hyperventilation syndrome. If there are significant findings on otoscopic examination, a diagnosis of otitis media, cholesteatoma, or mastoiditis should be considered.

The workup will depend on whether the patient has objective findings on otoscopic or neurologic examination. If local pathology is suspected, perhaps a tympanogram, x-ray of the mastoids and petrous bones, audiogram, or referral to an otolaryngologist are required. If there are neurologic findings, perhaps a CT scan or MRI of the brain and auditory canal is indicated along with a referral to a neurologist. It is wise to have a specialist on board before ordering an expensive workup.

● Other Useful Tests

1. Thyroid profile (vertigo from thyroid disease)
2. Electronystagmogram (Ménière disease)
3. Brainstem evoked potentials (MS)
4. Caloric testing (Ménière disease)
5. Drug screen (drug abuse)
6. Hallpike maneuvers (benign positional vertigo)
7. VDRL or fluorescent treponemal antibody absorption (FTA-ABS) test (neurosyphilis)

Case Presentation #17

A 36-year-old black woman presents with acute dizziness, which she describes as a sensation of turning in relation to her environment.

Question #1. Given the methods provided above, what would be your list of possible causes?

Further history reveals that she has not been on any medication recently and denies fever or a recent URI. There is, however, a history of similar attacks in the past associated with numbness of the left side of the face and weakness of the extremities.

Question #2. What is your list of possibilities now?

(See Appendix B for the answers.)

DOUBLE VISION

Most physicians know that double vision is a neurologic condition and may refer these cases immediately to a neurologist, but what about the cases of double vision with one eye closed? Surprisingly enough, this condition really does exist. Monocular diplopia results from dislocation of the lens (e.g., from injury and Marfan syndrome), the incipient stage of cataracts, corneal opacities, double pupils (from surgery or trauma), or hysteria. Fortunately for us but unfortunately for the patient, double vision is usually binocular and due to paralysis of the extraocular muscles. The causes can be recalled best by anatomically grouping them into those that involve the muscles themselves, those that involve the myoneural junction, those that involve the peripheral portion of the cranial nerve, and those that involve the nucleus of the cranial nerve in the brainstem and supranuclear causes.

1. **Extraocular muscle:** Using the mnemonic **MINT** the following differential can be developed.
   M—**Malformations** such as myotonic dystrophy and congenital opthalmoplegia belong here.
   I—**Inflammatory** conditions such as dermatomyositis and orbital cellulitis are considered here.
   N—**Neoplasms** of the orbit and exophthalmic goiter are classified here.

   T—**Trauma** suggests orbital fractures and contusions or lacerations of the muscles.
2. **Myoneural junction:** This suggests the important condition of myasthenia gravis.
3. **Peripheral portion of the cranial nerve:** Recall of these conditions is assisted by the mnemonic **VINCE.**
   V—**Venous** sinus thrombosis (cavernous sinus in this case) is suggested.
   I—**Inflammatory** conditions remind one of syphilis and tuberculous meningitis, postdiphtheritic neuritis, sphenoid sinusitis, petrositis, and increased intracranial pressure.
   N—**Neoplasms** suggest pituitary tumors, suprasellar tumors, nasopharyngeal carcinomas, chordomas, and sphenoid ridge meningiomas.
   C—**Congenital** lesions suggest aneurysms.
   E—**Endocrine** disorders suggest diabetic neuropathy, a common cause of sudden extraocular muscle palsy.
4. **Brainstem:** Recall of these conditions is best undertaken with the mnemonic **VINDICATE.**
   V—**Vascular** lesions include basilar artery thrombosis, hemorrhages, emboli, and aneurysms. Migraine may belong here, too.
   I—**Inflammatory** lesions include syphilis, tuberculosis, and viral encephalitis.
   N—**Neoplasms** include brainstem gliomas, metastatic carcinomas, and Hodgkin lymphoma.
   D—**Deficiency** diseases suggest Wernicke encephalopathy.
   I—**Intoxication** suggests botulism, bromide, and iodide poisoning.
   C—**Congenital** conditions suggest hydrocephalus and Arnold–Chiari malformation.
   A—**Autoimmune** disease suggests MS, postinfectious encephalitis, and lupus.
   T—**Traumatic** conditions suggest subdural hematomas, basilar skull fractures, and pontine hematomas.
   E—**Endocrine** reminds one of the increased incidence of basilar artery thrombosis in diabetes.
5. **Supranuclear causes (including cortical):** These recall a pineal tumor, the conjugate palsy of cerebral thrombosis or hemorrhage, the conjugate gaze in focal cortical epilepsy, and the dilated pupil in early herniation through the tentorium.

● Approach to the Diagnosis

This is similar to that for all neurologic disorders and depends on the association of other signs. Isolated palsies of the third (oculomotor) or sixth (abducens) nerve without pupillary changes suggest diabetic neuropathy, so a glucose tolerance test would be done. A thyroid profile is useful to rule out hyperthyroidism. An isolated palsy of the third nerve with pupillary changes (mydriasis) suggests an aneurysm and angiography is indicated. X-rays of the skull and orbits, a spinal tap, and CT scans would all be useful under certain circumstances, but a neurologist is in a better position to determine this. A cavernous sinus thrombosis is possible if the patient is febrile and has more than one cranial nerve palsy along with loss of the corneal

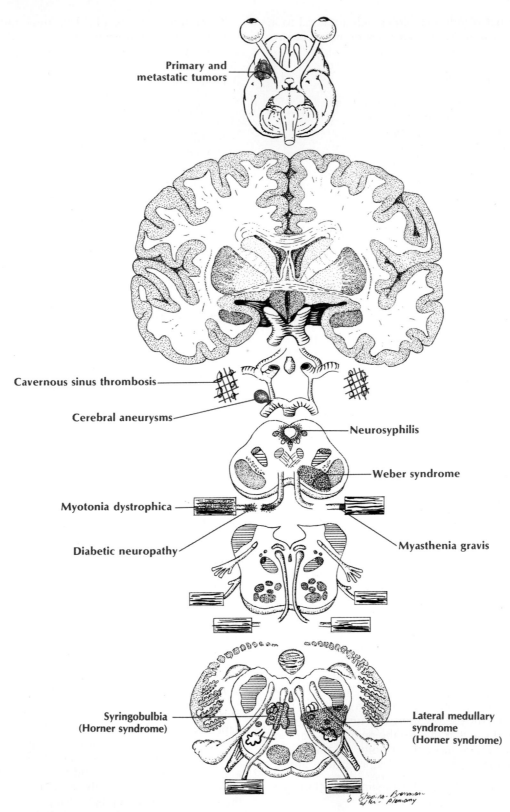

● **FIGURE 8** Double vision.

reflex, chemosis, ecchymosis, and distended retinal veins. Treatment should be started immediately.

● Other Useful Tests

1. VDRL or FTA-ABS test (neurosyphilis)
2. Sedimentation rate (cerebral abscess)
3. Tensilon test (myasthenia gravis)
4. Acetylcholine receptor antibody titer (myasthenia gravis)
5. X-ray of the skull and orbits (orbital abscess or tumor, brain tumors)
6. X-ray of the sinuses (trauma, sinusitis)
7. Visual field examination (MS)
8. Serum growth hormone, corticotropin, LH, and FSH levels (pituitary tumor)
9. CT scan of the brain and sinuses (brain tumor, abscess)
10. MRI of the brain (space-occupying lesion, MS)

Case Presentation #18

A 66-year-old white preacher complained of intermittent double vision for the past 6 months.

Question #1. Based on a review of the methods outlined above, what are your possible diagnoses at this point?

There is no history of headache, alcohol or drug use, or any other neurologic symptomatology. Neurologic examination revealed a left external rectus palsy and bilateral partial ptosis.

Question #2. What is your diagnosis at this point?

(See Appendix B for the answers.)

DROP ATTACKS

In drop attacks, the patient, usually elderly, experiences the sudden giving away of his or her legs and falls to the floor without loss of consciousness. The fact that the patient remains conscious distinguishes drop attacks from syncope or the vasovagal attack and epilepsy. Nevertheless, these attacks result from a temporary decrease in blood supply to centers in the brainstem responsible for muscle tone. Consequently, we can develop a differential diagnosis by following the arterial tree from the heart to the brainstem.

Heart: A coronary thrombosis and cardiac arrhythmias may cause drop attacks.
Aorta: Aortic stenosis and insufficiency may be the cause of recurring drop attacks.
Arteries: Focusing on the arteries in general we can recall orthostatic hypotension either related to drugs, anemia, or idiopathic type.
Vertebral–basilar arteries: Atherosclerotic narrowing of these arteries leads to transient cerebral ischemia and drop attacks.

This leaves a few conditions that may simulate drop attacks in elderly persons such as weak quadriceps muscles,

poor vision, postural instability from posterior column degeneration, and tripping over unseen objects.

● Approach to the Diagnosis

Basic workup includes a CBC, chemistry panel, urinalysis, carotid Doppler study, and electrocardiogram (ECG). The clinical picture and neurologic or cardiology consult will help determine if Holter monitoring or four-vessel cerebral angiography should be done.

● Other Useful Tests

1. ECG (cardiac arrhythmia)
2. MRI of the brain (basilar artery insufficiency)
3. Magnetic resonance angiography (orthostatic hypotension)
4. 24-hour blood pressure monitoring (hypotension)
5. 5-hour glucose tolerance test (hypoglycemia)

DWARFISM

A list of possible causes of dwarfism may be developed anatomically, physiologically, and biochemically. Visualizing the many organs of the body is an excellent way to recall the causes. Beginning with the **pituitary** one thinks of hypopituitarism and Lawrence–Moon–Biedl syndrome. The **thyroid** suggests cretinism. The **heart** suggests the many congenital anomalies there (e.g., tetralogy of Fallot) that are associated with dwarfism. The **GI tract** suggests the malabsorption syndrome and its many causes. The **pancreas** suggests cystic fibrosis. The **kidney** suggests chronic nephritis with renal rickets. The **bone** suggests rickets and achondroplasia. The **brain** suggests microcephaly and all the other causes of mental retardation (such as Down syndrome) that are associated with stunted growth. The **ovary** suggests Turner syndrome. (This method will not help recall the primordial dwarf and some of the other genetic dwarfs but it is a good start.)

Applying physiology and biochemistry, one must consider the intake of food and oxygen, its absorption and transport, and its uptake by the cells and excretion of waste products. For the regulation and promotion of this metabolic process, adequate vitamins and hormones are essential. With these processes in mind, one can recall the diseases that interfere with each.

Intake: Starvation and malnutrition cause dwarfism and various vitamin deficiency states, rickets being the most significant.
Absorption: Malabsorption syndromes may create dwarfism by preventing food and vitamins from getting into the body.
Transport: Congenital anomalies of the heart prevent distribution of oxygen and glucose to the cells.
Cell uptake: Impaired cell uptake of glucose in diabetes may cause a short stature; the bulging of the cells with glycogen in glycogen storage disease may do the same. Galactosemia is a possible cause. Reticuloendotheliosis and gargoylism may be recalled under this heading.

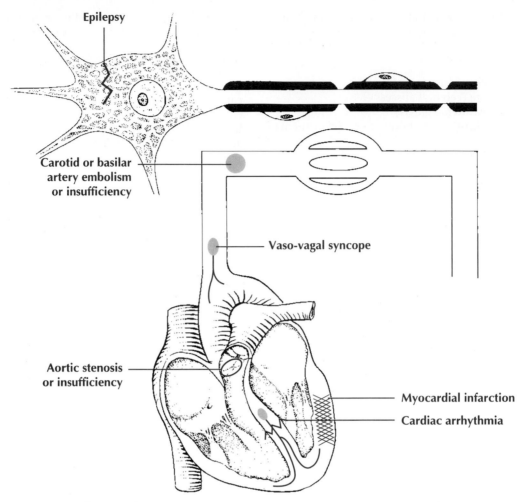

● **FIGURE 9** Drop attacks.

Excretion of waste products: This heading should help recall renal rickets.

Regulation: This heading helps recall the hormonal deficiency states: cretinism (deficiency of thyroxine), Turner syndrome (deficiencies of estrogen and progesterone), and hypopituitarism (deficiency of growth hormone). Poor function of all of the above would suggest progeria. The adrenal carcinomas may cause precocious puberty and premature closure of the epiphysis. The above method fails to include most of the genetic causes of dwarfism, so perhaps this group can be remembered by its exclusion.

● **Approach to the Diagnosis**

The workup of dwarfism should probably be done by an endocrinologist. Many of the causes are genetic and untreatable, but it would be a shame to miss cretinism, hypopituitarism, or Turner syndrome. Hypothyroidism can be distinguished by a delayed bone age. All of these have associated findings that should help to differentiate them, but hypopituitarism may be very subtle. Cystic fibrosis can be diagnosed by a sweat test. Down syndrome, Turner syndrome, and certain other genetic causes can be determined by a chromosomal analysis.

DYSARTHRIA AND SPEECH DISORDERS

Besides dysarthria, three other types of speech disorders should be considered here: dysphasia, cerebellar speech, and extrapyramidal speech. In each case, the anatomic location in the nervous system is fairly specific.

Dysarthria: This may be due to a lesion at the end organ (muscles of the mouth and tongue), the myoneural junction, the peripheral branches of the 5th (trigeminal) and 12th (hypoglossal) cranial nerves, the brainstem, or the cerebrum.

1. **End organ:** Hypertrophy of the tongue from myxedema, carcinoma of the tongue, and painful lesions of the mouth and tongue may cause speech difficulty. Inability to swallow may leave saliva and food in the mouth and interfere with speech. The facioscapulohumeral form of muscular dystrophy may cause dysarthria.
2. **Myoneural junction:** Myasthenia gravis, a treatable form of dysarthria, should always be ruled out.
3. **Peripheral nerve:** Hypoglossal nerve damage from trauma and severing of the motor portion of the trigeminal nerve in trauma and surgery are the principal lesions here.

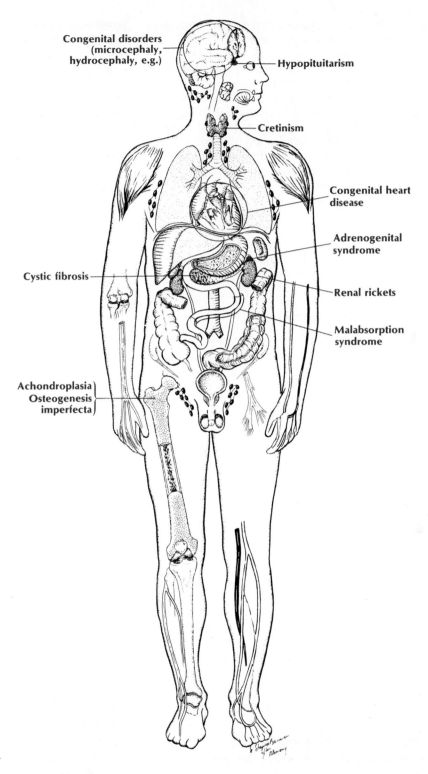

● **FIGURE 10** Dwarfism.

4. **Brainstem:** Poliomyelitis, Guillain–Barré syndrome, disseminated encephalomyelitis, brainstem gliomas, and basilar artery occlusions are the most important lesions to recall in this category.

5. **Cerebrum:** Any disorder that may cause hemiplegia from cerebral involvement may cause dysarthria and pseudobulbar palsy. Cerebral thrombi, emboli, or hemorrhages are perhaps the most significant of these.

Frontal lobe tumors or abscesses may be the cause here. Diffuse cerebral diseases such as alcoholism, Huntington chorea, and general paresis may cause dysarthria, but they are more likely to cause other speech disorders.

Cerebellar speech: This may be scanning or staccato (clipped). MS is often the first condition to consider, but the hereditary cerebellar ataxias (e.g., Marie ataxia), alcoholic cerebellar atrophy, syphilis, and cerebellar tumors may also be the cause.

Dysphasia: In this condition, words cannot be pronounced properly (motor dysphasia), there is difficulty naming objects (nominal aphasia), or the words cannot be placed properly in a sentence (syntactic aphasia). In determining the etiology, it is not important to know the exact location of the lesion in the cerebrum because any disease of the cerebrum may cause aphasia or dysphasia. Cerebral hemorrhages, thrombi, emboli, and tumors or other space-occupying lesions are the most important ones to remember. The others are listed on page 362 (memory loss).

Extrapyramidal speech: This is the monotone, rapid, dysarthric speech of paralysis agitans, but it may be found in cerebral palsy, Wilson disease, or Huntington chorea. The last two conditions may also have a jerky speech or dysarthria.

● Approach to the Diagnosis

Dysarthria without other symptoms or signs requires that myasthenia gravis be ruled out with a Tensilon test and psychometrics be done to rule out hysteria. In the presence of other neurologic signs, speech disorders require a thorough neurologic workup with an EEG, skull x-ray, and CT scan or MRI of the brain; a spinal tap or arteriogram may be indicated. The clinician should remember that dysarthria may be only the first sign of a serious neurologic disease such as MS, Wilson disease, lupus erythematosus, or chronic alcoholism; therefore, close follow-up is important.

● Other Useful Tests

1. Neurology consult
2. VDRL test (neurosyphilis)
3. Acetylcholine receptor antibody titer (myasthenia gravis)
4. Brainstem evoked potentials (MS)
5. Carotid scans (carotid insufficiency or thrombosis)
6. Serum copper and ceruloplasmin (Wilson disease)
7. Spinal tap (MS, neurosyphilis)
8. EEG (intermittent dysarthria, epilepsy)
9. Four-vessel cerebral angiography (cerebrovascular disease)
10. Drug screen (drug abuse)

DYSMENORRHEA (*SEE ALSO PREMENSTRUAL SYNDROME*)

Visualizing the parts of the female reproductive system (see figure), one can systematically formulate a differential diagnosis of this common malady. At the **cervix**, stenosis, cervical polyps, and other neoplasms may obstruct the egress of blood and induce dysmenorrhea. In the **uterus**, polyps, fibroids, adenomyosis, and deformities such as anteflexion, retroflexion, anteversion, or retroversion may be the cause. Pelvic congestion syndrome is a

possibility. Does the patient have an intrauterine device (IUD)? This may be the cause. The **tubes** may be involved by endometriosis, abscess, or ectopic pregnancy. The **ovaries** may be involved by the same processes as the tubes, but they should suggest the most common cause of dysmenorrhea: hormonal. Thus, any condition—thyroid, pituitary, or ovarian—that might disturb the cyclic output of estrogen and progesterone in the proper sequence may induce dysmenorrhea. Psychogenic disturbances are especially significant.

● Approach to the Diagnosis

The clinical approach to dysmenorrhea is simply to rule out significant organic disease by a thorough pelvic and rectal examination. If this can not be done (obesity, etc.), ultrasonography should be done. A smear and culture for gonococcus and *Chlamydia* should be done. If there is a negative examination and the pain is consistently relieved by nonsteroidal anti-inflammatory drugs (NSAIDs), nothing else needs be done. A course of contraceptives or progesterone in adequate doses may then be tried. Diuretics may be indicated if examination suggests pelvic congestion. Removal of an IUD may relieve the pain. When the aforementioned measures fail, a dilatation and curettage (D & C) may be indicated. A gynecologist may decide to do a culdoscopy, a peritoneoscopy, or an exploratory laparotomy.

● Other Useful Tests

1. Sonogram (pelvic inflammatory disease [PID], ectopic pregnancy)
2. Pregnancy test
3. Fern test and basal body temperature charting (endometriosis)
4. Gynecology consult
5. Psychiatric consult
6. Transvaginal ultrasonography

DYSPAREUNIA

Painful introduction of the male organ or pain during intercourse are both considered under this title. The mnemonic to use here is **MINT**. This can then be applied to the anatomic structures as we explore the genital tract. Of course, psychologic disturbances are probably the most common causes of this disorder. They are discussed after the anatomic causes.

M—Malformations include a disproportionately large or deformed male organ (not amusing to the man in this predicament), an unruptured or thick hymen, vaginal stenosis, a retroverted uterus, and prolapsed ovaries.

I—Inflammatory disorders include vulvitis and bartholinitis (often related to gonorrhea), various forms of vaginitis (bacterial, trichomoniasis, and moniliasis), and salpingo-oophoritis. (Note that an inflamed uterus and cervix are only infrequently associated with

D

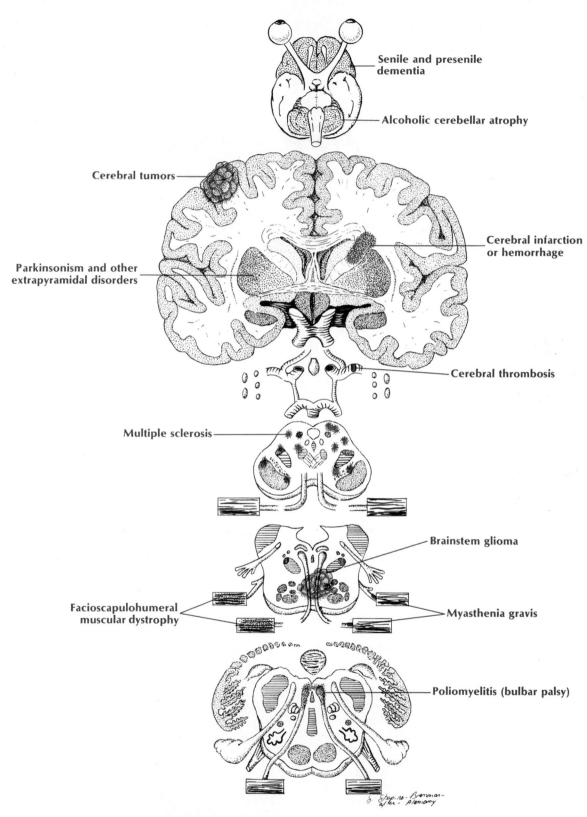

● **FIGURE 11** Dysarthria and speech disorders.

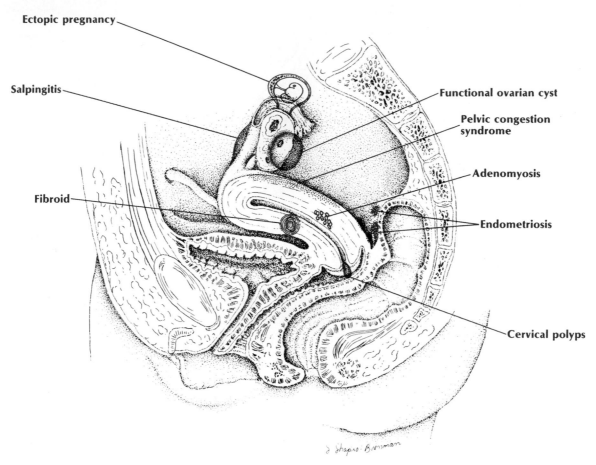

Ectopic pregnancy

Salpingitis

Fibroid

Functional ovarian cyst

Pelvic congestion syndrome

Adenomyosis

Endometriosis

Cervical polyps

● **FIGURE 12** Dysmenorrhea.

dyspareunia.) Inflammatory lesions of nearby structures are important. Thus, a urethral carbuncle, urethritis, cystitis, hemorrhoids, and anal fissures can cause dyspareunia.

N—**Neoplasms** causing dyspareunia are leukoplakia vulvitis, kraurosis vulvae, carcinoma of the vulva and vagina, ovarian cysts, and carcinoma. When uterine and cervical carcinomas extend beyond the genital tract, dyspareunia is present. Any neoplasm of the bladder and rectum that has extended into the genital tract will undoubtedly cause dyspareunia.

T—**Traumatic** disorders include too-frequent intercourse and masturbation. Introduction of the male organ before adequate foreplay has created a lubricated vagina is another cause. The male patient should be instructed in the gentle introduction of the organ.

Women in menopause may require lubricants to prevent local trauma, because the vagina remains dry even after sexual excitement because of lack of hormonal secretion.

Discovery of psychogenic causes often requires thorough psychoanalysis. A careful evaluation for sexual abuse must be done. Incest, guilt from masturbation, and latent homosexuality are a few of the problems that may be encountered.

● Approach to the Diagnosis

The approach to this diagnosis includes an examination of both male and female genital organs and counseling by an understanding physician if these examinations are negative.

● Other Useful Tests

1. Pregnancy test
2. Vaginal smear and culture
3. Urinalysis and culture
4. Sonogram (ectopic pregnancy, ovarian cyst, tubo-ovarian abscess)
5. Laparoscopy
6. Gynecology consult
7. Psychiatric consult

DYSPNEA, TACHYPNEA, AND ORTHOPNEA

Dyspnea is the subjective feeling of rapid or difficult breathing. The patient will often say: "I can't get my breath!" **Tachypnea** is the objective finding of a rapid respiratory rate, and may or may not be associated with

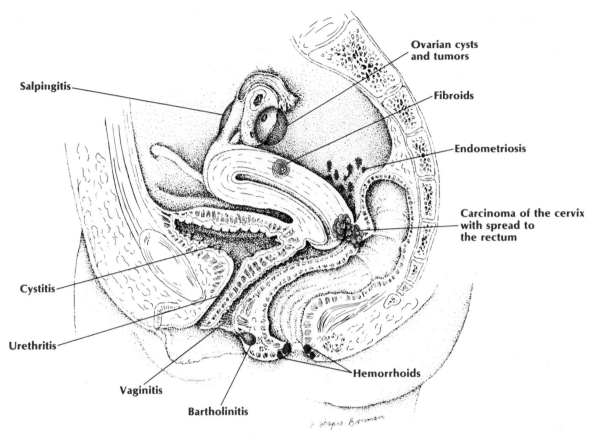

● **FIGURE 13** Dyspareunia.

the feeling of not being able to breathe properly. One is a symptom and the other is a sign, but the mechanisms for producing them are the same: inadequate oxygen for body needs or inability to excrete CO_2. A few other mechanisms that produce hyperventilation and tachypnea will be discussed later on in this chapter. The best basic science for developing a list of the causes of dyspnea and tachypnea is **pathophysiology**. Difficulty breathing or rapid breathing will develop when there is decreased intake of oxygen, impaired absorption of oxygen, inadequate perfusion of the lungs with blood, inability of the body to transport enough oxygen to the tissues, increased demand of the tissues for oxygen, and inability of the body to excrete CO_2 and other waste products of body metabolism. These are tabulated in Table 25.

Disorders of oxygen intake: In this category are the conditions that may block the respiratory passages such as laryngitis, foreign bodies, an aortic aneurysm or mediastinal tumor pressing on the trachea or bronchi, bronchial asthma, acute infectious bronchitis, and pulmonary emphysema. Also considered in this category are conditions that interfere with the "respiratory pump" (thoracic cage, thoracic and diaphragmatic muscles, and respiratory centers in the brain) such as kyphoscoliosis, Pickwickian syndrome, myasthenia gravis, Muscular dystrophy and other neuromuscular diseases, peritonitis, encephalitis, and brain tumors.

Disorders of oxygen absorption: Lobar pneumonia, sarcoidosis, silicosis, Berylliosis, and various causes of pulmonary fibrosis, and pulmonary edema are considered here. Oxygen diffusion across the alveolocapillary membrane is affected in all of these. Alveolar proteinosis, shock lung, and the adult respiratory distress syndrome must also be considered here.

Disorders of perfusion of the pulmonary capillaries: Pulmonary emboli, hemangiomas of the lungs, and congenital heart increases such as tetralogy of Fallot belong in this category. In all of these conditions unoxygenated blood bypasses the alveoli. Also included in this category are diseases with a ventilation–perfusion defect. In other words, some alveoli are being ventilated but not perfused with blood, while at the same time some alveoli are being perfused but not ventilated. Pulmonary emphysema and the various conditions associated with pulmonary fibrosis (e.g., pneumoconiosis) cause dyspnea on this basis, as well as other physiologic reasons mentioned above.

Disorders of oxygen transport: The tissues will not get oxygen if there is not enough blood to transport it, as in anemia and hemorrhagic shock; if there is not enough blood pressure to perfuse the tissues, as in vasomotor and cardiogenic shock; or if the heart pump fails, as in CHF from many causes. In methemoglobinemia and sulfhemoglobinemia, there may be enough blood, but it is unable to carry the oxygen.

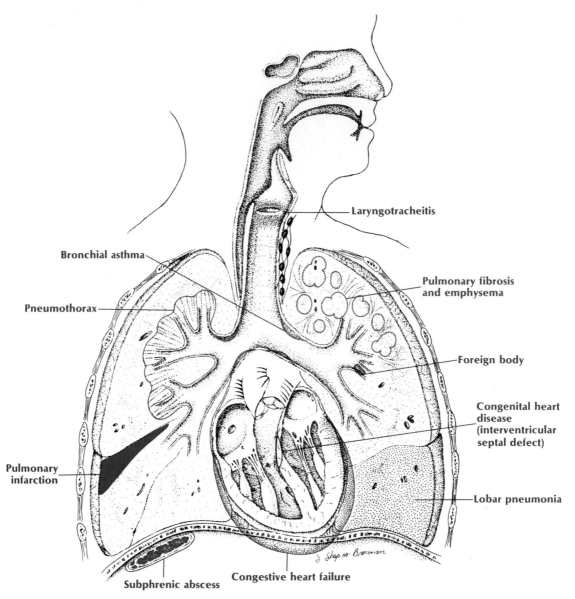

● FIGURE 14 Dyspnea and tachypnea.

Increased tissue oxygen demand: During exercise and nervous stress, and in febrile states, leukemia and other malignancies, and hyperthyroidism there is an increase in tissue metabolism; consequently, tachypnea may develop to increase the supply.

Inadequate excretion of CO_2 and other wastes of tissue metabolism: Inability to excrete CO_2 may occur without anoxia in pulmonary emphysema and other chronic obstructive lung diseases and initiate dyspnea, especially on exertion. Other wastes of tissue metabolism may cause an acidosis and stimulate the respiratory centers in this fashion. Lactic acidosis, diabetic acidosis, and uremia may cause dyspnea on this basis.

From the above discussion, it should be evident that the clinician can develop an excellent list of the causes of dyspnea and tachypnea with an understanding of the pathophysiology involved. A few conditions cannot be recalled with this method: hyperventilation syndrome, ingestion of acids (e.g., methyl alcohol poisoning) and drugs that stimulate the respiratory centers (such as amphetamines), and atmospheric reduction in oxygen tension.

● Approach to the Diagnosis

The history and physical examination will almost invariably disclose the cause of dyspnea. If acute respiratory distress syndrome (ARDS) is suspected, look for sepsis from an abdominal source and drug abuse. To confirm pulmonary disease one will order pulmonary function studies, a chest roentgenogram, and arterial blood gases. If routine pulmonary function studies are normal, more sophisticated studies such as the nitrogen washout test and perfusion and ventilatory scans may be necessary. To diagnose cardiac conditions, ordering an ECG and echocardiography are most useful.

TABLE 25 Dyspnea, Tachypnea, and Orthopnea

	V Vascular	I Inflammatory	N Neoplasm	D Degenerative	I Intoxication	C Congenital	A Allergic and Autoimmune	T Trauma	E Endocrine
Disorders of Oxygen Intake		Laryngitis Bronchitis	Bronchogenic carcinoma	Pulmonary emphysema	Pneumoconiosis Silo filler's disease	Muscular dystrophy Kyphoscoliosis Bronchiectasis	Bronchial asthma	Foreign body injury to ribs	
Disorders of Oxygen Absorption	Pulmonary edema	Pneumonia Tuberculosis Lung abscess	Alveolar carcinoma Metastatic carcinoma	Pulmonary emphysema and fibrosis	Lipoid pneumonia Toxic pneumonitis Shock lung	Atelectasis	Periarteritis nodosa Wegener granuloma Sarcoidosis Scleroderma	Pneumothorax	
Disorders of Perfusion	Pulmonary embolism		Hemangioma	Pulmonary fibrosis Pulmonary emphysema		Congenital heart disease			
Disorders of Transport	Congestive heart failure	Septicemia with shock		Aplastic anemia	Methemoglobinemia Shock from drugs and toxins	Sickle cell anemia Congenital heart disease	Shock	Hemorrhagic shock	Waterhouse–Friderichsen syndrome
Disorders of Increased Oxygen Demands	Polycythemia	Fever	Leukemia Hodgkin lymphoma Metastatic carcinoma						Hyperthyroidism
Disorders of Excretion of Carbon Dioxide and Other Wastes of Body Metabolism		Septicemia with lactic acidosis	Pulmonary emphysema		Uremia Lactic acidosis				Diabetic acidosis

Any patient with dyspnea and normal physical findings deserves a circulation time to rule out early CHF. A hemogram will diagnose anemias but it will not diagnose methemoglobinemia. A determination of the erythrocytes methemoglobin, arterial oxygen saturation, and diaphorase I test must be done.

● Other Useful Tests

1. CBC (anemia, polycythemia)
2. Sedimentation rate (pneumonia, subacute bacterial endocarditis [SBE])
3. Serial cardiac enzymes (acute myocardial infarction)
4. Sputum smear and culture (pneumonia)
5. Lung scan (pulmonary embolism)
6. Sputum for eosinophils (asthma)
7. Toxicology screen (drug abuse)
8. Echocardiogram (CHF, valvular heart disease)
9. Pulmonary angiogram (pulmonary embolism)
10. Trial of diuretics (CHF)
11. Forced vital capacity (FVC) with methacholine challenge (asthma)
12. B-type natriuretic peptide (BNP) assay (CHF)
13. Cardiac catheterization (CHF)
14. Spiral CT scan (pulmonary embolism)
15. Spirometry before and after bronchodilators (asthma)

Case Presentation #19

A 55-year-old white male electrician calls you asking if you would order an antibiotic for a cough he has had for 10 days. Over the phone you can tell he is short of breath. He denies chest pain or fever.

Question #1. Utilizing the methods discussed above, what are the possible causes of the cough and shortness of breath at this point?

You are concerned and decide to make a house call. On examination, you find that the patient is expectorating frothy, slightly blood-tinged sputum, has crepitant rales at both lung bases, cardiomegaly, and a rapid irregular heart rhythm with a pulse deficit.

Question #2. What is your diagnosis or diagnoses at this point?

(See Appendix B for the answers.)

DYSTOCIA

Both **physiology** and **anatomy** must be applied to develop the differential diagnosis of dystocia. An abnormally long

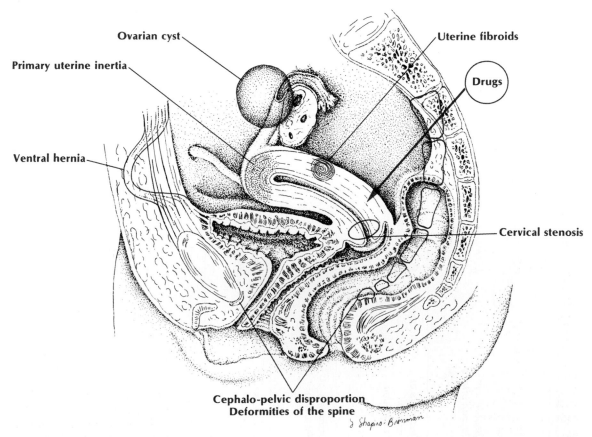

● **FIGURE 15** Dystocia.

D

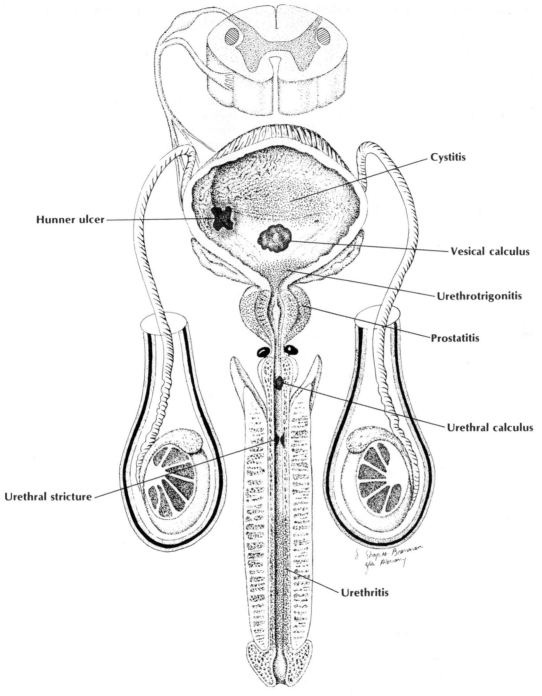

Cystitis

Hunner ulcer

Vesical calculus

Urethrotrigonitis

Prostatitis

Urethral calculus

Urethral stricture

Urethritis

● **FIGURE 16** Dysuria.

labor may result from inadequate abdominal muscle or uterine muscle contractions, obstruction of the birth canal, abnormalities of the fetus or placenta, and unusual positions of the fetus in the abdomen and pelvis.

1. **Inadequate abdominal muscle contractions:** This may be due to diastasis recti, ventral hernias, and obesity.
2. **Inadequate uterine muscle contractions:** This may result from malformations of the uterus, such as bicornuate uterus; multiple fibroids and other neoplasms of the uterus; drugs that inhibit uterine contractions, such

as morphine and other sedatives; and primary uterine inertia.
3. **Obstruction of the birth canal:** Look for ovarian cysts, uterine fibroids, cervical stenosis, deformities of the pelvis, impacted feces, and an enlarged bladder in this category.
4. **Abnormalities of the fetus:** This category includes large babies, polyhydramnios due to diabetes mellitus, hydrocephalus, abdominal neoplasms or ascites in the fetus, and twins or additional multiple births.

5. **Abnormal position of the fetus:** Breech presentation, transverse lie, face or brow presentation, and occipitoposterior presentations are included in this category.

● Approach to the Diagnosis

Thorough examinations, sonograms, x-rays of the abdomen for fetal size and position, and amniocentesis are all useful procedures to assist in the diagnosis.

DYSURIA

Dysuria is difficult or painful micturition. One could cover most of the causes simply by considering the **inflammatory** lesions of the genitourinary tract in ascending order. Thus, there may be urethritis or urethral carbuncle, trigonitis or prostatitis, cystitis, or pyelonephritis with associated cystitis. This would not, however, cover the disorders that frequently cause associated inflammation of the urinary tract or are associated with difficulty in voiding. To recall these, it is necessary to apply the mnemonic **MINT**.

M—Malformations would bring to mind meatal stricture, bladder neck obstruction by prostatic hypertrophy, median bar, and urethral strictures. Bladder and ureteral calculi should also be considered here.

I—Inflammatory conditions have already been considered. Intoxication should bring to mind drugs such as NSAIDs and cyclophosphamide, which causes cystitis.

N—Neoplasms of the prostate and bladder may cause difficulty in voiding or painful urination when secondary infection sets in. The **N** may also stand for neurologic conditions; one must not forget multiple sclerosis, poliomyelitis, diabetic neuropathy, and tumors of the spinal cord in the differential diagnosis of dysuria. These are also discussed in the section on incontinence on page 269.

T—Trauma suggests cystitis and trigonitis (honeymoon cystitis) caused by frequent or traumatic intercourse or by introduction of foreign bodies into the bladder, such as catheters.

● Approach to the Diagnosis

The approach to the diagnosis includes a urinalysis, urine cultures, smear and culture of any discharge, an IVP, voiding cystogram and cystoscopy, and cystometric examination. In women with "negative" cultures, *Chlamydia* urethritis must be considered and treated. In men with negative cultures, prostatic examination, massage, and evaluation of discharge are done. DNA probe testing of the urine is useful in detecting gonorrhea or Chlamydia and obviates the need for cultures. Massage of the prostate should be avoided in acute prostatitis. A 4-week trial of ciprofloxacin may help diagnose chronic prostatitis.

● Other Useful Tests

1. Cultures for gonorrhea and *Chlamydia*
2. Anaerobic cultures
3. Cultures for acid-fast bacilli
4. Urology consult
5. Gynecology consult
6. Four cup test (proatatitis)

Case Presentation #20

A 21-year-old male medical student presented to the student health service with fever and burning pain on urination.

Question #1. Applying the above methods, what would be your list of possible causes for this young man's problem?

History reveals that he was treated with penicillin 2 months ago for a urethral discharge that developed after a casual sexual encounter.

Question #2. What is your list of possibilities now?

_____

(See Appendix B for the answers.)

E

EARACHE

The analysis of earache is much like that of dysuria: It is **anatomic**, and **inflammation** accounts for the vast majority of causes. Thus, otitis externa would be like urethritis and otitis media like cystitis, and so forth.

Like cystitis, otitis media is often initiated by obstruction (e.g., swollen adenoids). Foreign bodies in the ear, like foreign bodies in the bladder, must always be looked for. Unlike dysuria, earache is often caused by referred pain. Thus, parotitis (e.g., mumps), temporomandibular joint (TMJ) syndrome, pharyngitis, and dental caries or abscesses may cause earache.

● Approach to the Diagnosis

The approach to the diagnosis requires ear, nose, and throat examination; culture of any discharge; and x-ray film of the mastoids, petrous bone, TMJs; and, in some cases, the sinuses and teeth. A careful neurologic examination is necessary in unexplained otalgia. Referral to an otolaryngologist or neurologist is probably best for the busy physician who is unable to find the cause on a routine examination.

● Other Useful Tests

1. Computed tomography (CT) scan of the mastoids (mastoiditis)
2. Magnetic resonance imaging (MRI) of the TMJs (TMJ syndrome)
3. Throat culture (streptococcal pharyngitis)
4. X-ray of the teeth (dental abscess)
5. Impedance tympanogram (otitis media)
6. Audiogram (otitis media)

EDEMA OF THE EXTREMITIES

Edema of the extremities is a common symptom. Most physicians, therefore, have an immediate working diagnosis when the patient walks into the office: Congestive heart failure (CHF) if the edema is bilateral and deep vein phlebitis if it is unilateral. Many times this is right. However, what if the heart and chest sound normal and there is a negative Homans sign? Obviously, before the physician questions the patient the clinician needs a more complete list of diagnostic possibilities. **Physiology** is the key to that list.

Fluid is passing from the blood compartment into the subcutaneous tissues and back again all the time. Why does it stay in the subcutaneous tissues? There are four main physiologic reasons and three minor ones.

1. **The pressure in the veins** may be so high that it overcomes the oncotic pressure of the albumin and other proteins in the blood. This is the explanation in phlebitis, venous thrombosis, pelvic tumors, centripetal obesity, and right-sided CHF (partially).
2. **The pressure in the arteries** may be so high that more fluid is pushed out than can be reabsorbed with normal oncotic pressure. This may be the case in acute glomerulonephritis and malignant hypertension.
3. **The level of serum albumin** may be so low that the oncotic pressure drops to a point where it cannot reabsorb all the fluid being driven out by the forward pressure of the arteries or backward pressure of the veins. This is seen in conditions in which either too little albumin is produced (cirrhosis of the liver) or too much albumin is lost in the urine (nephrotic syndrome of diabetes mellitus, lupus erythematosus, amyloidosis, and several other disorders of the kidney). It is also probably a component of the edema in beriberi and CHF.
4. **The lymphatic channels** that pick up any excess fluid that the veins cannot pick up may be blocked. This occurs notably in filariasis, Milroy disease, and lymphedema following mastectomy, but other conditions may also block the lymphatics.
5. **An abnormal protein** (mucoprotein) may be deposited in the tissues and lead to edema. This results in the nonpitting edema of hypothyroidism (myxedema).
6. **A reduction in tissue turgor pressure** may be responsible for the edema in older people and beriberi (vitamin B_1 deficiency).
7. **Retention of salt** as in primary and secondary aldosteronism is a minor factor, because most cases of aldosterone-secreting adenomas do not have significant edema.

It would be a serious omission not to mention local conditions such as cellulitis, ruptured Baker cysts, burns (especially sunburn), contusions, and urticaria that may cause edema, but these are usually obvious.

Edema is classified according to the anatomic site of origin and the mechanisms that are responsible in Table 26.

● Approach to the Diagnosis

Bilateral pitting edema of the lower extremities is usually due to CHF, nephrosis, or cirrhosis of the liver. Venous pressure and circulation time and serum BNP will rule out CHF, but echocardiography can be more definitive. Serum and urine osmolality can be helpful also. If there is nephrosis, there will be significant lowering

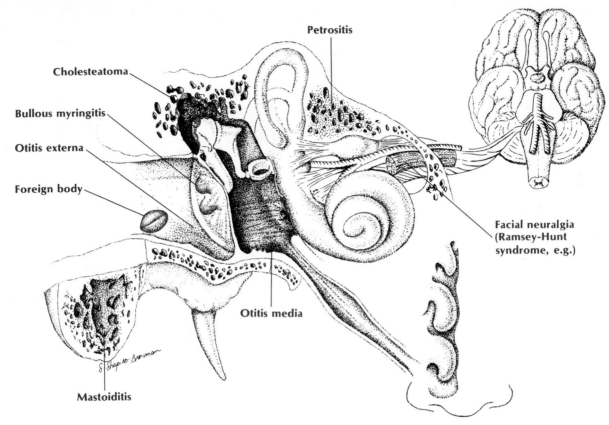

● **FIGURE 1** Earache.

of the serum albumin level and proteinuria. Liver function studies will usually confirm cirrhosis or liver disease, but ultrasonography can reveal ascites to assist in the diagnosis. Nonpitting edema of the lower extremities will usually be due to lymphatic obstruction, but hypothyroidism can be ruled out with a free thyroxine (T_4) or thyroid-stimulating hormone (TSH) assay. Unilateral edema of the lower extremities suggests deep vein thrombosis, which can be confirmed by Doppler ultrasound studies, plethysmography, or contrast venography. A CT scan of the chest will help diagnose constrictive pericarditis, which is rarely found today. Spirometry and arterial blood gas analysis will diagnose pulmonary emphysema with corpulmonale.

● **Other Useful Tests**

1. Complete blood count (CBC) (anemia)
2. Chemistry panel (nephrosis, cirrhosis)
3. Renal function test (nephritis, nephrosis)
4. Antinuclear antibody (ANA) analysis (collagen disease)
5. CT scan of the abdomen and pelvis (ovarian cyst or tumor)
6. Lymphangiogram (lymphedema)
7. CT scan of the chest (superior vena cava syndrome)
8. Serum protein electrophoresis (collagen disease, multiple myeloma)
9. Spiral CT venography (phlebitis)

Case Presentation #21

A 66-year-old white woman was found to have 4+ pitting edema on a routine checkup. There was no history of shortness of breath or chest pain. She admitted to consuming one to two glasses of wine before dinner almost daily for many years. She also has had Type II diabetes mellitus for 5 years managed on diet alone.

Question #1. What is your list of possibilities utilizing the methods described above?

Further history reveals that she has been treated with Timolol (a beta-adrenergic antagonist) for glaucoma the past few months. Physical examination reveals that, in addition to the pitting edema, she has mild cardiomegaly, crepitant rales at both bases, and mild hepatomegaly but no ascites. Her liver function tests were unremarkable.

Question #2. What is your diagnosis?

(See Appendix B for the answers.)

ELBOW PAIN

A painful elbow really does not require a detailed analysis of the anatomy to discover the various causes, almost all of which are bursal or bone and joint disorders. Of

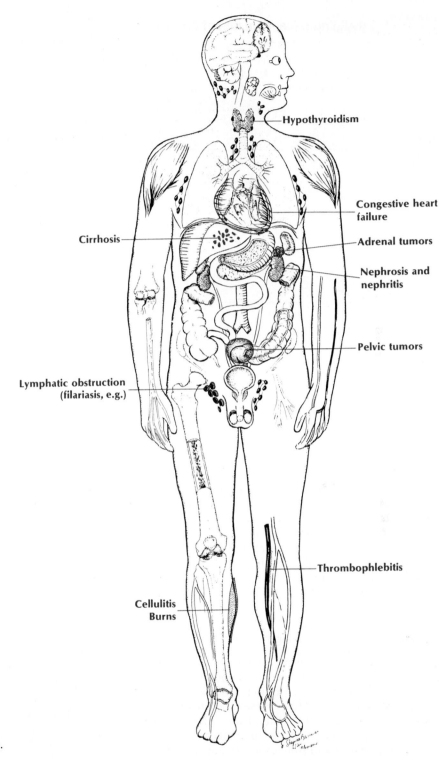

Hypothyroidism

Congestive heart
failure

Cirrhosis

Adrenal tumors

Nephrosis and
nephritis

Pelvic tumors

Lymphatic obstruction
(filariasis, e.g.)

Thrombophlebitis

Cellulitis
Burns

● **FIGURE 2** Edema of the extremities.

course, the skin may be involved by trauma and infection, just like the skin of the hands (see page 198). The arteries, veins, muscles, and nerves are rarely the cause of pain here. The simplest and most expedient approach is to use the mnemonic **MINT** and apply it to the bones, joints, and bursae.

M—Malformations are usually acquired, such as the Charcot joints of syphilis and syringomyelia. Bleeding into the joint in a hemophiliac is also classified here.

I—Inflammation should signal **bursitis**, particularly radiohumeral or lateral epicondylitis (popularly called tennis elbow) and olecranon bursitis. Medial epicondylitis

TABLE 26	Physiologic Mechanisms of Edema						
	Increased Venous Pressure	Increased Arterial Pressure	Decreased Serum Albumin	Lymphatic Obstruction	Abnormal Protein in Subcutaneous Tissue	Loss of Tissue Turgor	Aldosteronism
Congestive Heart Failure	√		√				√
Nephrosis			√				√
Cirrhosis	√		√				√
Pelvic Tumor	√						
Thrombophlebitis	√						
Filariasis				√			
Hypothyroidism					√		
Beriberi			√			√	
Malignant Hypertension		√					√
Acute Glomerulonephritis		√					√
Toxemia of Pregnancy		√	√				√

(golfer elbow) also occurs. One should also recall arthritis of the elbow joint, particularly rheumatoid arthritis, gout, and osteoarthritis. Surprisingly, rheumatic fever frequently affects the joint, and tuberculosis should be considered along with other forms of septic arthritis.

N—**Neoplasms** are unusual, but osteosarcomas and metastatic carcinomas nevertheless occur.

T—**Trauma** suggests fractures, dislocations, and elbow sprains.

● Approach to the Diagnosis

In the approach to the diagnosis, the traumatic conditions and arthritic disorders will probably stand out. A diagnostic dilemma occurs when the elbow looks normal and has good movement. Nevertheless, most of these cases are caused by tennis elbow, myositis, and fasciitis. Thus, a simple injection at the trigger point will assist the diagnosis and give the patient immediate and sometimes lasting relief. If this is unsuccessful, referral to an orthopedic surgeon is wise.

● Other Useful Tests

1. X-ray of the elbow (fracture)
2. CT scan or MRI of the elbow
3. Arthritis panel
4. X-ray of cervical spine (herniated disc)
5. Neurology consult

ENURESIS (BEDWETTING)

By following the innervation of the bladder from its termination to the spinal cord, brain, and "supratentorium," one can develop an extensive list of possibilities for this mischievous condition. Thus, **anatomy** is the key and the mnemonic **MINT** is the door.

Termination: The bladder and entire urinary tract should be suspect for pathology in any case of enuresis beyond the age of 6.

M—**Malformations** include phimosis, small urinary meatus, and vesicoureteral reflux.

I—**Inflammatory** conditions form the largest group and include balanitis, urethritis, cystitis, and pyelonephritis. If a child develops chronic nephritis at an early age, his or her bladder simply may be too small to retain the polyuria during sleep.

N—**Neoplasms** are an unlikely cause in children, but they occur in adults.

T—**Trauma** from a vesical calculus or other foreign bodies inserted into the bladder must also be considered. Postprostatectomy enuresis should be considered here in the adult.

Spinal cord: The following are included in this group:

M—**Malformations** such as spina bifida

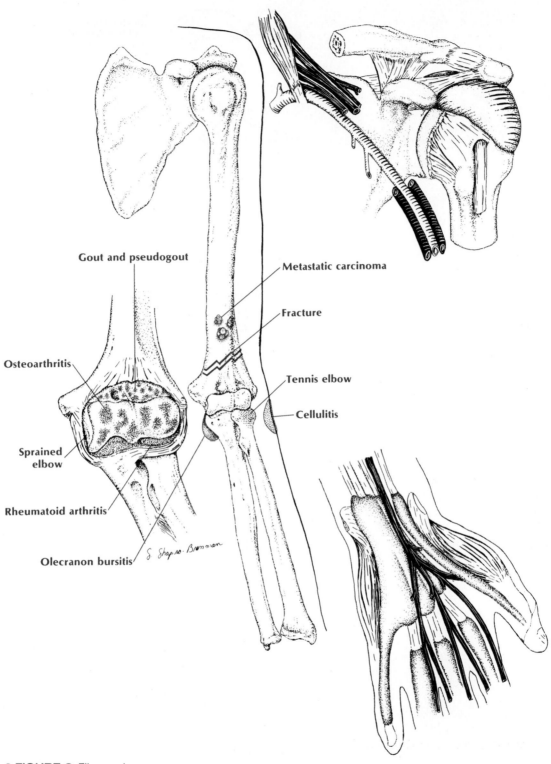

Gout and pseudogout

Metastatic carcinoma

Fracture

Osteoarthritis

Tennis elbow

Cellulitis

Sprained
elbow

Rheumatoid arthritis

Olecranon bursitis

S. Shapiro-Bronman

● **FIGURE 3** Elbow pain.

I—Inflammatory conditions such as poliomyelitis and transverse myelitis
N—Neoplasms such as spinal cord tumors
T—Traumatic conditions such as fracture, hematomyelia, and herniated discs

Brain: This is an important group of conditions to consider, if only briefly, because if the patient has a form of epilepsy, a cure may be easily obtained. Other neurologic conditions include mental retardation, multiple sclerosis, general paresis, brain tumors, and chronic encephalitides.

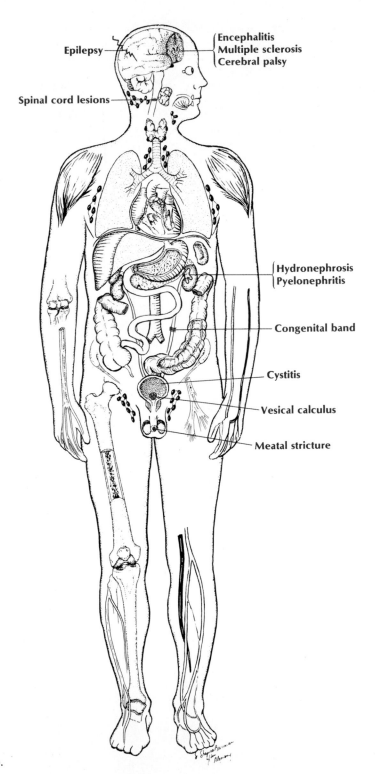

Epilepsy

Encephalitis
Multiple sclerosis
Cerebral palsy

Spinal cord lesions

Hydronephrosis
Pyelonephritis

Congenital band

Cystitis

Vesical calculus

Meatal stricture

● **FIGURE 4** Enuresis (bedwetting).

Supratentorium: A child may react violently to the pressure of toilet training by deliberately wetting the bed; this bedwetting may also be a way of getting back at generally strict parents or a way of getting their attention. Recent studies show that a child should not be considered a bedwetter until after the age of 6. Parents who put that label on a child too early may assure that the enuresis will continue for emotional reasons. Labeling the child as a bedwetter at any age is not a solution to, but an aggravation of, the problem.

● Approach to the Diagnosis

From the above discussion it should be obvious that simple bedwetting prior to age 6 may not require a workup at all. Look for a positive family history and beware of enuresis that develops after at least 6 months of remission (secondary enuresis). This may be a sign of sexual abuse. After that age a careful examination of the urine, including smear and culture for bacteria, should be done. An intravenous pyelogram and voiding cystogram are usually necessary. If these suggest a congenital lesion such as an ectopic ureter or are negative, cystoscopy may need to be done. An x-ray film for spina bifida and a sleep electroencephalogram (EEG) are probably worthwhile if urologic investigation is negative. If the workup is negative, reassure the patient that most children outgrow the problem by age 12.

● Other Useful Tests

1. Urology consult
2. Psychiatry consult
3. Examination of urinary sediment (urinary tract infection [UTI])
4. Sonogram (test for residual urine)
5. Cystometric tests (neurogenic bladder)
6. Psychometric testing (psychiatric disorder)

EPIPHORA

Epiphora is excessive tearing. It may be unilateral in which case there is usually obvious eye pathology, or it may be bilateral in which case it is psychogenic or related to the effects of drugs. The mnemonic **MINT** will help recall the most common causes.

M—Malformation brings to mind ectropion or entropion especially in elderly patients.

I—Inflammation suggests conjunctivitis, a corneal ulcer, or hordeolum.

N—Nervous system. This would bring to mind Bell palsy, migraine, and histamine cephalgia.

T—Trauma should prompt the recall of a corneal abrasion or foreign body. Trauma may also have caused obstruction of the lacrimal ducts.

● Approach to the Diagnosis

If the symptoms are bilateral, look for a history of drug use or emotional problems. If it is unilateral, careful examination of the eye before and after a drop of fluorescence is indicated. Continuous excessive tearing in one eye suggests dacryostenosis. This may turn up a foreign body, corneal ulcer, or conjunctivitis. If this is unremarkable, referral to an ophthalmologist is in order.

EPISTAXIS

The differential diagnostic approach to epistaxis is **anatomic** and **histologic**. Table 27 breaks the nasal passages into anatomic and histologic components and cross-indexes them with the various etiologies.

By far, the most common cause of epistaxis is **trauma** from nose picking. Many people are particularly vulnerable to this because of the closeness of Kiesselbach plexus of veins and capillaries to the surface of the septal mucosa. This cause can quickly be ruled out by nasoscopic examination of the anterior portion of the septum. This same area may be inflamed or ulcerated by various infections, particularly syphilis, tuberculosis, leprosy, and mucormycosis. Carcinomas in this area are uncommon, but the Schmincke tumor of the nasopharynx should not be forgotten; more important are allergic polyps, which usually do not bleed unless traumatized. Wegener midline granulomatosis is an autoimmune disease that may present with a bloody or nonbloody nasal discharge. It usually involves the sinuses, however, and must be differentiated from mucormycosis.

Other systemic diseases are prominent causes of epistaxis. Back pressure from obstructed veins in emphysema, asthma, and right heart failure must be considered. Arterial hypertension, from whatever etiology, is a common cause from middle age onward. Rheumatic fever and blood dyscrasias round out the picture.

Other miscellaneous causes of epistaxis are skull fracture and menopause. In most cases, adequate examination of the nasal septum discloses the diagnosis, and coagulation or nasal packing will suffice in treatment. The blood pressure should always be checked and, in recurrent cases, nasopharyngoscopy, coagulation studies, and a search for systemic disease must be made.

● Other Useful Tests

1. CBC (anemia, thrombocytopenia)
2. Chemistry panel (liver disease, renal disease)
3. Rumpel–Leede test (thrombocytopenia)
4. Liver function test (cirrhosis)
5. Prothrombin time (liver disease, vitamin K deficiency, drug effects)
6. Partial thromboplastin time (disseminated intravascular coagulation [DIC], hemophilia)
7. X-rays of the sinuses (neoplasm)
8. Nasopharyngoscopy (polyps, neoplasm)
9. Circulation time (CHF)
10. Arterial blood gas analysis (lung disease)
11. Platelet count (thrombocytopenia)
12. Bleeding time (thrombocytopenia, vascular purpura)

Case Presentation #22

A 42-year-old black man came to the emergency room because of persistent epistaxis. He had a history of smoking cigarettes for 30 years. History also revealed that he had several previous nosebleeds in the past 6 months but not this severe.

Question #1. What would be the possible causes of this man's difficulties utilizing the above-described methods?

Further history reveals he has had a chronic cough and mild shortness of breath for several years. Physical examination reveals sibilant and sonorous rales over both lungs and diminished alveolar breathing throughout.

Question #2. What is your diagnosis?

(See Appendix B for the answers.)

TABLE 27　Epistaxis

	V Vascular	I Inflammatory	N Neoplasm	D Deficiency	I Intoxication	C Collagen or Congenital	A Allergic and Autoimmune	T Trauma	E Endocrine
Anterior Septal Mucosa		Rhinitis Syphilis Leprosy Mucormycosis Tuberculosis	Carcinoma (rarely)				Midline granuloma and polyps Rhinitis	Nose-picking Foreign body	Menopause Menstruation
Sinuses		Tuberculosis Mucormycosis Viral sinusitis	Polyp Carcinoma				Midline granuloma and polyps Sinusitis		
Nasopharynx			Schmincke tumor Adenoid				Rheumatic fever	Skull fracture Foreign body	
Veins and Capillaries	Venous obstruction from emphysema, asthma, and congestive heart failure		Hemangioma			Kiesselbach plexus Telangiectasis			
Arteries	Hypertension								
Blood			Leukemia Polycythemia	Aplastic anemia	Heparin and warfarin therapy	Hemophilia and other coagulation defects	Thrombocytopenia		

EUPHORIA

Euphoria is characterized by a feeling of well-being, cheerfulness, and optimism. It can be constant or intermittent. It may be psychogenic or organic. The mnemonic **VINDICATE** will help recall the many causes of euphoria.

V—Vascular: Cerebral arteriosclerosis and stroke are rarely a cause of euphoria.

I—Inflammation: Aside from patients with general paresis or a frontal lobe abscess, euphoria is also rarely associated with an infectious disease process.

N—Neoplasm: This should bring to mind frontal lobe tumors in which the patient is not only euphoric but exhibits excessive jocularity, lack of insight, and poor memory for recent events.

D—Degenerative: In some cases of dementia, euphoria may present at the outset.

I—Intoxication: Drugs such as amphetamines, lysergic acid diethylamide (LSD), and corticosteroid may produce a euphoric state. Cocaine and other narcotics may do the same.

C—Congenital: Patients with cerebral palsy and other congenital disorders of the brain may exhibit euphoria.

A—Autoimmune: Multiple sclerosis is associated with euphoria in many cases.

T—Trauma: This brings to mind the euphoria associated with a concussion and posttraumatic neurosis.

E—Endocrine: Hyperthyroidism and Cushing syndrome may be associated with euphoria, but depression is much more likely.

Unfortunately, the mnemonic **VINDICATE** fails to remind us of psychogenic causes such as schizophrenia, manic–depressive psychosis, and psychopathic behavior disorders. Temporal lobe epilepsy may be associated with intermittent euphoria.

E

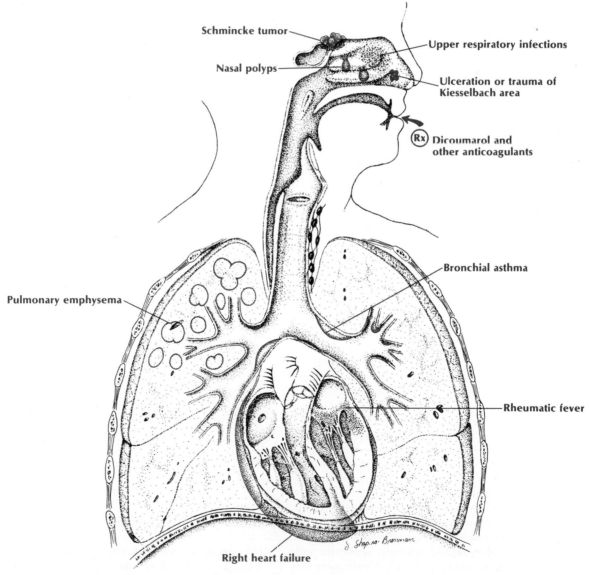

Schmincke tumor
Nasal polyps
Upper respiratory infections
Ulceration or trauma of Kiesselbach area
(Rx) Dicoumarol and other anticoagulants
Bronchial asthma
Pulmonary emphysema
Rheumatic fever
Right heart failure

● **FIGURE 5** Epistaxis.

● Approach to the Diagnosis

Look for a history of drug use or abuse. A careful mental status examination may suggest early Alzheimer disease or other forms of dementia. Neurologic examination may show bilateral pyramidal tract signs indicating multiple sclerosis or papilledema indicating a brain tumor.

A venereal disease research laboratory (VDRL) test or urine drug screen may suggest the diagnosis. A neurologic consult should be ordered before proceeding with expensive tests such as a CT scan or MRI. Perhaps a psychiatrist should be consulted early in the workup.

EXCESSIVE SWEATING

It is uncommon for patients to present with the chief complaint of excessive sweating (diaphoresis, hyperhidrosis); when they do, it is often hyperhidrosis of the hands and feet due to caffeine or nervous tension. Obese patients may complain of excessive sweating, especially under the armpits. What are the pathologic causes of sweating and how can they be recalled?

Physiology is the basic science most useful in developing a differential diagnosis. The sweat glands are under the control of the sympathetic nervous system; consequently, they respond to anything that increases the level of adrenalin in the body. Shock from any cause induces a reflex stimulation of the sympathetic nervous system and adrenal gland and an outpouring of adrenalin. Thus diaphoresis may be found in myocardial infarctions and CHF (cardiogenic shock); in pulmonary embolism, renal embolism, and peripheral embolism (vasomotor shock); and in bleeding peptic ulcer, pyloric obstruction with vomiting, cholera, intestinal obstruction, and other forms of shock due to a drop in blood volume. Acute labyrinthitis or seasickness causes sweating by neurogenic shock pathways.

The adrenalin level may also be increased in the body in hypoglycemic states. Thus, a patient with diabetes in insulin shock will sweat, whereas a patient with diabetes in acidosis will not. Islet cell adenomas cause diaphoresis during the hypoglycemic attacks. Hepatic hypoglycemia, glycogen storage disease, and hypopituitarism may all be associated with excessive sweating on the same basis. Excessive adrenalin output is the cause of diaphoresis in pheochromocytomas. It may be the cause in hyperthyroidism also, although another mechanism discussed below is undoubtedly involved.

Hypermetabolism causes excessive sweating by hypothalamic stimulation of the sweating center to assist in the cooling of the body. Thus, any cause of fever is associated with sweating (the sweating induces a drop in temperature). Most notable of these causes are rheumatic fever, pulmonary tuberculosis, and septicemia. An abscess large enough to cause fever will probably cause sweating. Hypermetabolism in hyperthyroidism is largely responsible for the continuous sweating, although excessive adrenalin is involved too. Neoplasms, especially leukemia and metastatic carcinoma, are associated with sweating on the same basis.

A miscellaneous group of conditions associated with diaphoresis that are also due to physiologic mechanisms include neurocirculatory asthenia, chronic anxiety neurosis, menopause; and various drugs, including camphor, morphine, and ipecac. Organophosphate intoxication may produce excessive sweating by allowing excessive accumulation of acetylcholine at the synaptic junction.

● Approach to the Diagnosis

Pinpointing the diagnosis involves a search for other symptoms and signs of the above conditions. A chest x-ray film to rule out pulmonary tuberculosis is especially important in a patient presenting with night sweats. Accurate charting of the temperature will indicate those cases due to fever. Urine vanillylmandelic acid (VMA) levels and a thyroid profile will spot pheochromocytomas and hyperthyroidism. A 36- to 48-hour fast with frequent glucose determinations will help diagnose insulinomas and other hypoglycemic states. Because this is not usually the major presenting symptom, the workup will usually center on another symptom. Asking about caffeine ingestion will often spot the cause without expensive laboratory testing.

● Other Useful Tests

1. CBC (anemia, infection)
2. Sedimentation rate (infection)
3. Rheumatoid arthritis test
4. Serum insulin assay (insulinomas)
5. C-peptide (insulinomas)
6. Urine cultures (pyelonephritis)
7. Blood culture (subacute bacterial endocarditis [SBE])
8. Chemistry panel (liver disease, kidney disease)
9. Drug screen (drug abuse)
10. Psychometric testing (chronic anxiety neurosis)

Case Presentation #23

A 39-year-old white man complained of recurrent episodes of diffuse sweating and palpitations for several months.

Question #1. What would be your list of possible causes based on your understanding of the physiology of this symptom as outlined above?

Further questioning reveals that the episodes are associated with throbbing headaches. His physical examination is unremarkable except for a blood pressure of 180/110.

Question #2. What is your diagnosis now?

(See Appendix B for the answers.)

EXOPHTHALMOS

The mnemonic **VINDICATE** is a useful and quick way to recall the causes of exophthalmos (for enophthalmos, see the section on ptosis, page 356).

E

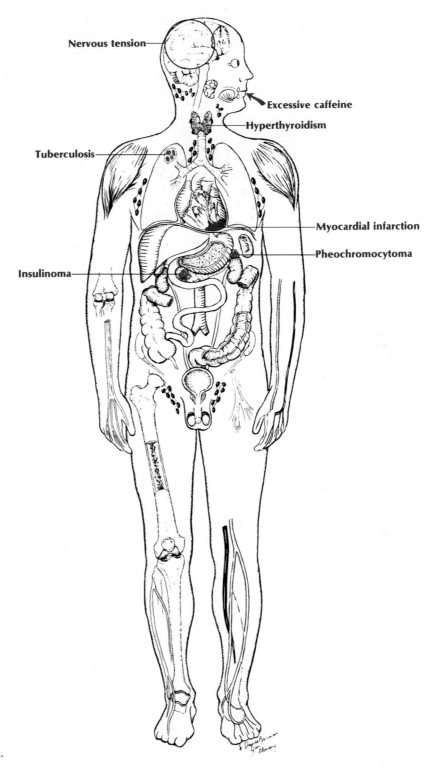

● **FIGURE 6** Excessive sweating.

V—Vascular disorders include a carotid–cavernous fistula and cavernous sinus thrombosis.

I—Inflammatory diseases recall orbital cellulitis, osteomyelitis, and sinusitis.

N—Neoplasms suggest hemangiomas, lymphangiomas, sarcomas, metastatic carcinomas, and nervous system tumors such as sphenoid ridge meningiomas.

D—Deficiency diseases suggest the retroorbital hemorrhages of scurvy. **Degenerative** diseases suggest the apparent exophthalmos of facial palsy associated with progressive muscular atrophy and dystrophy in many forms.

I—Intoxication suggests the exophthalmos that develops or progresses on treatment in hyperthyroidism.

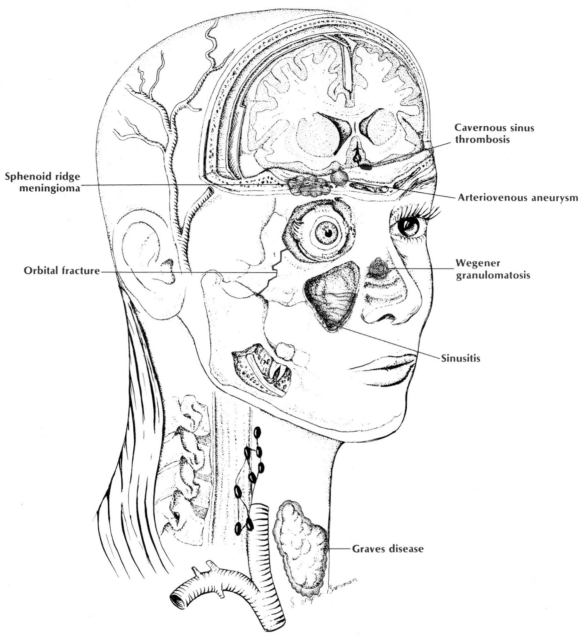

● **FIGURE 7** Exophthalmos.

Idiopathic diseases such as Paget disease and fibrous dysplasia of the skull must also be considered.

C—**Congenital** brings to mind hydrocephalus, Hand–Schüller–Christian disease, meningoceles, and cleido-cranial dysostosis, all of which cause exophthalmos. In this category, one should also include the genetic exophthalmos of blacks.

A—**Autoimmune** disorders suggest Wegener granulomatosis.

T—**Trauma** suggests orbital fractures and hematomas, which will cause proptosis in many cases.

E—**Endocrine** disorders suggest that the most significant cause of exophthalmos is Graves disease.

If exophthalmos can be classified as a result of a mass, then the causes can be recalled by the methods applied to any mass. The mass may be air (orbital emphysema), fluid (orbital abscess), blood (e.g., hematomas from trauma, scurvy, hemophilia), a foreign substance (e.g., echinococ-cal cyst), or hypertrophy of one of the tissues around the orbit. The latter can be developed by a histologic analysis. Thus, **fat** may hypertrophy or multiply in Hand–Schüller–Christian disease and in exophthalmic goiter. **Blood vessels** may become hypertrophied in cavernous sinus thrombosis, carotid–cavernous fistulas, and aneurysms and will undergo hyperplasia in hemangiomas. **Lymph tissue** and **connective tissue** may form sarcomas or granulomas. **Bone** may swell with a periosteitis and may undergo hyperplasia in Paget disease, osteomas, metastatic carcinoma, and meningiomas. **Nerve tissue** may undergo hyperplasia in neurofibromatosis.

● Approach to the Diagnosis

Because bilateral exophthalmos is usually due to hyperthyroidism, a thyroid profile must be done. The most useful in this profile are the total T_4 level by immunoassay, the free thyroxine index, and the radioiodine (RAI) uptake and scan. A total triiodothyronine (T_3) test by immunoassay should be done to exclude T_3 thyrotoxicosis. Because bilateral exophthalmos can occur without hyperthyroidism, testing for thyrotropin receptor antibody and peroxidase antibodies must be done if thyroid function tests are negative. With exophthalmos, chemosis, and ecchymosis, the patient should be hospitalized for a workup of cavernous sinus thrombosis and a neurologist consulted. When there is unilateral exophthalmos, ultrasonography and angiography will rule out carotid–cavernous fistula and a cystic lesion. A CT scan or MRI of the brain and orbits will rule out tumors and abscesses. It is wise to consult a neurologist, ophthalmologist, or endocrinologist to assist in this workup.

EXTREMITY, HAND, AND FOOT DEFORMITIES

Most deformities of the extremities are due to neurologic or joint diseases, but because there are some exceptions to this rule the clinician needs a method for easy recall of all the causes when faced with the complaint. The mnemonic **VINDICATE** provides the key.

V—Vascular disease includes arteriosclerosis, Buerger disease, and Raynaud syndrome, which may lead to gangrene or loss of a foot or digit.

I—Inflammatory diseases that deserve special mention include the deformities of poliomyelitis, osteomyelitis, and septic arthritis. Syphilis of the bone causes the saber shin, rarely seen today.

N—Neurologic disorders cover the largest group of deformities. The beefy red hand of syringomyelia, the wrist and foot drop of peripheral neuropathy (especially lead poisoning), the claw hand and foot of amyotrophic lateral sclerosis or progressive muscular atrophy, the preacher hand of myotonic dystrophy, and the tight fisted, flexed, and pronated hand of hemiplegia are the most important ones. Friedreich ataxia causes a hammer toe, and Charcot–Marie–Tooth disease causes a stork leg.

D—Degenerative diseases include the degenerative neurologic diseases mentioned above and degenerative osteoarthritis. Deficiency diseases include the bowlegs of rickets. Paget disease causes bowing and hypertrophy of the tibia.

I—Intoxication should remind one of the toxic neuropathies such as lead and arsenic, but it also brings to mind the Dupuytren contractures of alcoholic cirrhosis.

C—Congenital disorders form another large group. Many of the disorders in this group have been mentioned under neurologic disorders. However, congenital dislocation of the hip, talipes, equinovarus or valgus, and calcaneovarus or valgus should be remembered. These are often signs that a congenital lesion exists elsewhere.

Hallux valgus is a frequent deformity of the toes. Pes planus and pes cavus belong in this category, although they are not nearly as significant. The deformities of Marfan syndrome (long fingers with syndactyly), Down syndrome (e.g., short fingers and simian crease), Laurence–Moon–Biedl syndrome, and achondroplasia are mentioned here.

A—Autoimmune diseases include the spindle deformities of lupus erythematosus and rheumatoid arthritis; the gangrene, autoamputation, and smooth, swollen hands of scleroderma; and the gangrene of periarteritis nodosa.

T—Traumatic lesions need little prompting to recall, but Pott fracture with eversion of the foot and fracture of the neck of the femur that causes eversion of the entire leg are noteworthy. Dislocations of various joints should be easy to spot, but the mallet or baseball finger of ruptured tendons is tricky.

E—Endocrine disorders include the large hands of acromegaly, the short fingers of cretinism and pseudohypoparathyroidism, and the swollen hands of myxedema. The *accoucheur* hand ("pelvic exam hand") of tetany is appropriate to mention here.

● Approach to the Diagnosis

It is usually a simple matter to decide whether the deformity is due to neurologic disease or to joint or bone disease. An x-ray film of the hands or feet may be useful in acromegaly and many congenital disorders. Referral to an orthopedic or neurologic specialist is usually indicated if bone or neurologic involvement is probable. An arthritis workup can be done (see page 276) if joint disease is the cause of the deformity.

EXTREMITY MASS

When the clinician tries to recall the causes of a mass in the extremities, he or she should consider the **anatomy**. As the clinician dissects downward from the skin, he or she encounters the subcutaneous tissue, veins, muscles, ligaments, bursae, arteries, lymph nodes, nerves, bones, and joints. The common lesions causing a mass in each of these should easily come to mind.

1. **Skin:** Common lesions to consider here are sebaceous cysts, lipomas, and cellulitis. Other skin masses are considered on page 396.
2. **Subcutaneous tissue:** Rheumatic or rheumatoid nodules, tophi of gout, lipomas, and contusions are common.
3. **Veins:** Dilated veins (varicoceles) and thrombophlebitis present as mass lesions.
4. **Muscles and ligaments:** Contusions, nodules in myofascitis, ganglions, and partial or complete rupture of muscle (e.g., rupture of the rectus femoris) are typical masses originating in the muscles and ligaments. Myositis ossificans may present with nodular masses.
5. **Bursae:** The bursae may be involved by gout, trauma, or rheumatic conditions and swell with fluid.

E

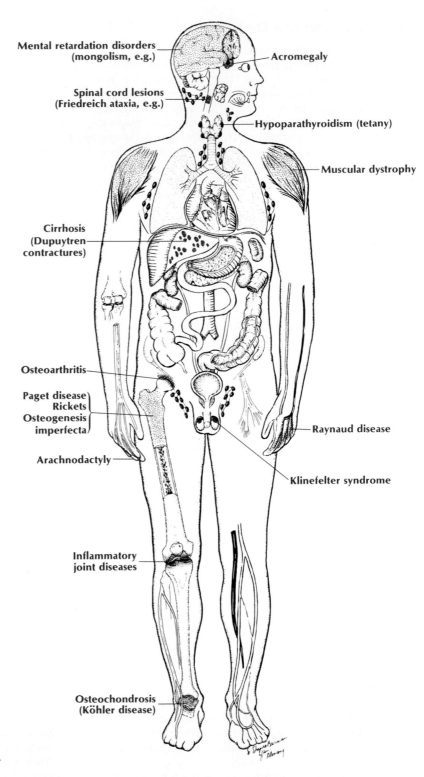

● **FIGURE 8** Extremity, hand, and foot deformities.

6. **Arteries:** Aneurysms are the most likely cause of an extremity mass originating from the arteries. Severe arteriosclerosis may cause confusion occasionally.

7. **Lymph nodes:** Tuberculous adenitis, adenitis secondary to infections in the distal portion of the extremity, and metastatic tumors may cause enlargement of the lymph nodes.

8. **Nerves:** Traumatic neuromas, neurofibromas, and hypertrophy of the nerve in Dejerine–Sottas disease are typical "masses" arising from the peripheral nerve.

9. **Bone:** Trauma may lead to fractures and subperiosteal hematomas, callus formation following the fracture, or secondary osteomyelitis, all of which may cause a mass. Primary osteomyelitis, tuberculosis of the bone, syphilis of

E

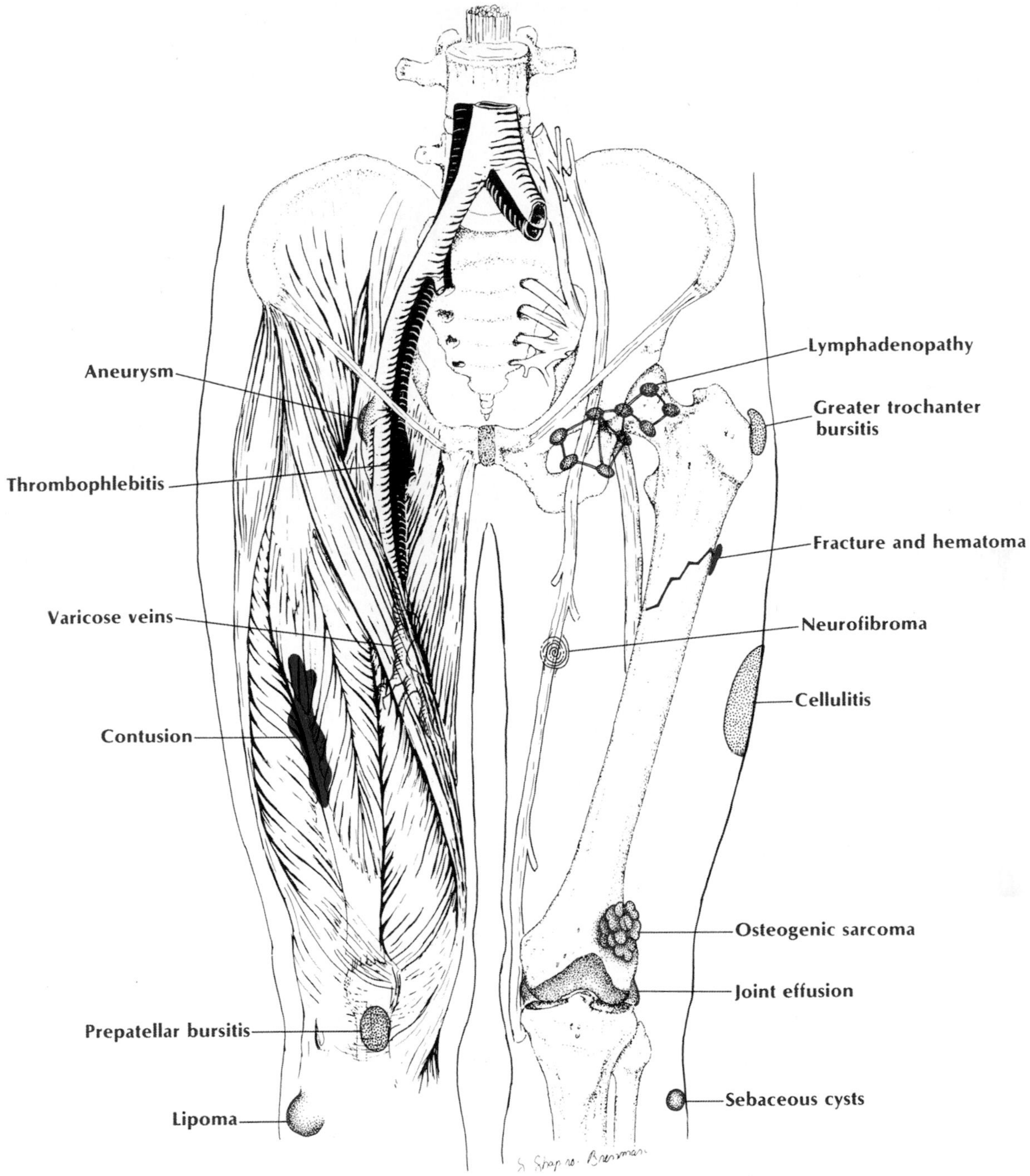

● **FIGURE 9** Extremity mass.

the bone, rickets, and acromegaly may cause bone masses. Typical tumors affecting the bone are chondromas, exostoses (osteomas), osteogenic sarcomas, fibrosarcomas, and metastatic carcinomas, but there are several others. Paget disease may present as an enlargement of the bone.

● Approach to the Diagnosis

Because the extremities are not considered vital areas, the primary method of diagnosing the cause of a mass is exploration and biopsy. This is all well and good when the lesion is on the skin or subcutaneous tissue; however, when the mass is in the deeper tissues, it is wise to utilize diagnostic tests to determine what the mass is before exploration. If the mass is suspected to be a varix or aneurysm, ultrasonography can be extremely useful in defining it. If the mass is attached to or thought to originate in bone, x-rays of the area and bone scans are useful. If it is uncertain what tissue the mass originates from, a CT scan can be used to help define it. Before ordering any of the above tests, it is best to consult a general or orthopedic surgeon to help select the most appropriate test for the case at hand.

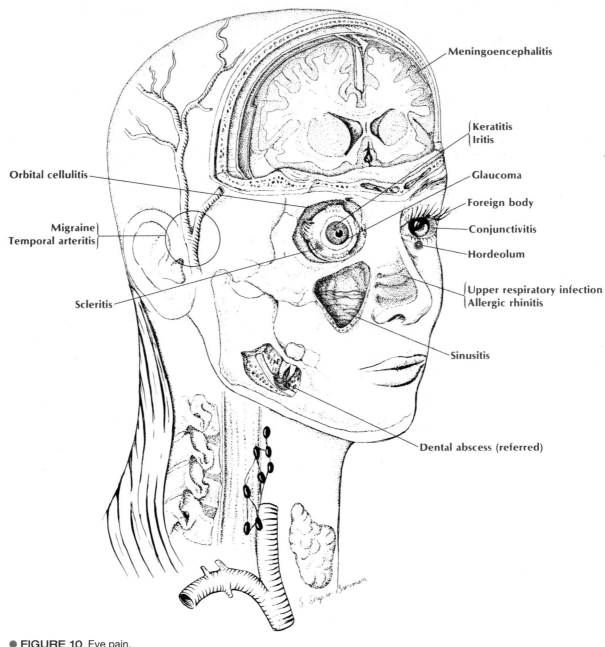

Meningoencephalitis

Keratitis
Iritis

Orbital cellulitis

Glaucoma

Foreign body

Migraine
Temporal arteritis

Conjunctivitis

Hordeolum

Upper respiratory infection
Allergic rhinitis

Scleritis

Sinusitis

Dental abscess (referred)

● **FIGURE 10** Eye pain.

● Other Useful Tests

1. CBC (abscess)
2. Sedimentation rate (cellulitis)
3. Tuberculin test (cold abscess)
4. Serum protein electrophoresis (multiple myeloma)
5. Skeletal surgery (metastatic neoplasm)
6. Arteriogram (aneurysm)
7. Phlebogram (varix)
8. Lymphangiogram (Hodgkin lymphoma, lymph node metastasis)
9. Exploratory surgery

EYE PAIN

Applying the mnemonic **MINT** to the various anatomic parts of the eye will aid in systematically developing a list of diagnostic possibilities for eye pain.

M—Malformations most certainly suggest glaucoma and all the refractive disorders (e.g., astigmatism, myopia, hypermetropia).
I—Inflammation accounts for most cases. One anatomically recalls conjunctivitis, Sjögren syndrome, keratitis, scleritis, corneal ulcers, iridocyclitis, and optic neuritis.

Do not forget inflammation of the orbit. Vasculitis from temporal arteritis must be considered with obstruction of the retinal veins or arteries.

N—**Neoplasms** are unlikely causes but must be considered.

T—**Trauma** should suggest abrasions and foreign bodies, particularly those of the cornea.

Eye pain, like earache, may be referred. Cerebral neoplasms, migraine, and sinusitis may all present with orbital or retroorbital pain. An additional category of etiologies that is not common in earache is systemic disease. Any febrile disease may cause bilateral eye pain, particularly viral influenza.

● Approach to the Diagnosis

The approach to the diagnosis of eye pain involves a careful search for inflammation of the various anatomic structures; then a drop or two of fluorescent dye is inserted and the cornea inspected for lacerations, herpes ulcers, and foreign bodies. Finally, tonometry may be done. Referral to an ophthalmologist is often necessary, but the astute clinician will want to x-ray the sinuses, ask about a history of migraine, do a visual field, and rule out systemic diseases beforehand.

● Other Useful Tests

1. Smear and culture of exudate (conjunctivitis)
2. Smear for eosinophils (allergic conjunctivitis)
3. Histamine test (cluster headaches)
4. Sedimentation rate (temporal arteritis)
5. X-ray of sinuses (sinusitis)
6. Visual fields (glaucoma)
7. Slit lamp examination (iritis)
8. CT scan of brain (tumors, abscess)
9. Temporal artery biopsy (temporal arteritis)
10. Therapeutic trial of beta blockers (migraine)

Case Presentation #24

A 56-year-old white woman complained of headache and pain in the right eye for 3 days associated with nausea and vomiting.

Question #1. Applying the methods presented above, what is your list of possibilities?

Further questioning reveals that she has also noticed blurring of vision in the right eye associated with halos around objects. There is no history of previous attacks and her neurologic examination is normal.

Question #2. What diagnosis would you consider now?

(See Appendix B for the answers.)

E

F

FACE MASS

To develop a list of possible causes of a face mass, let us turn to anatomy. The face is composed of skin, subcutaneous tissues, muscle, bone, teeth, the sinuses, salivary glands, arteries, veins, and nerves. Applying the mnemonic **VINDICATE** to each one of these structures, we can come up with an excellent list of possibilities:

Skin and subcutaneous tissues—Carbuncles, cellulitis, sebaceous cysts; lipomas, carcinomas, angioneurotic edema, etc.

Muscle—Myositis, myomas, hypertrophy

Bone—Osteomas, metastatic tumor, multiple myelomas, osteomyelitis

Teeth—Dental abscess, neoplasm

Sinuses—Wegener midline granuloma, mucormycosis, neoplasm

Salivary glands—Mumps, tumors, calculus, Mikulicz syndrome, Sjögren syndrome

Arteries and veins—Hemangiomas, arteriovenous fistula

Nerves—Neuroma, neurofibromatosis

● Approach to the Diagnosis

If infection is suspected, smears and cultures of exudates should be done. X-rays of the skull, sinuses, and jaw may be helpful. A computed tomography (CT) scan will be more definitive. If neoplasm or granuloma is suspected, a biopsy or excision will be necessary. If there is still doubt about the etiology, an oral surgeon or otolaryngologist should be consulted.

● Other Useful Tests

1. Complete blood count (CBC) (infection)
2. Sedimentation rate (abscess, osteomyelitis)
3. Chest x-ray (tuberculosis, Wegener granulomatosis)
4. Chemistry panel (multiple myeloma)
5. Blood cultures (osteomyelitis)
6. x-Ray of the teeth (dental abscess)
7. Trial of epinephrine and antihistamines (angioneurotic edema)
8. Sialography (salivary gland duct calculus)
9. Cytoplasmic antineutrophil cytoplasmic antibody (C–ANCA) test (Wegener granulomatosis)
10. Rheumatoid arthritis (RA) test, anti-Ro (SSA) antibodies (Sjögren syndrome)

FACIAL PAIN

Visualize the structures of the face in a systematic fashion to develop a differential diagnosis of facial pain. With the **skin,** herpes zoster and carbuncles come to mind. Next, the **internal maxillary artery** suggests histamine cephalalgia and arteritis, just as the **nerves** suggest trigeminal neuralgia, herpes zoster, and the atypical facial neuralgias encountered in multiple sclerosis, Wallenberg syndrome, and other central nervous system conditions. These will almost invariably be associated with other neurologic findings. With reference to the **bones,** one should recall temporomandibular joint (TMJ) syndrome, sinusitis, and dental caries or abscesses. An elongated styloid process may cause facial pain (Eagle syndrome). Disorders of the eye that cause face pain are included in the section on eye pain (see page 164).

Of course, one could apply the mnemonic **VINDICATE** to the differential diagnosis and come up with an extensive list. Thus, **V—Vascular** conditions suggest histamine cephalalgia; **I—Inflammatory** conditions suggest herpes zoster, sinusitis, and dental abscesses; and **N—Neoplasms** suggest Schmincke tumors, carcinoma of the tongue, and so forth. This procedure, however, is more involved than is necessary.

● Approach to the Diagnosis

The approach to the diagnosis of face pain includes a careful history and physical examination with a good neurologic examination. The sinuses are transilluminated, and x-rays may be performed. The teeth and occlusion are examined carefully and possibly x-rayed. A histamine test may be indicated to rule out histamine cephalalgia. The busy physician may want to refer the patient to a neurologist immediately, but this will obviously take away the challenge.

● Other Useful Tests

1. Therapeutic trial of sumatriptan (migraine)
2. Therapeutic trial of carbamazepine (Tegretol) (trigeminal neuralgia)
3. Temporal artery compression (migraine)
4. Sedimentation rate (temporal arteritis)
5. x-Rays of the TMJ (TMJ syndrome)
6. CT scan of the brain (tumors)
7. CT scan of the sinuses (sinusitis)
8. Nasopharyngoscopy
9. Magnetic resonance imaging (MRI) of the TMJ (TMJ syndrome)

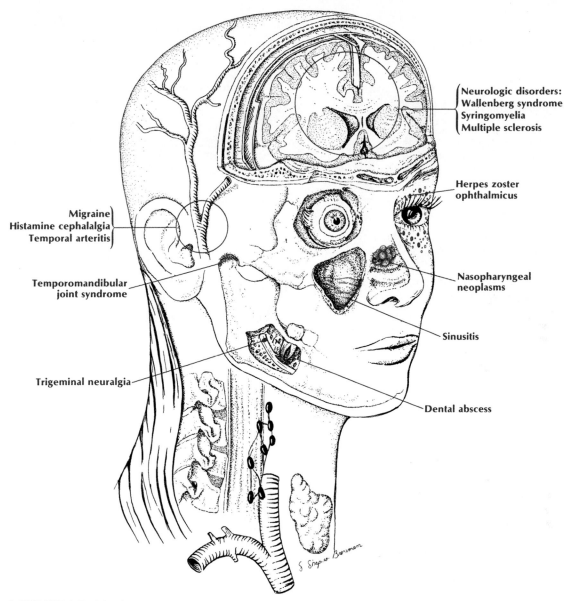

● FIGURE 1 Facial pain.

Case Presentation #25

A 28-year-old white man stops you as you are coming out of church because he is concerned about acute pain in his left cheek that developed in the past 24 hours. He also complains of a nasal discharge and blocking of his left nasal passage.

Question #1. Utilizing your knowledge of anatomy, what would be your list of possible causes for this man's problem?

On examination, his temperature is 102.1°F, and his maxillary sinus fails to transilluminate.

Question #2. What is your diagnosis now?

(See Appendix B for the answers.)

FACIAL PARALYSIS

A facial palsy is usually considered to be Bell palsy and it frequently is. Nevertheless, the clinician who begins treatment without ruling out other possibilities will eventually get burned. **Anatomy** is the key to recalling these possibilities before the patient leaves the office. Follow the facial nerve from its origin along its pathway to its termination, and all the causes should come to mind.

Origin: Diseases of the brain and brainstem are considered here. They are usually distinguished from Bell palsy by the presence of other neurologic findings. The mnemonic **ANITA** will help recall them in an organized fashion.

A—Arterial diseases include aneurysms, emboli, thromboses, and hemorrhages. Occlusion of the posterior inferior cerebellar artery will cause a peripheral facial palsy,

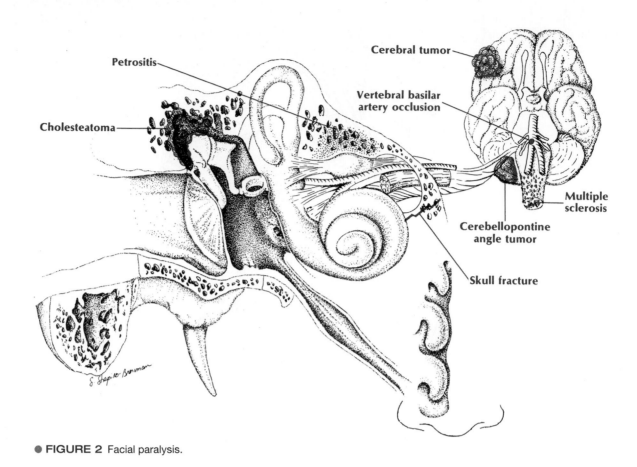

● **FIGURE 2** Facial paralysis.

but it can easily be distinguished from Bell palsy by the presence of a Horner syndrome, hoarseness, ataxia, and crossed hemianalgesia.

N—**Neoplasms** include gliomas and the cerebellopontine angle tumor or acoustic neuroma.

I—**Inflammation** suggests neurosyphilis, tuberculosis, brain abscess, and encephalitis.

T—**Trauma** helps recall skull fractures and epidural and subdural hematomas.

A—**Autoimmune** disease suggests multiple sclerosis, the collagen diseases, and early Guillain–Barré syndrome.

Pathway: The facial nerve has a long pathway, and along that path, it can be destroyed by the following:

A—**Arterial** aneurysms

N—**Neoplasms** such as acoustic neuromas and parotid gland tumors

I—**Inflammatory** conditions like herpes zoster (Ramsey–Hunt syndrome), petrositis, mastoiditis, and cholesteatomas

T—**Trauma** such as basilar skull fractures and otologic surgery

A—**Autoimmune** disease such as Bell palsy, or uveoparotid fever

Termination: The site of termination of the facial nerve should suggest myasthenia gravis, muscular dystrophy, and facial hemiatrophy. These rarely present with an isolated facial palsy.

● Approach to the Diagnosis

The clinical picture will frequently help to determine the cause of facial paralysis. Peripheral facial palsy as occurs in Bell palsy involves the forehead muscles and there is difficulty in closing the eyelid, whereas central facial palsy involves the face and lips and there is often associated hemiplegia or monoplegia. When there is exclusively a peripheral facial palsy without hearing loss or other neurologic signs, Bell palsy should be strongly suspected, although diabetes and myasthenia gravis need to be excluded. A bilateral peripheral nerve palsy should make one consider Guillain–Barré syndrome as well as Lyme disease; be on the lookout for paralysis of the extremities as well. Bilateral facial palsy is also seen in myotonic dystrophy and myasthenia gravis. A "Bell palsy" with hearing loss and an aural discharge should prompt consideration of mastoiditis and petrositis. If there is hearing loss without a discharge, the possibility of an acoustic neuroma or cholesteatoma must be entertained. The association of a central facial palsy with hemiplegia brings up a host of possibilities including subdural hematoma, brain abscess, brain tumor, and cerebrovascular accident. The workup of these conditions is considered on page 218.

If the patient has clinical Bell palsy, one could start a therapy without a workup, but it is wise to get an x-ray of the skull and mastoids to rule out mastoiditis and petrositis and a glucose tolerance test to rule out diabetes.

An acetylcholine receptor antibody titer or Tensilon test would only be ordered if the palsy were intermittent or there were other cranial nerve signs. If a middle ear infection or acoustic neuroma is suspected, the patient needs x-rays of the mastoids and petrous bones and a CT scan or MRI of the brain and auditory canal.

● Other Useful Tests

1. CBC (ear infection)
2. Sedimentation rate (ear infection)
3. Venereal disease research laboratory (VDRL) test (neurosyphilis)
4. Cultures of ear discharge (otitis)
5. Audiogram and caloric tests (petrositis, acoustic neuroma)
6. Posterior fossa myelogram (acoustic neuroma)
7. Electromyogram (EMG) (Bell palsy)
8. Lyme disease antibody titer (Lyme disease)
9. Blood lead level (lead neuropathy)
10. Spinal tap (Guillain–Barré syndrome)
11. Serologic tests (enzyme-linked immunosorbent assay [ELISA]) for Lyme disease

Case Presentation #26

A 21-year-old Hispanic man complained of acute onset of swelling of the right side of his face. Examination revealed weakness of the right facial muscles and inability to close his right eye.

Question #1. Utilizing the methods presented above, what would you consider in the differential diagnosis at this point?

A neurologist is consulted and his examination shows weakness of the left facial muscles as well. Furthermore, there is mild weakness and loss of sensation in all four extremities and diminished deep tendon reflexes.

Question #2. What is your list of possibilities now?

(See Appendix B for the answers.)

FACIES, ABNORMAL

A list of possible causes of abnormal facies can best be arrived at by thinking of the endocrine, cardiovascular, nervous, and skeletal systems.

Endocrine system: This would bring to mind the coarse facial features of myxedema and cretinism, the proptosis of hyperthyroidism, the moon face of Cushing syndrome, and the square protruding jaw of acromegaly. It would also suggest the Peter Pan face of hypopituitarism.

Cardiovascular system: This should prompt the recall of the malar flush in mitral stenosis and the cyanosis of congenital heart disease. Facial edema is seen in superior vena cava syndrome and nephritis.

Nervous system: This should suggest the masked face of Parkinsonism, the hatchet-shaped face of myotonic dystrophy, the snarl of myasthenia gravis, and the drawing

of the face to one side in Bell palsy with flattening of the nasolabial fold. It should also suggest the expressionless face and often drooling mouth of bulbar and pseudobulbar palsy and sarcastic smile of patients with tetanus.

Skeletal system: This would bring to mind the protruding forehead of Paget disease and the wide separation of the eyes in hypertelorism.

Aside from these disorders it is well to recall the flushing of the face in alcoholism, Cushing syndrome, carcinoid syndrome, and menopause as well as the waxy nonwrinkled face of scleroderma and the oriental appearance of the face in mongolism.

● Approach to the Diagnosis

Obviously, the workup of abnormal facies will depend on what disease is suggested by the facial appearance combined with other abnormalities of the physical and neurologic examination. A careful history will be helpful in many cases.

FAILURE TO THRIVE

Failure to thrive is germane to the pediatric patient who is not growing adequately or fails to gain weight and appears emaciated. The physiologic model of intake, absorption, transport, and utilization will help develop a differential diagnosis.

Intake: Intake of food may be impaired by social conditions of poverty, malnutrition, and child abuse. It may also be impaired by chronic anxiety and depression or other psychiatric disorders. Finally, the patient may not eat because of a neurologic disorder such as microcephaly, hydrocephalus, cerebral palsy, or other disorders associated with mental retardation (see page 295).

Absorption: Absorption of food may be impaired by malabsorption syndrome and fibrocystic disease.

Transport: This topic brings to mind chronic anemia and congenital heart disease especially when associated with hypoxemia.

Utilization: Utilization of food is impaired in diabetes mellitus, hypothyroidism, pituitary insufficiency, galactosemia, and uremia.

Several chronic infectious diseases are associated with failure to thrive. The child may also come from an abnormal gestation where the mother suffered alcoholism, drug abuse, or chronic illness.

● Approach to the Diagnosis

Routine diagnostic workup should include a CBC, sedimentation rate, urinalysis, urine culture, chemistry panel, sweat test, stool for quantitative fat, chest x-ray, and electrocardiogram (ECG). Bone age x-rays are helpful in determining growth retardation. At this point, it is helpful to consult a pediatrician before ordering expensive diagnostic tests. When studies are negative, consider constitutional growth delay as the cause.

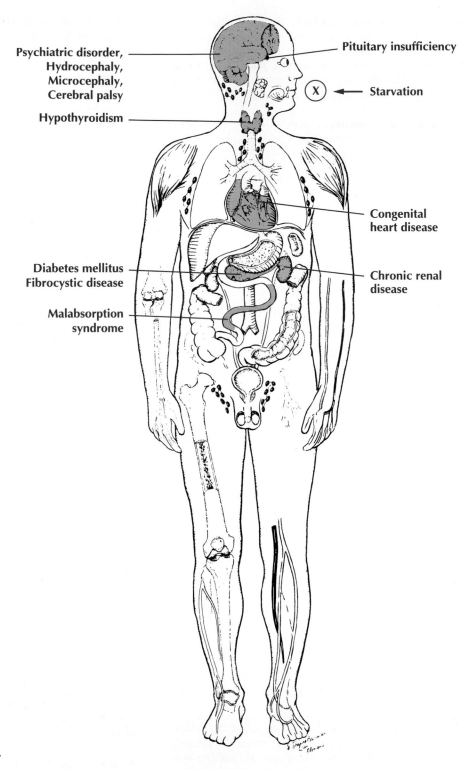

Psychiatric disorder,
Hydrocephaly,
Microcephaly,
Cerebral palsy

Pituitary insufficiency

Starvation

Hypothyroidism

Congenital
heart disease

Diabetes mellitus
Fibrocystic disease

Chronic renal
disease

Malabsorption
syndrome

● **FIGURE 3** Failure to thrive.

● Other Useful Tests

1. D-xylose absorption test (malabsorption syndrome)
2. Stool for ova and parasites (intestinal parasites)
3. Serum growth hormone (pituitary insufficiency)
4. Somatomedin-C level (pituitary insufficiency)
5. Overnight dexamethasone suppression test (adreno-genital syndrome)
6. Thyroid profile (myxedema)
7. CT scan of the brain (hydrocephalus, etc.)
8. MRI of the brain (hydrocephalus)
9. Neurology consult
10. Orthopedic consult
11. Endocrinology consult
12. Buccal smear for Barr bodies (Turner syndrome)
13. Karyotyping (Turner syndrome)

FASCICULATIONS

This sign is generally considered pathognomonic for anterior horn cell or root disease. It may occur, however, in certain cases of peripheral neuropathy, in electrolyte disturbances, and in myasthenia gravis, especially under treatment. It is also found in healthy states, most commonly in the twitching of the orbicularis oculi muscle from nervous tension or eyestrain. Fasciculations must be distinguished from fibrillations that are not visible, are detected only with EMG, and are caused by muscle disease. The causes can easily be recalled by visualizing the anterior horn cells and nerves and applying the mnemonic **VINDICATE** to this area.

V—**Vascular** conditions include anterior spinal artery occlusion and intermittent claudication from peripheral vascular disease.
I—**Inflammatory** diseases include poliomyelitis, viral encephalomyelitis, tetanus, syphilis, and diphtheria.
N—**Neoplasm** suggests intramedullary tumors of the cord such as ependymomas, and extramedullary tumors such as meningioma, Hodgkin lymphoma, metastatic carcinoma, and multiple myeloma must be considered.
D—**Degenerative** diseases are the most important causes of fasciculations. They include progressive spinal muscular atrophy, amyotrophic lateral sclerosis, Werdnig–Hoffmann disease, and syringomyelia.
I—**Intoxication** includes lead poisoning and alcoholism.
C—**Congenital** disorders suggest Werdnig–Hoffmann disease, spondylolisthesis, and other anomalies of the spinal cord that may compress the anterior horn and roots.
A—**Autoimmune** disorders recall transverse myelitis, myasthenia gravis (under treatment), periarteritis nodosa, and Guillain–Barré syndrome.
T—**Trauma** suggests herniated discs and fractures that compress the anterior horn or roots.
E—**Endocrine** and metabolic diseases include hypoparathyroidism and other causes of tetany, magnesium deficiency and other electrolyte disturbances, diabetic myelopathy, and hypothyroid myopathy (more commonly the cause of fibrillations which can only be detected by EMG).

● Approach to the Diagnosis

Deciding on the cause of fasciculations will usually be based on other neurologic symptoms and signs. Muscular atrophy without sensory changes suggests progressive muscular atrophy, whereas atrophy and fasciculations with sensory changes suggest syringomyelia, peripheral neuropathy, and root compression (e.g., a herniated disc). Treatable neurologic disorders should be considered first. Thus, x-rays of the spine, spinal fluid analysis, and MRI should be performed to rule out a space-occupying lesion. EMG is useful in detecting which level is involved and in following the progress of the disease. Serum electrolytes, calcium, phosphorus, and magnesium levels are useful in selected disorders.

● Other Useful Tests

1. Blood lead level (lead poisoning)
2. Glucose tolerance test (diabetes mellitus)
3. Serum protein electrophoresis (polyclonal gammopathy)
4. Antinuclear antibody (ANA) analysis (collagen disease)
5. Nerve conduction velocity (NCV) test (peripheral neuropathy)
6. Free thyroxine and sensitive thyroid-stimulating hormone (S-TSH) levels (hypothyroid myopathy)
7. Acetylcholine receptor antibody titer (myasthenia gravis)
8. CT scan of the thoracic or lumbar spine (space-occupying lesion)
9. MRI of the cervical, thoracic, or lumbar spine (space-occupying lesion)
10. Neurology consult
11. Muscle biopsy

FEVER

The differential diagnosis of fever is best developed using **physiology** first and **anatomy** second.

Physiology: Increased heat in the body is caused by increased production or decreased elimination or dysfunction of the thermoregulatory system in the brain. Increased production of heat occurs in conditions with increased metabolic rate such as hyperthyroidism, pheochromocytomas, and malignant neoplasms. Poor elimination of heat may occur in congestive heart failure (CHF) (poor circulation through the skin) and conditions where the sweat glands are absent (congenital) or poorly functioning (heat stroke). Most cases of fever are caused by the effect of toxins on the thermoregulatory centers in the brain. These toxins may be exogenous from drugs, bacteria (endotoxins), parasites, fungi, rickettsiae, and virus particles, or they may be endogenous from tissue injury (trauma) and breakdown (carcinomas, leukemia, infarctions, and autoimmune disease).

Anatomy: With the etiologies suggested by the mnemonic **VINDICATE**, one can apply anatomy and the various organ systems and make a useful chart (see Table 28). The infections should be divided into the **systemic diseases** that affect more than one organ, such as typhoid, brucellosis, tuberculosis, syphilis, acquired immunodeficiency syndrome (AIDS), leptospirosis, Lyme disease, and bacterial endocarditis, and the **localized diseases** that usually affect the same specific organ, such as infectious hepatitis, subacute thyroiditis, pneumococcal pneumonia, and cholera. It is wise to divide the localized infectious diseases into the "**itises**" (e.g., pneumonitis, hepatitis, and prostatitis) and the **abscesses** (dental abscess, empyema, perinephric abscess, liver abscess, and subdiaphragmatic abscess).

Also, when the physician attempts to recall the specific infections, he or she can group them into six categories beginning with the smallest organism and working up to the largest as follows: viruses, rickettsiae, bacteria, spirochetes, fungi, and parasites. Endogenous toxins released by infarctions of various organs form another convenient

Table 28 Fever

	V Vascular	I Inflammatory	N Neoplasm	D Degenerative	I Intoxication	C Congenital	A Autoimmune Allergic	T Trauma	E Endocrine Metabolic
Brain	Occlusion Infarction Hemorrhage	Meningitis Encephalitis Abscess Epidural abscess	Glioma Metastasis		Pyrogen Endotoxin Heat stroke	Ruptured aneurysm	Collagen disease	Epidural and sub-dural hematomas Cerebral contusion	Pituitary tumor
Ear, Nose, and Throat		Otitis media Mastoiditis Petrositis Dental abscess							
Lungs	Pulmonary infarction	Pneumonia Lung abscess Empyema Tuberculosis	Carcinoma			Bronchiectasis	Wegener granulomatosis Periarteritis nodosa Lupus erythematosus	Contusion Hemorrhage	
Heart	Myocardial infarction	Myocarditis Subacute bacterial endocarditis					Collagen disease	Hemopericardium Contusion	
Liver and Biliary Tract	Budd–Chiari syndrome Pyelophlebitis	Hepatitis Amebic abscess Cholangitis Cholecystitis Diaphragmatic abscess	Hematoma Metastasis Hodgkin lymphoma		Alcoholic cirrhosis Toxic hepatitis Calculus		Collagen disease	Contusion Laceration	
Pancreas		Pancreatitis Pancreatic cyst	Carcinoma						Diabetes mellitus

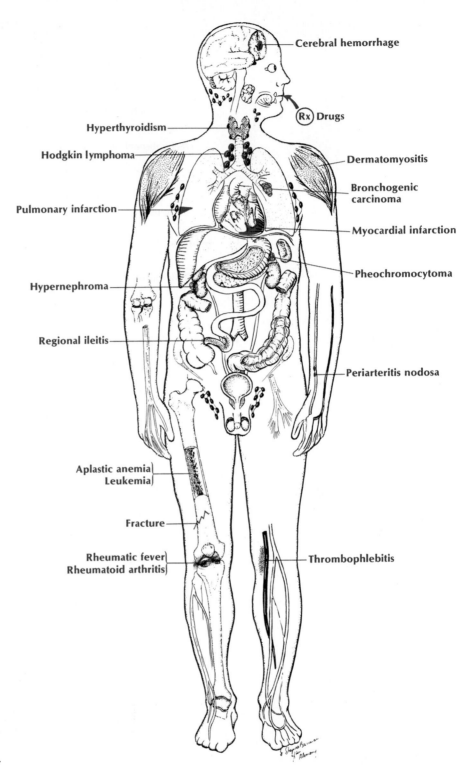

Cerebral hemorrhage

Rx Drugs

Hyperthyroidism

Hodgkin lymphoma

Dermatomyositis

Bronchogenic carcinoma

Pulmonary infarction

Myocardial infarction

Pheochromocytoma

Hypernephroma

Regional ileitis

Periarteritis nodosa

Aplastic anemia
Leukemia

Fracture

Rheumatic fever
Rheumatoid arthritis

Thrombophlebitis

● **FIGURE 4** Fever, noninfectious causes.

F

group. Finally, the most common neoplasms to cause fever (by tissue breakdown) are illustrated on page 172.

● Approach to the Diagnosis

There are certain things to remember when a patient with fever is approached. First, a mild elevation up to 100.5°F (38°C) rectally may be normal in some people. Second, one should rule out malingering by the patient or incorrect recording by hospital personnel. A normal sedimentation rate is found in factitious fever. Finally, psychogenic disorders must be ruled out.

The duration and severity of the fever are important. If possible, a careful chart of the fever should be made with

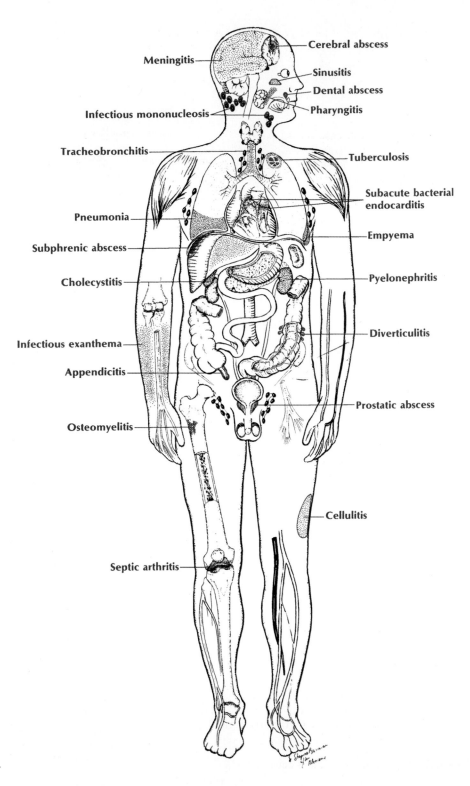

● **FIGURE 5** Fever, infectious causes.

the patient off all drugs (especially aspirin and steroids). Conditions with intermittent or relapsing fever such as brucellosis, malaria, and Mediterranean fever will be elucidated in this fashion (see Table 28).

The association with other symptoms is important. Fever, right upper quadrant pain, and jaundice suggest cholecystitis or cholangitis, whereas fever with right-sided flank pain suggests pyelonephritis. After taking a few moments to jot down the differential diagnosis before launching into the history and physical examination, one can question and examine the patient more appropriately. The differential diagnosis will also lead to more appropriate use of laboratory testing. A serum procalcitonin will distinguish bacterial infections from viral infections.

● Other Useful Tests

1. CBC (infectious disease, leukemia)
2. Urinalysis (urinary tract infection [UTI])
3. Sedimentation rate (infectious disease, collagen disease)
4. Chemistry panel (liver disease, renal disease)
5. Smear and culture of discharge from any body orifice or skin (e.g., abscess)
6. Blood cultures (septicemia, bacterial endocarditis)
7. Urine culture (pyelonephritis)
8. Bone marrow smear and culture (subacute bacterial endocarditis [SBE])
9. Stool for ova and parasites (e.g., amebiasis)
10. Blood smear for parasites and spirochetes (e.g., malaria)
11. Febrile agglutinins (*Salmonella*, brucellosis)
12. Monospot test (infectious mononucleosis)
13. Cold agglutinins (*Mycoplasma pneumoniae*)
14. ANA (collagen disease)
15. Serum protein electrophoresis (multiple myeloma, collagen disease)
16. Sickle cell preparation (sickle cell crisis)
17. Urine porphobilinogen (porphyria)
18. Fibrin index (Mediterranean fever)
19. *Trichinella* skin test or serology (trichinosis)
20. Acute- and convalescent-phase sera for viral studies
21. Spinal fluid analysis (meningitis)
22. Urine for etiocholanolone (etiocholanolone fever)
23. Tuberculin test
24. Fungal skin test
25. Frei test (lymphogranuloma venereum)
26. Kveim test (sarcoidosis)
27. Angiotensin-converting enzyme level (sarcoidosis)
28. Chest x-ray (tuberculosis, pneumonia)
29. Flat plate of the abdomen (liver, spleen size, peritonitis stones)
30. X-ray of hands (sarcoidosis)
31. Gallbladder ultrasound (cholelithiasis)
32. Intravenous pyelogram (IVP) (hypernephroma, renal calculi)
33. Barium enema (neoplasm, diverticulitis)
34. CT scan of abdomen and pelvis (abscess)
35. CT scan of chest and mediastinum (abscess, neoplasm)
36. Bone scan (osteomyelitis, metastatic tumor)
37. X-ray of teeth (dental abscess)
38. Indium scan (abscess)
39. Liver biopsy (hepatic neoplasm, hepatitis, abscess)
40. Lymph node biopsy (inflammation, metastatic neoplasm)
41. Muscle biopsy (collagen disease, trichinosis)
42. Human immunodeficiency virus (HIV) antibody titer (AIDS)
43. Antistreptolysin-O (ASO) titer (rheumatic fever)
44. Epstein–Barr virus (EBV) immunoglobulins (infectious mononucleosis)
45. Transesophageal echocardiography (endocarditis)
46. ELISA (Lyme disease)

Case Presentation #27

A 16-year-old white boy is referred to you with a history of sore throat and intermittent fever for 10 days. He was treated with penicillin by his family physician 1 week ago but failed to respond. On inspection, he is found to have a rash of the trunk and extremities.

Question #1. Utilizing the methods discussed above, what is your list of possibilities at this point?

Further examination discloses generalized lymphadenopathy and mild splenomegaly.

Question #2. What is your diagnosis now?

(See Appendix B for the answers.)

FLANK MASS

A flank mass is usually renal in origin. However, if the clinician immediately focuses on the kidney, he or she may be sadly mistaken because one forgets the other significant organs in the area. By realizing the anatomy of the area, the clinician will not be readily fooled. Starting with the abdominal wall, there may be a tumor, hematoma, or hernia. Penetrating deeper, one encounters the kidney and adrenal gland. Disorders of the kidney may be recalled by the mnemonic **MINT**.

M—**Malformations** include hydronephrosis, solitary cysts, and polycystic kidneys.
I—**Inflammation** brings to mind a perinephric abscess and tuberculosis.
N—**Neoplasms** help to recall Wilms tumors and hypernephroma.
T—**Trauma** leads one to consider a hematoma or laceration of the kidney.

Looking at the adrenal gland, one need only recall the tumors of this gland such as a neuroblastoma, adrenocortical carcinoma, or pheochromocytoma. Surprisingly, other organs located near the flank may be palpated as a flank mass. In the right flank an enlarged liver (see page 220). As in the right upper quadrant, a carcinoma or collection of stool can be palpated in the flank. A pancreatic cyst or neoplasm may also present as a left flank mass. Rarely an ovarian cyst or tumor may present as a flank mass. Moving into the retroperitoneal area, we again may find hematomas of the wall of the flank, bony tumors, and retroperitoneal sarcomas.

● Approach to the Diagnosis

The history of trauma will be helpful in narrowing the diagnosis. If the mass is painful, it is more likely due to trauma or inflammation. If it is painless, a neoplasm or congenital malformation is more plausible. Obviously,

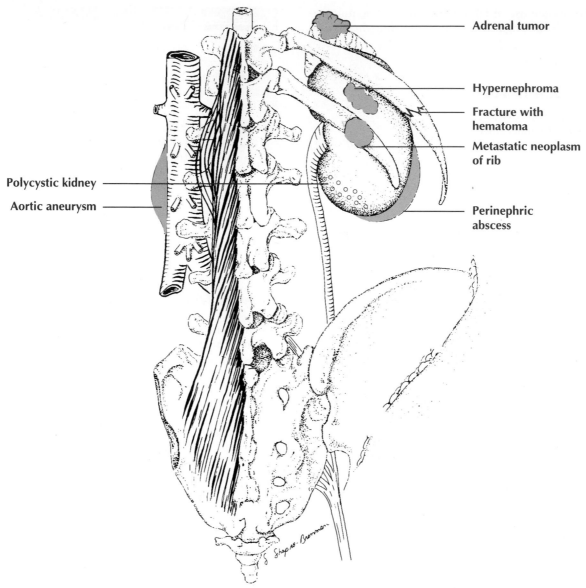

Adrenal tumor

Hypernephroma

Fracture with hematoma

Metastatic neoplasm of rib

Perinephric abscess

Polycystic kidney

Aortic aneurysm

● **FIGURE 6** Flank mass.

if there is fever a perinephric abscess, pyonephrosis, or tuberculosis is more likely. Turning to the laboratory, a CBC, urinalysis, urine culture and colony count, chemistry panel, and sedimentation rate should be ordered. x-Ray diagnosis may be made with an IVP, but a more definitive diagnosis can be established with a CT scan of the abdomen. It is wise to consult a urologist before ordering any x-ray procedure to help decide which is the most cost-effective approach.

● **Other Useful Tests**

1. Sonogram (neoplasm, cyst)
2. VDRL test (aneurysm)
3. Renal angiogram (aneurysm, hemorrhage)
4. Cystoscopy and retrograde pyelography (hydronephrosis, neoplasm)
5. Exploratory surgery

Case Presentation #28

A 46-year-old male executive was found to have a large right flank mass on routine physical examination. His blood pressure was 190/110 mm Hg.

Question #1. Visualizing the anatomy of the right flank and cross-indexing each structure with the etiology classification, what would be your list of possible causes at this point?

Further history reveals the patient has noted painless hematuria on a couple of occasions but is otherwise asymptomatic. Physical examination is unremarkable aside from the large nontender mass in the right flank. Laboratory studies show polycythemia and microscopic hematuria.

Question #2. What is your list of possibilities now?

(See Appendix B for the answers.)

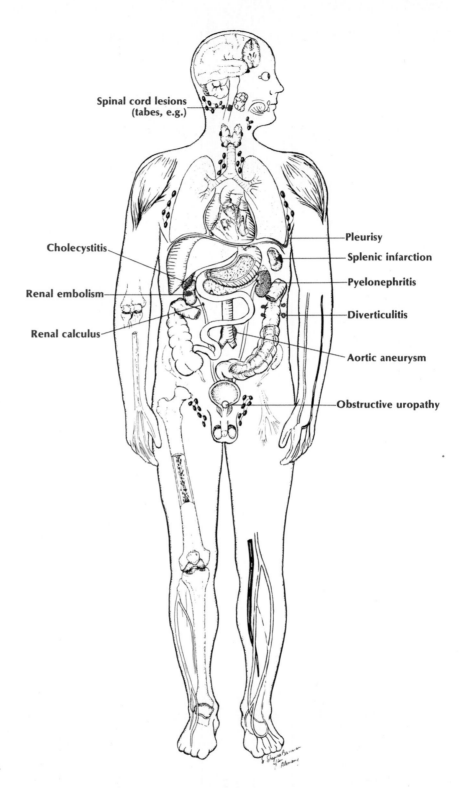

Spinal cord lesions
(tabes, e.g.)

Cholecystitis

Renal embolism

Renal calculus

Pleurisy

Splenic infarction

Pyelonephritis

Diverticulitis

Aortic aneurysm

Obstructive uropathy

● **FIGURE 7** Flank pain.

FLANK PAIN

Most cases of flank pain are associated with inflammation of the kidney. As is shown in Table 29, however, jumping to that conclusion in any given case may be hazardous.

In addition to the kidney (pyelonephritis and perinephric abscess), inflammation of the **skin** (herpes zoster), the **colon** (diverticulitis and colitis), the **gallbladder** (cholecystitis), and the **spine** (epidural abscess and Pott disease) may also cause flank pain. The mnemonic **VINDICATE** also suggests several vascular disorders that are significant causes of flank pain such as aortic aneurysms, embolic nephritis, and mesenteric thrombosis. Neoplasms of the kidney and colon are less likely to produce pain unless they are complicated by infection. However, trauma of the kidney and spine and renal calculi—whether due to hyperparathyroidism, idiopathic etiologies,

TABLE 29 Flank Pain

	V Vascular	I Inflammatory	N Neoplasm	D Degenerative	I Intoxication Idiopathic	C Congenital Acquired Malformation	A Autoimmune	T Trauma	E Endocrine
Skin		Cellulitis Herpes zoster						Contusion Laceration	
Muscle and Fascia		Trichinosis				Hernia	Dermatomyositis	Contusion	
Colon	Mesenteric thrombosis	Colitis	Carcinoma			Diverticulitis Appendix	Ulcerative colitis Granulomatous colitis	Contusion Laceration	
Gallbladder		Cholecystitis Cholangitis	Carcinoma						
Adrenal Gland									Hemorrhage Infarction Tumor
Kidney	Embolism Thrombosis	Pyelonephritis Perinephric abscess	Wilms tumor Hypernephroma		Gout Toxic nephritis Crush syndrome	Obstruction Infection due to malformation	Periarteritis nodosa Vasculitis of other cause	Contusion Laceration	Calculus due to hyperparathyroidism
Aorta	Aneurysm							Rupture	
Vena Cava	Thrombosis								
Spine		Osteomyelitis Tuberculosis	Metastatic carcinoma	Osteoarthritis			Marie–Strümpell disease	Fracture Herniated disc	
Spinal Cord and Nerves	Anterior spinal artery occlusion	Tabes dorsalis Myelitis Epidural abscess	Spinal cord tumor		Arsenic poisoning Porphyria	Syringomyelia	Guillain–Barré syndrome	Hematoma	

or hyperuricemia—are important causes. Neoplasms of the spinal cord and tabes dorsalis must also be considered.

● Approach to the Diagnosis

The diagnosis of flank pain usually involves careful examination of the urine and a urine culture, an IVP, and plain films of the abdomen and spine. If these are negative, bone scans, arteriogram, and other tests listed below may be required. CT has eliminated the need for exploratory laparotomy in many cases. Noncontrast helical CT scan has the greatest specificity for renal stones (95% to 100%).

● Other Useful Tests

1. Urology consult
2. Neurology consult
3. CBC
4. Chemistry panel (uremia, renal calculi)
5. CT scan of the abdomen and pelvis (neoplasms, stones, hemorrhage abscess)
6. x-Rays of the thoracolumbar spine (bone metastasis, herniated disc)
7. MRI of the thoracic spine (neoplasms, herniated disc)
8. Sonogram (renal cyst)
9. Urine for acid-fast bacillus (AFB) smear and culture (tuberculosis)
10. Cystoscopy and retrograde pyelography (malformations, neoplasm)
11. Protein electrophoresis (multiple myeloma)

Case Presentation #29

A 36-year-old black woman complained of severe left flank pain for 3 days. She denies fever, dysuria, or hematuria.

Question #1. Utilizing the methods discovered above, what would be your list of possibilities at this point?

Physical examination is unremarkable except for hyperesthesia and hyperalgesia in the distribution of T_{12} dermatome on the left. Urinalysis is negative.

Question #2. What diagnosis would you consider most likely now?

(See Appendix B for the answers.)

FLASHES OF LIGHT

Flashes of light usually result from involvement of the retina, optic nerve, optic cortex, or the arterial circulation to these areas.

1. **Retina:** Conditions of the retina to be considered in this symptom are exudative choroiditis, retinal detachment, venous thrombosis, and embolism.
2. **Optic nerve:** Optic neuritis at the onset may cause flashes of light. Multiple sclerosis is prone to present this way.
3. **Optic cortex:** Transient ischemic attacks in the posterior cerebral circulation and epileptic auras may cause this symptom.

4. **Arterial circulation to the eye and brain:** Migraine, cerebral thrombosis, and emboli present with this symptom.

● Approach to the Diagnosis

This is similar to the workup of blurred vision (see page 76).

FLATULENCE AND BORBORYGMI

Flatulence is increased output of gas by mouth or rectum. Borborygmi are audible sounds of hyperperistalsis of gas. Both are caused by similar physiologic mechanisms. The increase of gas in the intestinal tract depends on three physiologic mechanisms:

1. **Increased intake of air:** This is probably one of the most frequent causes of flatulence and borborygmi. Aerophagia in neurosis is a well-known psychogenic cause. However, compulsive eating, compulsive drinking, excessive smoking, or excessive talking may produce the same effect. All of us take in a certain amount of air when we swallow food or liquids. When we overeat, however, or when we drink too much, the amount of gas taken in may exceed our ability to absorb it. Salesmen and public speakers have an additional problem because talking increases salivation and swallowing, and frequently air is swallowed between sentences.

   Some people have a particular beverage they are fond of, such as cola, coffee, or alcohol. Excessive drinking of these beverages entails the swallowing of excess air. In addition, some of these beverages release gas after ingestion (carbonated beverages especially), which causes flatulence. Reflux esophagitis is a frequent cause.
2. **Increased production of gas in the intestinal tract:** In acute bacterial gastroenteritis (e.g., *Salmonella* and *Shigella*), gas-producing organisms multiply and produce excess gas. The diarrhea or vomiting associated with these disorders usually makes the diagnosis easy. A more obscure cause of increased production of gas is chronic mild intestinal obstruction leading to excessive bacterial overgrowth. Adhesions, intestinal polyps, regional ileitis, and the various causes of paralytic ileus (e.g., anticholinergic drugs, tranquilizers, uremia, and chronic anoxia) cause increased gas production by this mechanism. Gas production is also increased when bacteria are allowed to accumulate in large numbers in chronic intestinal disorders. The blind loop syndrome, diverticulitis, and Meckel diverticulum fall into this category. Some types of irritation in the intestinal tract cause a mild paralytic ileus and allow bacteria to multiply and ferment: Esophagitis and hiatal hernia, chronic gastritis, ulcers, regional ileitis, and ulcerative and mucous colitis may cause mild paralytic ileus on this basis.

   When the amount of digestive juices is insufficient to digest food, more food is available for bacterial fermentation. Thus, in chronic atrophic gastritis, the reduced level of hydrochloric acid leaves undigested food for bacterial action. In cholecystitis and partial bile duct obstruction or liver disease, there are insufficient bile acids for digestion and more food is left for bacterial fermentation. In chronic pancreatitis, the reduction in pancreatic enzymes causes the same problem. Lactase deficiency leaves food for fermentation.

3. **Decreased absorption of gas:** Malabsorption syndromes cause this condition. In acute gastroenteritis, the swollen inflamed intestines cannot absorb the gas. Intestinal motility may be so rapid that there is not enough time for absorption. In celiac disease, the atrophied villi cannot pick up food and gas, and these are passed through the intestines. Intestinal parasites may preempt food from absorption and produce excessive gas in their own digestive processes.

● Approach to the Diagnosis

If excessive food, beverages, or air swallowing from nervous tension or talking can be excluded, reflux esophagitis and diverticulitis must be considered. Upper gastrointestinal (GI) series, esophagram, small-bowel

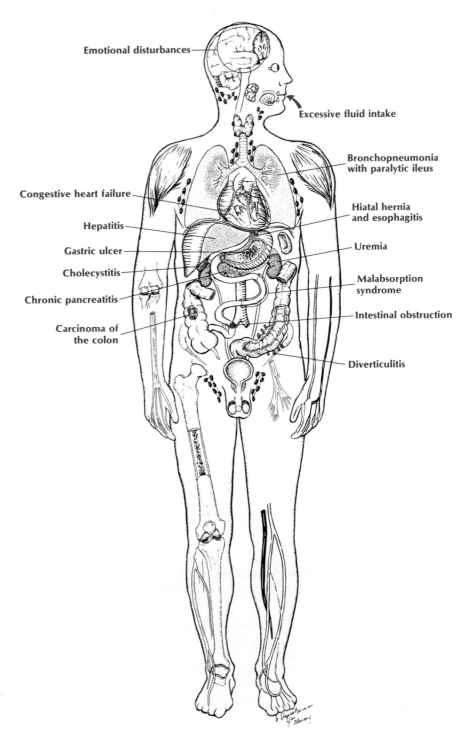

Emotional disturbances

Excessive fluid intake

Bronchopneumonia with paralytic ileus

Congestive heart failure

Hiatal hernia and esophagitis

Hepatitis

Uremia

Gastric ulcer

Cholecystitis

Malabsorption syndrome

Chronic pancreatitis

Intestinal obstruction

Carcinoma of the colon

Diverticulitis

● **FIGURE 8** Flatulence and borborygmi.

series, and sigmoidoscopy with a barium enema should be done. A gallbladder series is also ordered. If these findings are questionable, a more definitive diagnosis may be made with endoscopy. Stools for ova, parasites, blood, and cultures should be done. When the outcome is still uncertain, evaluation of the adequacy of the intestinal digestive secretions is worthwhile. Gastric analysis with Histalog and duodenal analysis for bicarbonate, bile, and pancreatic enzymes is done. A lactose tolerance test should be done. If the digestive secretions are adequate, a small-bowel biopsy may be necessary to exclude a malabsorption syndrome. Xylose absorption is a good screening test for this.

● Other Useful Tests

1. Amylase and lipase levels (chronic pancreatitis)
2. Stool for trypsin (chronic pancreatitis)
3. Quantitative stool fat (malabsorption syndrome)
4. Liver function test (chronic hepatic disease)
5. Urine 5-hydroxyindole acetic acid (5-HIAA) (carcinoid syndrome)
6. Esophagoscopy (reflux esophagitis)
7. Gastroscopy (gastric ulcer, neoplasm)
8. Colonoscopy (diverticulitis, colitis)
9. Analysis of flatus (aerophagia, carbohydrate intolerance)
10. Hydrogen breath test (carbohydrate intolerance, bacterial overgrowth)
11. Schilling test (pernicious anemia)
12. Therapeutic trial of proton pump inhibitors (reflux esophagitis)

Case Presentation #30

A 67-year-old white man complained of increasing burping, indigestion, and hiccoughs for the past year. His appetite has decreased and he has lost 15 lb during that time. There is also occasional constipation. Physical examination is unremarkable except for pale conjunctiva and a smooth tongue.

Question #1. What would your list of possibilities be at this point?

An upper GI series and barium enema were unremarkable. His stools tested negative for occult blood. Hemoglobin was 7.2 g.

Question #2. What are the most likely diagnoses at this point?

(See Appendix B for the answers.)

FLUSHED FACE (PLETHORA)

Not everyone with a red face should be classified as an alcoholic. The causes of this symptom can best be established with the help of **physiology**. A flushed face may result from an increased amount of circulating blood (polycythemia) or from any factor that may dilate the blood vessels in the face.

Polycythemia may be primary, as in polycythemia vera, or secondary, as in Cushing syndrome, unilateral renal disease, hypernephroma, and pulmonary or cardiovascular disease associated with chronic anoxia. Capillary dilatation may result from serotonin output in carcinoid syndrome, from vasomotor instability of menopause, from chronic alcoholism (which causes direct capillary dilatation), from sunburn or any burn that damages the capillaries and precapillary arterioles so that they cannot contract, and from mitral stenosis, where the back pressure from the heart causes congestion of the capillaries. It is less commonly found in the use of belladonna, alkaloids, histamine headaches (usually unilateral), and cirrhosis of the liver, but it is common in chronic skin diseases of the face such as acne rosacea.

● Approach to the Diagnosis

The clinical picture will often point to the diagnosis. For example, a flushed face with obesity would suggest Cushing syndrome. A flushed face with a heart murmur would suggest mitral stenosis or a right to left shunt with polycythemia. A flushed face with wheezing would suggest pulmonary emphysema. A flushed face and chronic diarrhea would prompt one to consider a carcinoid syndrome.

The initial workup should include a CBC, chemistry panel, arterial blood gas analysis, urinalysis, chest x-ray, and ECG. If carcinoid syndrome is suspected, a urine test for 5-HIAA is ordered. If alcoholism is suspected, a blood alcohol level can be done. If menopause is suspected, serum follicle-stimulating hormone (FSH) and luteinizing hormone levels should be ordered. If Cushing syndrome is suspected, a serum cortisol level and a cortisol suppression test could be done. If systemic mastocytosis is suspected, a skin or muscle biopsy may be done.

● Other Useful Tests

1. Blood volume (polycythemia vera)
2. Serum erythropoietin level (primary and secondary polycythemia)
3. Serum gastrin level (gastrinoma)
4. Pulmonary function tests (pulmonary emphysema)
5. 24-hour vanillylmandelic acid test (pheochromocytoma)
6. Bone marrow examination (polycythemia vera)

Case Presentation #31

A 46-year-old white woman complained that for the past year she has had increasing episodes of flushing of the face and neck, especially during exercise or stress.

Question #1. What diagnosis should you entertain considering the physiology involved in this symptom?

Further history reveals that she has had chronic diarrhea for a couple of years as well. Physical examination revealed telangiectasias of the face and neck and mild hepatomegaly.

Question #2. What is your diagnosis now?

(See Appendix B for the answers.)

FOOT, HEEL, AND TOE PAIN

Many patients presenting with pain in the foot or toes have joint disease (see pages 276 and 278 for a discussion of these differentials). Other anatomic components of the foot and toes may cause pain as well, so a consideration of the differential diagnosis of foot and toe pain must include diseases of these structures.

Let us develop our list by moving from the skin inward. Many of these conditions are illustrated on page 184 (see Table 30). Painful conditions of the **skin** include warts, calluses, bunions, and corns, conditions often caused by bad posture and poor-fitting shoes. Ingrown toenails may be found. Herpes zoster in this location is unusual. Moving to the **subcutaneous tissue** and **fascia**, cellulitis and plantar fasciitis are suggested. In plantar fasciitis, a spur of the

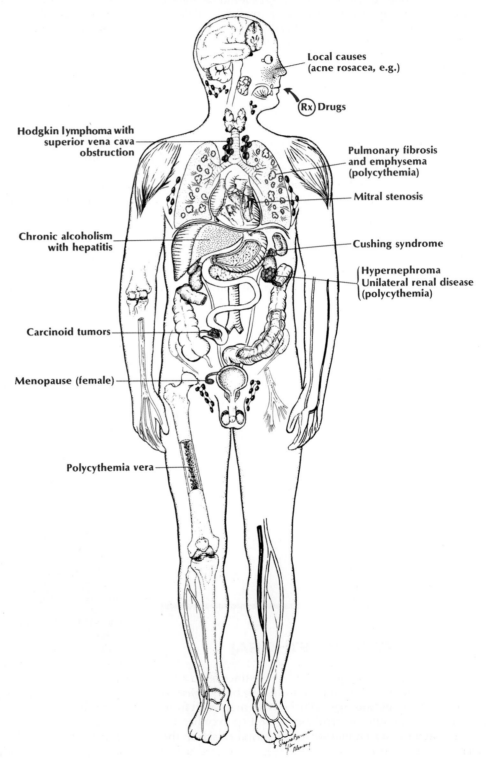

Local causes
(acne rosacea, e.g.)

Rx Drugs

Hodgkin lymphoma with
superior vena cava
obstruction

Pulmonary fibrosis
and emphysema
(polycythemia)

Mitral stenosis

Chronic alcoholism
with hepatitis

Cushing syndrome

Hypernephroma
Unilateral renal disease
(polycythemia)

Carcinoid tumors

Menopause (female)

Polycythemia vera

● **FIGURE 9** Flushed face (plethora).

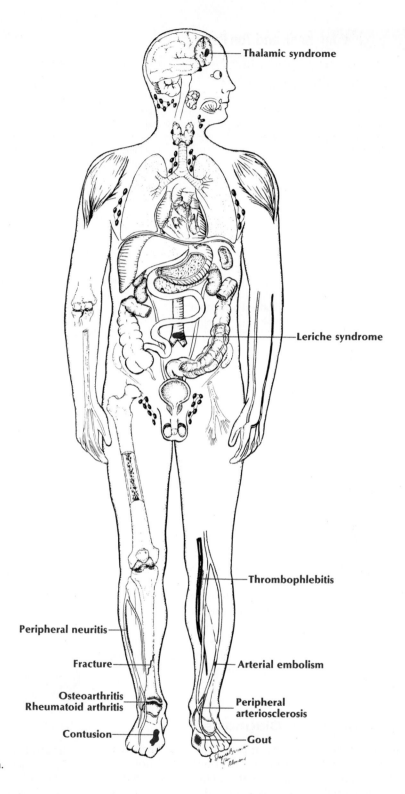

Thalamic syndrome

Leriche syndrome

Thrombophlebitis

Peripheral neuritis

Arterial embolism

Fracture

Osteoarthritis
Rheumatoid arthritis

Peripheral
arteriosclerosis

Contusion

Gout

● **FIGURE 10** Foot, heel, and toe pain.

F

calcaneus will be found on the x-ray. Achilles bursitis and tendonitis are suggested in this layer. These conditions are often associated with Reiter syndrome and ankylosing spondylitis. The **veins** may be involved by phlebitis and hemorrhage.

The **arteries** may be inflamed in Buerger disease and periarteritis nodosa; they are painfully obstructed in the arteriolar sclerosis of diabetes mellitus and arteriosclerosis. Emboli may be a cause of foot pain. Raynaud disease may also affect the foot. The **nerves** of the foot may be involved by the many causes of peripheral neuropathy, as well as herniated lumbosacral discs and cauda equina tumors; the radiation of the pain should suggest the latter two conditions. Trapping of the plantar tibial nerve may

TABLE 30	**Foot, Heel, and Toe Pain**				
	M **Malformation**	**I** **Inflammation**	**N** **Neoplasm**	**T** **Trauma**	**S** **Systemic Disease**
Skin	Ingrown toenail	Herpes zoster Cellulitis		Callus Bunion	
Subcutaneous Tissue and Fascia		Cellulitis Plantar fasciitis			
Arteries		Vasculitis Erythromelalgia		Hemorrhage Contusion Aneurysm	Diabetes Periarteritis nodosa Buerger disease
Veins	Varicose vein	Thrombophlebitis		Hemorrhage	Buerger disease
Nerves	Hypertrophic polyneuritis Peroneal muscular atrophy Plantar entrapment syndrome Fabrys disease	Tuberculosis of spine	Neuroma Cauda equina tumor	Contusion Compression Laceration	Diabetic neuropathy
Bones	Pes planus Pes cavus Talipes equinovarus	Osteomyelitis Kohler disease	Primary and metastatic neoplasms	Fracture	Hyperparathyroidism Sickle cell anemia
Joints		Rheumatoid arthritis Gout Osteoarthritis Pseudogout		Traumatic synovitis	Gout Rheumatic fever Reiter syndrome

cause pain just like the carpal tunnel syndrome in the hand. Metatarsalgia may be caused by a plantar digital neuroma. Morton neuromas are most commonly found in the second and third interdigital space. Tracing the arteries centrally will suggest Leriche syndrome, whereas tracing the nerves centrally will suggest a thalamic syndrome.

Finally, the **bones** may be involved by fractures, by deformities such as pes planus, pes cavus, talipes equinovarus, and hallux valgus and by many postural defects. Kohler disease is aseptic bone necrosis in the calcaneus (considered in the section on joint pain, page 276). Stress fractures, Achilles tendonitis, and tarsal tunnel syndrome are common in runners.

● Approach to the Diagnosis

Special considerations in the approach to the diagnosis of foot pain include examining the shoes for abnormal areas of wear and tear, measuring the arches, palpating the joints for maximal tenderness, and ordering laboratory tests for joint disease (page 278). Nerve blocks and lidocaine injections in the plantar fascia and other areas of maximum tenderness will assist in diagnosis. Abnormal weight distribution is diagnosed by quantitative scintigraphs. A therapeutic trial of proper-fitting shoes and arches may be indicated. Weight control is essential in the obese. Referral to a podiatrist or orthopedic surgeon is often necessary.

● Other Useful Tests

1. x-Ray of the feet (fracture, dislocation)
2. Doppler studies (arterial and venous insufficiency)
3. Bone scan (osteomyelitis, fracture)
4. EMG and NCV (peripheral neuropathy)
5. Angiogram (arteriosclerosis)
6. Venogram (deep vein thrombosis)
7. CT scan (fracture, tumor)
8. MRI (stress fracture)
9. CT scan or MRI of lumbar spine (herniated disc)
10. Arthritis panel

Case Presentation #32

A 58-year-old man complained of sudden onset of pain in his left foot. There is no history of trauma.

Question #1. Utilizing anatomy, what would be your differential diagnosis at this point?

Further questioning reveals that he is on hydrochlorothiazide, but there is no history of diabetes, heart disease, or back pain. Physical examination reveals erythema, swelling, and exquisite tenderness of the first metatarsophalangeal joint. The peripheral pulses are good.

Question #2. What is your diagnosis now?

(See Appendix B for the answers.)

FOREHEAD ENLARGEMENT

Anatomy will help to recall the causes of forehead enlargement. Before the history and physical examination create a biased point of view, sit down and make a list of the possibilities.

1. **Skin and subcutaneous tissues**—Myxedema, cretinism, cellulitis, hematomas
2. **Bone**—Paget disease, fibrous dysplasia, leontiasis ossea, rickets, congenital syphilis, ivory exostosis, acromegaly, and metastatic carcinoma
3. **Central nervous system**—Hydrocephalus and meningioma

● Approach to the Diagnosis

The history and physical examination will often point to the diagnosis: the nonpitting edema of hypothyroidism, the protruding jaw of acromegaly, and the disproportionate enlargement of the head compared to the facial bones in hydrocephalus. Plain films of the skull will be helpful in the diagnosis of rickets, Paget disease, acromegaly, and meningiomas. A CBC, sedimentation rate, TSH and free thyroxine (T_4) index, and chemistry panel should be ordered. A neurologist should be consulted before ordering expensive diagnostic tests such as a CT scan or MRI.

FREQUENCY AND URGENCY OF URINATION

Frequency of urination may be due to polyuria (increased output of urine), obstruction to the output of urine (requiring frequent voiding to get the urine out) because the net capacity of the bladder is reduced, or irritative lesions in or near the urinary tract.

Polyuria: Increased output of urine is discussed on page 345, but, in summary, it may be caused by pituitary diabetes insipidus, nephritis, diabetes mellitus, hyperthyroidism, hyperparathyroidism, or nephrogenic diabetes insipidus.
Obstruction of the bladder: This may be mechanical, as occurs in bladder neck obstruction due to prostatic hypertrophy, prostatitis, median bar hypertrophy, urethral stricture, and bladder calculi; or it may be due to a neurogenic bladder, as occurs in poliomyelitis, parasympatholytic drugs, tabes dorsalis, multiple sclerosis, other spinal cord lesions, and diabetic neuropathy.
Irritative lesions of the urinary tract: Infection, calculus, or neoplasm of the bladder, kidney, ureters, or urethra may do this. Chronic or acute prostatitis is sometimes the culprit. Inflammation anywhere in the pelvis (vaginitis, hemorrhoids, diverticulitis, appendicitis, or salpingitis) may also cause this.

● Approach to the Diagnosis

This is no problem. Examine a drop of unspun urine under the microscope. More than one or two motile bacteria per high-power field is diagnostic of UTI. If this is negative, be sure to do a rectal and vaginal examination. Then culture the urine, catheterize for residual urine, and do an IVP and voiding cystogram. A cystoscopy may be necessary. If these are negative for abnormal findings, it is a good idea to collect a 24-hour specimen; if the amount of urine exceeds 5 L, check the response to pitressin. Special cultures for *Chlamydia* should be done if all else fails. The workup of polyuria (see page 345) can proceed further, if necessary.

● Other Useful Tests

1. Prostatic massage and examination of exudate (prostatitis)
2. Fishberg concentration test (chronic nephritis)
3. CT scan of the brain (pituitary tumor)
4. Serum antidiuretic hormone (ADH) (diabetes insipidus)
5. Hickey–Hare test (diabetes insipidus)
6. Cystometric studies (neurogenic bladder)
7. Circulation time (CHF)

Case Presentation #33

A 26-year-old white woman complains of frequency of urination for the past 2 weeks. There is no dysuria, fever or chills, or flank pain. She had a similar episode 2 years ago.

Question #1. Utilizing anatomy and physiology, what would be your list of possibilities at this point?
Further questioning reveals that she had an attack of double vision at age 19 which cleared spontaneously in 3 weeks. Review of systems revealed that she has had intermittent stiffness in her legs for several months. Neurologic examination revealed hyperactive reflexes in both lower extremities and a spastic ataxic gait.

Question #2. What is your diagnosis now?

(See Appendix B for the answers.)

FRIGIDITY

Frigidity may be due to an organic cause, in which case the differential diagnosis is similar to dyspareunia (see page 140), or it may be functional. The **organic** causes can be recalled with the mnemonic **MINT**.

M—**Malformations** include a hood clitoris or imperforate hymen, vaginal stenosis, hermaphroditism, retroverted uterus, and Turner syndrome.
I—**Inflammation** suggests vaginitis, bartholinitis, endometritis, or salpingitis.
N—**Neoplasms** recall neoplasms of the vagina, cervix, uterus, and ovary; endometriosis; and neurologic conditions such as multiple sclerosis or peripheral neuropathy (diabetes).
T—**Trauma** includes introduction of a large male organ, masturbation, or previous rape, in addition to the emotional trauma discussed below. Unfortunately, this does not include the numerous hormonal causes of frigidity (e.g., menopause, hypopituitarism, Stein–Leventhal syndrome, and adrenal tumors). Obesity would seem

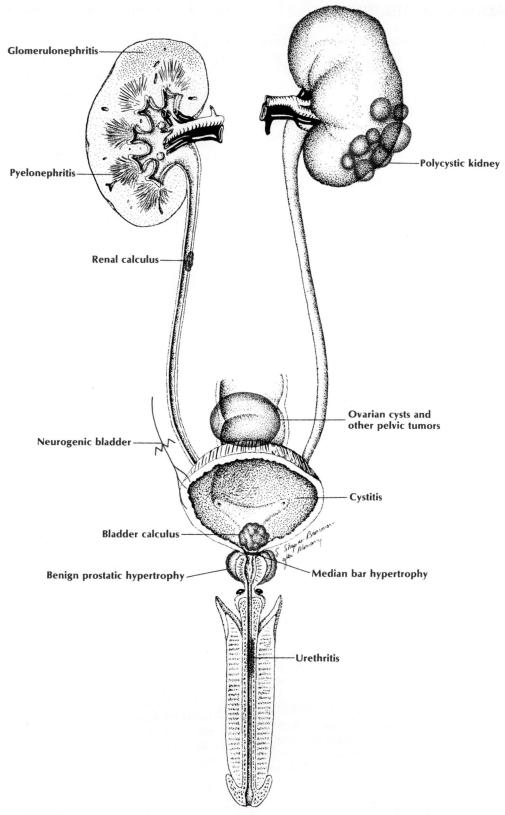

● **FIGURE 11** Frequency and urgency of urination.

to be another "organic" cause of frigidity, but this may simply be another sign of a functional disorder.

Functional or psychogenic causes of frigidity include all the neuroses and psychoses, especially schizophrenia and endogenous depression, as well as specific feelings of fear or hostility related to intercourse. These may be grouped into conscious or unconscious feelings.

Conscious fears include a fear of pregnancy or, if pregnant, fear of damage to the fetus. It would also include fear of not being able to consummate the marriage and have a child. Another important conscious fear that many women have is that they will not be able to satisfy the husband or that they themselves will not reach a climax. Conscious hostility may be based on a disgust for male superiority or anger at the husband for the way he treats her parents or other relatives or for his lack of respect for her. She may be disgusted because his lack of technique or premature ejaculation prevents her from reaching orgasm.

Unconscious fears include repressed anxiety from previously being raped in childhood, repressed anxiety from previous incest, and repressed guilt that sex is dirty. Unconscious hostility may come from a castration complex or a reluctance to identify with the feminine role.

● Approach to the Diagnosis

The approach to the diagnosis here is to examine the patient and husband for organic causes and perhaps even do FSH, estradiol, and other hormone blood levels. Estrogen replacement therapy may be indicated in menopause. If no organic cause can be found, referral to a psychiatrist or sex therapist is indicated. A reassuring, personable, and interested physician, however, may be quite capable of determining the psychologic cause, especially if it is in the conscious mind.

● Other Useful Tests

1. Careful pelvic and rectovaginal examination (pelvic mass)
2. Sonogram (tubo-ovarian abscess)
3. Laparoscopy (pelvic mass)
4. Chromosomal analysis (e.g., Turner syndrome)
5. Vaginal smear and culture (pelvic inflammatory disease)
6. Psychometric testing (e.g., anxiety, depression)
7. Gynecology consult

F

G

GAIT DISTURBANCES

The anatomic location of the lesion in a gait disturbance depends on the type of disturbance.

1. **Spastic gait:** In this type of lesion, both feet shuffle along the floor in short steps and the legs are close together moving in a scissors-like fashion. Spastic gait is caused by lesions of both pyramidal tracts anywhere from the lower spinal cord to the brain stem and brain. The principal disorders are the following:
   A. **In the cord:** Multiple sclerosis, amyotrophic lateral sclerosis, spinal cord tumors, syringomyelia, and cervical trauma or spondylosis
   B. **In the brainstem:** Tumors, basilar artery thrombosis, multiple sclerosis, platybasia, and progressive lenticular degeneration
   C. **In the brain:** Cerebral arteriosclerosis, cerebral palsy, general paresis, and senile or presenile dementia
2. **Hemiplegic gait:** One foot is dragged above the floor, swinging out in a semicircular fashion. This is due to involvement of only one pyramidal tract, usually in the brain. Cerebral hemorrhage, thrombosis, emboli, and space-occupying lesions may be the culprits. Multiple sclerosis, early cervical cord tumor, or disc may do the same.
3. **Steppage gait:** Because of the weakness of dorsiflexion of both feet, the patient has to lift the foot high to avoid tripping. The lesion is a diffuse peripheral neuropathy that may be caused by lead intoxication, alcoholism, diabetes, porphyria, perineal muscular atrophy, or a cauda equina tumor. There are many other causes of peripheral neuropathy discussed on page 437.
4. **Limping gait:** Pain in one lower extremity due to bone disease, sciatica, hip disease, knee joint disease, or ankle and foot disorders of all types may cause favoring of the painful limb and quickening of the stride on that side so the victim can get back on the healthy limb. Osteoarthritis of the hip or knee, a herniated disc, an osteoarthritic spur of the heel, a sprained ankle, and fracture of any of the bones of the limb are typical conditions causing this type of gait. In children, consider child abuse.
5. **Ataxic gait:** The gait is wide-based, clumsy, and staggering. An ataxic gait may be sensory or cerebellar. Sensory ataxia is due to a lesion of the dorsal columns, such as tabes dorsalis, pernicious anemia, or a spinal cord tumor. In sensory ataxia, the patient walks carefully with his eyes fixed on the ground. Cerebellar ataxia is due to involvement of the spinocerebellar tracts and cerebellum. This occurs in hereditary cerebellar ataxia, Friedreich ataxia,

cerebellar tumors, multiple sclerosis, and alcoholic cerebellar atrophy. In a cerebellar ataxia, the patient reels about when walking, and it is not much more difficult to walk with the eyes closed. Multiple sclerosis and syringomyelia may involve the dorsal columns, pyramidal and spinocerebellar tracts, or cerebellum, producing a mixed spastic–ataxic gait.

6. **Muscular dystrophy gait:** This is wide-based with a pelvic tilt forward as if the patient is trying to "show off," but the feet are lifted from the ground with difficulty and there is waddling or rolling from side to side.
7. **Extrapyramidal disease gait:** The gait is short-stepped and spastic, and the feet shuffle along the ground. The patient may tilt forward with the trunk and head bent toward the ground, causing acceleration (propulsion); at times, the reverse may occur (retropulsion). In Huntington chorea, the gait is clownish and grotesque, as if the patient were drunk but playing games.

● Approach to the Diagnosis

The workup depends on the presence or absence of other neurologic signs. If a peripheral nerve lesion is suspected, a workup for diabetes and a careful history for alcoholism and porphyria are expected. A suspected spinal cord lesion requires x-rays of the spinal column, spinal tap, Schilling test, and possibly a myelogram or magnetic resonance imaging (MRI). When the lesion is believed to be in the brain or brain stem, an MRI or computed tomography (CT) scan is almost axiomatic before a spinal tap or other radiocontrast studies are considered. A neurologist or neurosurgeon can best decide how the workup should be conducted.

● Other Useful Tests

1. Complete blood count (CBC) (pernicious anemia)
2. Sedimentation rate (epidural abscess, collagen disease)
3. Fluorescent treponemal antibody absorption (FTA-ABS) test (neurosyphilis)
4. Tuberculin test (tuberculosis of the spinal column)
5. Chemistry panel (muscle disease, cirrhosis)
6. Serum protein electrophoresis (multiple myeloma)
7. Blood lead level (lead neuropathy)
8. Antinuclear antibody (ANA) analysis (collagen disease)
9. Rheumatoid arthritis (RA) test
10. Serum B_{12} and folate levels (pernicious anemia)
11. Urine porphobilinogen (porphyria)
12. 24-hour urine for creatinine and creatine (muscular dystrophy)
13. Muscle biopsy (muscular dystrophy, collagen disease)

G

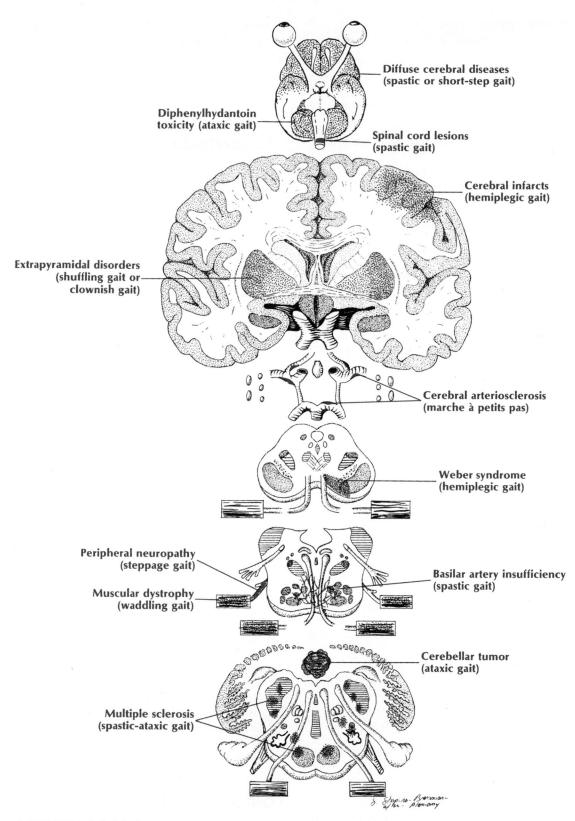

Diffuse cerebral diseases
(spastic or short-step gait)

Diphenylhydantoin
toxicity (ataxic gait)

Spinal cord lesions
(spastic gait)

Cerebral infarcts
(hemiplegic gait)

Extrapyramidal disorders
(shuffling gait or
clownish gait)

Cerebral arteriosclerosis
(marche à petits pas)

Weber syndrome
(hemiplegic gait)

Peripheral neuropathy
(steppage gait)

Basilar artery insufficiency
(spastic gait)

Muscular dystrophy
(waddling gait)

Cerebellar tumor
(ataxic gait)

Multiple sclerosis
(spastic-ataxic gait)

● **FIGURE 1** Gait disturbances.

Case Presentation #34

A 42-year-old black man complained of difficulty walking and weakness of all four extremities which had become progressively worse over the last 3 years. He denied any pain, numbness, or tingling, but his vision had also deteriorated somewhat in the same period of time.

Question #1. Utilizing the methods discussed above, what is your differential diagnosis?

Neurologic examination revealed weakness, atrophy, and diminished reflexes of all extremities. There were bilateral cataracts and testicular atrophy.

Question #2. What is your diagnosis?

(See Appendix B for the answers.)

GANGRENE

The mnemonic **VINDICATE** will help formulate a useful list of possible causes of gangrene.

V—Vascular: Gangrene is seen in peripheral arteriosclerosis, Buerger disease, thrombosis of the large arteries such as the femoral artery, thrombosis of the terminal aorta, and arterial embolism.

I—Infection: Gas gangrene is typically produced by *Clostridium perfringens* and other clostridia. Streptococci, peptostreptococci, and staphylococci can produce progressive bacteria-synergistic gangrene.

N—Neoplasm and neurological: Cryoglobulinemia and multiple myeloma are associated with the Raynaud phenomenon producing gangrene in the fingers. Peripheral neuropathy, syringomyelia, transverse myelitis, and tabes dorsalis may be associated with gangrene.

D—Degenerative diseases are not generally associated with gangrene.

I—Intoxication should bring to mind the gangrene associated with the use of ergot alkaloids.

C—Congenital disorders are not usually associated with gangrene.

A—Autoimmune disease: Lupus erythematosus, scleroderma, periarteritis nodosa, and RA may be associated with the Raynaud phenomenon and gangrene.

T—Trauma: Laceration of a major artery to an extremity or pressure from splints may cause gangrene. Extreme cold will produce gangrene from frostbite.

E—Endocrine disorders bring to mind the well-known diabetic gangrene.

● Approach to the Diagnosis

All patients should have a CBC, sedimentation rate, venereal disease research laboratory (VDRL) test, chemistry panel, and serum protein electrophoresis. In cases of Raynaud phenomenon, an ANA and RA titer should also be done. Allen's test is also helpful. Aerobic and anaerobic cultures of exudates from the wound should also be taken. Plain x-rays of the area involved are recommended. If an embolism or obstruction of the large arteries is suspected, contrast angiography needs to be done. An ice water test, Sia water test, and serum immunoelectrophoresis will be useful in cases of the Raynaud phenomenon. A rheumatology consult is wise.

GIGANTISM

The differential of this symptom can be developed physiologically by overactivity or underactivity of an endocrine gland. Thus, overactivity of the pituitary gland (as in eosinophilic adenomas of the pituitary) causes gigantism from too much growth hormone, whereas underactivity of the testicles (as in Klinefelter syndrome) produces a tall individual because the inadequate secretion of testosterone delays closure of the epiphysis. Tumors of the adrenal cortex, testicle, and pineal gland may produce macrogenitosomia or prepubertal gigantism by stimulation of overgrowth by androgens and estrogens only to lead to ultimate dwarfism by premature closure of the epiphysis. Primary gigantism is like the gigantism of plants and flowers; genetic arachnodactyly is also a genetic form of gigantism, although it is a true disease and is associated with dislocation of the lens.

● Approach to the Diagnosis

The approach to the diagnosis of these conditions is simple. Radioimmunoassay (RIA) studies of hormone levels are now readily available, and x-rays of the skull with CT scans and tomography will allow a diagnosis. Referral to an endocrinologist may be wise from the start, especially because potentially tall girls may want endocrine therapy to close the epiphysis early.

● Other Useful Tests

1. Serum growth hormone (pituitary adenoma)
2. Serum corticotropin, luteinizing hormone (LH), and follicle-stimulating hormone (FSH) levels (pituitary adenoma)
3. Serum testosterone (Klinefelter syndrome, adrenal tumors, and hyperplasia)
4. Serum dihydrotestosterone and dehydroepiandrosterone sulfate (adrenal tumor and hyperplasia)
5. Urine hydroxyproline level (Marfan syndrome)
6. Urine homocystine level (homocystinuria)
7. Chromosomal analysis (Klinefelter syndrome)
8. MRI of the pituitary (microadenoma)
9. Testicular biopsy (Klinefelter syndrome)

GIRDLE PAIN

Girdle pain is defined as radicular pain radiating around the trunk and anatomically would almost invariably signify involvement of the intercostal nerves or roots. The mnemonic **MINT** should bring to mind the commonest causes of this symptom.

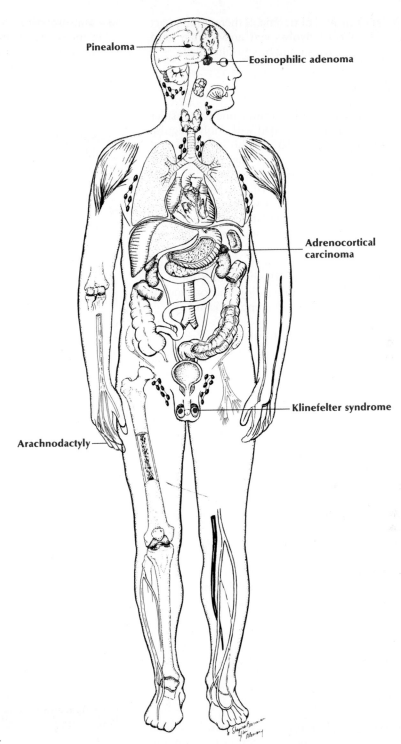

Pinealoma

Eosinophilic adenoma

Adrenocortical carcinoma

Klinefelter syndrome

Arachnodactyly

● **FIGURE 2** Gigantism.

M—**Malformation** would suggest syringomyelia.

I—**Inflammation** should suggest herpes zoster, tabes dorsalis, or epidural abscess.

N—**Neoplasm** prompts the recall of the spinal cord tumor involving the dorsal root.

T—**Trauma** would suggest not only vertebral or rib fractures but also a herniated thoracic disc, which although rare must be considered in the differential diagnosis.

Two conditions that may not be suggested by this mnemonic are multiple sclerosis and subacute combined degeneration of the spinal cord associated with pernicious anemia.

● **Approach to the Diagnosis**

Routine laboratory tests such as a CBC, sedimentation rate, VDRL, and chemistry panel should be done but may not be revealing. Plain x-rays of the spine and ribs should be ordered especially if there is a history of trauma. If there is long tract or other signs of spinal cord involvement, an MRI may need to be done, but a neurologist should be consulted first.

GLYCOSURIA

The finding of glycosuria should prompt one to consider first the conditions that are associated with faulty **regulation** of the blood sugar and sugar metabolism. First and foremost on that list is diabetes mellitus. However, the differential must include many other endocrine disorders; focusing on the endocrine glands will prompt recall of most of these. Visualizing the pituitary will prompt recall of acromegaly, visualizing the adrenal gland will remind one of Cushing syndrome and pheochromocytoma, and visualizing the thyroid will prompt recall of hyperthyroidism. Finally, visualizing the pancreas will remind one of diabetes mellitus and glucagonoma. The clinician should be careful not to forget renal glycosuria (idiopathic or Fanconi syndrome) and starvation in the differential diagnosis.

● Approach to the Diagnosis

The investigation of glycosuria should include a glucose tolerance test, chemistry panel, and electrolyte panel. A clinical history of polyuria, polyphagia, weakness, and weight loss will be helpful. If there are clinical features of one of the endocrine diseases listed above, various tests for these disorders and an endocrinology consult should be ordered.

● Other Useful Tests

1. Free thyroxine (T_4) (hyperthyroidism)
2. T_3 assay (hyperthyroidism)
3. Radioactive iodine uptake and scan (thyroid adenoma)
4. Plasma cortisol (Cushing syndrome)
5. Overnight dexamethasone suppression test (Cushing syndrome)
6. Serum growth hormone (acromegaly)
7. 24-hour urine for catecholamine, vanillylmandelic acid, or metanephrine (pheochromocytoma)
8. Skull x-ray (pituitary adenoma)
9. CT scan of the brain (acromegaly)
10. CT scan of the abdomen (pancreatic neoplasm, glucagonoma)

GROIN MASS

A mass of the groin found on routine examination is most likely an enlarged lymph node. In contrast, when the patient presents with a groin mass for diagnosis, it is probably a hernia. But why diagnose by probability? A systematic approach will avoid misdiagnoses and should make medicine more fun.

Visualize the anatomy of the groin. There are skin, subcutaneous tissue, and the inguinal and femoral canals; underneath these are the saphenous and femoral veins, the femoral artery and nerve, and lymph nodes. In the next layer are the psoas and iliac muscles and the bones and ligaments of the hip joints. Apply the mnemonic **MINT** to these structures, and the following list of possibilities may be arrived at.

M—**Malformations** suggest inguinal and femoral hernias in the fascia, hydroceles, and undescended testicles in the inguinal canal. A saphenous varicocele and iliac aneurysm are also malformations to consider.

I—**Inflammatory** lesions include cellulitis, acute adenitis (usually secondary to venereal disease or skin disease) and chronic adenitis secondary to tuberculosis or a systemic disease (see page 292). In addition, tuberculosis may cause a psoas abscess, there may be thrombophlebitis of the saphenous or femoral vein (especially postpartum), or there may be arthritis (RA, gout, or osteoarthritis) of the joint. Finally, osteomyelitis of the hip bones must be considered.

N—**Neoplasms** suggest skin tumor (see page 381), lipoma, tumor of the lymph node such as Hodgkin lymphoma and metastatic tumor, and sarcoma of the bone.

T—**Trauma** includes a perforation of the femoral vein or artery, contusion and fracture, or dislocation of the hip.

● Approach to the Diagnosis

Obviously, the approach to diagnosis involves differentiating enlarged lymph nodes from other conditions. Hernias are usually reducible; if they are not, they are extremely tender, and the patient often experiences gastrointestinal (GI) complaints. They do not transilluminate, and bowel sounds can often be heard over them. The location of inguinal hernias above the inguinal ligament should help differentiate them from lymph nodes and femoral hernias, which are below the inguinal ligament. Lymphadenitis will usually be associated with a lesion on the genitalia (e.g., chancre) or the lower extremity. Exploratory surgery and lymph node biopsy may be necessary to make a definitive diagnosis. Phlebography may be necessary to rule out venous thrombosis and angiography to rule out aneurysm.

● Other Useful Tests

1. CBC (abscess)
2. Tuberculin test (psoas abscess)
3. Protein electrophoresis (multiple myeloma)
4. X-rays of the hips (metastatic tumor, multiple myeloma)
5. VDRL test (chancre with regional lymphadenitis)
6. Small-bowel series (hernia)
7. Lymphangiogram (neoplasm of the lymph glands)
8. Sonogram (saphenous varix, aneurysm)

Case Presentation #35

A 34-year-old pilot was found on a routine physical examination to have a mass in his right groin.

Question #1. Utilizing anatomy, what possible diagnoses would you consider at this point?

On further examination, the mass was reducible and situated above the Poupart ligament.

Question #2. What is your diagnosis now?

(See Appendix B for the answers.)

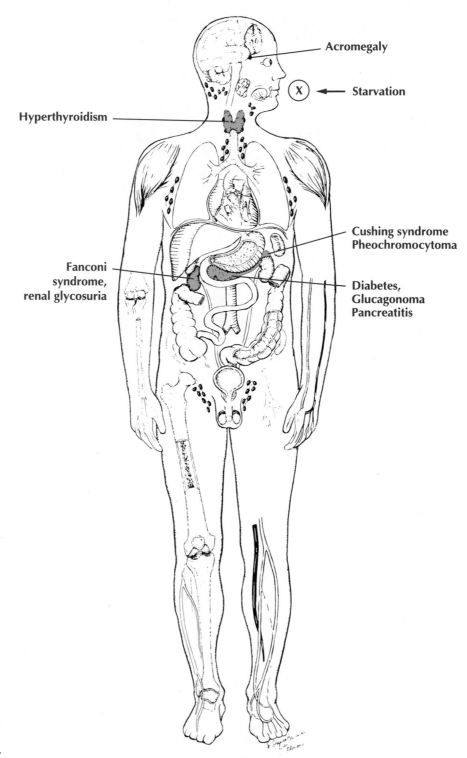

● **FIGURE 3** Glycosuria.

G

GROIN PAIN

The anatomic components of the groin consist of the skin, subcutaneous tissue, fascia, lymph nodes, the femoral nerve, arteries and veins, and, underneath, the hip bones. With these components in mind, it should be easy to develop a differential diagnosis of groin pain because most of the lesions are inflammatory or traumatic.

The **skin** is affected by intertrigo, scabies, furuncles, and herpes zoster, among other things. The **subcutaneous tissue** may be involved by cellulitis and a tuberculous abscess. When the **fascia** is weak or torn, femoral or inguinal hernias

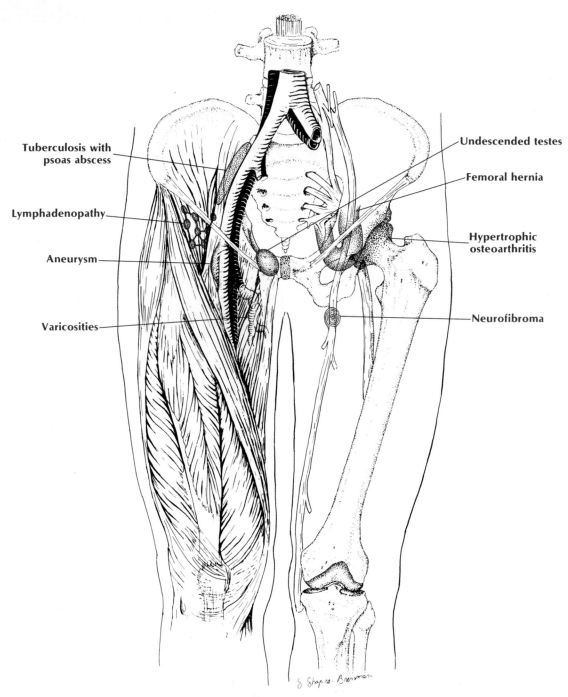

● **FIGURE 4** Groin mass.

develop. More likely causes of groin pain are inflamed **lymph nodes** that may be from any venereal disease (such as gonorrhea or chancroid) or infections of other portions of the genitalia. The **femoral nerve** may be affected by viral neuritis, diabetic neuropathy, and disease of the spine (fracture, disc, or tumors). The **femoral artery** may be involved by a thrombosis, embolism, or dissecting aneurysm, whereas the **vein** may be thrombosed. Finally, the underlying **hip bones** can be involved by any form of arthritis and by infections or metastatic tumors of the bone. Fractures and other traumatic disorders affect the bones of the hip also.

It would be a gross omission if referred pain to the groin were not considered. Pain may be referred to the groin in pyelonephritis, renal colic, regional ileitis, appendicitis, salpingitis, and many other abdominal disorders.

● **Approach to the Diagnosis**

In the approach to the diagnosis of groin pain, a mass or tender structure is usually present in the groin. If the mass is a lymph node, careful examination of the genitalia and lower extremities will often show the cause, but a urethral or vaginal smear and culture may be necessary to show gonorrhea. Investigation of the genitourinary tract and the GI tract for causes of referred pain is then undertaken. If the mass is reducible, a hernia is likely and referral to a surgeon is in order. Incarcerated hernias, of course, demand immediate referral.

● Other Useful Tests

1. Tuberculin test
2. Sonogram (cystic mass)
3. Flat plate of abdomen (hernia with intestinal obstruction)
4. X-ray of hip (fracture, osteomyelitis)
5. CBC (abscess)
6. Bone scan (tumor, osteomyelitis)
7. Angiogram (aneurysm)
8. Phlebogram (saphenous varix)
9. Exploratory surgery (hernia, tumor)
10. Biopsy (tumor)
11. CT scan (tumor, abscess)

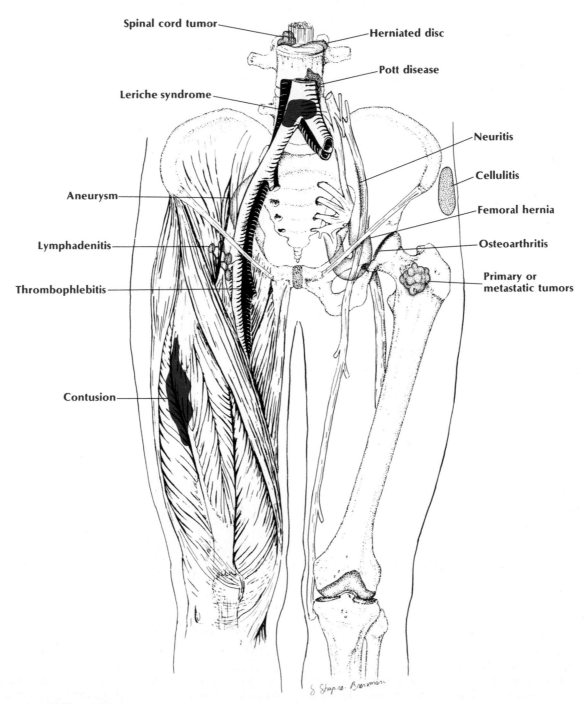

● **FIGURE 5** Groin pain.

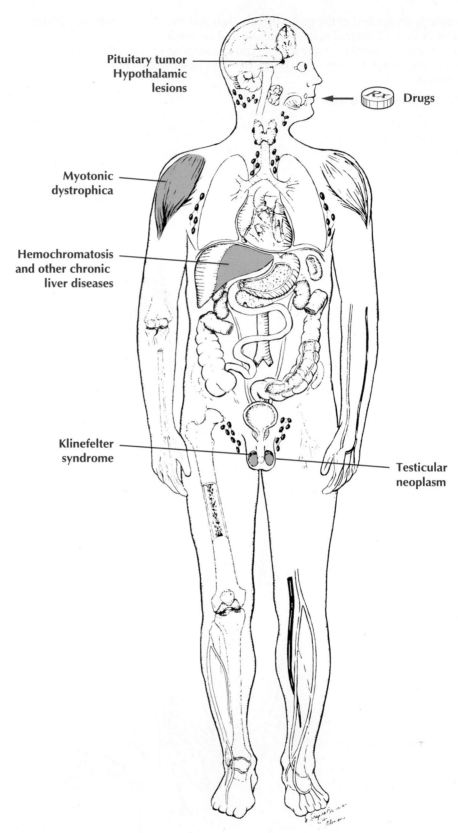

Pituitary tumor
Hypothalamic
lesions

Drugs

Myotonic
dystrophica

Hemochromatosis
and other chronic
liver diseases

Klinefelter
syndrome

Testicular
neoplasm

● **FIGURE 6** Gynecomastia.

A 38-year-old carpenter complained of intermittent pain in his right groin for several months. The pain was so severe he had to quit work for the past 2 weeks. Physical examination failed to disclose a mass in his right groin, but there was slight tenderness on palpation.

Question #1. Utilizing anatomy, what is your differential diagnosis?

Neurologic examination reveals diminished sensation to touch, pain in the right L$_1$ dermatome, and precipitation of the pain by coughing or sneezing.

Question #2. What is your diagnosis now?

(See Appendix B for the answers.)

GYNECOMASTIA

Because gynecomastia is produced by a hormonal disturbance, the many causes of this disorder can be recalled by using the physiologic model of intake, production, transport, regulation, destruction, or excretion.

Intake: Obviously if one takes estrogen or other feminizing hormones, gynecomastia may result. Injections of human chorionic gonadotropin (HCG) as are used in the treatment of obesity may cause gynecomastia. Not so obvious is the gynecomastia resulting from ingestion of methyl testosterone and desoxycorticosterone. Taking drugs such as amphetamines, tricyclic antidepressants, methadone, and isoniazid may also cause this disorder.

Production: The production of estrogen or estrogen-like substances is increased in testicular tumors such as seminomas, Sertoli cell tumors, and adrenal tumors. The production of prolactin or HCG is increased in pituitary tumors and carcinoma of the lung. Several drugs including phenothiazines, marijuana, reserpines, and methyldopa increase prolactin production. Carcinoma of the lung may also increase HCG production. Production of testosterone and other androgens or androgen-producing substances is decreased in Klinefelter syndrome, advancing age, mumps orchitis, hypothalamic lesions, liver disease, and neurologic disorders such as myotonic dystrophy, syringomyelia, and Friedreich ataxia. Testosterone production is also reduced in pseudohermaphroditism and congenital adrenal hyperplasia.

Transport: Plasma proteins that carry hormones are reduced in starvation, and many debilitating states reduce testosterone activity and availability leading to gynecomastia.

Regulation: The regulation of the ratio of circulating estrogen and androgen may be affected in hyperthyroidism, hypothyroidism, renal failure, and dialysis. Drugs such as spironolactone, digitalis, griseofulvin, cimetidine, and cannabis antagonize androgens causing gynecomastia. Benign gynecomastia is a common condition in adolescent boys.

Destruction: In liver diseases such as hemochromatosis, cirrhosis, carcinoma, and hepatitis there may be increased conversion of testosterone to estrogen. The same mechanism may occur in hyperthyroidism.

● Approach to the Diagnosis

It is important to find out if the patient has been taking alcohol or drugs of any kind. On physical examination, the physician may find bronze skin (a sign of hemochromatosis), a testicular mass, neurologic signs (suggesting, e.g., Friedreich ataxia, myotonic dystrophy, paraplegia), or abnormal secondary sex characteristics (suggesting Klinefelter syndrome or pseudohermaphroditism). The laboratory workup should include a thyroid profile, liver profile, serum prolactin, urine drug screen, serum iron and iron-binding capacity, and serum FSH, LH, testosterone, and estradiol. Referral to an endocrinologist may be wise before ordering these expensive tests.

● Other Useful Tests

1. Buccal smear for Barr bodies (Klinefelter syndrome)
2. Serum cortisol (Cushing syndrome)
3. Cortisol suppression test (Cushing syndrome)
4. Rapid corticotropin test (congenital adrenal hyperplasia)
5. β-HCG (pituitary tumor, neoplasm of lung)
6. Neurology consult
7. Chest x-ray (Carcinoma of the lung)

A 46-year-old diabetic man complained of swelling of his breasts for the past 4 months. He denies taking any drugs other than insulin for his diabetes.

Question #1. Utilizing your knowledge of physiology, what is your differential diagnosis?

Physical examination revealed hepatomegaly and testicular atrophy.

Question #2. What is your diagnosis now?

(See Appendix B for the answers.)

G

H

HALITOSIS AND OTHER BREATH ODORS

What are the various causes of bad breath and how can they be recalled with ease? The best method is to visualize the respiratory and upper gastrointestinal (GI) tree, because this is where the substances (mucus, sputum, and vomitus or regurgitant material) that produce these odors may be found.

In the **mouth**, pyorrhea due to poor dental care and infection may cause halitosis. A stomatitis (e.g., aphthous) may also be a cause. Sinusitis and atrophic rhinitis are causes in the **nasal passages**. Anyone who has a friend with large tonsils knows that this is a frequent cause, especially when the tonsils become infected. Any form of pharyngitis may also cause halitosis. Carcinoma and tuberculosis (TB) of the larynx and lower respiratory tract may cause halitosis. More likely causes are bronchiectasis and lung abscess.

Proceeding down the **esophagus** to the **stomach**, one should recall the accumulation of food in diverticula, cardiospasm of the esophagus, and the frequent foul odor of chronic membranous or granulomatous esophagitis associated with a hiatal hernia. Carcinoma of the esophagus may also cause obstruction and allow putrefaction of food that accumulates there. A chronic gastritis or gastric carcinoma may also cause halitosis.

A sweet odor to the breath may be found in diabetes mellitus and alcoholism. Uremia will often present with an ammoniac and urinous odor to the breath, whereas the breath of hepatic coma may be fishy (fetor hepatis). The feculent odor of a gastrocolic fistula and late states of intestinal obstructions should also be recalled. A garlic odor is found in many poisonings (arsenic, organophosphates, etc.).

● Approach to the Diagnosis

The workup of bad breath involves a careful examination of the mouth and nasal passages. If this is negative, chest and sinus x-rays and upper GI series with barium swallow should be done. If the studies are still unrewarding, then endoscopy of the respiratory and upper GI tract would be indicated. Appropriate liver and renal function tests will be ordered when uremia or hepatic coma is suspected. If pyorrhea is suspected, refer the patient to a dentist.

HALLUCINATIONS

A hallucination is seeing, hearing, touching, smelling, or tasting something that is not there. Auditory hallucinations without evidence of mental deterioration usually indicate schizophrenia, but epilepsy, drug toxicity, and brain tumors

must be excluded. Visual hallucinations are often the sign of drug or alcohol intoxication, but occasionally they occur in schizophrenia. Hallucinations with mental deterioration should prompt the recall of the differential diagnosis for memory loss (see page 295). When faced with a hallucinating patient, think of the mnemonic **MINT**, and a list of possibilities can be recalled easily.

M—**Mental** disease brings to mind schizophrenia, manic depressive psychosis, and paranoid states.

I—**Intoxication** and **inflammation** suggest alcoholism, cannabis, lysergic acid diethylamide, bromism, various other drugs, and encephalitis, cerebral abscess (temporal lobe especially), and syphilis. The **I** should also suggest **idiopathic** disorders such as epilepsy, presenile dementia, and arteriosclerosis.

N—**Neoplasm** suggests brain tumors. A tumor of the occipital lobe may present with visual hallucinations, whereas a tumor of the temporal lobe causes auditory hallucinations or uncinate fits (i.e., bad smells). A tumor of the parietal lobe may present with tingling or other paresthesias of the body.

T—**Trauma** should suggest concussions, epidural or subdural hematomas, and depressed skull fractures.

● Approach to the Diagnosis

In the workup of hallucinations, it is essential to get a drug history from a relative or friend if not from the patient. Ask about a family history of epilepsy or head trauma. A drug screen should be ordered. If there is no mental deterioration, referral to a psychiatrist may be done but an electroencephalogram (EEG) may still be indicated. A therapeutic trial of 100 mg of thiamine IV should be done if Wernicke encephalopathy or Korsakoff syndrome is suspected. With mental deterioration, a neurologist should be consulted. When there is doubt about mental deterioration, psychologic testing may be done. Computed tomography (CT) or MRI scans, EEGs, skull x-ray films, and arteriograms may be necessary in selected cases.

HAND AND FINGER PAIN

Visualize the anatomy when a patient presents with pain in the hand or fingers (Table 31). The **skin** may show contact dermatitis, fungal infection, furuncle, cellulitis, or traumatic lesion. An insignificant wound may be infected; if there are streaks going up the arm, lymphangitis has complicated the picture. Herpes zoster rarely occurs in this area. Underneath the skin, the many **tendon sheaths** and **fascial pockets** are inviting sites for infection following a minor wound, but the swelling is obvious. One space particularly well known, the pulp space at the tip of the finger (usually

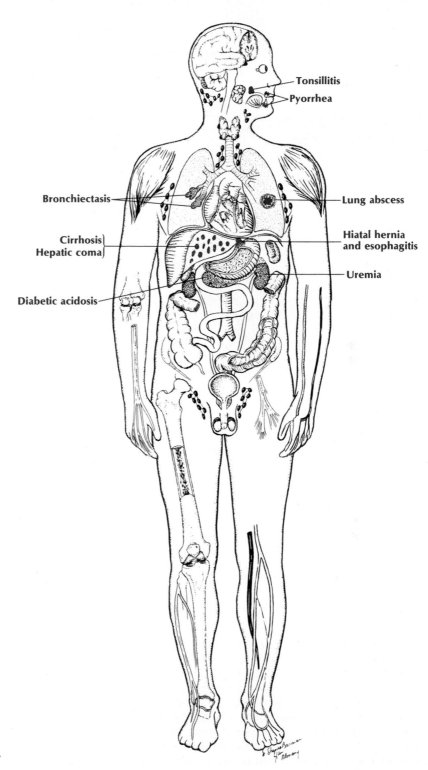

Tonsillitis
Pyorrhea
Bronchiectasis
Lung abscess
Cirrhosis
Hepatic coma
Hiatal hernia
and esophagitis
Uremia
Diabetic acidosis

● **FIGURE 1** Halitosis and other breath odors.

the index finger), may develop a felon. A paronychial infection that involves the nail is very painful. A hematoma under the nail is perhaps even more painful.

The **arteries** of the hand may go into intermittent painful spasms in the Raynaud phenomenon, which occurs for example in macroglobulinemia, menopause, and rheumatoid arthritis (RA). It also occurs in a primary form called Raynaud disease. This is an extremely painful condition

associated with cold, blue hands (intermittently) and gangrene (ultimately). The collagen diseases and Buerger disease may cause a vasculitis of the arteries and the Raynaud phenomenon. Finally, peripheral arterial emboli may occur here, but they are more frequent in the lower extremities.

Surprisingly, the **veins** of the hand do not frequently develop thrombophlebitis, except in the hospitalized patient on frequent intravenous therapy. This may not

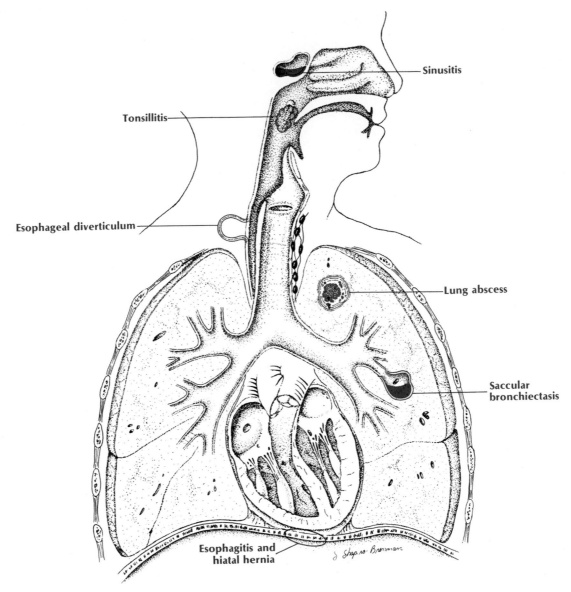

● **FIGURE 2** Halitosis and other breath odors.

be unusual when one realizes that varicose veins are uncommon in the upper extremities. Buerger disease also may involve the veins of the hand. The **tendons** are sometimes trapped in their sheaths and cause pain. De Quervain stenosing tenosynovitis of the extensor pollicis tendon is a common form. Ruptured tendons of the fingers such as mallet finger should be obvious. The **muscles** of the hands are not commonly involved in myositis but are frequently traumatized and contused, particularly in contact sports.

Trapping of the **median nerve** in the carpal tunnel is a well-known cause of pain in the hand and fingers, particularly in the thumb, index, and middle fingers. Sensory changes involve these and the medial half of the ring finger; there may be significant atrophy of the thenar eminence with the Tinel sign. The Phalen test is usually positive also. Remember that the **ulnar nerve** may be trapped in Guyon's canal also, causing pain in the little finger and associated

sensory changes. The carpal tunnel syndrome may be caused by multiple myeloma, amyloidosis, acromegaly, RA, menopause, and a host of other conditions.

Symptoms similar to those of the carpal tunnel syndrome may come from high up the peripheral nerve tract. Compression of the **brachial plexus** by a cervical rib, a scalenus anticus muscle, or the clavicle (so-called costoclavicular compression syndrome) may be the culprit. Chronic bursitis or arthritis of the shoulder may ultimately lead to a causalgia, as will a peripheral nerve injury, and create pain in the hand and fingers. The frozen shoulder following pneumonia, myocardial infarctions, and other chest conditions can do the same. The brachial plexus may also be involved by Pancoast tumors.

At a third site, compression of the **cervical nerve roots** by a herniated disc, cervical spondylosis, TB, and primary and metastatic tumors may be the cause of hand and/or finger pain. Cord conditions like syringomyelia and

TABLE 31 Hand and Finger Pain

	V Vascular	I Inflammatory	N Neoplasm	D Degenerative and Deficiency	I Intoxication	C Congenital	A Autoimmune Allergic	T Trauma	E Endocrine
Skin	Periarteritis nodosa Gangrene	Carbuncle Ulcers Folliculitis Herpes zoster	Carcinoma				Contact dermatitis Erythema multiforme	Contusion	
Fascia, Ligaments, Tendon Sheaths, Subcutaneous Tissue		Felon Abscess Cellulitis Tendon sheath infection	Sarcoma		De Quervain stenosing tenosynovitis	Ganglion	Scleroderma	Hematoma Contusion Ruptured tendon	Pseudogout
Arteries	Arteriosclerosis Norwegian pulseless disease	Subacute bacterial endocarditis	Macroglobulinemia			Buerger disease	Vasculitis Rheumatoid arthritis	Laceration Contusion	Menopause
Veins		Thrombophlebitis				Buerger disease			
Muscles		Myositis							
Peripheral Nerves (Carpal Tunnel)		Multiple myeloma				Amyloidosis Rheumatoid arthritis		Laceration Contusion	Myxedema Acromegaly Diabetes mellitus
Brachial Plexus	Ischemic neuritis Myocardial infarction	Bursitis Arthritis Pneumonia	Pancoast tumor		Scalenus anticus syndrome	Cervical rib		Costoclavicular compression	
Spinal Cord and Cervical Roots		Tuberculosis	Primary or metastatic tumors of cord	Cervical spondylosis Syringomyelia			Rheumatoid spondylitis	Herniated disc Fracture	
Bone		Gonococcal arthritis		Osteoarthritis	Gout		Rheumatoid arthritis Lupus erythematosus	Fracture Sprain Contusion	

H

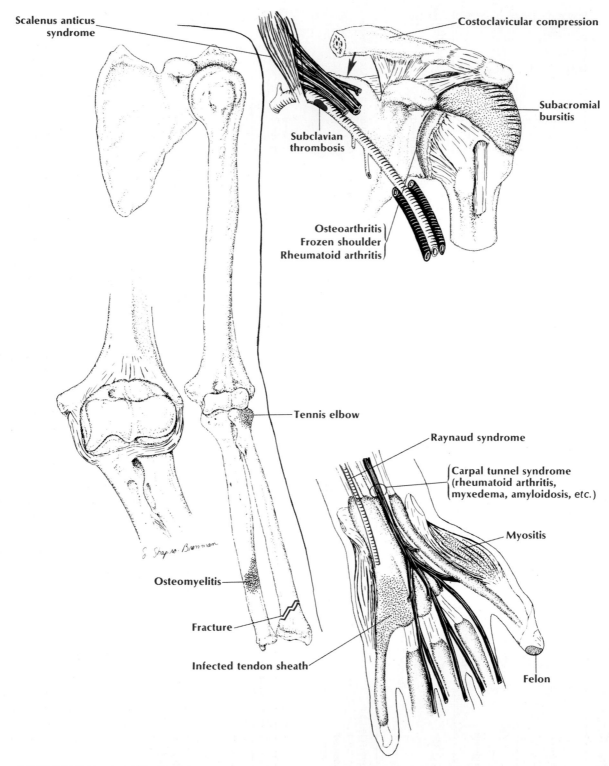

● **FIGURE 3** Hand and finger pain.

brain stem involvement of the thalamus by embolism or thrombosis may occasionally cause pain in the hand, but in the latter condition, there is usually an accompanying leg pain.

In the deepest penetration of our dissection of the hand, we encounter the most common structures that cause hand pain, the **bones** and **joints**. The bones may be fractured, dislocated, or contused or the joints may be sprained, but if the joints are painful, arthritis is the most likely cause. This may be RA, osteoarthritis, gout, or gonococcal arthritis. More rarely, it is associated with psoriatic arthritis, lupus erythematosus, and other systemic diseases.

● Approach to the Diagnosis

In diagnosis, most of these conditions will be obvious on inspection. The difficulty arises when the hand looks normal. Then one must check for the following:

1. Carpal tunnel syndrome by tapping the volar aspect of the wrist (Tinel sign)
2. Brachial plexus neuralgia and scalenus anticus syndrome by Adson tests
3. Causalgia by stellate ganglion block to see if pain is relieved
4. Cervical spine disease by a roentgenogram, possibly a myelogram or magnetic resonance imaging (MRI), and nerve blocks of the various roots. Referral to a neurologist is often necessary. In early RA, the joints may be normal on inspection, but pain and stiffness of the hands and fingers in the morning is an excellent clue.
5. Pain over the radial aspect of the wrist which is aggravated by flexing the thumb and applying ulnar deviation is most likely de Quervain tenosynovitis. This is called the Finkelstein test.
6. Tenderness in the anatomical snuffbox may indicate a scaphoid fracture. A plain x-ray may be normal and only a bone scan will demonstrate the fracture.

● Other Useful Tests

1. Arthritis panel
2. Antinuclear antibody (ANA) test (lupus erythematosus)
3. Electromyogram (EMG) and nerve conduction velocity (NCV) test (carpal tunnel syndrome)
4. X-ray of hand (arthritis)
5. Cold response test (Raynaud phenomenon)
6. Muscle biopsy (collagen disease)
7. Serum protein electrophoresis (macroglobulinemia, multiple myeloma)
8. Exploratory surgery
9. Nail fold capillary loop dilatation and dropout (Raynaud disease)
10. Therapeutic trial of a steroid and xylocaine injection (carpal tunnel syndrome)

Case Presentation #38

A 33-year-old Filipino female secretary complained of pain, numbness, and tingling in both hands for several months.

Question #1. Utilizing your knowledge of anatomy, what would be your differential diagnosis?

Neurologic examination revealed diminished sensation to touch and pain in the thumb and index fingers bilaterally and a positive Tinel sign at the wrists.

Question #2. What is your diagnosis now?

(See Appendix B for the answers.)

HEADACHES

This symptom is best analyzed by using **anatomy**, as seen in Tables 32 and 33, but differentiation by pathophysiology is interesting, particularly in muscle traction headaches and migraines.

Moving by layers from the **skin** to the center of the brain is the local application of the anatomic process. Thus, sunstroke is a cause of headache originating in the sunburnt skin, as is herpes zoster. Abscesses of the scalp are uncommon but significant causes of head pain. Moving to the **muscles**, one encounters the most common cause of headache, muscle traction headache, which may be secondary to other conditions (e.g., migraine or eyestrain), or primarily due to nervous tension or constantly holding the head in one position. Fibromyositis (usually of rheumatic etiology) may also cause a headache.

The next most common type of headache, migraine, originates from the **superficial arteries**. It usually involves the superficial temporal arteries, but it can involve the internal carotid arteries (Horton cephalalgia or cluster headaches), the occipital artery, and the intracranial arteries (e.g., hemiplegic migraine). Temporal arteritis and hypertension are two other important causes of headache originating from the **extracranial arteries**. The adjacent superficial **nerves** are a less common but important cause of headache. Occipital neuralgia may result from inflammation or compression of either the minor or major occipital nerve, and is often involved secondarily in muscle contraction headaches. This cause is established by blocking these two nerves (medially and laterally). Trigeminal neuralgia is no less important.

Moving to deeper layers, one encounters the **skull**, where osteomyelitis (e.g., tuberculous or syphilitic), primary and metastatic carcinomas, cranial stenosis, Paget disease, and skull fractures are important causes of headache. The **temporomandibular joint** (TMJ) is the origin of headache in the TMJ syndrome (usually caused by malocclusion) and RA. Important causes of headache affect the **cervical spine**. Cervical spondylosis is a major cause in elderly persons, but RA, spondylitis, spinal cord tumors, and metastatic disease of the vertebrae are also etiologies to consider.

Several common causes of headache come to mind when considering the organs of the head. Thus, the **eyes** are affected by refractive errors, astigmatism, and glaucoma, all etiologies of headache. The **ear** is affected by otitis media, mastoiditis, acoustic neuromas, and cholesteatomas. The **nose** is affected by infectious rhinitis, allergic rhinitis, Wegener granulomatosis, nicotine toxicity, fractures, and deviated septum, all causes of headache. Sinusitis (both the purulent and the vacuum type), sinus polyps, and tumors make checking the nasal sinuses important in analyzing the cause of headaches. Chronic sinusitis is almost never a cause of headache. Finally, the **teeth** should be investigated for caries, abscesses, and fillings that may be too close to the nerve root.

Intracranially there are very important but less common causes of headache. The **meninges** are the site of

H

TABLE 32 Headache—Extracranial and Cranial

	V Vascular	I Inflammatory	N Neoplasm	D Degenerative and Deficiency	I Intoxication Idiopathic	C Congenital	A Autoimmune Allergic	T Trauma	E Endocrine
Skin		Herpes zoster Abscess (scalp)			Sunstroke				
Muscle and Fascia					Muscle traction headache Fibromyositis				
Superficial Arteries	Migraine				Migraine Histamine cephalalgia		Temporal arteritis		
Superficial Nerves		Occipital neuralgia			Trigeminal neuralgia Sphenopalatine ganglion neuralgia				
Skull		Tuberculosis Osteomyelitis	Osteomas Metastatic carcinoma Multiple myeloma		Paget disease Cranial stenosis Hyperostosis frontalis			Skull fracture	Hyperparathyroidism
Temporomandibular joint					TMJ syndrome	Malocclusion	Rheumatoid arthritis		
Cervical Spine		Tuberculosis	Cord tumor Metastasis	Osteoarthritis	Cervical spondylosis		Rheumatoid arthritis		
Sinuses		Sinusitis	Sinus tumor or polyp		Vacuum sinus headache Caffeine withdrawal		Allergic sinusitis	Fracture	
Eyes	Retinal artery or vein occlusion	Uveitis Retinitis Scleritis	Orbital tumor		Glaucoma Refraction error	Glaucoma Astigmatism	Uveitis Scleritis	Orbital trauma Corneal erosion	
Ears		Otitis media Mastoiditis Petrositis	Acoustic neuroma Cholesteatoma					Basilar fracture	
Teeth		Abscess		Dental caries				Irritation of nerve root by filling	
Nose	Wegener granulomatosis	Rhinitis Mucormycosis	Schmincke tumor		Toxic rhinitis (e.g., nicotine)	Deviated septum	Allergic rhinitis	Broken nose	

TABLE 33 Headache—Intracranial

	V Vascular	I Inflammatory	N Neoplasm	D Degenerative and Deficiency	I Intoxication Idiopathic	C Congenital	A Autoimmune Allergic	T Trauma	E Endocrine
Meninges	Subarachnoid hemorrhage	Meningitis Cystic hygroma Epidural abscess Rocky Mountain spotted fever	Meningioma Hodgkin lymphoma		Hydrocephalus Meningocele	Hydrocephalus Other congenital disorders		Subdural and epidural hematoma Lumbar puncture headache	
Cerebral Arteries	Hemorrhage Thrombosis Embolism					Aneurysm A-V anomaly	Arteritis		
Cerebral Veins		Venous sinus thrombosis						Subdural hematoma	
Cranial Nerves					Trigeminal and glossopharyngeal neuralgia		Optic neuritis		
Brain	See above Hypertensive encephalopathy	Lues Encephalitis Parasite Tuberculoma Cerebral abscess	Primary and metastatic tumors		Benign intracranial hypertension Bromism Alcoholism Other drugs Gout			Concussion Contusion Postconcussion syndrome	Pituitary tumor Acromegaly
Systemic Disease	Hypertension CHF	Fever of any cause	Leukemia Hodgkin lymphoma Metastasis		Lead poisoning Drugs Uremia Jaundice Lodide toxicity		Collagen disease		Diabetic acidosis Goiter Menstrual tension Menopause Hypothyroidism

CHF, congestive heart failure; A–V, arteriovenous.

H

subarachnoid hemorrhages, subdural and epidural hematomas, meningitis, and hydrocephalus. Missing one of these causes is a grave error. The **cerebral arteries** are the site of cerebral hemorrhages, thrombosis, and emboli, as well as aneurysms and arteriovenous anomalies. The **cerebral veins**, especially the venous sinuses, may become inflamed and thrombosed, producing a headache. The **cranial nerves** are the site of trigeminal neuralgia mentioned above and glossopharyngeal neuralgia.

Although the **brain** itself is not tender, lesions of the brain cause increased intracranial pressure or traction on other painful structures, such as the intracranial arteries, venous sinuses, or nerves. A third of the cases of brain tumors present with a headache. Encephalitis produces a headache by the associated fever or meningeal irritation. Concussions, pituitary tumors, toxic encephalopathy from alcohol, bromides, and other substances are important causes, in addition to the cerebral hemorrhage, thrombosis, and emboli already mentioned. The various systemic diseases shown in Table 33 are too numerous to mention here, but fever of any etiology is an important cause and must not be forgotten, although this symptom is usually obvious.

● Approach to the Diagnosis

The patient presenting with a history of headaches is an exciting diagnostic challenge. If one approaches the challenge simply on the basis of what is common, the patient most likely has migraine or muscle traction headache. But, wait a minute! Shouldn't we look for serious conditions such as brain tumor, meningitis, or subarachnoid hemorrhage to avoid a serious mistake and a malpractice suit? First, check for nuchal rigidity to rule out meningitis and subarachnoid hemorrhage. Next, do a careful neurologic examination to rule out a brain tumor or other space-occupying lesion. These steps are particularly important in a patient who is experiencing his or her first serious headache. If there is nuchal rigidity or focal neurologic signs, it is wise to immediately refer the patient to a neurologist or neurosurgeon for further workup and possible hospitalization. The specialist will probably order a CT scan of the brain and follow that with a spinal tap if a subarachnoid hemorrhage or meningitis is suspected. It is clear that a CT scan should be done prior to a spinal tap if there are focal neurologic signs or papilledema. One other condition that must be considered in acute headache (particularly in elderly persons) is temporal arteritis. A sedimentation rate will usually be positive, but a neurology consult is axiomatic so that steroids can be started immediately.

In the patient with chronic or recurring headaches and no neurologic findings, it is wise to see the patient during the attack. Migraine and histamine headaches can be diagnosed by the response to sumatriptan by mouth or injection. If the headaches are due to chronic allergic or infectious rhinitis, relief can be had by spraying the turbinates with phenylephrine. Muscle traction headaches will often be relieved by occipital nerve blocks supporting the diagnosis. Compression of the superficial temporal artery will often relieve migraine temporarily supporting that diagnosis. Compression of the jugular veins will often give relief to patients with post spinal tap headaches.

If the patient is seen between headaches, certain prophylactic measures may help establish the diagnosis. For migraine, β-blockers may be prescribed; if the headaches are prevented, there is good support for the diagnosis. A course of corticosteroids may be initiated in patients with histamine (cluster) headaches to help establish the diagnosis. Muscle relaxants and/or tricyclic drugs may be given to help diagnose muscle contraction headaches.

The diagnostic workup of chronic headaches might include a CT scan of the brain, x-rays or CT scans of the sinuses, x-rays of the cervical spine, and routine blood work. Certainly if headache persists after careful follow-up, these need to be done.

● Other Useful Tests

1. Neurology consult
2. Sedimentation rate (temporal arteritis)
3. X-ray of the teeth (dental abscess)
4. MRI of the brain (brain tumor)
5. Spinal fluid analysis (meningitis, subarachnoid hemorrhage)
6. 24-hour blood pressure monitoring (pheochromocytoma)
7. 24-hour urine catecholamines (pheochromocytoma)
8. Tonometry (glaucoma)
9. MRI of the TMJs (TMJ syndrome)
10. Allergy skin tests (allergic rhinitis)
11. Temporal artery biopsy (temporal arteritis)

Case Presentation #39

A 28-year-old white woman comes to your office with the chief complaints of continuous generalized headache and nausea for 3 days. The patient has also experienced occasional vomiting. She was seen in the emergency room the night before and was diagnosed with migraine, given a shot, and sent home.

Question #1. Utilizing anatomy, what is your differential diagnosis at this point?

On examination, the patient was found to have nuchal rigidity but no focal neurologic signs. Her temperature is 100.2°F, and her blood pressure is 110/70 mmHg.

Question #2. What is your diagnosis now?

(See Appendix B for the answers.)

HEAD DEFORMITIES

The best method to recall the causes of head deformities is to think of the mnemonic **VINDICATE**.

V—Vascular suggests Cooley anemia and the enlargement of head and cheekbones with a small bridge of the nose.

I—Infection recalls syphilis in which the head assumes the shape of a hot cross bun.

N—Neurologic disease includes microcephaly (small underdeveloped brain) and hydrocephaly (due to several

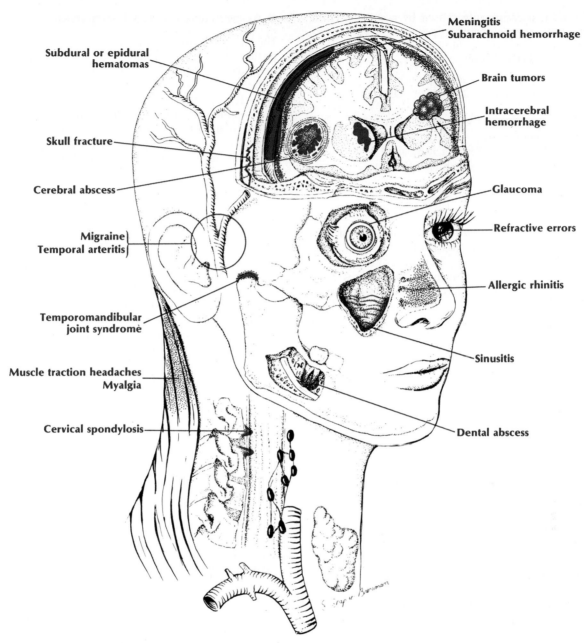

Subdural or epidural
hematomas

Skull fracture

Cerebral abscess

Migraine
Temporal arteritis

Temporomandibular
joint syndrome

Muscle traction headaches
Myalgia

Cervical spondylosis

Meningitis
Subarachnoid hemorrhage

Brain tumors

Intracerebral
hemorrhage

Glaucoma

Refractive errors

Allergic rhinitis

Sinusitis

Dental abscess

● **FIGURE 4** Headache.

causes); the most important diseases from a treatable standpoint are subdural hematomas, brain abscesses, and neoplasms. Cerebral palsy also should be included here.

D—Deficiency disease suggests rickets, in which the head is elongated, square, and flattened at the vertex.

I—Idiopathic disease recalls Paget disease. There is symmetric enlargement (occasionally a triangular shape) because the bones of the face do not enlarge. In facial hemiatrophy, one side of the head is smaller than the other.

C—Congenital disorders include scaphocephaly (elongated from front to back), oxycephaly or tower skull, hypertelorism (increased breadth of the skull and eyes far apart), mongolism, and brachycephaly.

A—Achondrodysplasia suggests a large head with a broad nose and prognathism.

T—Trauma recalls injury to the skull, causing edema (caput succedaneum), hematomas, and fractures.

E—Endocrine disorders such as acromegaly, myxedema, and cretinism cause a large head. Acromegaly is usually easily distinguishable by the protruding jaw.

● Approach to the Diagnosis

Obviously, the most important thing in the workup of this symptom is a good neurologic examination and a skull x-ray film. Other studies will be dictated by the findings of the above. A blood count and morphology study will be worthwhile if Cooley anemia is suspected and Wassermann or fluorescent treponemal antibody absorption (FTA-ABS) test if congenital syphilis is suspected. Positional head deformity is most commonly caused by a child sleeping frequently in the supine position.

● Other Useful Tests

1. Chemistry panel (rickets, Paget disease)
2. Serum 25-OHD and 1,25-(OH)2 D3 (vitamin D deficiency)
3. Sickle cell preparation (sickle cell anemia)
4. Bone scan (Paget disease)
5. Serum growth hormone level (acromegaly)
6. CT scan of brain (acromegaly, meningioma)

HEAD MASS

A localized mass on the head is usually a skin lesion, a lesion of the bone, or a protrusion of intracranial tissue through the bone. An extensive discussion of skin masses may be found on page 381, but most head masses originating from the skin are sebaceous cysts, carbuncles, or lipomas. Lesions of the skull that may present as focal lesions are metastatic tumors, multiple myeloma, osteitis fibrosa cystica (hyperparathyroidism), and osteomas. Brain tumors, subdural hematomas, and epidural abscesses may cause proliferation of the bone over the lesion and produce a mass. Congenital meningoceles and meningoencephaloceles may protrude through defects in the skull, producing large focal lesions in the midline.

● Approach to the Diagnosis

The approach to the diagnosis includes excision or biopsy of skin lesions, skull x-rays, CT scans, bone scans, and, if necessary, a bone biopsy. A neurosurgeon should be consulted before ordering expensive diagnostic tests.

HEARTBURN

True heartburn (see also sections on indigestion, page 264 and anorexia, page 55) may be defined as a burning pain in the substernal area or midepigastrium, which is usually increased by swallowing and which is almost invariably due to esophagitis from gastric reflux. There are other causes, however, and the problem for the diagnostician is how best to recall these in the clinical situation. From an etiologic standpoint **inflammation** is almost invariably the culprit, although myocardial infarction or angina pectoris are two frequent causes that are not inflammatory.

Anatomically, the best approach is to move in a target-like fashion from the intrinsic portion of the esophagus and stomach peripherally. Thus, in the **first zone**, one encounters esophagitis, gastritis, and gastric ulcers. In the **second zone**, one encounters hiatal hernia (which, of course, predisposes to esophagitis), pericarditis, mediastinitis, and gastrojejunostomy complications. In the **third zone**, one visualizes cholecystitis (which probably induces a bile esophagitis), pancreatitis, myocardial infarction or coronary insufficiency, pleurisy, and intestinal obstruction. In the **fourth zone**, one recalls systemic diseases such as uremia, severe emphysema, cirrhosis, and congestive heart failure (CHF) (which probably causes gastritis or gastric ulcers).

● Approach to the Diagnosis

The approach to the diagnosis of heartburn is similar to that of any GI complaint, but a few clinical tricks will help decide whether it is intrinsic or extrinsic, especially if the upper GI series is negative. Always order an esophagram. If the patient has the pain when in your office, administer a tablespoon or two of lidocaine (xylocaine viscous). If the patient gets relief in 5 to 10 minutes, the heartburn is probably caused by esophagitis. Further confirmation can be obtained by a Bernstein test. In this test, solutions of normal saline and 0.10 normal HCl are administered by intravenous tubing into the lower esophagus, alternating one with the other. If the patient invariably experiences pain when the 0.10 normal HCl is administered, esophagitis is confirmed. Esophagoscopy and gastroscopy will reveal most intrinsic lesions with certainty, but occasionally they are normal in esophagitis. Manometric studies of the esophagus are the best way to diagnose esophageal reflux. If the episodes are frequent but relatively brief, a trial of nitroglycerin may diagnose angina pectoris. Coronary insufficiency may also be confirmed by an exercise tolerance test. Cholecystogram and liver and pancreatic function studies may also be indicated.

● Other Useful Tests

1. Ambulatory pH monitoring (esophageal reflux)
2. Gallbladder sonogram (cholecystitis)
3. Thallium scan (coronary insufficiency)
4. Acid barium swallow (esophagitis)
5. Therapeutic trial of nitroglycerin (coronary insufficiency)
6. Holter monitoring (coronary insufficiency)
7. Coronary angiogram (coronary insufficiency)
8. Therapeutic trial of proton pump inhibitors (reflux esophagitis)

Case Presentation #40

A 48-year-old black man complained of recurrent substernal burning pain radiating to his jaw for several months. He has a history of smoking 2 packs of cigarettes a day for 30 years and consumes alcohol in moderation.

Question #1. Utilizing your knowledge of anatomy and histology, what is your differential diagnosis?

The pain is only occasionally relieved by antacids but can be precipitated by exercise. Physical examination is unremarkable except for a blood pressure of 155/110 and grade two arteriosclerotic retinopathy.

Question #2. What is your diagnosis now?

(See Appendix B for the answers.)

HEMATEMESIS AND MELENA

Hematemesis means vomiting or regurgitation of frank bright red blood or coffee-ground material that is positive

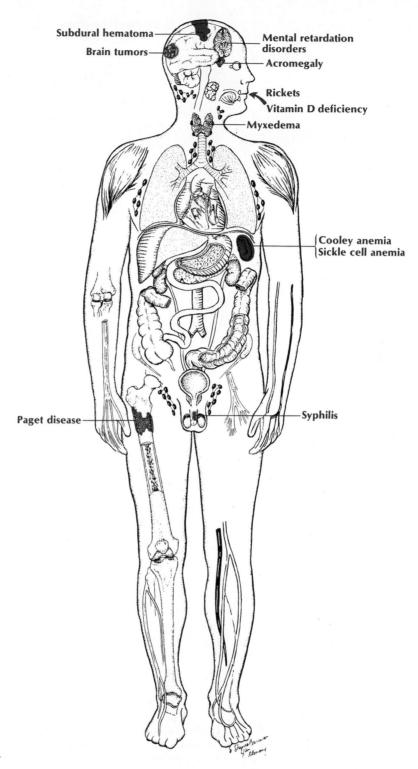

● **FIGURE 5** Head deformities.

for occult blood. It may be differentiated from hemoptysis because it usually gives an acidic reaction to nitrazine paper. It may be swallowed blood from any site in the oral cavity or nasopharynx, thus careful examination of these areas must be done. Melena is the passage of black tarry stools.

The differential diagnosis of hematemesis, like that for bleeding from other body orifices, is best developed with

the use of **anatomy**. Thus, beginning with the esophagus and working down to the ligament of Treitz and at the same time cross-indexing each structure with the various etiologies, one can make a chart like Table 34.

The major causes are illustrated on pages 208 and 211. In the esophagus the most common causes are varices, reflux esophagitis, carcinoma, and the Mallory–Weiss

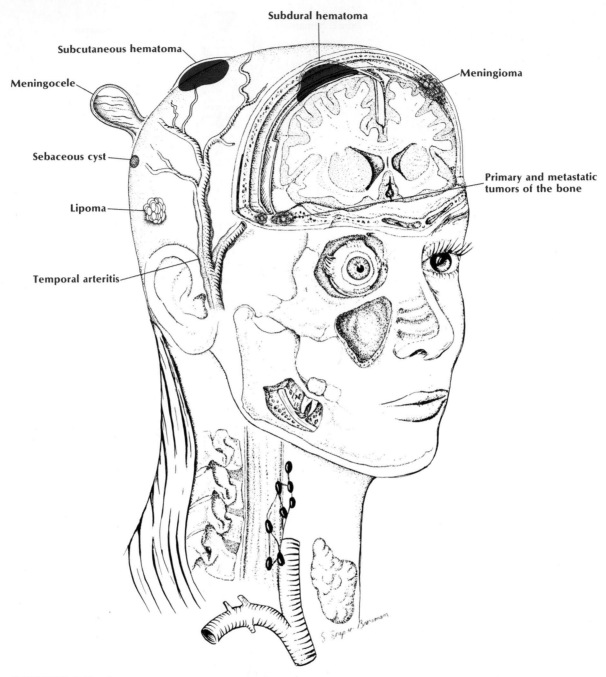

Subdural hematoma

Subcutaneous hematoma

Meningocele

Meningioma

Sebaceous cyst

Primary and metastatic
tumors of the bone

Lipoma

Temporal arteritis

● **FIGURE 6** Head mass.

syndrome. One should not forget foreign bodies or irritants such as lye, especially in children. Barrett esophagitis and ulcers caused by ectopic gastric mucosa are rare congenital causes of hematemesis. Finally, aortic aneurysms, mediastinal tumors, and carcinomas of the lung may ulcerate through the esophagus and bleed.

In the **stomach**, inflammation, especially gastritis and ulcers, is a prominent cause. Aspirin or alcohol, however, is often the cause. Varices of the cardia of the stomach may bleed. Carcinomas and **hereditary telangiectasis** are less common causes. Duodenal ulcers are usually the cause of bleeding from the duodenum, but occasionally neoplasms

and regional ileitis may be involved. Ulceration of gallstones through the gallbladder and duodenal wall is another rare cause of bleeding from this site. The pancreas is included in the drawing because occasionally one encounters gross hematemesis during acute hemorrhagic pancreatitis when blood pours out of the duct and is vomited.

Trauma is an important cause of bleeding from all the aforementioned sites, especially following intubation or surgery. Blood dyscrasias associated with coagulation disorders should be looked for immediately whenever a focal cause of hematemesis cannot be found, especially if bleeding is massive.

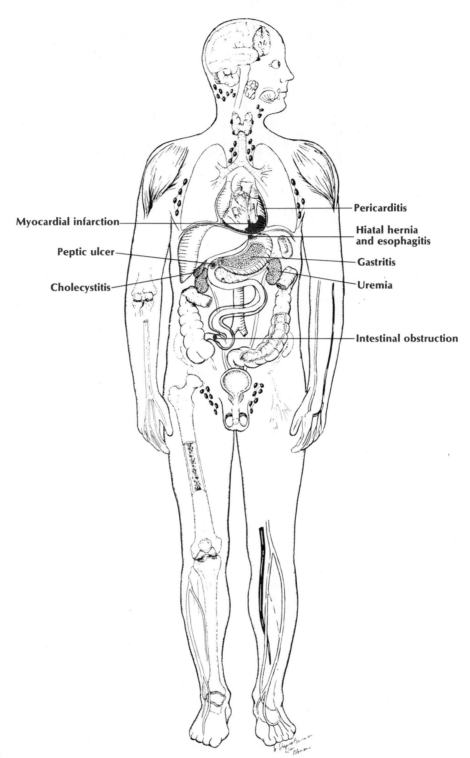

Myocardial infarction
Peptic ulcer
Cholecystitis

Pericarditis
Hiatal hernia and esophagitis
Gastritis
Uremia
Intestinal obstruction

● **FIGURE 7** Heartburn.

● Approach to the Diagnosis

When confronted with solid evidence of hematemesis, the clinician should not waste valuable time on a thorough history and physical examination when endoscopy is more important in both diagnosis and therapy. Ordering a type and cross for multiple units of blood, coagulation studies, and the other tests listed below should also be done immediately in most cases. History of alcoholism, use of aspirin and other drugs, and previous ulcers or esophageal disease is important to get while preparing for endoscopy and other emergency procedures. Patients without massive or recent acute hematemesis or melena may be approached with traditional methods. A history of vomiting nonhemorrhagic gastric fluid before the onset of hematemesis is helpful in diagnosing a Mallory–Weiss syndrome. Remember black stools can be caused by Pepto-Bismal, iron, spinach, or licorice ingestion.

TABLE 34 **Hematemesis and Melena**

	V Vascular	I Inflammatory	N Neoplasm	D Degenerative and Deficiency	I Intoxication	C Congenital	A Autoimmune Allergic	T Trauma	E Endocrine
Esophagus	Esophageal varices Aortic aneurysm	Reflux esophagitis Ulcer Trypanosomiasis cruzi	Carcinomas of esophagus and lung		Lye and other irritants Foreign body	Hiatal hernia Esophagitis	Scleroderma	Foreign body Nasogastric tube Mallory–Weiss syndrome	
Stomach	Cardiac varices Ruptured aneurysm	Gastritis Gastric ulcer	Carcinoma	Atrophic gastritis	Alcoholic gastritis, aspirin, and other drugs (e.g., arsenic)	Hereditary telangiec-tasis		Perforation and laceration surgery	Zollinger–Ellison syndrome
Duodenum		Ulcer					Regional ileitis	Perforation and laceration surgery	Zollinger–Ellison syndrome
Pancreas		Acute pancreatitis (hemorrhagic)							
Blood			Leukemia Polycythemia	Aplastic anemia Vitamin K deficiency	Warfarin Heparin Other drugs	Hemophilia and other hereditary coagulation disorders	ITP Collagen disease and other causes of thrombocytopenia		

ITP, idiopathic thrombocytopenic purpura.

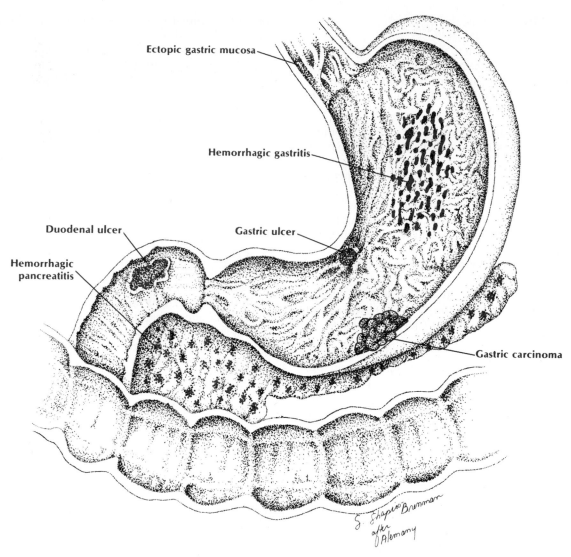

Ectopic gastric mucosa

Hemorrhagic gastritis

Duodenal ulcer

Gastric ulcer

Hemorrhagic
pancreatitis

Gastric carcinoma

H

● **FIGURE 8** Hematemesis and melena.

● Other Useful Tests

1. Complete blood count (CBC) (anemia of blood loss)
2. Chemistry panel (liver disease, kidney disease)
3. Stool for occult blood (ulcer, neoplasm, diverticulitis)
4. Gastric analysis (ulcer, neoplasm)
5. Liver function tests (esophageal varices)
6. Upper GI series and esophagram (reflux esophagitis, ulcer, esophageal carcinoma, gastric carcinoma)
7. Coagulation studies (e.g., blood dyscrasias, hemophilia)
8. Barium enema (colon neoplasm, diverticulitis)
9. Small-bowel series (neoplasm, diverticulitis)
10. CT scan of abdomen (neoplasm)
11. Colonoscopy (colon neoplasm, bleeding diverticulum)
12. Arteriogram (mesenteric thrombosis)
13. Fluorescein dye string test (to determine site of occult bleeding)
14. Nuclear scan (to detect bleeding)
15. Breath test and stool antigen for *Helicobacter pylori* (peptic ulcer)
16. Ultrasonography (esophageal varices)

Case Presentation #41

A 36-year-old black woman is brought to the emergency room with a chief complaint of hematemesis. She denies any previous episodes of hematemesis and only drinks on social occasions.

Question #1. Utilizing your knowledge of anatomy of the upper GI tract and physiology, what would be the possible causes of hematemesis in this woman?

Further history reveals that she had three episodes of vomiting food and bile-stained material prior to the hematemesis. Her physical examination was unremarkable except for pale conjunctiva.

Question #2. What is your diagnosis now?

(See Appendix B for the answers.)

HEMATURIA

Using the **anatomic** approach, the physician can arrive at most of the causes of hematuria (Table 35). One need only visualize the urinary tract and proceed from the kidney on down to get a differential list. Let us apply the mnemonic **VINDICATE** to the kidney.

V—**Vascular** diseases make one think of embolic glomerulonephritis, renal vein thrombosis, and subacute bacterial endocarditis SBE).

I—**Infectious** causes of hematuria are pyelonephritis (infrequently) and renal TB.

N—**Neoplasms** that may present with hematuria are hypernephromas and papillomas and carcinomas of the renal pelvis. Wilms tumors present with hematuria less frequently.

D—**Degenerative** diseases rarely present with hematuria as in other organ systems.

I—**Intoxicants** such as sulfa drugs (that lead to nephrocalcinosis), mercury poisoning, and blood transfusion reactions are common causes of gross or microscopic hematuria.

C—**Congenital** lesions such as polycystic kidneys and medullary sponge kidneys cause hematuria and predispose to stones and infections that may present with hematuria.

A—**Autoimmune** conditions such as acute and chronic glomerulonephritis, Goodpasture disease, Wegener midline granulomatosis, and lupus erythematosus commonly present with hematuria.

T—**Trauma** to any organ causes hemorrhages, and the kidney is no exception. Hematuria after automobile or other accidents should signal the need for hospitalization, intravenous pyelogram (IVP), and close observation of vital signs. Hematuria may present with a crush injury to any muscle or a burn. Injury to muscle (rhabdomyolysis) may also cause a positive urine dipstick test for blood because of myoglobin released by the muscle.

E—**Endocrine–metabolic** diseases caused by stones. Most calcium stones are not caused by hyperparathyroidism, but it should always be considered a possibility. Urate stones are usually caused by gout, and cystine stones are always associated with congenital cystinuria.

Ureter: Stones, papillomas, and congenital defects (contributing to stones) are the most likely causes here.

Bladder: Vascular disease is infrequently a cause, but cystitis (especially acute or "honeymoon" type) is a common cause. Stones, neoplasms (papillomas and transitional cell carcinomas), and foreign bodies are the next most likely causes. Trauma should not be forgotten, especially because of the numerous instances of various instruments being introduced into the bladder.

Prostate: Neoplasms of the prostate occasionally cause hematuria, but most other etiologic conditions (prostatitis) are rarely associated with gross or microscopic hematuria.

Urethra: Stones, neoplasms, and infections of the urethra may all cause hematuria, but very infrequently.

Using **biochemistry** as the basic chemistry, do not forget the coagulation disorders that may cause hematuria. Thus hematuria is often found in idiopathic thrombocytopenia purpura and in almost any disorder in which the platelet count drops below 40,000 cells/mm². Hemophiliacs may present with hematuria. Patients given too much warfarin (Coumadin) will often get hematuria. Fibrinolysins and afibrinogenemia will also cause hematuria.

From this exercise, it should be evident that arriving at the causes of hematuria is not difficult if one visualizes the anatomy of the urinary tree and then considers each etiologic category in this light.

● Approach to the Diagnosis

The clinical picture will point to the diagnosis in many cases. If there is a history of abdominal trauma, a contusion or laceration of the kidney or bladder should be suspected. Massive trauma anywhere prompts a tentative diagnosis of crush syndrome. This will cause myoglobinuria as well as hematuria. Purpura or bleeding from other sites suggests a coagulation disorder. Severe colicky pain in the abdomen suggests kidney stone. A long history of hypertension suggests polycystic kidneys, renal artery stenosis, or glomerulonephritis. A history of fever and rheumatic valvular disease suggests SBE with renal embolism. Painless hematuria in an otherwise healthy-looking adult suggests neoplasm, whereas painful hematuria with frequency and dysuria suggests cystitis. Hematuria and a flank mass would make a neoplasm or polycystic kidney likely.

The initial workup should include a CBC, urinalysis, urine culture, chemistry panel, flat plate of the abdomen to assess the presence of stones and kidney size, and personal examination of the urinary sediment. If a renal calculus is suspected, a noncontrast helical CT scan is ordered immediately, and a urologist consulted. A three-glass test will help to localize the site of the bleeding. If there is blood in the initial specimen only, the urethra is probably the site of bleeding. If the blood is primarily in the final specimen, the bladder is most likely the site of bleeding. Equal blood discoloration in all specimens points to a renal lesion.

If renal TB is suspected, an acid-fast bacillus (AFB) smear and culture is done. If collagen disease is suspected, an ANA analysis and anti–double-strand DNA antibody titer is ordered.

If a renal carcinoma is suspected, a CT scan of the abdomen is probably the best study to order, but the advice of a urologist ought to be sought. Ultrasonography is useful in differentiating cysts from tumors. If a bladder neoplasm is suspected, cystoscopy will be done. If renal artery embolism or thrombosis is suspected, renal angiography may need to be done to clearly make the diagnosis.

● Other Useful Tests

1. Chest x-ray (TB, Goodpasture disease)
2. Tuberculin test (TB)
3. Strain urine for stones

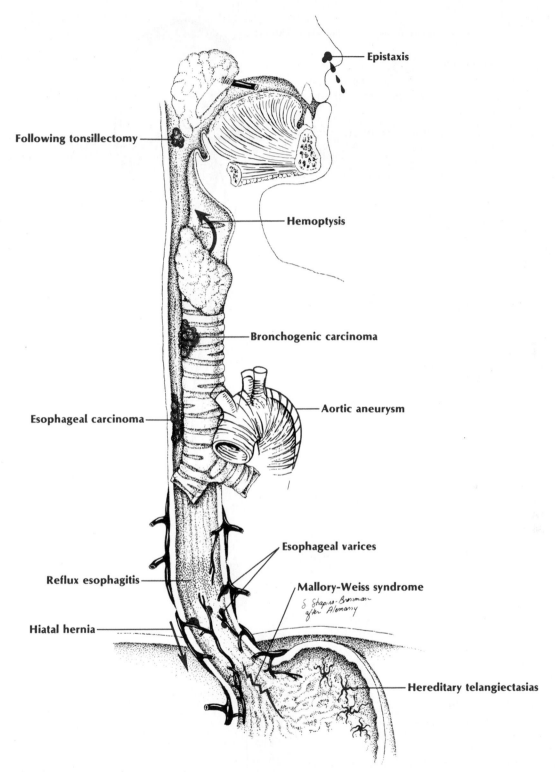

Epistaxis

Following tonsillectomy

Hemoptysis

Bronchogenic carcinoma

Esophageal carcinoma

Aortic aneurysm

Esophageal varices

Reflux esophagitis

Mallory-Weiss syndrome

Hiatal hernia

Hereditary telangiectasias

● **FIGURE 9** Hematemesis and melena.

4. Serum complement (acute glomerulonephritis, lupus)
5. AntistreptolysinO(ASO)titer(acuteglomerulonephritis)
6. Addis count (glomerulonephritis)
7. Blood cultures (SBE)
8. Coagulation studies (hemophilia, collagen disease, allergic purpura)

9. Plasma haptoglobins (hemolytic anemias)
10. Coombs test (hemolytic anemias)
11. Platelet count (thrombocytopenic purpura)
12. Renal biopsy (chronic nephritis, neoplasm)
13. Surgical exploration

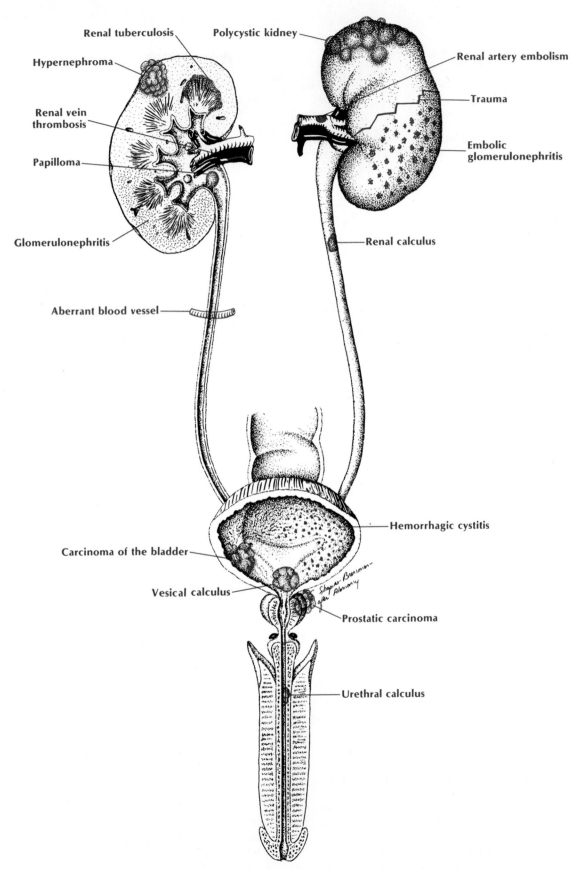

● **FIGURE 10** Hematuria.

TABLE 35   Hematuria

	V Vascular	I Inflammatory	N Neoplasm	D Degenerative and Deficiency	I Intoxication	C Congenital	A Autoimmune Allergic	T Trauma	E Endocrine and Metabolic
Kidney	Embolic glomerulonephritis Renal vein thrombosis Subacute bacterial endocarditis	Pyelonephritis Renal TB	Hypernephromas Papillomas Carcinomas Wilms tumor		Sulfa drugs Mercury poisoning Blood transfusion reaction	Polycystic kidney Medullary sponge kidney Congenital lesion	Acute and chronic glomerulonephritis Goodpasture disease Wegener midline granulomatosis Lupus erythematosus	Crush injury to muscle Burn Laceration	Stones (uric acid, calcium phosphate, cystine)
Ureters			Papilloma			Congenital bands (e.g., aberrant vessels)			Stones (see above)
Bladder		Cystitis Hunner ulcer Foreign body	Papilloma Transitional cell carcinoma					Ruptured bladder (e.g., from instruments)	Stones (see above)
Prostate		Prostatitis	Carcinoma						
Urethra		Infections of urethra (e.g., gonorrhea)	Neoplasm						Stones (see above)

H

Case Presentation #42

A 31-year-old white man presents to the emergency room with severe right flank pain and a specimen of bloody urine. He is begging for a shot to relieve the pain.

Question #1. Utilizing your knowledge of anatomy of the urinary tract, what is your differential diagnosis?

The patient is given a shot of Demerol and admitted to the hospital. Physical examination aside from exquisite tenderness in the right flank is unremarkable. Complete workup including an IVP is negative. Repeated urinalysis reveals grossly bloody urine. However, on catheterization a normal specimen of urine is obtained.

Question #2. What is your diagnosis now?

(See Appendix B for the answers.)

HEMIANOPSIA

To develop a list of possible causes of hemianopsia, trace the fibers of the optic nerve through the optic chiasma, optic tract, optic radiation, and optic cortex and apply a mnemonic such as **VINDICATE** to prompt the recall of the conditions affecting each level.

Optic chiasma: Vascular—aneurysm; **inflammatory**—syphilis, arachnoiditis; **neoplasm**—pituitary adenoma, suprasellar cysts, meningiomas; **congenital**—hydrocephalus; **autoimmune**—multiple sclerosis; **trauma**—gunshot wound; **endocrine**—pituitary tumors, pseudotumor cerebri.

Optic tract: Aneurysm, arachnoiditis, brain stem tumors, gunshot wounds, and multiple sclerosis.

Optic radiations: Hemorrhage or infarct of the internal capsule (as occurs in the thalamic syndrome), parietal and temporal lobe tumors, lupus erythematosus, and multiple sclerosis.

Optic cortex: Posterior cerebral artery embolism or thrombosis, occipital lobe tumors, abscess, or hematoma.

● Approach to the Diagnosis

A careful outline of the field defect by a tangent screen or perimetry is essential. An ophthalmologist should be consulted to do this. A bitemporal hemianopsia suggests a pituitary tumor warranting a CT scan or MRI. The finding of hair loss, weight loss, and/or loss of secondary sexual characteristics points to a pituitary tumor as the cause. It is wise to order a 24-hour urine gonadotropin and other tests of pituitary function.

Long tract signs suggest a vascular, neoplastic, or demyelinating lesion in the brain stem or cerebral cortex. A neurologist should be consulted before ordering expensive diagnostic tests.

● Other Useful Tests

1. Venereal disease research laboratory (VDRL) (syphilis)
2. Visual evoked potentials (VEPs) (multiple sclerosis)
3. Spinal tap (syphilis, multiple sclerosis, pseudotumor cerebri)
4. ANA (collagen disease)
5. Four-vessel cerebral angiography (posterior cerebral artery thrombosis)

HEMIPLEGIA

Hemiplegia is paralysis of one side of the body and is almost invariably the result of damage to the pyramidal tract somewhere along its course from the upper cervical cord to the cerebral cortex. Recall of the many causes can be facilitated by the mnemonic **VITAMIN**.

V—**Vascular** disease would help recall cerebral hemorrhage, thrombosis, and embolisms. When these occur in the vertebral–basilar artery distribution, quadriparesis or paraplegia is more common. Aneurysm and arteriovenous malformation can be associated with paraplegia. Anterior spinal artery occlusions are more likely to be associated with paraplegia.

I—**Inflammatory** disease would suggest cerebral abscess, cortical vein thrombophlebitis, encephalomyelitis, viral encephalitis, and some form of meningitis.

T—**Trauma** brings to mind epidural, subdural, and intracerebral hematomas resulting from trauma. Although uncommon, a high cervical cord lesion due to a fractured cervical spine with cord compression may cause hemiplegia.

A—**Autoimmune** disorders that may cause hemiplegia include multiple sclerosis, possible Schilder disease, and collagen disorders.

M—**Malformation** brings to mind porencephalic cysts, cerebral agenesis, and Sturge–Weber syndrome.

I—**Intoxication** is not likely to cause hemiplegia, but ischemia would suggest the transient ischemia of carotid stenosis and migraine.

N—**Neoplasms** of brain (causing hemiplegia) include meningiomas, gliomas, and metastatic carcinoma. An early meningioma of the high cervical cord may rarely be associated with hemiplegia. **N** for **neurosis** will help to recall the hemiplegia of conversion hysteria.

● Approach to the Diagnosis

The history is very important in determining the diagnosis of hemiplegia. An acute onset without a history of trauma would suggest a cerebral embolism, hemorrhage, or thrombosis, whereas a gradual onset would indicate a possible neoplasm or other space-occupying lesion. Intermittent occurrence of hemiplegia might suggest migraine, multiple sclerosis, or carotid artery insufficiency. A history of fever may indicate a cerebral abscess or subacute bacterial endocarditis. The physical examination may also be helpful. A carotid bruit points to carotid stenosis. A cardiac arrhythmia suggests cerebral embolism. Hypertension points to cerebral hemorrhage. A central facial palsy or other cranial nerve signs indicate a brain or brain stem lesion as opposed to a cervical cord insult. The initial diagnostic workup would include a CBC, sedimentation rate, VDRL, ANA, and chemistry panel.

More definitive studies such as a CT scan or MRI will almost certainly be necessary, but a neurologist should be consulted first. If a vascular lesion is suspected, MRI, a carotid duplex scan, and four-vessel cerebral angiography may be indicated. Blood cultures would be helpful in ruling out bacterial endocarditis. Spinal fluid analysis should be done if multiple sclerosis or neurosyphilis is suspected.

● Other Useful Tests

1. Endocarditis (cerebral embolism)
2. Electrocardiogram (ECG) (myocardial infarction with mural thrombosis, atrial fibrillation)

3. Somatosensory evoked potential (SSEP), brain stem–evoked potential (BSEP), VEP (multiple sclerosis)
4. Echocardiography (dilated myocardiopathy)

HEMOPTYSIS

True **hemoptysis** must be distinguished from **epistaxis** (see page 155) and hematemesis (see page 208). If the blood is bright red and alkaline (use nitrazine paper to test) and the nasal passages and posterior pharynx are clear, then it is probably hemoptysis.

Anatomy is the basic science to apply to develop a differential diagnosis of hemoptysis. Beginning at the **larynx** and working down the trachea, bronchi, and alveoli, one can quickly recall the major causes of hemoptysis using the cross-index of the various etiologies as in Table 36. Laryngitis is an infrequent cause of hemoptysis, but laryngeal carcinoma

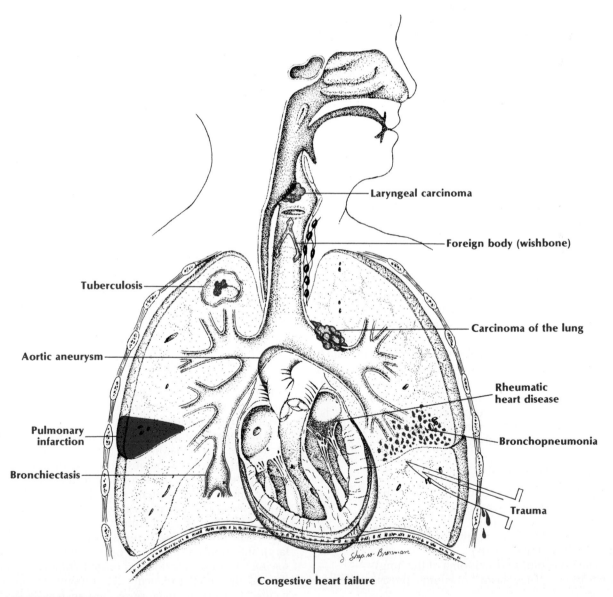

● **FIGURE 11** Hemoptysis.

may cause it. TB of the larynx used to be a common cause but it is not often seen today. A foreign body such as a chicken bone lodged in the larynx or **trachea** should always be considered, especially in children. Additional etiologies of hemoptysis that one might encounter in the trachea are ulceration and rupture of an aortic aneurysm or a carcinoma of the esophagus with a tracheoesophageal fistula. Hereditary telangiectasia may lead to hemoptysis anywhere along the tracheobronchial tree. In the **bronchi**, carcinoma, TB, and bronchiectasis become prominent causes. These are probably the most common causes of chronic hemoptysis in the adult.

In the **alveoli** the acute causes of hemoptysis—pneumonia (pneumococcal and Friedlander, especially), and pulmonary embolism or infarctions—are encountered. CHF may cause a foamy hemoptysis. Carcinoma, TB, fungi, parasites, and trauma are also important. Collagen diseases, Goodpasture syndrome, and primary hemosiderosis should be looked for in the elusive cases.

● Approach to the Diagnosis

The differential diagnosis of hemoptysis can be narrowed considerably by the clinical picture. Acute hemoptysis with chest pain would suggest pulmonary embolism. A chronic cough with occasional hemoptysis suggests neoplasm, TB, or bronchiectasis. Hemoptysis with chills and fever suggests pneumonia, but one should always keep pulmonary embolism in mind. Hemoptysis with dyspnea, edema, or cardiomegaly suggests mitral stenosis or CHF. The sputum is usually foamy in cases of CHF. Hemoptysis with purpura or bleeding from other sites should suggest a systemic disease or coagulation disorder.

The initial workup of hemoptysis includes a CBC, urinalysis, sedimentation rate, chemistry panel, sputum smear and culture, ECG, and chest x-ray. If a pulmonary embolism is suspected, arterial blood gas analysis and a lung scan are ordered. Pulmonary angiography may also be necessary. If routine studies and the clinical picture suggest pneumonia, nothing more may need to be done other than a careful follow-up. If CHF is suspected, a circulation time may be done, but a cardiology consult and echocardiogram would be more definitive. What would you do if it was your heart?

If a bronchogenic neoplasm or bronchiectasis is suspected, a pulmonary consult and bronchoscopy would be ordered. Bronchiectasis can be identified with a CT scan of the chest also. If TB is suspected, a tuberculin test is performed, and sputum is cultured for AFB and possibly Guinea pig inoculation performed.

● Other Useful Tests

1. Papanicolaou smears of sputum (neoplasm)
2. Coagulation studies (see page 65)
3. Apical lordotic views (TB)
4. Spirometry (chronic bronchitis and emphysema, CHF)
5. ECG (CHF, mitral stenosis)
6. Scalene node biopsy (carcinoma of the lung)
7. Lung biopsy (neoplasm, pneumoconiosis, collagen disease)
8. Coccidioidin skin test

9. Histoplasmin skin test
10. Blastomycin skin test
11. Circulatory antiglomerular antibodies

Case Presentation #43

A 41-year-old nurse presents with a history of intermittent blood-streaked sputum for the past 2 months. She is a 20-year smoker and has had a chronic cough which has become more and more productive in the past 2 years. She was hospitalized 1 year ago for bronchopneumonia.

Question #1. Utilizing anatomy, what would be your list of most likely diagnoses at this time?

She denies fever, chills, or weight loss. Physical examination reveals a few sibilant and sonorous rales over both lungs but is otherwise unremarkable. A 24-hour sputum collection revealed a volume of 5 oz.

Question #2. What is your diagnosis now?

(See Appendix B for the answers.)

HEPATOMEGALY

Two key words to think of here are **histology** and **obstruction**: The analysis of the differential diagnosis of hepatomegaly is best begun with a histologic breakdown of the liver tissue (Table 37). Thus, there are **parenchymal cells** that can be involved by toxic or inflammatory hepatitis. A variety of drugs (e.g., isoniazid) and toxins (e.g., carbon tetrachloride) can cause toxic hepatitis. Infectious hepatitis is most commonly caused by a virus (type A or B; which is usually transfusion-transmitted but may be transmitted by fecal–oral route) or by infectious mononucleosis.

Beginning with the smallest organism (virus) and working up to the largest, one must consider brucellosis, TB (bacteria), syphilis, leptospirosis (spirochetal), amebiasis, amebic abscess, schistosomiasis, hydatid cysts (parasites), histoplasmosis, actinomycosis, and other systemic mycoses (fungi). When considering the **supporting tissue**, do not forget lupoid hepatitis, periarteritis nodosa, sarcoidosis, and cirrhosis. In addition, because the liver contains von Kupffer cells, any disease causing proliferation of the reticuloendothelial system may produce hepatomegaly. Myeloid metaplasia and Gaucher disease are good examples of this.

The **hepatic veins** may be involved with a thrombosis and lead to hepatomegaly (Budd–Chiari syndrome). The **portal veins** may be obstructed by thrombophlebitis (pyelophlebitis), usually secondary to infection elsewhere in the gut. **Portal lymphatics** involved in Hodgkin lymphoma may cause hepatomegaly. From the **bile canaliculi** down to the hepatic and common bile ducts, obstruction may occur from stones, neoplasms (pancreatic or ampullary), infection (cholangitis), or parasites (e.g., *Clonorchis sinensis)*. Chlorpromazine and related drugs cause obstruction of the small canaliculi and present an obstructive picture. Pancreatitis may cause the pancreas to swell and produce bile duct obstruction and hepatomegaly.

TABLE 36   Hemoptysis

	V Vascular	I Inflammatory	N Neoplasm	D Degenerative and Deficiency	I Intoxication and Idiopathic	C Congenital	A Autoimmune Allergic	T Trauma	E Endocrine Metabolic
Larynx		Laryngitis especially TB	Carcinoma Polyp		Laryngitis Smoke			Foreign body	
Trachea	Aortic aneurysm	Tracheitis	Carcinoma and adenomas Esophageal carcinoma		Tracheitis from smoke	Hereditary telangiectasis		Foreign body	
Bronchi	Ruptured bronchial vein	Chronic bronchitis and TB Viral influenza	Carcinoma and bronchial adenomas			Bronchiectasis		Foreign body	Carcinoid
Alveoli	Pulmonary embolism Congestive heart failure	Tuberculosis Pneumonia Fungus Parasite	Carcinomas, primary and metastatic	Pulmonary fibrosis Scurvy	Sarcoidosis	Sickle cell anemia Kartagener syndrome Primary hemosiderosis	Collagen disease Wegener granuloma Goodpasture disease	Biopsy, fracture Perforation and contusion	
Blood		Sepsis with disseminated intravascular coagulopathy	Leukemia Polycythemia Lymphoma	Aplastic anemia Vitamin K deficiency	Drug Warfarin sodium Heparin	Coagulation defect (hemophilia)	Thrombocytopenia		

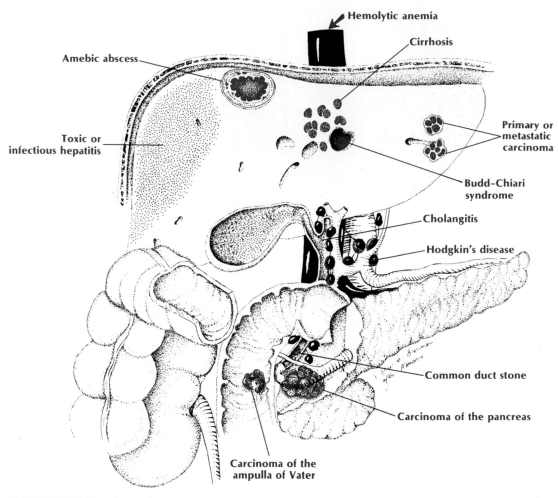

● **FIGURE 12** Hepatomegaly.

The **parenchymal cells** can respond in other ways to various etiologic agents to cause hepatomegaly. In diabetes and alcoholism, they may undergo fatty degeneration and infiltration. They may become hyperplastic in cirrhosis or neoplasm-causing hepatomas. Metastatic carcinoma is a common cause of hepatomegaly. Supporting tissue may proliferate to form a sarcoma. Edema of the liver with hepatomegaly results from chronic CHF. Infiltration with amyloid or glycogen may cause hepatomegaly; CHF and infectious hepatitis cause a tender liver, which distinguishes them from other forms of hepatomegaly. Extrinsic conditions causing apparent hepatomegaly, but which is really only displacement of the liver, are diaphragmatic abscess and pulmonary emphysema. In hemolytic anemias, the liver may be enlarged because of the increased load on the reticuloendothelial tissue (both in liver and spleen) to dispose of the damaged red cells.

● **Approach to the Diagnosis**

The clinical picture will help to distinguish many causes of hepatomegaly. Shortness of breath, pitting edema, and hepatomegaly suggest CHF. Chronic cough, wheezing, jugular vein distention, hepatomegaly, and pitting edema suggest

pulmonary emphysema and cor pulmonale. Fever, tender hepatomegaly, and jaundice suggest viral hepatitis or cholangitis. Hepatomegaly and ascites with a history of heavy alcohol intake suggest alcoholic cirrhosis. Hepatomegaly with gross or occult blood in the stool would suggest metastatic neoplasm of the GI tract. Asymptomatic hepatomegaly is probably related to congenital cystic disease, metastasis, or alcoholism.

The initial workup will involve a CBC, urinalysis, sedimentation rate, chemistry panel, amylase and lipase levels, and a flat plate of the abdomen. If viral hepatitis is suspected, a hepatitis profile should be done. If CHF is suspected, a circulation time and spirometry is an inexpensive method of confirming the diagnosis. A chest x-ray and ECG need to be ordered also. If obstructive jaundice is suspected, endoscopic retrograde cholangiopancreatography may be done, but a CT scan of the abdomen should probably be done first. A CT scan of the abdomen will also identify primary and metastatic carcinoma of the liver. The many infectious diseases that are associated with hepatomegaly will need antibody titers, blood smears, or skin tests to reveal the diagnosis. Hemolytic anemias require blood smears, sickle cell preparation, serum haptoglobins, and hemoglobin electrophoresis to get a definitive diagnosis.

TABLE 37 Hepatomegaly

	V Vascular	I Infection	N Neoplasm	D Degenerative	I Intoxication	C Congenital	A Autoimmune	T Trauma	E Endocrine
Parenchyma		Viral hepatitis Infectious mononucleosis Amebiasis	Hepatoma Metastatic carcinoma	Fatty liver	Alcoholism Carbon tetrachloride Drugs	Cystic disease Hamartoma	Lupoid Hepatitis	Contusion Laceration	Hyperthyroidism
Supporting Tissue			Sarcoma			Gaucher disease Hemolytic anemias	Periarteritis nodosa Myeloid metaplasia		
Veins	Hepatic vein thrombosis	Pyelophlebitis							
Arteries	Hepatic artery ligation							Hepatic artery ligation	
Lymphatics			Hodgkin lymphoma						
Bile Ducts		Cholangitis *Clonorchis sinensis*	Papilloma Ampullary carcinoma Pancreatic carcinoma		Milk causing bile inspissation	Biliary atresia		Stone	Stone (diabetes mellitus)
Cholangioles		Bacterial cholangitis	Cholangioma		Thorazine Birth control pills	Dubin–Johnson syndrome			Pregnancy

H

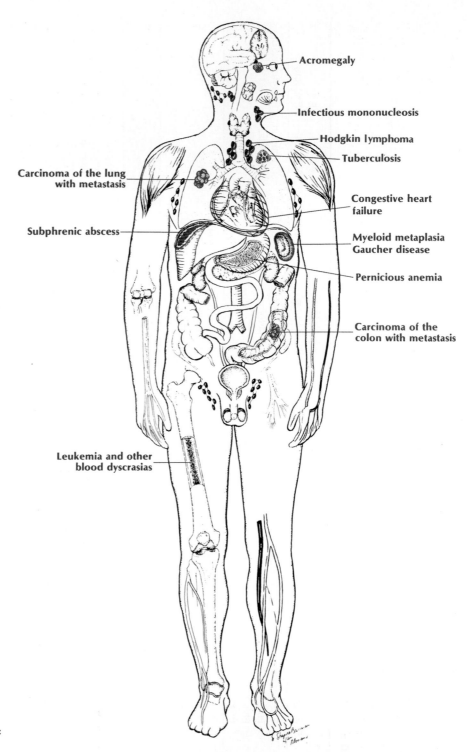

Acromegaly

Infectious mononucleosis

Hodgkin lymphoma

Tuberculosis

Carcinoma of the lung with metastasis

Congestive heart failure

Subphrenic abscess

Myeloid metaplasia Gaucher disease

Pernicious anemia

Carcinoma of the colon with metastasis

Leukemia and other blood dyscrasias

● **FIGURE 13** Hepatomegaly, systemic causes.

Amebic abscess can be elucidated by a CT scan, but an antibody titer will assist in the definitive diagnosis. Venography will reveal hepatic vein thrombosis.

● **Other Useful Tests**

1. Febrile agglutinins (typhoid fever, brucellosis)
2. Monospot test (infectious mononucleosis)
3. Serum iron and iron-binding capacity (hemochromatosis)
4. Serum copper and ceruloplasmin (Wilson disease)
5. ANA analysis (lupoid hepatitis, collagen disease)
6. Stool for occult blood (metastatic malignancy)
7. Stool for ova and parasites (amebic abscess, cysticercosis and other parasites)
8. Bone marrow examination (hemolytic anemias, leukemia, myeloid metaplasia)
9. GI series and barium enema (metastatic neoplasm)
10. Sonogram (hepatic cyst, gallstones, abscess)
11. Laparoscopy (cirrhosis, metastatic neoplasm)

12. Liver biopsy (cirrhosis, hepatitis, metastatic carcinoma)
13. Serum α-fetoprotein (hepatoma)
14. Mitochondrial antibody titer (biliary cirrhosis)

Case Presentation #44

A 28-year-old Puerto Rican man presents with weight loss and loss of appetite. Physical examination reveals hepatosplenomegaly.

Question #1. Utilizing your knowledge of histology, what is your differential diagnosis?

There is no history of alcoholism, drug use, or jaundice. However, he had one episode of hematemesis 3 months ago. There is only mild splenomegaly. A diagnostic workup revealed slight leucopenia with a relative eosinophilia and anemia but no blood in the stool. Serum iron and iron-binding capacity were normal.

Question #2. What is your list of diagnostic possibilities now?

(See Appendix B for the answers.)

HICCOUGHS

A list of causes of this common symptom is best developed by considering the **anatomy** of the structures associated with the phrenic nerve at its origin, along its pathway, and at its termination. Applying the mnemonic **MINT** to these structures allows one to arrive at a fairly complete list of possibilities.

Origin: Impulses transmitted along the phrenic nerve originate in the brainstem and spinal cord, so diseases of these structures must be considered.

M—Malformations to be considered are hydrocephalus and kernicterus.

I—Inflammatory and **intoxicating** conditions that are possible causes are encephalitis, toxic encephalopathy (e.g., alcohol, bromides, drugs, and uremia), and, in the spinal cord particularly, tabes dorsalis. Meningitis may be associated with persistent hiccoughs. Epidemic hiccoughs are probably a form of encephalitis.

N—Neoplasms of the brain may cause hiccoughs, especially when they are associated with increased intracranial pressure.

T—Traumatic lesions include concussions and hematomas. Supratentorial conditions (such as neurosis) may be associated with hiccoughs, but this is present only during the waking hours and the patient eats surprisingly well.

Pathway: Along the pathway of the phrenic nerve, mediastinal and chest conditions are important.

M—Malformations such as aortic aneurysm, dermoid cyst, and enlarged heart from whatever cause should be considered.

I—Inflammatory lesions such as pericarditis, mediastinitis, pneumonia, and pleurisy are equally important.

N—Neoplasm here, particularly Hodgkin lymphoma and bronchogenic carcinoma, may cause hiccoughs.

T—Trauma, particularly penetrating wounds of the chest causing pneumothorax and hemopneumothorax, is often associated with hiccoughs.

Termination: The most common causes of hiccoughs are found in the diaphragm.

M—Malformations include hiatal hernia, pyloric obstruction, and Barrett esophagitis.

I—Inflammation suggests reflux or bile esophagitis, gastritis, hepatitis, cholecystitis, peritonitis, and subphrenic abscess.

N—Neoplasms include esophageal carcinoma, carcinoma of the stomach, retroperitoneal Hodgkin lymphoma, and sarcoma.

T—Trauma includes hemoperitoneum from ruptured spleen or liver, ruptured viscus, or ruptured ectopic pregnancy. One other group of causes is the reflex stimulation of the phrenic nerve from organs far beneath the diaphragm. For example, carcinoma of the uterus or colon without metastasis may occasionally cause hiccoughs.

● **Approach to the Diagnosis**

The usual reaction to a patient with hiccoughs is "They'll get over them regardless of what we do so why worry about them?" If, however, one puts oneself in the position of the patient, it behooves one to be certain that a grave condition such as uremia or subdiaphragmatic abscess is not present. Relief with Pepto-Bismal or xylocaine viscus suggests the cause is reflux esophagitis. In the otherwise healthy patient, esophagoscopy and gastroscopy often reveal a reflux esophagitis or gastritis. Cholecystograms, liver and pancreatic function studies, spinal tap, and brain and total body scan have their place in individual cases.

● **Other Useful Tests**

1. CBC (anemia, chronic infection)
2. Chemistry panel (uremia, cirrhosis)
3. Esophagram (reflux esophagitis)
4. Upper GI series (gastritis, gastric ulcer)
5. Gallbladder ultrasound (cholelithiasis)
6. CT scan of the abdomen (e.g., subdiaphragmatic abscess)
7. ECG (pericarditis)
8. Bernstein test (reflux esophagitis)
9. Ambulatory pH monitoring (reflux esophagitis)

Case Presentation #45

A 44-year-old white male street cleaner presented with recurrent hiccoughs and weight loss. Physical examination revealed slight hepatomegaly, tremor, and rigidity.

Question #1. Utilizing the methods discussed above, what would be your differential diagnosis at this point?

After hospitalization, he was observed to have intermittent fever and chills and a white blood cell count of 18,900; a chest x-ray revealed an elevated right diaphragm. Serum copper and ceruloplasmin were normal.

Question #2. What is your diagnosis now?

(See Appendix B for the answers.)

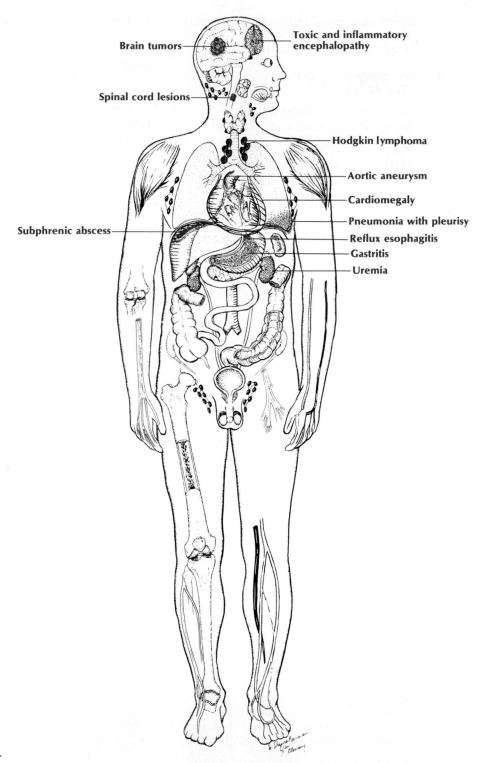

Brain tumors

Toxic and inflammatory
encephalopathy

Spinal cord lesions

Hodgkin lymphoma

Aortic aneurysm

Cardiomegaly

Pneumonia with pleurisy

Reflux esophagitis

Gastritis

Uremia

Subphrenic abscess

● **FIGURE 14** Hiccoughs.

HIP PAIN

When confronted with a case of hip pain in an adult, the clinician is most likely to think of fracture or joint inflammation such as osteoarthritis, realizing however that there are many other possibilities (Table 38). How can the clinician think of them on the spot? **Anatomy** is the key. The hip is composed of skin, muscle, bursa, ligament, joint, and bone. It is also supplied by nerves, arteries, and veins. Looking at each of these structures in terms of etiology, skin should prompt the recall of herpes zoster, and muscle should prompt the recall of contusion or sprain. The bursa should allow one to recall greater trochanter bursitis—a common and easily treated form of hip pain. Thinking of the ligaments, consider sprain. Iliotibial band syndrome is a common cause of hip pain in runners. Visualizing the joint would prompt consideration of osteoarthritis, gout, and RA as well as congenital dislocation of the joint, slipped femoral epiphysis, Legg–Perthes disease, and rheumatic fever. Visualizing the bone should prompt recall of fracture and primary and metastatic tumors. Visualizing the nerves, one should think of the sciatic nerve and consider a herniated lumbar disc, cauda equina tumor, or sciatic neuritis (which is rare). Considering the arteries and veins may prompt one to think of avascular necrosis.

● Approach to the Diagnosis

The history and physical examination will allow differentiation of many of the conditions listed above. For example, the history of trauma suggests sprain, fracture, or contusion. Remember that fractures of the hip can occur in elderly persons without a history of trauma. A positive straight leg raise (SLR) test suggests a herniated disc or other cauda equina pathology. X-rays of the hip and lumbosacral spine will help rule out fracture or osteoarthritis, but CT scan, bone scan, or MRI may be necessary. If x-rays and laboratory examinations are negative, a trial of lidocaine injections into the greater trochanter bursa or other trigger points may be diagnostic.

● Other Useful Tests

1. CBC (infection)
2. Chemistry panel (metastatic neoplasm)
3. Urinalysis (multiple myeloma, gout)
4. Sedimentation rate (osteomyelitis, arteritis)
5. RA tests
6. ANA analysis (collagen disease)
7. Joint fluid analysis (all types of arthritis)
8. Tuberculin test (TB of the joint)
9. Bone biopsy (neoplasm)
10. Exploratory surgery

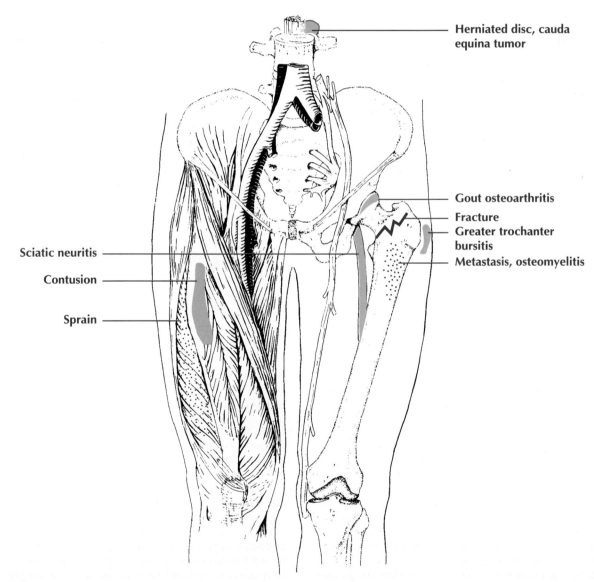

● FIGURE 15 Hip pain.

TABLE 38   **Hip Pain**

	M Malformation	I Inflammation	N Neoplasm	T Trauma
Skin		Herpes zoster		Contusion
Muscle		Myositis		Contusion
Bursa		Greater trochanter bursitis		Contusion
Ligaments				Sprain
Joint	Congenital dislocation	Rheumatoid arthritis Osteoarthritis Gout		Contusion Hemorrhage
Bone		Osteomyelitis	Primary or metastatic neoplasm	Fracture Avascular necrosis
Nerves		Neuritis	Cauda equina tumor	Herniated disc

Case Presentation #46

A 56-year-old white woman complained of increasing left hip pain which began 3 months ago and had gradually gotten worse. There is no history of trauma, fever or chills, and no numbness or tingling of the extremities. She had a mastectomy for breast cancer 5 years previously.

Question #1. Utilizing anatomy, what would be your differential diagnosis at this point?

Physical examination is unremarkable except for tenderness of the greater trochanter bursa and a positive Patrick sign. The SLR test is negative, and there are no focal neurologic signs. Plain films of the spine and hip are negative.

Question #2. What is your diagnosis now?

(See Appendix B for the answers.)

HIRSUTISM

The vast majority of women presenting to the clinician with excessive hair on the face or body are normal and healthy. Nevertheless, one should be alert to the pathologic consequences of this symptom.

Anatomy is the best basic science to use in recalling the various causes. Simply by visualizing the endocrine glands and proceeding from the head caudally, one may come up with the most significant pathologic causes of hirsutism. If these are ruled out, the patient most likely has idiopathic hirsutism and nothing needs to be done.

Pituitary: Acromegaly and a basophilic adenoma of the pituitary may cause hirsutism.

Thyroid: Congenital and juvenile hypothyroidism are associated with hirsutism but not virilism.

Adrenal gland: Adrenal carcinomas, adenomas, and hyperplasia may all be associated with hirsutism. With the exception of Cushing syndrome, there is usually virilism as well. Congenital adrenal hyperplasia may become manifest at puberty, in which case there will be both hirsutism and virilism.

Ovary: Polycystic ovary syndrome (Stein–Leventhal syndrome) will be recalled by visualizing this endocrine gland. It is second only to idiopathic hirsutism in frequency. There is usually no virilism, but it does occur occasionally. However, obesity and hypomenorrhea are common. The ovary is also the site of arrhenoblastomas, hilus cell tumors, and luteomas that may cause hirsutism. There is usually associated virilism with these tumors. Ovarian failure (menopause) may also be associated with hirsutism, but there is no associated virilism.

Anatomy will not be useful in recalling the many drugs that may produce hirsutism. These include phenytoin, diazoxide, minoxidil, anabolic steroids, androgens, and glucocorticoids. Hirsutism may also be found in porphyria, anorexia nervosa, and the Cornelia de Lange syndrome (Amsterdam dwarfism).

● Approach to the Diagnosis

Clinically it is most important to look for obesity and virilism. A history of hypomenorrhea or amenorrhea is also important. The workup initially should include serum cortisol or 24-hour urine 17-hydroxycorticoids or 17-ketosteroids, and a thyroid profile. A skull x-ray and flat plate of the abdomen may be helpful. A cortisone suppression test may be required. Ultrasonography of the ovaries may reveal a neoplasm or polycystic ovaries. An endocrinologist should be consulted before proceeding with CT scans of the brain, abdomen, and pelvis. A pituitary microadenoma may only be found by an MRI of the pituitary.

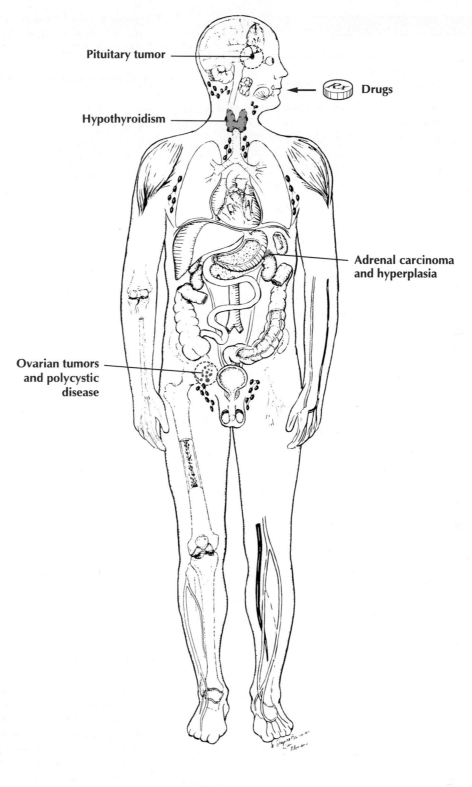

Pituitary tumor

Drugs

Hypothyroidism

Adrenal carcinoma
and hyperplasia

Ovarian tumors
and polycystic
disease

● **FIGURE 16** Hirsutism.

● Other Useful Tests

1. Serum follicle-stimulating hormone (FSH) and luteinizing hormone (LH) assay (acromegaly or polycystic ovary syndrome)
2. Serum growth hormone assay (acromegaly)
3. Laparoscopy (polycystic ovaries)
4. Thyrotropin level (hypothyroidism)
5. Selective venous sampling of adrenal veins for androgens (adrenal carcinoma)
6. Isotope scanning of adrenal glands (Cushing syndrome)
7. Exploratory surgery
8. Serum prolactin level (pituitary tumor)
9. Serum testosterone

Case Presentation #47

A 19-year-old, 6-month-pregnant Hispanic woman complained of increasing hair growth on her face. Otherwise, she is doing well aside from increasing obesity.

Question #1. Utilizing anatomy and physiology, what would be your differential diagnosis?

Physical examination revealed a male escutcheon, enlarged clitoris, and purple striae of the abdomen. An MRI revealed a mass in the right adrenal cortex.

Question #2. What is your diagnosis now?

(See Appendix B for the answers.)

HOARSENESS

Neuroanatomy provides the most useful basic science in developing a list of causes for hoarseness. Hoarseness may occur from involvement of the larynx, myoneural junction of the vocal cord muscles, vagus nerve, or the brainstem. When these structures are cross-indexed with the many etiologies suggested by the mnemonic **VINDICATE**, a chart like Table 39 can be prepared.

The **larynx** may be involved with acute infections such as diphtheria and influenza and with chronic infections such as TB and syphilis. It may also be involved with allergy, neoplasms, and chronic trauma from overuse of the voice. Smoking and alcohol are common causes of hoarseness. Hypothyroidism and acromegaly may present with hoarseness.

The **myoneural junctions** prompt the recall of myasthenia gravis, whereas the peripheral portion of the vagus nerve prompts the recall of the greatest number of disorders; thyroid tumors and surgery to the thyroid, mediastinal tumors, and aortic aneurysms are only a few. Lead and diphtheria may cause neuritis to this nerve. The **intracranial portions of the vagus nerve** may be involved by basilar artery aneurysms, basilar meningitis, platybasia, and foramen magnum tumors.

In the **brainstem**, the nucleus ambiguus is involved in poliomyelitis, ependymomas, Wallenberg syndrome, syringomyelia, and amyotrophic lateral sclerosis. Multiple sclerosis and gliomas may involve the roots of the ambiguus nucleus as they pass through the brain stem white matter.

● Approach to the Diagnosis

A careful examination of the larynx with a laryngoscope or the fiberoptic bronchoscope is essential. The indirect laryngeal mirror is difficult to use and probably should be discarded by those unfamiliar with its use. If no local disease is found, evidence of vagal nerve palsy will be noted by the cord paralysis. A chest x-ray, thyroid function tests, blood lead level, and Tensilon test may be necessary to diagnose recurrent laryngeal involvement. Intracranial lesions will demonstrate other neurologic signs. A skull roentgenogram, CT scan, and spinal tap will probably give valuable clues to their cause. X-ray films of the cervical spine, an RA test, and arteriogram may be necessary.

● Other Useful Tests

1. CBC (anemia, infection)
2. Sedimentation rate (inflammation)
3. Tuberculin test (TB)
4. VDRL test (syphilis of the vocal cords)
5. Nose and throat culture (pharyngitis)
6. Sputum culture (pneumonia)
7. AFB culture (TB)
8. Acetylcholine receptor antibody titer (myasthenia gravis)
9. C1 esterase inhibitor level (angioneurotic edema)
10. Allergy skin test
11. Otolaryngology consult
12. CT scan of the mediastinum (mediastinal tumor)
13. Aortogram (aortic aneurysm)
14. Radioiodine (RAI) uptake and scan (thyroid tumor)
15. MRI of the neck
16. Esophagoscopy (reflux esophagitis)

Case Presentation #48

A 48-year-old white woman complained of hoarseness which was intermittent at first but had become steady in the past 4 months. She has a history of heavy smoking and moderate alcohol consumption.

Question #1. Utilizing your knowledge of anatomy and neuroanatomy, what would be your list of possibilities?

Physical examination reveals thickening of the hair, skin, and nails but is otherwise unremarkable. Fiberoptic laryngoscopy was negative for mass or ulceration of the vocal cords.

Question #2. What is your diagnosis now?

(See Appendix B for the answers.)

HORNER SYNDROME

Horner syndrome results from a lesion anywhere along the sympathetic pathways from the brain stem to the spinal cord; then from the spinal cord to the sympathetic chain of the thorax; then to the cervical sympathetic system including the stellate ganglion and superior cervical ganglion giving off fibers around the carotid arteries. If we picture this neuroanatomy, we can recall most of the causes of Horner syndrome.

Brain stem: Wallenberg syndrome (posterior inferior cerebellar artery thrombosis)

Spinal cord: Syringomyelia spinal cord tumors, neurosyphilis

Thorax: Carcinoma of the lung or esophagus, Hodgkin lymphoma, aortic aneurysm, mediastinitis

TABLE 39 Hoarseness

	V Vascular	I Inflammatory	N Neoplasm	D Degenerative and Deficiency	I Intoxication and Idiopathic	C Congenital	A Autoimmune Allergic	T Trauma	E Endocrine
Larynx		Viral upper respiratory infection Diphtheria Syphilis Tuberculosis Sinusitis Epiglottitis	Singers node Polyp Carcinoma		Smoking Alcohol Gout	Laryngeal web	Angioneurotic edema Cricothyroid arthritis	Overuse of voice Foreign body Fracture	Hypothyroidism Acromegaly
Myoneural Junction					Anectine Cholinergic drugs		Myasthenia gravis		
Vagus Nerve: Extracranial Portion	Aortic aneurysm Mitral stenosis	Mediastinitis Tuberculosis Sarcoid Diphtheria	Hodgkin lymphoma Bronchogenic carcinoma Esophageal carcinoma		Idiopathic paralysis Lead neuropathy	Platybasia		Thyroid surgery	Thyroid carcinoma Reidel struma
Vagus Nerve: Intracranial Portion	Aneurysm Jugular vein thrombosis	Syphilis Tuberculosis Meningitis	Tumor of ganglion Foramen magnum tumor				Multiple sclerosis		
Brain Stem	Wallenberg syndrome Basilar artery insufficiency	Encephalitis Poliomyelitis Syringobulbia Syphilis	Brain stem glioma Metastasis	Amyotrophic lateral sclerosis					

H

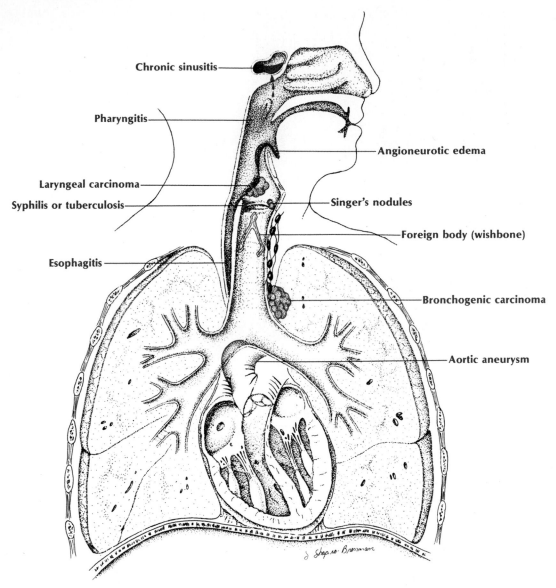

● **FIGURE 17** Hoarseness.

Cervical sympathetics: Laryngeal carcinoma, thyroid carcinoma, cervical rib, brachial plexus neuralgia or trauma
Carotid artery chain: Migraine, cluster headaches, carotid thrombosis

● Approach to the Diagnosis

A history of headaches would suggest migraine or cluster headaches as the cause. The finding of long tract signs (e.g., pyramidal tract) would suggest a brain stem or cord lesion. Hemiplegia would point to a carotid artery thrombosis. A mass in the neck suggests a Pancoast tumor or thyroid carcinoma. Pain in the neck or upper extremities without a mass should suggest brachial plexus neuralgia, scalenus anticus syndrome, or Pancoast tumor. X-rays of the chest and cervical spine are indicated in all cases without other neurologic signs. When there are other neurologic signs, an MRI of the brain or spinal cord must be done. A neurologist should be consulted.

● Other Useful Tests

1. VDRL (neurosyphilis)
2. Carotid duplex scan (carotid artery thrombosis)
3. CT scan of the mediastinum (mediastinal tumor)
4. SSEP (brachial plexus neuralgia)
5. Histamine test (cluster headaches)
6. Aortography (aortic aneurysm)
7. Mediastinoscopy (mediastinal tumor)

HYPERCALCEMIA

Hypercalcemia may result from disorders of calcium storage, intake, regulation, and transport.

Storage: Storage of calcium is in the bone. It follows that diseases that invade the bone will cause excessive release of calcium. Thus, metastatic carcinoma will cause an

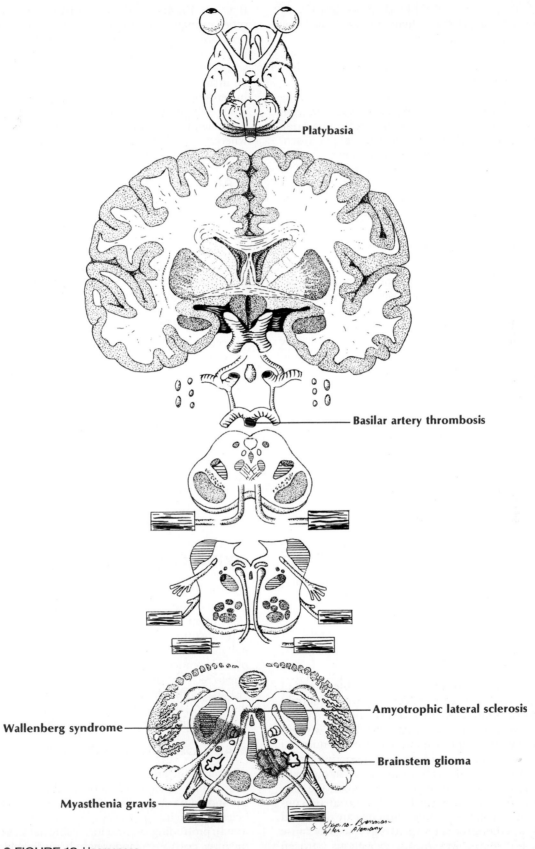

Platybasia

Basilar artery thrombosis

Amyotrophic lateral sclerosis

Wallenberg syndrome

Brainstem glioma

Myasthenia gravis

● **FIGURE 18** Hoarseness.

H

elevation of calcium in the blood. Paget disease, by increasing the osteoclastic activity in the bone, may cause an elevated calcium level.

Intake: Increased intake of calcium usually does not cause hypercalcemia, but when associated with the milk–alkali syndrome or hypervitaminosis D, it may.

Regulation: Excessive secretion of parathyroid hormone (PTH) by the parathyroid gland or ectopic PTH secretion by a neoplasm elsewhere will cause hypercalcemia. Look for type 1 and type 11 multiple endocrine neoplasm syndrome in patients with parathyroid adenomas.

Transport: Half the calcium in the blood is transported by protein. It follows that the conditions with increased plasma protein (such as multiple myeloma and Boeck sarcoid) may be associated with hypercalcemia.

● Approach to the Diagnosis

A history of neoplasm or clinical evidence of bone disease should alert one to the possibility of metastatic neoplasm. Symptoms of polyuria, polydipsia, weakness, pathologic fracture, and weight loss should suggest hyperparathyroidism. Hypercalcemia may also present with pancreatitis. Serial calcium, phosphorus, and alkaline phosphatase levels and serum PTH assay and skeletal survey should pin down the diagnosis of hyperparathyroidism and metastatic neoplasm. A bone scan will also be helpful in identifying metastasis. A cortisone suppression test will help differentiate hyperparathyroidism from metastasis. The serum calcium will not be lowered by cortisone in hyperparathyroidism.

● Other Useful Tests

1. CBC (myelophthisic anemia)
2. Sedimentation rate (neoplasm)
3. Chemistry profile (hyperparathyroidism)
4. Free thyroxine (T_4) (hyperthyroidism)
5. Serum 25-hydroxy-calciferol (25-COH) vitamin D (hypervitaminosis D)
6. Protein electrophoresis (sarcoidosis, multiple myeloma)
7. MRI of the neck (parathyroid adenoma)
8. Endocrinology consult

HYPERCHOLESTEROLEMIA

Anatomy is the key to forming a list of possible causes of hypercholesterolemia. If we consider the **liver**, it should prompt recall of primary biliary cirrhosis, hepatoma, glycogen storage disease, and obstructive jaundice. If we consider the kidney, it should facilitate recall of uremia and the nephrotic syndrome. Considering the endocrine glands should facilitate recall of diabetes mellitus, acromegaly, hypothyroidism, Cushing disease, insulinoma, and isolated growth hormone deficiency. Two other groups of conditions associated with hypercholesterolemia are drugs and the primary hyperlipoproteinemias. Drugs that may cause an elevated cholesterol level include exogenous estrogen and corticosteroids, thiazides, and β-adrenergic blocking agents. The primary hyperlipoproteinemias include types

II-a, II-b, III, and V. These can be differentiated from the other primary hyperlipoproteinemias by determining the presence of chylomicrons and elevated triglycerides. Types II-a and II-b hyperlipoproteinemia are not associated with elevated chylomicrons. Type II-b is associated with an increased triglyceride, whereas type II-a is not. Type III hyperlipoproteinemia is associated with both chylomicrons and an elevated triglyceride level. Type I hyperlipoproteinemia is not associated with an increased cholesterol, whereas type V is associated with chylomicrons and an increase of both cholesterol and triglyceride levels.

● Approach to the Diagnosis

One should look for a family history of lipoproteinemia as well as determine what drugs the patient is taking. On examination, one should look for tendon xanthomas. As mentioned above, lipoprotein electrophoresis should be done as well as a lipid profile and overnight refrigeration of plasma to look for lactescence (a sign of chylomicrons). An endocrinology consult will be helpful.

● Other Useful Tests

1. CBC
2. Sedimentation rate
3. Chemistry panel (liver disease, kidney disease)
4. Urinalysis (nephrosis)
5. Liver profile (biliary cirrhosis, obstructive jaundice)
6. Thyroid profile (hypothyroidism)
7. Antimitochondrial antibody titer (biliary cirrhosis)
8. 24-hour urine protein level (nephrosis)
9. Liver biopsy (cirrhosis)
10. Renal biopsy (nephrosis)
11. Consult with metabolic disease specialist
12. CT scan of the abdomen (Cushing syndrome, renal disease, liver disease)

HYPERGLYCEMIA

To form a list of diagnostic possibilities in a case of hyperglycemia, one needs only to think of the endocrine glands. Considering the pancreas should prompt the recall of diabetes mellitus and glucagonomas. Considering the adrenal gland would prompt the recall of Cushing disease and pheochromocytoma. Visualizing the pituitary should help one to recall acromegaly and basophilic adenoma, whereas visualizing the thyroid should prompt the recall of hyperthyroidism. Other considerations in hyperglycemia are starvation and drug-induced hyperglycemia.

● Approach to the Diagnosis

Obviously, the first thing to do is repeat the blood sugar test after fasting. If the result is borderline, a glucose tolerance test should be done. Clinical evaluation for a history of diabetes, hypertension (Cushing disease and pheochromocytoma), protruding jaw and increasing hat size (acromegaly), polyuria, polydipsia, and weight loss (diabetes mellitus and hyperthyroidism) is important. Further workup depends on which endocrine disorder is being considered.

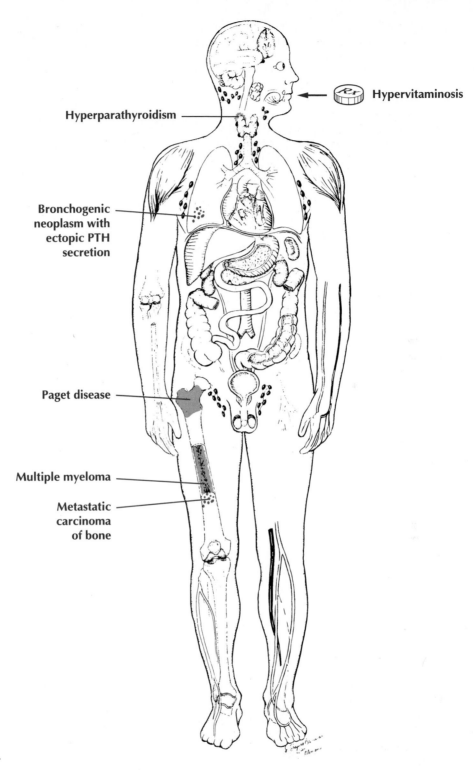

Hypervitaminosis

Hyperparathyroidism

Bronchogenic
neoplasm with
ectopic PTH
secretion

Paget disease

Multiple myeloma

Metastatic
carcinoma
of bone

● **FIGURE 19** Hypercalcemia.

● Other Useful Tests

1. CBC (Cushing syndrome)
2. Sedimentation rate (pancreatitis)
3. Chemistry panel (diabetic acidosis)
4. Plasma insulin level (diabetes mellitus)
5. Urinalysis and urine culture (pyelonephritis)
6. Glycosylated hemoglobin (diabetes mellitus)
7. Growth hormone assay (acromegaly)
8. Plasma cortisol level (Cushing syndrome)
9. Dexamethasone suppression (Cushing syndrome)
10. 24-hour urine catecholamine level or vanillylmandelic acid (VMA) (pheochromocytoma)
11. T_4 and thyrotropin (hyperthyroidism)
12. CT scan of the abdomen (Cushing syndrome)
13. Endocrinology consult

H

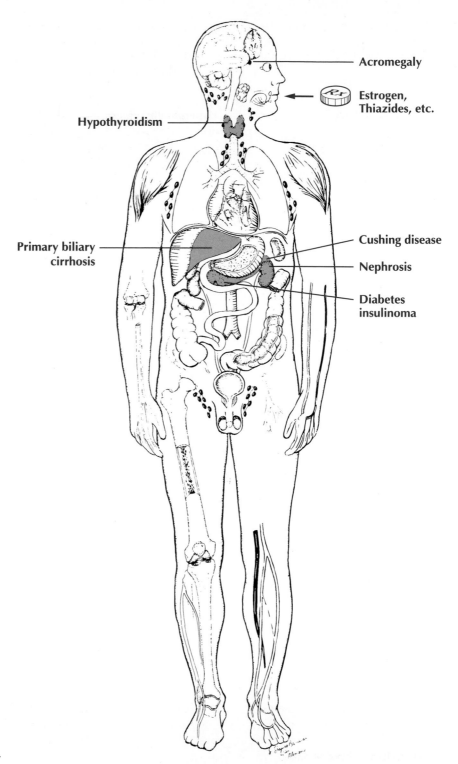

● **FIGURE 20** Hypercholesterolemia.

HYPERKALEMIA

When confronted with a laboratory report of an unexpected elevated potassium level, the first thing to do in most cases is to repeat the test. The increased potassium may be due to hemolyzed blood or excessively tight tourniquet used to draw the blood. If these causes can be ruled out, one can recall most of the causes by thinking of the physiologic mechanisms of excretion and regulation.

Excretion: Acute renal failure causes retention of potassium. This may be caused by drugs, heavy metals, transfusion, shock, dehydration, glomerulonephritis, or obstructive uropathy.

Regulation: The exchange of potassium and hydrogen ions for sodium in the distal tubule is regulated by the hormone aldosterone. Consequently, in Addison disease this mechanism is partially shut down causing the retention of potassium. Various diuretics such as triamterene and the spironolactones may do the same thing. Metabolic acidosis, especially diabetic acidosis, may be associated with hyperkalemia because the potassium moves out of the cell in exchange for hydrogen ions to buffer the acidosis.

● Approach to the Diagnosis

Most helpful in the diagnosis will be laboratory tests to rule out renal failure and Addison disease. Thus a CBC, urinalysis, chemistry panel, renal function tests, plasma cortisol, 24-hour urine aldosterone level, and serial electrolytes may be necessary. As a precaution, it may be wise to hold all but critical drugs until the diagnosis is certain.

● Other Useful Tests

1. Corticotropin stimulation test (Addison disease)
2. Cystoscopy and retrograde pyelography (obstructive uropathy)
3. CT scan of abdomen (renal disease, neoplasm)
4. Renal biopsy (renal disease)
5. Nephrology consult
6. Endocrinology consult
7. Plasma renin level (Addison disease)

HYPERMENORRHEA

The causes of hypermenorrhea or excessive menstrual bleeding can be easily recalled by simply applying the mnemonic **MINTS**.

M—Malformations include bicornuate uterus, congenital ovarian cysts, endometriosis, ectopic pregnancies, and retained placenta.

I—Inflammation recalls cervicitis, endometritis, and pelvic inflammatory disease.

N—Neoplasms include fibroids, carcinoma, and polyps of the cervix and endometrium. One should also not forget choriocarcinoma, hydatidiform moles, and hormone-producing tumors of the ovary.

T—Trauma includes perforation of the uterus, excessive intercourse during the menses, and introduction of foreign bodies into the uterus.

S—Systemic diseases include anemia and the coagulation disorders such as hemophilia, idiopathic thrombocytopenic purpura, and scurvy. Also in this category are lupus erythematosus and endocrine disorders, especially hypothyroidism and dysfunctional uterine bleeding from disproportion in the output of estrogen and progesterone by the ovary.

● Approach to the Diagnosis

The diagnosis includes a thorough pelvic examination, CBC, coagulation studies, thyroid function tests, and perhaps other endocrine tests. Ultrasonography is ordered next. If all these are normal, a trial of estrogen or progesterone supplementation or a dilatation and curettage (D & C) may be indicated. Culdoscopy, peritoneoscopy, and a hysterosalpingogram may be necessary before

performing an exploratory laparotomy and, if necessary, a hysterectomy. A gynecologist or endocrinologist will be helpful in solving the diagnostic dilemma in many cases.

Case Presentation #49

An 18-year-old Puerto Rican woman complained of increasing and prolonged periods for the past 14 months. She had also experienced arthralgias, weight loss, and fatigue. Her pregnancy test is negative.

Question #1. Utilizing physiology, what would be your list of possibilities at this point?

Physical examination revealed pale conjunctiva, a rash on her cheeks, and a palpable spleen. The vaginal examination was unremarkable. The Rumple–Leeds test was positive.

Question #2. What is your diagnosis now?

(See Appendix B for the answers.)

HYPERNATREMIA

If an electrolyte profile shows an elevated sodium level, the **physiology** model of intake, regulation, and excretion may be applied to develop a list of possibilities. However, the focus should be on water intake, transport, regulation, and excretion because this will help recall most of the possibilities.

Intake: When water intake is diminished in dehydration states, the sodium level increases.

Regulation: Antidiuretic hormone (ADH) allows for the retention of water by the distal tubule. When this hormone is reduced or absent, as in pituitary diabetes insipidus, hypernatremia results. Furthermore, if the kidney does not respond to ADH, as in renal diabetes insipidus, hypernatremia results. Aldosterone hormone promotes increased reabsorption of sodium in the distal tubule in primary aldosteronism, causing hypernatremia. However, this may be counterbalanced by an increased ADH secretion and water retention causing the sodium to return to normal.

Excretion: Sodium excretion may be reduced in acute renal failure but, because water is retained as well, the plasma sodium is not usually increased. Other causes of hypernatremia include the administration of normal and hypertonic saline, prolonged vomiting, and heat exhaustion.

● Approach to the Diagnosis

Dehydration can be diagnosed clinically by the tenting of the skin, mushy eyeballs, and concentrated urine. Laboratory workup includes serial electrolytes, chemistry panel, serum and urine osmolality, serum ADH, plasma renin, 24-hour urine aldosterone level, and consultation

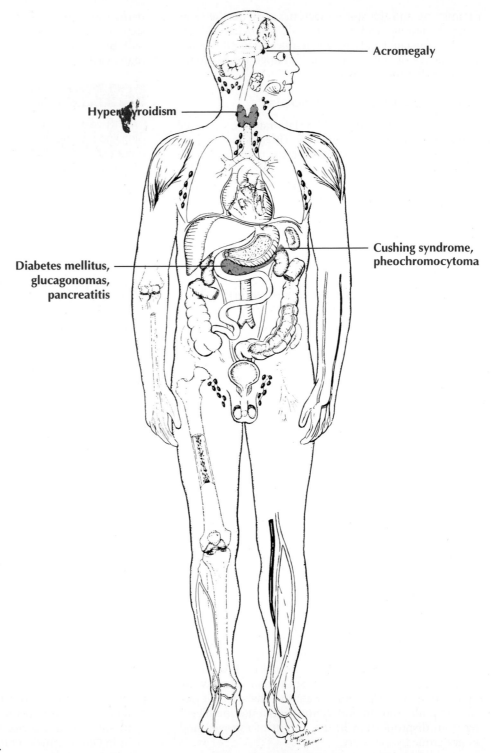

Acromegaly

Hyperthyroidism

Cushing syndrome,
pheochromocytoma

Diabetes mellitus,
glucagonomas,
pancreatitis

● **FIGURE 21** Hyperglycemia.

with an endocrinologist or a nephrologist. It is wise to withhold all noncritical drugs until a diagnosis is certain.

HYPERTENSION

With the emphasis placed on the diagnosis and treatment of hypertension in the past 20 years, every physician has a good knowledge of the causes of hypertension. The list, nevertheless, may be incomplete. If consideration is to be given only to the treatable disorders, then one simply needs to remember the cardiovascular system, adrenal gland, and kidney and apply the mnemonic **VINDICATE** to develop a list of the causes (Table 40). It is more instructive, however, to apply **physiology** in developing a differential.

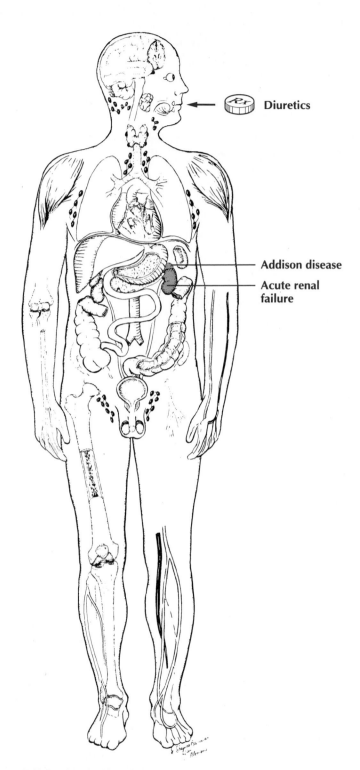

Diuretics

Addison disease

Acute renal failure

● FIGURE 22 Hyperkalemia.

Because blood pressure is maintained by an adequate blood volume, an adequate cardiac output, and appropriate vasomotor tone, it follows that hypertension may result from an increase in any one or more of these three factors.

1. **Increased blood volume:** This results in most cases from an increase in sodium in the blood from primary aldosteronism (adrenal tumors) or from secondary aldosteronism (renovascular hypertension from glomerulonephritis and other primary renal diseases or obstruction of the renal arteries by atherosclerotic plaques or fibromuscular hyperplasia). Administration of corticosteroid drugs may cause hypertension by the same mechanism. Polycythemia vera is often associated with moderate hypertension because of increased red cell mass.

2. **Increased cardiac output:** This mechanism accounts for the systolic hypertension in hyperthyroidism, aortic insufficiency, patent ductus arteriosus, arteriovenous shunts, and Paget disease. Excessive intake of caffeinated beverages (coffee, coke, tea, chocolate, etc.) is a common cause of systolic hypertension.

3. **Increased vasomotor tone:** Increased output of epinephrine and norepinephrine as occurs in pheochromocytoma is one example of this type of hypertension. Administration of sympathomimetic drugs is another. Essential hypertension is probably based on this mechanism, but increased total body sodium leading to an increased blood volume may also be a pathophysiologic mechanism. Unfortunately, this approach omits dissecting aneurysm and coarctation of the aorta, two important causes of hypertension. Systolic hypertension without a corresponding increase in diastolic pressure should be taken seriously especially in the elderly.

● Approach to the Diagnosis

Take the blood pressure yourself to be sure the hypertension is real; 24-hour blood pressure monitoring is now available. The workup of hypertension includes a family history, serial electrolytes, urinalysis and urine culture, metabolic panel, lipid panel, TSH, ECG, and chest x-ray. A complete hypertensive workup is not usually performed today unless there is no family history of hypertension, the hypertension does not respond to treatment, there are other symptoms suggesting a surgical lesion (e.g., paroxysmal headaches), or there is sudden onset of hypertension in a known normotensive individual.

● Other Useful Tests

1. Serum cortisol level (adrenal tumor or hyperplasia)
2. Dexamethasone suppression test (adrenal tumor or hyperplasia)
3. Plasma renin level (renovascular hypertension)
4. 24-hour urine aldosterone (aldosterone-producing tumor)
5. Cystoscopy and retrograde pyelography (tumor or malformation of the urinary tract)
6. Renal angiogram (renal artery stenosis)
7. CT scan of abdomen (hypernephroma)
8. Glucagon stimulation test (pheochromocytoma)
9. Magnetic resonance angiography (MRA) (renal artery stenosis)
10. Ultrasonography (hydronephrosis)

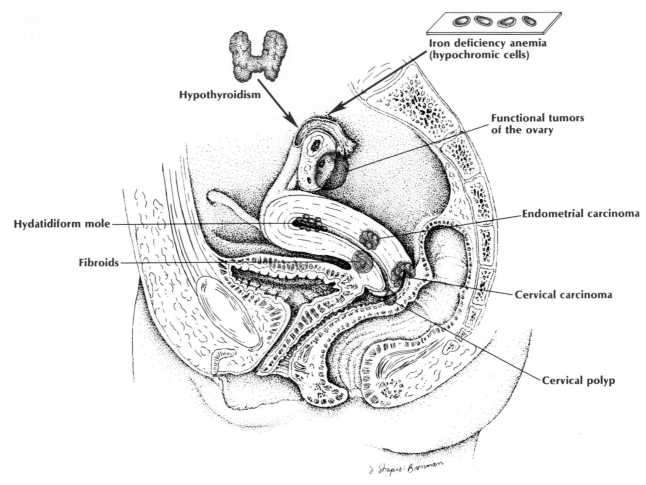

Hypothyroidism

*Iron deficiency anemia
(hypochromic cells)*

*Functional tumors
of the ovary*

Hydatidiform mole

Endometrial carcinoma

Fibroids

Cervical carcinoma

Cervical polyp

● **FIGURE 23** Hypermenorrhea.

Case Presentation #50

A 42-year-old white male executive complained of fatigue, frequent muscle cramps, and frequency of urination at the time of his annual physical examination. His blood pressure was 188/115 mm Hg but, otherwise, his physical examination was unremarkable. His family history is negative for hypertension.

Question #1. What is your differential diagnosis at this point?

Urinalysis and 24-hour urine catecholamines were normal, but serial serum electrolytes repeatedly showed hypokalemia.

Question #2. What is your diagnosis now?

(See Appendix B for the answers.)

HYPERTRIGLYCERIDEMIA

In developing a list of possible causes of hypertriglyceridemia, first consider **anatomy**, particularly the kidney, liver, and endocrine glands. The kidney should remind one of the nephrotic syndromes which are associated with elevated triglyceride and cholesterol levels. The liver should remind one of obstructive jaundice. Looking at the endocrine glands, consider the pancreas and immediately diabetes mellitus and insulinomas come to mind. Considering the thyroid gland, hypothyroidism comes to mind. Considering the adrenal gland, Cushing syndrome will not be forgotten. Finally, consider the pituitary gland and acromegaly will be recalled. Other causes of secondary hypertriglyceridemia include drugs such as thiazide diuretics and β-adrenergic blocking agents, exogenous estrogen, and corticosteroids. If the above conditions have been excluded, the clinician must consider the primary hyperlipoproteinemias; the triglycerides are elevated in type I, II-b, III, IV, and V. These may be further differentiated by looking at the chylomicron and cholesterol levels. In type I, there is marked elevation of chylomicrons but the cholesterol is normal. In type II-b, the chylomicrons are normal but the cholesterol is elevated. In types III and V, the chylomicrons and cholesterol are both elevated, whereas in type IV only the triglyceride is increased and the plasma is clear.

● Approach to the Diagnosis

Clinical examination may show eruptive xanthomas, tendon xanthomas, and arcus senilis of the cornea in the

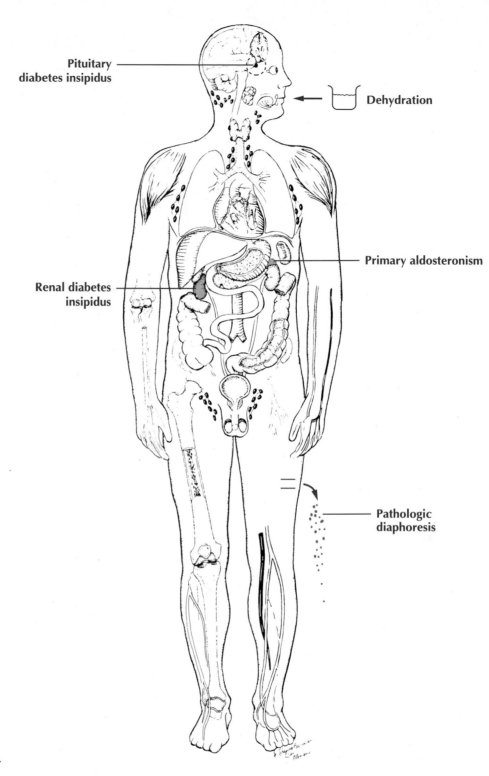

Pituitary
diabetes insipidus

Dehydration

Primary aldosteronism

Renal diabetes
insipidus

Pathologic
diaphoresis

● **FIGURE 24** Hypernatremia.

primary hyperlipoproteinemias. There may be a clear family history also. Laboratory studies that need to be done include a liver profile, thyroid profile, serum protein electrophoresis, and lipoprotein electrophoresis. Free plasma cortisol will help rule out Cushing syndrome, whereas a growth hormone assay will help rule out acromegaly. Overnight refrigeration of plasma will help differentiate the primary hyperlipoproteinemias.

● **Other Useful Tests**

1. CBC and urinalysis (nephrosis)
2. Sedimentation rate (hepatitis)
3. Chemistry profile (liver disease, kidney disease)
4. Exercise tolerance test (coronary arteriosclerosis)
5. Liver biopsy (biliary cirrhosis)
6. Skull x-ray (acromegaly)

H

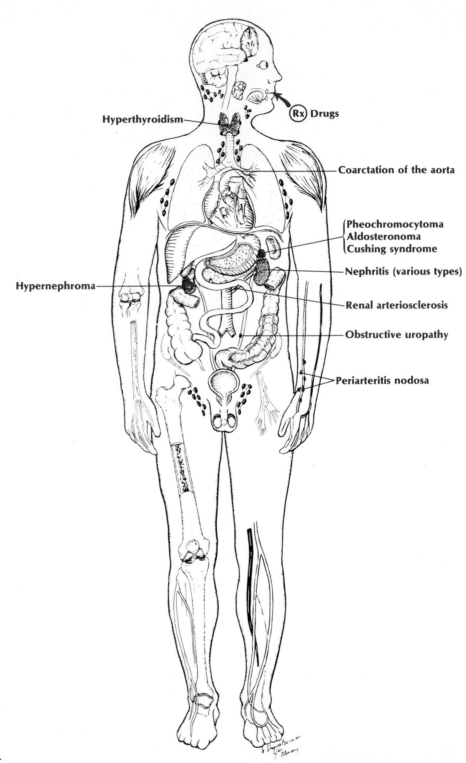

Hyperthyroidism

Rx Drugs

Coarctation of the aorta

Pheochromocytoma
Aldosteronoma
Cushing syndrome

Nephritis (various types)

Hypernephroma

Renal arteriosclerosis

Obstructive uropathy

Periarteritis nodosa

● **FIGURE 25** Hypertension.

7. Endocrinology consult
8. Glucose tolerance test (acromegaly, diabetes, Cushing syndrome)
9. Plasma insulin assay (insulinoma)
10. C-peptide level (insulinoma)
11. Consultation with a metabolic disease specialist

HYPOACTIVE REFLEXES

Diffuse hypoactive reflexes are of no significance in otherwise healthy individuals; however, **anatomy** is the key to recalling the many pathologic causes of hypoactive reflexes. Visualizing the reflex arc (see figure on page 246), we have

TABLE 40 Hypertension

	V Vascular	I Inflammatory	N Neoplasm	D Degenerative	I Intoxication	C Congenital	A Allergic and Autoimmune	T Trauma	E Endocrine
Cardiovascular System		Aortic insufficiency	Polycythemia vera Intracranial tumor	Atherosclerosis Medionecrosis	Sympathomimetics Exogenous corticosteroid Porphyria	Coarctation of the aorta Patent ductus Essential hypertension	Polyarteritis nodosa	A-V fistula Intracranial hemorrhage	Hyperthyroidism Acromegaly
Adrenal Gland			Pheochromocytomas Cushing disease Primary aldosteronism						Adrenocortical hyperplasia
Kidney	Atherosclerotic plague of renal artery (stenosis)	Pyelonephritis Renal TB	Hypernephroma Multiple myeloma		Toxic nephritis Toxemia of pregnancy	Polycystic kidney Hydronephrosis Other anomalies	Glomerulonephritis Vasculitis		Kimmelstiel–Wilson syndrome

A-V, arteriovenous.

H

the spinal cord nerve roots, peripheral nerves, myoneural junction, and muscle. Now we simply think of the various diseases that may affect each one of these structures and we have an extensive list of possibilities.

Spinal cord: Diminished reflexes are seen in poliomyelitis, syringomyelia, Werdnig–Hoffman syndrome, muscular atrophy, and pernicious anemia with subacute combined degeneration. Spinal cord concussion, transection, or hemorrhage may cause hypoactive reflexes at first.

Nerve roots: Diffusely hypoactive reflexes may be found in Guillain–Barré syndrome and tabes dorsalis, both of which affect the nerve roots. Focal loss of reflexes may occur in herniated disc, cauda equina tumor, spinal stenosis, abscess, TB, multiple myeloma, and fracture.

Peripheral nerves: Peripheral neuropathy is associated with diffuse hypoactive reflexes. There are several causes including alcoholism, diabetes, drugs, malnutrition, Charcot–Marie–Tooth disease, porphyria, hereditary hypertrophic neuritis, lead intoxication, and collagen disease. Focal involvement may be seen in brachial plexus neuritis, sciatic neuritis, and mononeuritis multiplex.

Myoneural junction: This should bring to mind myasthenia gravis.

Muscle: Generalized decrease in reflexes may be seen in dermatomyositis, advanced muscular dystrophy, myotonic dystrophica, and McArdle syndrome.

● Approach to the Diagnosis

The differential diagnosis will depend on the presence or absence of other signs. If there is an acute onset of diffuse hypoactive reflexes and weakness, poliomyelitis Guillain–Barré syndrome, toxic peripheral neuropathy, and polymyositis must be considered in the differential diagnosis. A gradual onset of diffuse weakness and hypoactive reflexes is more consistent with muscular atrophy, tabes dorsalis, pernicious anemia, and muscular dystrophy. Abnormal sensory findings would point to pernicious anemia, tabes dorsalis, and peripheral neuropathy whereas the absence of abnormal sensory findings would suggest muscular atrophy, muscular dystrophy, or myasthenia gravis. Focal loss of reflexes suggests a herniated disc, especially if there is associated radicular pain. Focal hypoactive reflexes of the lower extremities require plain films of the lumbosacral spine, EMG and NCV studies, and an MRI or CT scan of the lumbar spine. Isolated hypoactive reflexes in the upper extremities require an x-ray of the cervical spine, MRI of the cervical spine, and NCV and EMG of the upper extremities. Diffuse hypoactive reflexes merit an extensive laboratory workup including a CBC, urinalysis, chemistry panel, serum B_{12} and folic acid, ANA, glucose tolerance test, blood lead level, urine for porphobilinogen, human immunodeficiency virus (HIV) antibody titer, and serum protein electrophoresis. A spinal tap should be done if Guillain–Barré syndrome is suspected. An EMG and NCV study should also be done if peripheral neuropathy or muscular dystrophy is suspected. A muscle biopsy may be needed in muscular dystrophy and dermatomyositis.

● Other Useful Tests

1. Anti–double-stranded DNA (lupus)
2. Thyroid profile (hypothyroidism)
3. Immunoelectrophoresis (macroglobulinemia)
4. Kveim test (sarcoidosis)
5. Drug screen (drug-induced neuropathy)
6. Quantitative urine niacin and thiamine (pellagra, beriberi)

Case Presentation #51

A 49-year-old white man complained of increasing weakness and fatigue of all four extremities. Neurologic examination disclosed hypoactive reflexes in the upper extremities. There were bilateral Babinski signs.

Question #1. Utilizing your knowledge of neuroanatomy, what is your differential diagnosis?

Additional history reveals that he has had pain and stiffness in the neck and difficulty walking for several months. A neurologist found diminished sensation to touch and pain in the right C6 dermatome.

Question #2. What is your diagnosis now?

(See Appendix B for the answers.)

HYPOALBUMINEMIA

The physiologic model of intake, absorption, transport, production, regulation, and excretion will help develop a list of causes of hypoalbuminemia.

Intake: Starvation and anorexia nervosa are recalled in this category.

Absorption: Poor absorption of dietary protein in the malabsorption syndrome is recalled in this category.

Transport: In CHF there is failure to eliminate water, causing hemodilution and, consequently, hypoalbuminemia.

Production: Albumin is produced in the liver, so chronic liver disease such as cirrhosis will be recalled in this category.

Regulation: Hyperthyroidism will cause the breakdown of plasma protein leading to hypoalbuminemia.

Excretion: In this category, one will recall the nephrotic syndrome or chronic renal failure, where protein is lost in the urine, and protein-losing enteropathy in which protein is lost in the stool from a villous adenoma.

Miscellaneous conditions: These include metastatic neoplasm and infectious diseases such as TB that are associated with hypermetabolic states.

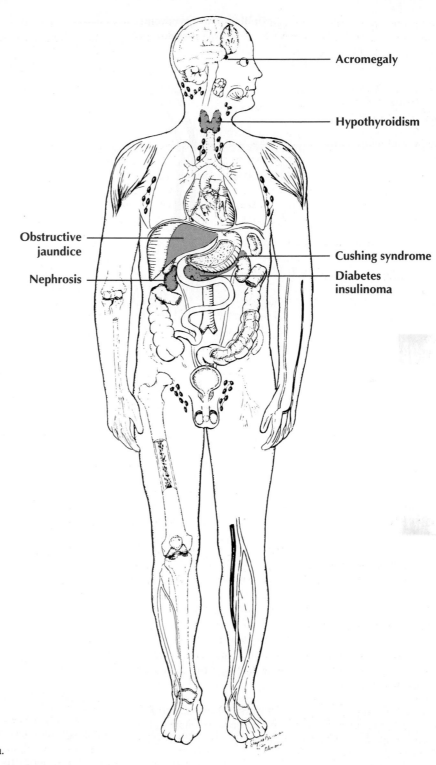

● FIGURE 26 Hypertriglyceridemia.

● Approach to the Diagnosis

Clinically, look for weight loss, jaundice, or anemia. Laboratory workup usually includes CBC, urinalysis, 24-hour urine protein level, chemistry panel, protein electrophoresis, chest x-ray, and ECG.

● Other Useful Tests

1. Liver function tests (cirrhosis)
2. Renal function tests (nephrosis)
3. ECG (CHF)
4. Arm-to-tongue circulation time (CHF)

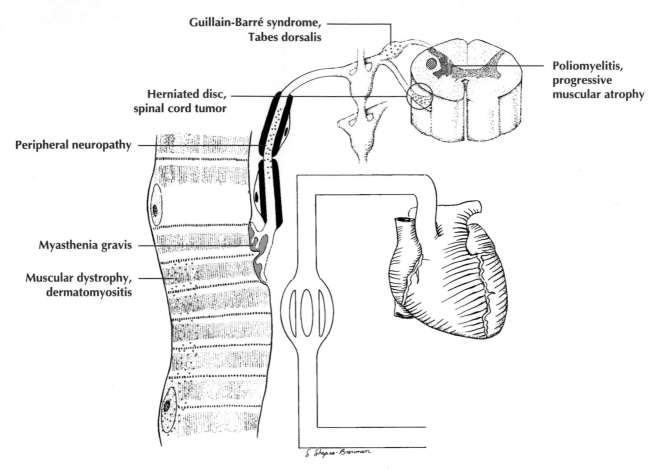

Guillain-Barré syndrome,
Tabes dorsalis

Poliomyelitis,
progressive
muscular atrophy

Herniated disc,
spinal cord tumor

Peripheral neuropathy

Myasthenia gravis

Muscular dystrophy,
dermatomyositis

S. Shapiro-Brennman

● **FIGURE 27** Hypoactive reflexes.

5. CT scan of the abdomen (liver disease, renal disease, neoplasm)
6. Liver biopsy (cirrhosis)
7. Kidney biopsy (nephritis)
8. Nephrology consult
9. Hepatology consult

HYPOCALCEMIA

The **physiologic** model of intake, absorption, transport, regulation, and excretion lends itself well to developing a list of possible causes of hypocalcemia.

Intake: Poor dietary intake of calcium is not often seen in developed countries. However, poor intake of vitamin D may be the cause. Vitamin D facilitates the absorption of calcium.

Absorption: Malabsorption syndrome is often associated with hypocalcemia.

Transport: Anything that lowers the plasma protein may be associated with hypocalcemia. Consequently, nephrotic syndrome, cirrhosis of the liver, malnutrition, and malabsorption syndrome may all produce hypocalcemia on this basis.

Regulation: Hypocalcemia is associated with pseudohypoparathyroidism, where the kidney fails to respond to PTH. In hypoparathyroidism, there is decreased or absent PTH, causing hypocalcemia.

Excretion: In chronic nephritis, hypocalcemia occurs because the kidney cannot excrete phosphates. More phosphates are excreted in the stool, blocking calcium absorption and lowering serum calcium. Secondary hyperparathyroidism results and aggravates the situation. In contrast, with renal tubular acidosis, the kidneys do not reabsorb calcium and phosphorus from the glomerular filtrate, causing hypocalcemia. Secondary hyperparathyroidism results here also. Long-term diuretic therapy may induce the same picture.

● Approach to the Diagnosis

Determining the serum phosphate and alkaline phosphatase levels will facilitate differentiating the causes of hypocalcemia. The phosphates and alkaline phosphatase are elevated in chronic nephritis, but only the alkaline phosphatase is elevated in renal tubular acidosis and malabsorption syndrome. Only the phosphorus is elevated in hypoparathyroidism and pseudohypoparathyroidism. Hypoparathyroidism can be distinguished by a low serum PTH assay result.

● Other Useful Tests

1. CBC (malabsorption syndrome)
2. Sedimentation rate (nephritis, acute pancreatitis)

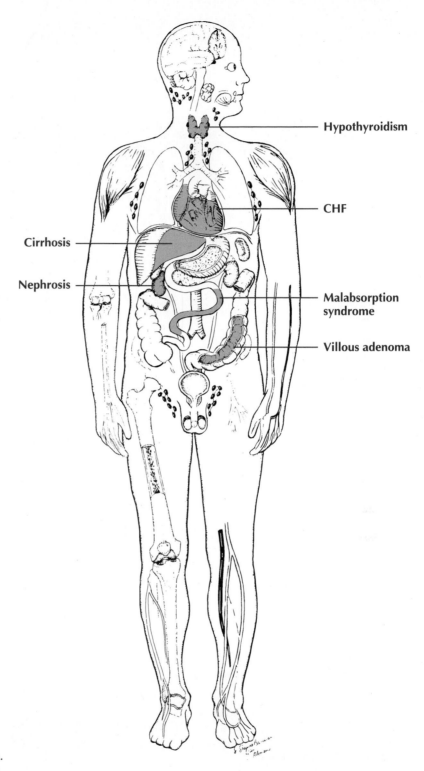

● **FIGURE 28** Hypoalbuminemia.

3. Chemistry profile (uremia)
4. Urinalysis (chronic nephritis; renal tubular acidosis)
5. 24-hour urine calcium (hypoparathyroidism)
6. Skeletal survey (rickets)
7. D-xylose absorption test (malabsorption syndrome)
8. Serum protein electrophoresis (nephrosis)
9. Ellsworth–Howard test (pseudohypoparathyroidism)

10. Bone biopsy (rickets, osteomalacia)
11. Endocrinology consult

HYPOGLYCEMIA

A list of possibilities for hypoglycemia may be had simply by thinking of the **endocrine glands**. Consequently,

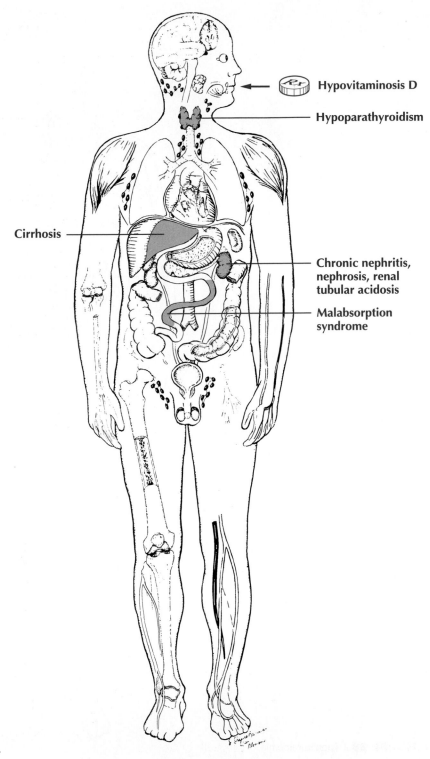

Hypovitaminosis D

Hypoparathyroidism

Cirrhosis

Chronic nephritis, nephrosis, renal tubular acidosis

Malabsorption syndrome

● **FIGURE 29** Hypocalcemia.

thinking of the pancreas, one could recall insulinoma. Thinking of the adrenal gland, one would recall Addison disease. Considering the pituitary, one would remember hypopituitarism, and the thyroid hypothyroidism. Unfortunately, a few conditions may be overlooked by this method alone. If none of the above diagnoses seem to fit, the patient may have glycogen storage disease, cirrhosis, or functional hypoglycemia. Diabetics with hypoglycemia

may be taking too much insulin, or their doses of oral hypoglycemic agents may be too high.

● **Approach to the Diagnosis**

The clinical picture may fit one of the endocrine disorders mentioned above. If not, the laboratory can be of tremendous assistance. A glucose tolerance test will help diagnose

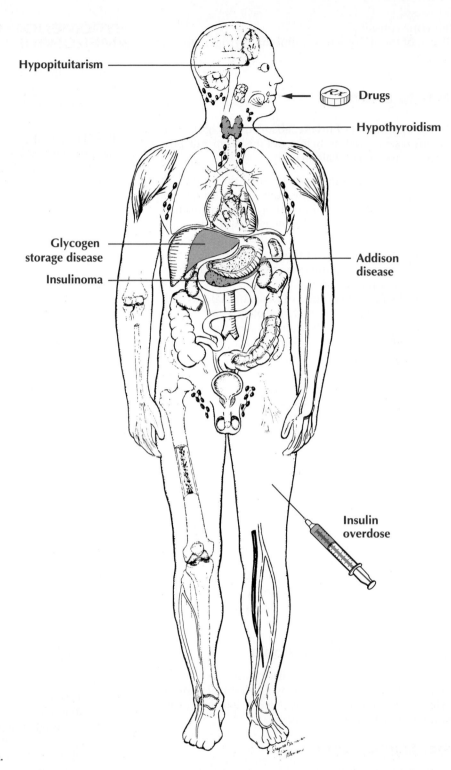

Hypopituitarism

Drugs

Hypothyroidism

Glycogen
storage disease

Insulinoma

Addison
disease

Insulin
overdose

● **FIGURE 30** Hypoglycemia.

functional hypoglycemia. Hospitalization for a 72-hour fast while taking frequent blood sugar tests will help to diagnose an insulinoma.

● **Other Useful Tests**

1. CBC
2. Urinalysis
3. Chemistry panel (advanced liver disease)
4. Liver profile (cirrhosis)
5. Thyroid profile (hypothyroidism, hypopituitarism)
6. Plasma cortisol level (Addison disease)
7. Serum growth hormone assay (hypopituitarism)
8. C-peptide level (insulinoma)
9. Plasma insulin assay (insulinoma)
10. Tolbutamide tolerance test (insulinoma)

11. Endocrine consult
12. CT scan of the abdomen (insulinoma, glycogen storage disease)

HYPOKALEMIA

The **physiologic** model of **intake**, **absorption**, **regulation**, and **excretion** serves well to help recall the diagnostic possibilities in a case of hypokalemia.

Intake: Potassium enters the body through the GI tract. It follows that starvation and anything else that interferes with the intake of potassium (such as vomiting or diarrhea) will cause depletion of body potassium. In addition, potassium is secreted in the GI tract in the digestive juices. This mechanism contributes to the depletion of potassium in pyloric obstruction, intestinal obstruction, and diarrhea of many causes.

Absorption: The poor absorption of water and salts in malabsorption syndrome leads to hypokalemia.

Regulation: The hormone aldosterone activates the kidney to reabsorb large amounts of sodium in exchange for potassium and hydrogen ion. Consequently, when the adrenal cortex secretes large amounts of this hormone, as in primary aldosteronism, there is associated hypokalemia. Hypokalemia is also associated with secondary aldosteronism as occurs in malignant hypertension, renal artery stenosis, and Bartter syndrome.

Excretion: In chronic renal failure of many causes, there is damage to the distal tubules of the kidney so that reabsorption of potassium is impaired; therefore, hypokalemia results. Diuretics such as hydrochlorothiazide may inhibit the distal tubular reabsorption of potassium, causing hypokalemia. Hypokalemia develops in renal tubular acidosis because of a renal tubular defect causing more sodium to be absorbed in exchange for potassium, which creates a potassium deficit. Metabolic alkalosis also enhances the secretion of potassium in exchange for sodium to conserve hydrogen ion, causing hypokalemia.

● Approach to the Diagnosis

A history of vomiting, diarrhea, or use of diuretics will be helpful in determining the cause of hypokalemia. However, serial electrolytes, chemistry panel, and a 24-hour urine potassium level will be most useful.

● Other Useful Tests

1. CBC (infection, septicemia)
2. Urinalysis (chronic nephritis)
3. Plasma renin level (aldosteronism)
4. 24-hour urine aldosterone level (primary aldosteronism)
5. Plasma cortisol level (Cushing syndrome)
6. D-xylose absorption test (malabsorption syndrome)
7. Endocrinology consult
8. Nephrology consult

HYPOMENORRHEA AND AMENORRHEA

Combining the **anatomy** of the female genital tract with the **endocrine system** will key in on the major sources of absent or diminished menstrual flow. It is perhaps best to begin at the bottom and work upward to the head.

1. **Female genital tract:** Such congenital anomalies as an imperforate hymen, imperforate vagina, cervical stenosis, double uterus, or the complete absence of any one or more of these organs would obviously cause amenorrhea. Radiation therapy may destroy the endometrium so that it cannot respond to female hormones. Pregnancy is the most common cause of amenorrhea, and it must be considered the cause of sudden onset of amenorrhea in an apparently healthy woman until proven otherwise. Excessive blood levels of endogenous or exogenous estrogen or progesterone will cause amenorrhea. The tubes should immediately suggest an ectopic pregnancy as the cause, although spotting and metrorrhagia are frequent in these cases.

2. **Ovary:** The mnemonic **MINTS** serves well in subdividing the causes here.

   M—Malformations of the ovary include Turner syndrome (where the ovaries are reduced to a fibrotic, pea-sized nodule), Stein–Leventhal syndrome, and other congenital cysts. Acquired malformations suggest the atrophy of menopause, which may occur as early as the late 20s.

   I—Intoxication includes the ovarian dysfunction of exogenous hormones, irradiation, chronic alcoholism, or drug addiction. **I** for **inflammation** helps to recall autoimmune oophoritis. **I** for **idiopathic** helps to recall idiopathic ovarian failure.

   N—Neoplasms of the ovary frequently cause amenorrhea, especially if they secrete hormones or are bilateral. The arrhenoblastomas, granulosa cell and theca cell tumors, and cystadenocarcinomas must be considered in this category.

   T—Trauma as a cause of amenorrhea is well known, but this is generally due to diffuse body trauma such as an automobile crash, severe burns, or extensive surgery. Direct trauma to the ovary merely reminds one that oophorectomy can cause amenorrhea. Emotional trauma is probably a more common cause of amenorrhea than any of the above.

   S—Systemic disease suggests the amenorrhea of leukemia, Hodgkin lymphoma, chronic nephritis, fever, and severe malnutrition.

3. **Thyroid:** It is well known that hyperthyroidism causes hypomenorrhea or amenorrhea and hypothyroidism causes hypermenorrhea; however, the exact reverse may occur.

4. **Adrenal gland:** Visualizing this organ should stimulate the recall of amenorrhea in the adrenogenital syndrome of adrenal hyperplasia or carcinomas and in Addison disease.

5. **Pituitary gland: MINT** is a useful mnemonic here also.

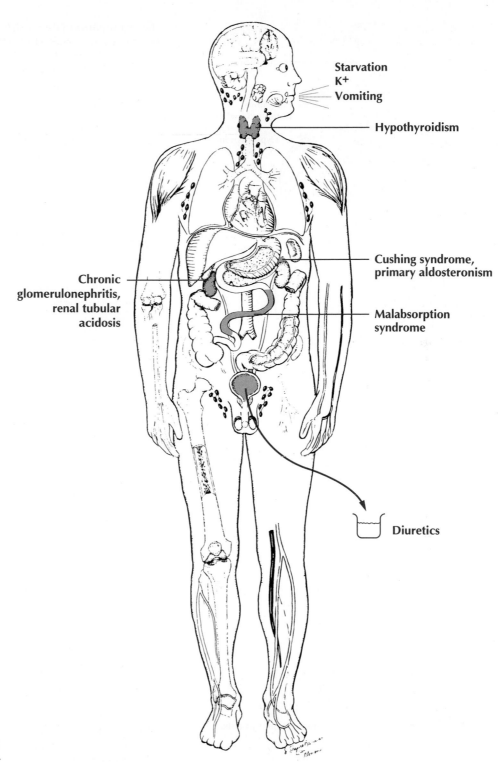

Starvation
K+
Vomiting

Hypothyroidism

Cushing syndrome,
primary aldosteronism

Malabsorption
syndrome

Chronic
glomerulonephritis,
renal tubular
acidosis

Diuretics

● **FIGURE 31** Hypokalemia.

M—Malformations here are Fröhlich syndrome and Chiari–Frommel syndrome, but perhaps more important is the reduced output of pituitary hormone in many states of congenital mental retardation and brain damage.

I—Inflammation suggests the hypopituitarism of sarcoid and TB.

N—Neoplasm suggests the largest group of causes of hypopituitarism, including chromophobe adenomas and basophilic adenomas.

T—Trauma recalls the hypopituitarism of postpartum hemorrhage and amniotic fluid emboli or Sheehan syndrome.

H

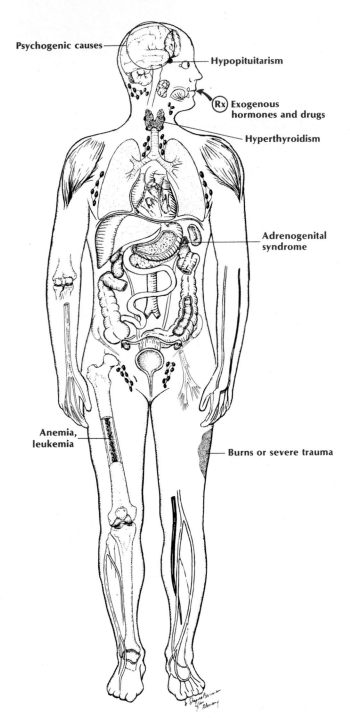

Psychogenic causes
Hypopituitarism
(Rx) Exogenous hormones and drugs
Hyperthyroidism
Adrenogenital syndrome
Anemia, leukemia
Burns or severe trauma

● **FIGURE 32** Hypomenorrhea and amenorrhea, systemic causes.

● Approach to the Diagnosis

Obviously the first thing to do is rule out pregnancy both by examination and a pregnancy test, preferably the serum β-subunit human chorionic gonadotropin (HCG). One must keep an ectopic pregnancy in mind even if the examination is normal and plan follow-up examinations and ultrasonography should the situation warrant. Altered secondary sex characteristics should be noted. If

the examination fails to show evidence of pregnancy, congenital anomalies, or tumors of the ovaries, the physician should order thyroid function studies, a Wassermann test, CBC, and sedimentation rate. If these tests are normal, a gynecologist should be consulted. The gynecologist may give a test dose of intramuscular progesterone to prove that the endometrium functions well. He or she may do a D & C first. Then serum or urine FSH, LH, and prolactin levels are done; if the FSH level is high, the ovary is probably the site of the trouble. If the levels are low, even after gonadotropin-releasing factor (GRF) is administered, the pituitary is responsible. X-rays of the skull, CT scans, culdoscopy, and exploratory laparotomy all share their place in the workup.

Case Presentation #52

A 34-year-old white mother of three complained of amenorrhea and weight loss. A pregnancy test was negative. She has been under a lot of emotional distress for several months and has lost her appetite.

Question #1. Utilizing your knowledge of anatomy and physiology, what is your differential diagnosis?

Further history reveals that she had a postpartum hemorrhage following her last delivery, and the amenorrhea began at that time. Review of systems reveals that she had loss of axillary and pubic hair and insignificant lactation following her last delivery.

Question #2. What is your diagnosis now?

(See Appendix B for the answers.)

HYPONATREMIA

The **physiologic** model of **intake, absorption, transport, regulation,** and **excretion** lends itself well to developing a list of possible causes of hyponatremia.

Intake: A limited intake of sodium by itself does not usually cause hyponatremia. However, in disorders of the GI tract that cause vomiting or diarrhea, there is often associated hyponatremia. Consequently, pyloric obstruction, cholera, viral gastroenteritis, intestinal obstruction, acute ulcerative colitis, and bacterial dysentery lead to hyponatremia.

Absorption: Absorption of sodium through the intestinal wall is inhibited in malabsorption syndrome, causing hyponatremia.

Transport: In CHF, there is decreased perfusion of the glomeruli, leading to retention of both sodium and water. There is also inappropriate secretion of ADH, causing a greater retention of water than sodium, and thus dilutional hyponatremia is known to occur.

Regulation: The hormone aldosterone regulates the reabsorption of sodium by the kidney; when this is absent, as in Addison disease and other conditions associated with adrenal insufficiency, there is hyponatremia. Diuretics

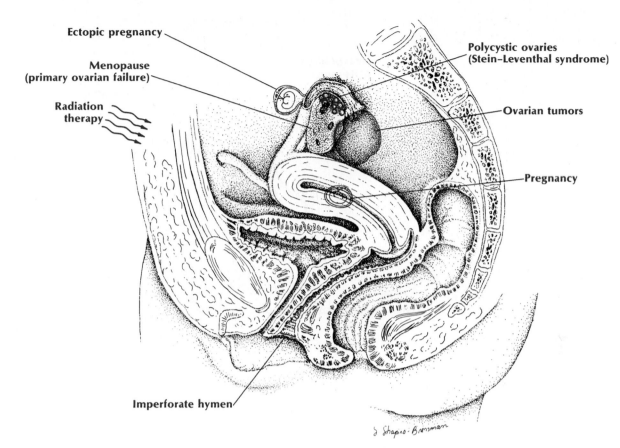

● **FIGURE 33** Hypomenorrhea and amenorrhea, local causes.

also interfere with the reabsorption of sodium by the kidney, leading to hyponatremia, which is desirable as long as it is not taken to extreme. In the syndrome of inappropriate ADH secretion, more water than sodium is retained, causing hyponatremia. This syndrome is found in carcinoma of the lung, porphyria, Guillain–Barré syndrome, postoperatively, and other pulmonary and neurologic disorders.

Excretion: Excess sodium is excreted via the kidney. Consequently, in renal failure one would consistently expect salt retention and hypernatremia. In fact, the opposite usually occurs. In **acute renal failure**, hyponatremia results because more water than sodium is retained, and there is often vomiting that contributes to the hyponatremia because the patient usually replaces the water without adequate salt replacement. In **chronic renal failure**, there is often hyponatremia because reabsorption of sodium by the distal tubules is impaired. In **renal tubular acidosis**, hyponatremia occurs because of the interference with the exchange of the hydrogen ion for sodium. Sodium is secreted by the sweat glands. It follows that hyponatremia is found in pathologic diaphoresis and heat exhaustion.

● **Approach to the Diagnosis**

The history may reveal causes of hyponatremia such as the use of diuretics, CHF, malabsorption syndrome, or chronic renal failure. Symptoms of vomiting or diarrhea should also alert one to a GI disorder as the cause. Laboratory tests such as a chemistry panel, serial electrolytes, plasma cortisol, serum and urine osmolality, spot urine sodium, and blood volume may be very helpful.

● **Other Useful Tests**

1. CBC (infection, Addison disease)
2. Urinalysis (acute or chronic nephritis)
3. Serum ADH assay (diabetes insipidus)
4. Plasma renin (aldosteronism)
5. Arterial blood gases (shock, CHF)
6. Endocrinology consult
7. Nephrology consult
8. 24-hour urine aldosterone (Addison disease)
9. Corticotropin stimulation test (Addison disease)

HYPOTENSION AND SHOCK

Many patients are told that they have a low blood pressure and are even treated for it when that blood pressure may be entirely normal for them. Asymptomatic hypotension may not be pathologic at all. At any rate, an expensive investigation into the causes of "hypotension" would seem unnecessary if the systolic pressure is above 80 mm Hg, especially when the patient is asymptomatic.

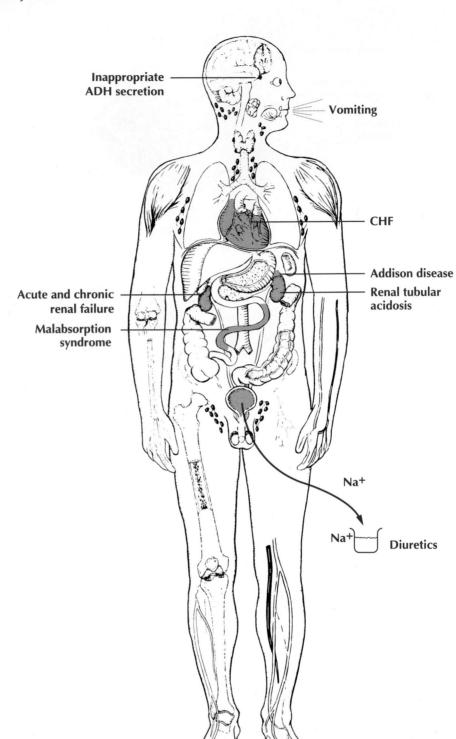

● **FIGURE 34** Hyponatremia.

The differential diagnosis of both hypotension and shock is best developed using **physiology**. There are three things that are necessary to sustain the blood pressure at the normal level: adequate blood volume, adequate cardiac output, and adequate tone in the arteries and arterioles. Alteration of any of these may produce hypotension.

Low blood volume may result from any of the following conditions:

1. Hemorrhagic shock such as acute upper GI bleeding
2. Chronic blood loss (e.g., peptic ulcer) or anemia of decreased production (such as aplastic anemia) or increased destruction (hemolytic anemias)

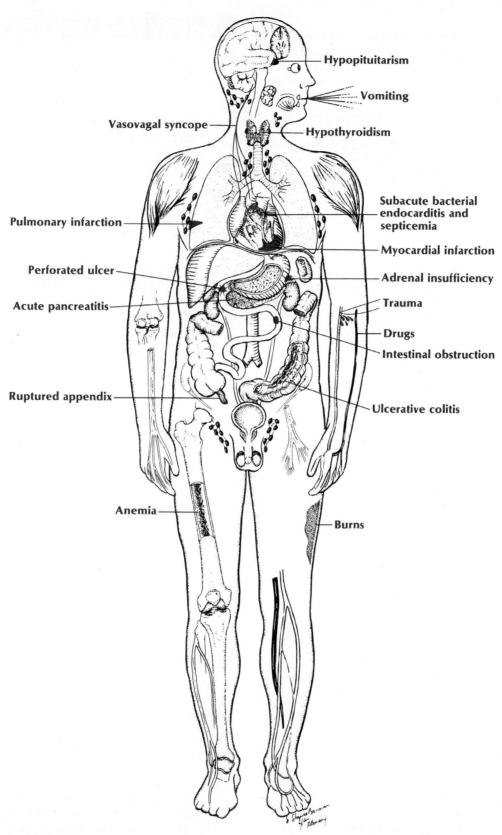

● **FIGURE 35** Hypotension and shock.

3. Dehydration
4. Decreased sodium chloride (NaCl) in blood from pituitary and adrenal insufficiency, diuretics, diarrhea or vomiting, chronic nephritis, or severe diaphoresis
5. Decreased albumin in the blood from nephrosis, cirrhosis, and malnutrition or malabsorption syndrome

Any one of the conditions listed above may be associated with hypotension.

Decreased cardiac output usually results from CHF of many causes and from myocardial infarction. Many valvular lesions (e.g., mitral stenosis) may manifest hypotension without overt heart failure. Cor pulmonale may lead to hypotension from a decreased cardiac output.

Decreased arterial tone (e.g., vasomotor shock) occurs in the following conditions:

1. When the sympathetic nerves are blocked by antihypertensive drugs (e.g., α-methyldopa, guanethidine, and pentolinium tartrate), by diabetic neuropathy, or after a sympathectomy.
2. When there is increased vagal stimulation, as in neurogenic shock (common faint) and late stages of increased intracranial pressure.
3. When toxins are introduced into the bloodstream from necrotic tissue, bacteria, or drugs that act directly on the arterioles. Toxic shock in young menstruating women is caused by staph or strep toxins from infected vaginal tampons.

Examples of the last type of hypotension are pulmonary infarction (necrotic tissue), toxins, septicemia (bacterial toxins), and hydralazine therapy.

● Approach to the Diagnosis

The workup of shock must be vigorous with emergency CBC, blood cultures, blood gases, ECG, electrolytes, blood urea nitrogen (BUN), and type- and cross-match of blood at the same time that vigorous antishock measures are applied. Checking the GI tract for blood loss with a rectal and nasogastric tube can be both diagnostic and therapeutic. To work up chronic hypotension, one should not forget venous pressure and circulation times (to diagnose decreased cardiac output and CHF), serial electrolytes and cortisol levels (to rule out adrenal insufficiency), and sedimentation rate and cultures of various body fluids (to exclude a chronic infectious disease, e.g., TB).

● Other Useful Tests

1. Blood volume study (dehydration, hypovolemic shock)
2. Electrolytes (Addison disease)
3. 24-hour blood pressure monitoring
4. ECG (CHF, valvular heart disease)
5. Visual field examination (pituitary tumor)
6. Thyroid profile (hypothyroidism)
7. CT scan of the brain (pituitary tumor)
8. Drug screen (drug or alcohol abuse)
9. Echocardiography

Case Presentation #53

A 52-year-old white man complained of generalized fatigue, weight loss, and occasional diarrhea for the past year. His blood pressure was 75/50 mm Hg. He was treated for pulmonary TB several years ago.

Question #1. What is your differential diagnosis considering the physiology of hypotension?

Your examination shows diffusely increased skin pigmentation and induration of the testicles.

Question #2. What is your diagnosis now?

(See Appendix B for the answers.)

HYPOTENSION, ORTHOSTATIC

In this condition, there is a drop in blood pressure of 20 mm or more on standing. The causes are similar to those discussed under "hypotension" plus disorders of the autonomic nervous system such as diabetic neuropathy and Shy–Dragger syndrome.

● Approach to the Diagnosis

A tilt table test is the best way to diagnose this disorder. Blood volume studies, echocardiography, a glucose tolerance test, serum ACTH, and cortisol may need to be ordered as well as a neurology consult.

HYPOTHERMIA

Subnormal temperature is not usually a presenting finding, but when it is found in cases of coma, hypothyroidism (myxedema coma) is the first thing to rule out. Understanding the cause of this sign is best approached from a **physiologic** standpoint. There are three basic reasons why a temperature drops: absolute decrease in metabolic rate, decreased circulation to the area where the temperature is being recorded, and disorders of the thermoregulatory center in the brain.

1. **Decreased metabolic rate:** Hypothyroidism and hypopituitarism are the principal conditions that fall into this category. Senility, starvation, and chronic inanition may cause hypothermia due to a decreased metabolic rate. Diabetes mellitus may cause hypothermia because of poor cellular absorption of glucose.
2. **Poor circulation:** Shock from any cause (hypovolemia, cardiogenic, or neurogenic) falls into this category. Hemorrhagic shock, dehydration, CHF, and adrenal insufficiency are all probably based on this mechanism. With poor circulation, there is tissue anoxia and a reduced metabolism in the skin and mucosa where the temperature is taken.
3. **Disorders of the thermoregulatory center:** Cerebral thrombosis and hemorrhage, certain pituitary tumors,

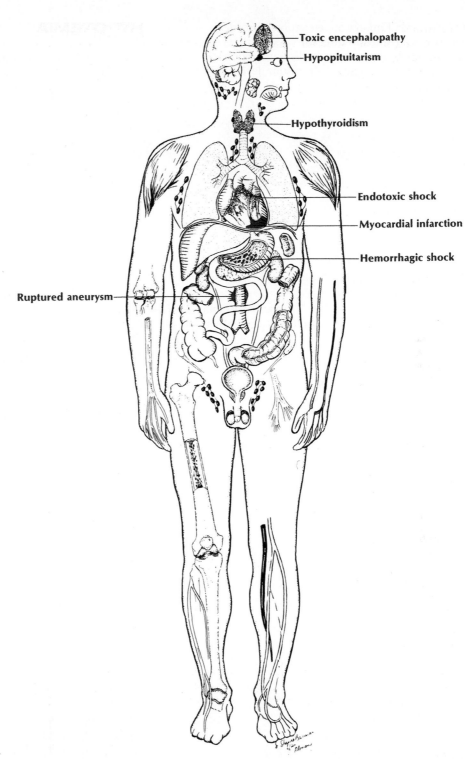

● **FIGURE 36** Hypothermia.

and toxic suppression of this center by barbiturates, alcohol, opiates, and general anesthesia all fit into this category. Any case of prolonged coma may cause hypothermia on this basis.

● **Approach to the Diagnosis**

Establishing a definitive diagnosis of hypothermia depends heavily on the interpretation of other symptoms and signs.

A good history is invaluable as well as laboratory studies including fasting blood sugar (FBS), thyroid functions, electrolytes, BUN, and drug screens; in selected cases, a spinal tap may be useful.

● **Other Useful Tests**

1. CBC (anemia)
2. Chemistry panel (uremia, liver disease)

3. ECG (myocardial infarction, electrolyte disorder)
4. Serum cortisol (Addison disease)
5. CT scan of the brain (tumor, cerebral infarction)
6. Serum FSH, LH, and growth hormone levels (pituitary insufficiency)

HYPOXEMIA

In developing the list of possible causes of hypoxemia, the physiologic model of intake, absorption, transport, regulation, and excretion is most useful.

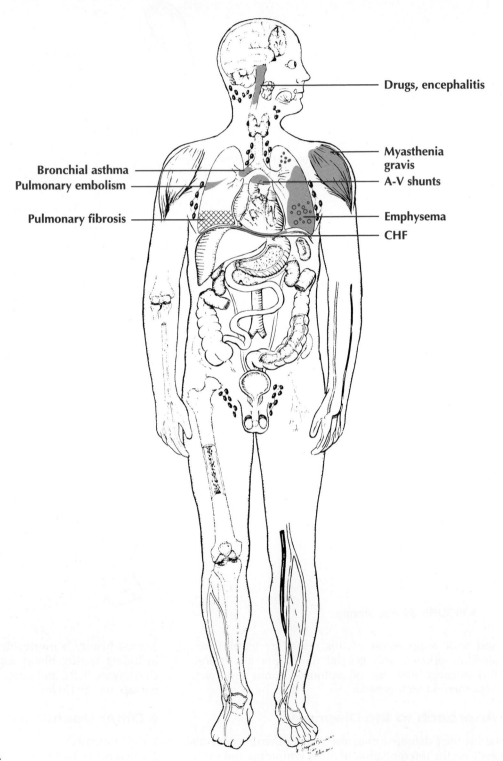

Drugs, encephalitis

Myasthenia gravis

A-V shunts

Bronchial asthma

Pulmonary embolism

Emphysema

CHF

Pulmonary fibrosis

● **FIGURE 37** Hypoxemia.

Intake: Both upper airway obstruction (laryngotracheitis, foreign body) and lower airway obstruction (bronchial asthma, emphysema) may inhibit the intake of oxygen, causing hypoxemia. In addition, conditions that affect the chest wall such as kyphoscoliosis, ankylosing spondylitis, and myasthenia gravis reduce the intake of oxygen by decreasing the vital capacity.

Absorption: Absorption of oxygen in the lungs may be inhibited by atelectasis, pneumothorax, or pneumonia where the alveolar sacs are blocked or collapsed or by a diffusion defect as occurs in Hamman–Rich disease, silicosis, sarcoidosis, and scleroderma. Absorption is also impeded by a pulmonary embolism or pulmonary hemangioma, which interferes with the perfusion of a segment of a lung. Large venous–arterial shunts such as tetralogy of Fallot can produce the same picture.

Transport: The cardiovascular system transports oxygen to the tissue. When blood flow is slowed because of CHF or shock, oxygen is not picked up in the lungs and transported to the tissues fast enough to keep pace with the demand, resulting in hypoxemia. CHF also decreases absorption by the accumulation of fluid in the lungs, blocking the diffusion of oxygen across the alveoli.

Regulation: Respirations are regulated by the central nervous system. Consequently, drugs such as phenobarbital that decrease the respiratory rate cause hypoxemia. Diseases that affect the respiratory center such as poliomyelitis or Guillain–Barré syndrome can suppress respiration, causing hypoxemia.

Excretion: Blocking the excretion of oxygen does not cause hypoxemia. However, blockage of the excretion of carbon dioxide, as in pulmonary emphysema and asthmatic bronchitis, contributes to hypoxemia by not allowing the blood to pick up oxygen in exchange for carbon dioxide.

● Approach to the Diagnosis

The clinical picture of obstructive lung disease is usually obvious. Other causes of hypoxemia may require more extensive laboratory evaluation to diagnose. It is most important to study the arterial blood gases. An increased carbon dioxide level suggests pulmonary emphysema or asthma. Pulmonary function tests can assist in the diagnosis of these conditions as well. If the carbon dioxide level is normal or decreased, a perfusion or defusion defect must be looked for. A lung scan will help rule out a pulmonary embolism. A chest x-ray will help reveal pneumothorax, atelectasis, sarcoidosis, and pulmonary fibrosis. An arm-to-tongue circulation time will help rule out CHF. A consult with a pulmonologist or cardiologist is always wise when faced with hypoxemia.

● Other Useful Tests

1. CBC (shock, infection)
2. Urinalysis (collagen disease)
3. Sedimentation rate (infection)
4. Chemistry panel (shock, myocardial infarction)
5. Blood volume (shock, CHF)
6. Sulfhemoglobin and methemoglobin (sulfhemoglobinemia, methemoglobinemia)
7. Carboxyhemoglobin (carbon monoxide poisoning)
8. Serial ECGs and cardiac enzymes (myocardial infarction)
9. CT scan of the chest (pulmonary aneurysm, bronchiectasis)
10. Lung biopsy (neoplasm, pulmonary fibrosis)
11. Bronchoscopy (neoplasm, bronchiectasis)

H

I

IMPOTENCE

Impotence is now more commonly referred to as erectile dysfunction. Impotence may be due to local end-organ disease, dysfunction of the peripheral nerve pathways, disease of the spinal cord or brain, pituitary and other endocrine disorders, and supratentorial disorders. Thus, recall of the various causes is based on both **anatomy** and **physiology**.

1. **End-organ disorders:** These include phimosis, paraphimosis, prostatitis, prostate carcinoma, and Peyronie disease. The blood supply to the penis may be affected by arteriosclerosis of the dorsal penile arteries or the terminal aorta (Lariche syndrome).
2. **Peripheral nerve disorders:** Diabetic neuropathy is a common cause in this category, but alcoholic neuropathy and other neuropathies may occasionally cause impotence.
3. **Spinal cord disorders:** Transverse myelitis, poliomyelitis, compression fractures, spinal cord tumors, multiple sclerosis, and tabes dorsalis are important disorders to be considered here.
4. **Disorders of the brain:** In addition to general paresis, brain tumors, vascular occlusions, and arteriosclerosis, degenerative diseases such as Alzheimer disease, senile dementia, and Schilder disease will cause impotence.
5. **Pituitary and other endocrine disorders:** Impotence is found in pituitary tumors, acromegaly, testicular atrophy from hemochromatosis, mumps, Klinefelter syndrome, Cushing disease, and hypothyroidism. Hyperprolactinemia is associated with impotence.
6. **Supratentorial disorders:** Recent studies suggest that less than 10% of cases of impotence are caused by psychiatric disorders. After years of marriage and intercourse with the same sexual partner, one's libido may decline considerably. The first time the male patient has trouble reaching an erection, he begins to believe he is "over the hill." If he should happen to acquire a young mistress, he may find convincing proof that his impotence is psychologic.

Sometimes, in search of variety in his sexual life, a married man may decide to find a new sexual partner. When the moment of truth arrives, he may be unable to get an erection because of the associated guilt involved.

Premature ejaculation is common under these circumstances also. After his first failure, the fear of a repeated performance may make him impotent not only in extramarital relations but also in marital relations.

Young men, whether married or unmarried, may "fall into impotence" quite by accident because of alcoholic intoxication. As Shakespeare correctly surmised, "alcohol provokes the desire, but it takes away the performance."

Under the influence of alcohol, the inspired lover may fail miserably. When sober once more, he may begin a pattern of failure to get an erection simply because of the fear that it will happen again and he will be embarrassed beyond belief.

Some other supratentorial causes of impotence are endogenous: depression, schizophrenia, latent homosexuality, repressed hostility toward the partner, and fear of pregnancy. It is important to note that all of the above psychologic causes may occur in the female patient as well as the male. There are many more causes too numerous to mention in a book of this scope.

● Approach to the Diagnosis

A history of drug or alcohol abuse is important. Many drugs can cause impotence, especially the antihypertensives. A careful examination of the external genitalia, the prostate, and secondary sex characteristics is essential. The laboratory workup may include a glucose tolerance test, blood testosterone, free testosterone and cortisol levels, thyroid function studies, a spinal tap, a skull x-ray, and a chromosomal analysis. A nocturnal penile tumescence study is performed to rule out organic causes. If the physical examination is normal, it may be wise to administer psychometric tests or to refer the patient to a psychiatrist before doing an extensive endocrine and neurologic workup. A sympathetic physician may be able to find the supratentorial cause and cure it with a few long discussions with the patient. A female physician may have more success in this area than a male.

● Other Useful Tests

1. Serum follicle-stimulating hormone (FSH) and luteinizing hormone (LH) levels (pituitary or gonadal insufficiency)
2. Sperm count (testicular atrophy)
3. Penile blood pressure (Leriche syndrome, arteriosclerosis)
4. Spinal tap (multiple sclerosis, neurosyphilis)
5. Computed tomography (CT) scan of the brain (pituitary tumor)
6. Testicular biopsy (testicular atrophy)
7. Cystometric studies (neurogenic bladder)
8. Doppler sonogram of dorsalis penis artery (arteriosclerosis)
9. Drug screen (drug abuse)
10. Interview of spouse
11. Nerve conduction velocity (NCV) and electromyogram (EMG) (peripheral neuropathy)
12. Serum prolactin
13. 4-week therapeutic trial of antibiotics (chronic prostatitis)
14. Therapeutic trial of oral sildenafil or a prostadil injection

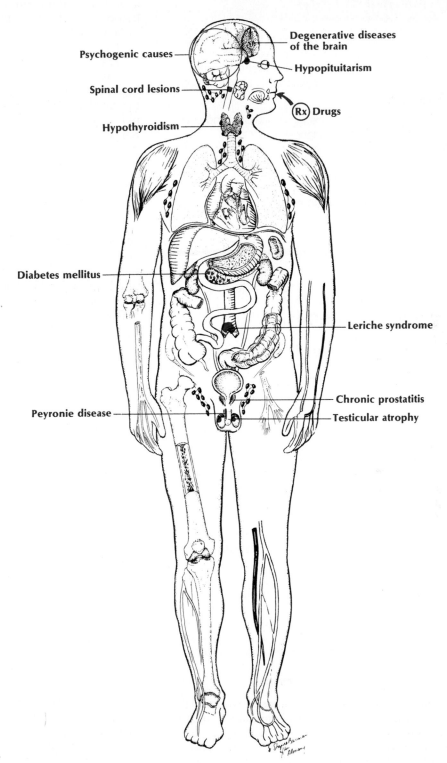

● **FIGURE 1** Impotence.

INCONTINENCE, FECAL

Anatomy will serve us well in recalling the various causes of fecal incontinence. The pathway of voluntary control of this function begins in the cerebrum and travels through the brain stem, spinal cord, and nerve roots, to the "end organ," which is the rectal sphincter.

Cerebrum: This should help recall the incontinence of Alzheimer disease, normal pressure hydrocephalus, and other causes of organic brain syndrome. It will also prompt the recall of the incontinence in functional psychosis and epilepsy.

Brainstem and spinal cord: This would bring to mind trauma, multiple sclerosis, transverse myelitis, syringomyelia, and brainstem and spinal cord tumors in which there is loss of voluntary control due to pyramidal tract damage.

Nerve roots: This should prompt the recall of cauda equina tumors, tabes dorsales, and spinal stenosis.

Rectal sphincter: Primary rectal sphincter incompetence leads to the release of small amounts of stool associated with anal fissures, hemorrhoids, and postoperative incontinence following a fistulectomy or episiotomy.

● Approach to the Diagnosis

Before beginning an expensive diagnostic workup, pay attention to the history and physical examination. Is there a small volume of stool? Look for an anal fissure, hemorrhoids, or other causes of sphincter incompetence. If the incontinence is sporadic, look for organic brain syndrome, epilepsy, or functional psychosis. If the neurologic examination reveals pathologic or hyperactive reflexes in the lower extremities, consider a spinal cord or brain stem lesion. If there are hypoactive reflexes in the lower extremities, consider the possibility of cauda equina tumor or tabes dorsalis. Careful digital examination will often reveal

a local cause. If the sphincter is tight, consider a spinal cord lesion. If it is flaccid, consider a lesion of the cauda equina or nerve roots.

Patients with signs of mental deterioration need a CT scan or MRI of the brain. Normal pressure hydrocephalus can be excluded by radioactive cisternography. Patients with hyperactive reflexes in the lower extremities need a CT scan or MRI of the suspected level of spinal cord involvement, whereas patients with hypoactive reflexes require an MRI of the lumbar spine or myelography. Anorectal manometry and defecography will assist in the diagnosis of anal and rectal sphincter dysfunction. A neurologist or gastroenterologist may need to be consulted.

INCONTINENCE, URINARY

Incontinence may be due to loss of voluntary control of urination, in which case neurologic disorders are usually the cause, or it may result from overflow of a distended bladder (overflow incontinence), in which case the cause may be bladder neck obstruction or a flaccid neurogenic bladder. Stress incontinence occurs on coughing or straining and is due to damage to the urethra or pelvic floor from pregnancy and delivery.

1. **Loss of voluntary control:** The neurologic causes include multiple sclerosis, neurosyphilis, syringomyelia, encephalitis, cerebral arteriosclerosis, frontal lobe tumors and abscesses, senile dementia, and transverse myelitis from trauma or infection. The local causes are a cystocele (often following a hysterectomy) and a damaged urethral sphincter from prostatectomy.
2. **Bladder neck obstruction:** Benign prostatic hypertrophy, chronic prostatitis, prostate carcinoma, median bar hypertrophy, vesical calculus, and urethral stricture are important mechanical causes of obstruction.
3. **Flaccid neurogenic bladder:** Drugs such as atropine, tranquilizers, and anesthetics and diseases of the cauda equina and nervi erigentes such as diabetic neuropathy, poliomyelitis, tabes dorsalis, and cauda equina tumors will cause a flaccid neurogenic bladder with overflow incontinence.

● Approach to the Diagnosis

First, exclude stress incontinence with a pad test. Perineal pads are weighed before and after walking and stress for 30 minutes. An increase in weight identifies urine loss. Catheterization and examination, smear, and culture of the urine are essential at the outset. Cystoscopy and cystometric studies are often needed. Surgical repair of a cystocele or a parasympathomimetic drug in cases of a flaccid neurogenic bladder and oxybutynin (Ditropan) for spastic neurogenic bladders may be all that is necessary. A neurologist and urologist often need to cooperate in the diagnosis and treatment of these unfortunate individuals.

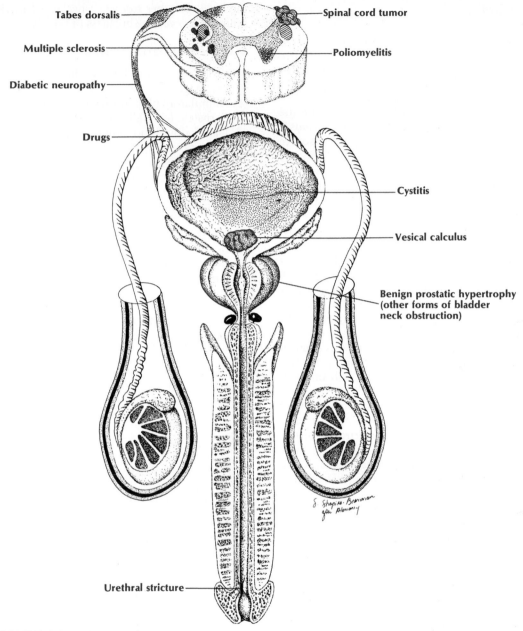

Tabes dorsalis

Multiple sclerosis

Diabetic neuropathy

Drugs

Spinal cord tumor

Poliomyelitis

Cystitis

Vesical calculus

Benign prostatic hypertrophy
(other forms of bladder
neck obstruction)

Urethral stricture

● **FIGURE 2** Incontinence, urinary.

● Other Useful Tests

1. Q tip test (stress incontinence)
2. Sonogram (test for residual urine)
3. Catheterization for residual urine (bladder neck obstruction)
4. CT scan of the lumbar spine (cauda equina tumor)
5. NCV and EMG (neuropathy)
6. Magnetic resonance imaging (MRI) of the brain and spinal cord (e.g., multiple sclerosis)
7. Psychometric testing (dementia)
8. Serum FSH and LH (menopause)
9. Trial of estrogen therapy
10. Transrectal ultrasound (benign prostatic hyperplasia)

Case Presentation #55

A 48-year-old white woman is brought to your office by her daughter who complains that she is getting forgetful and frequently wets herself. She is planning to admit her to a nursing home. She denies that her mother abuses drugs but admits she consumes a moderate amount of alcohol and falls occasionally.

Question #1. Utilizing your knowledge of neuroanatomy, what is your differential diagnosis?

You observe that the patient has a wide-based ataxic gait.

Question #2. What is your diagnosis now?

(See Appendix B for the answers.)

INDIGESTION

This is a vague term, and if the patient is put on the spot, he or she will usually describe the problem as heartburn, regurgitation of water brash, fullness in the stomach, or frequent belching following meals. Usually the patient's appetite is not affected, nor is there any weight loss.

The causes are easy to arrive at by merely asking the question, "Why would food cause these symptoms?" Obviously, the food or drink ingested may be the source of irritation: spicy foods, coffee and other caffeinated beverages, alcohol, excessive fried food (which actually suppresses the secretion of gastric juice and slows gastric emptying), and insufficiently masticated food. The patient may sometimes be allergic to a particular food. Air swallowing from nerves is a frequent cause of belching, especially in talkative individuals.

The upper gastrointestinal (GI) tract may be already irritated with reflux esophagitis from a hiatal hernia, gastritis, or gastric or duodenal ulcer, or it may be partially obstructed by a carcinoma of the esophagus or stomach or by a pyloric ulcer. Chronic appendicitis and regional ileitis may cause partial obstruction or paralytic ileus. There may be diminished secretion of GI juices in pernicious anemia, cholecystitis, cholelithiasis, hepatitis, chronic pancreatitis, or pancreatic carcinoma, or in patients with previous gastrectomies.

There may be a systemic illness that is associated with GI irritation or paralytic ileus. In this category, one must consider congestive heart failure (CHF), electrolyte disturbances such as hypokalemia (diuretics) or hyperkalemia (Addison disease), abdominal angina, migraine, and epilepsy. Anemia and diabetic acidosis may produce similar symptoms.

Is there another way of recalling these conditions that may be simpler? Yes, the application of the "target" method to the anatomy of the internal organs. In the "bull's-eye," one would think of the esophagus and stomach (esophagitis, esophageal carcinoma, gastritis, gastric ulcer, and gastric carcinoma); in the next circle one would consider gallbladder, pancreatic, liver, and heart diseases; and, in the final circle, kidney, central nervous system (CNS), and other systemic diseases and hormonal alterations.

A third approach is simply to apply the mnemonic **MINT** to the organs of the upper abdomen. It is recommended that the reader applies this method as an exercise. Table 41 applies the mnemonic **VINDICATE** to the same organs.

● Approach to the Diagnosis

The association of other symptoms and signs is important. If there is relief by antacids, esophagitis, gastritis, or an ulcer may be present. If there is blood in the stool, one should suspect an ulcer or carcinoma. Radiographic studies in the form of an upper GI series, esophagram, cholecystogram, and barium enema are usually indicated. A gastric analysis, esophagoscopy, and gastroscopy often need to be done. Awareness that a systemic disease such as an electrolyte disturbance or uremia may be the cause will suggest

the need for other studies, especially if there are systemic symptoms, fever, or shortness of breath.

● Other Useful Tests

1. Esophageal motility studies (cardiospasm, reflux esophagitis)
2. Ambulatory pH monitoring (reflux esophagitis)
3. Bernstein test (reflux esophagitis)
4. Gallbladder sonogram (cholecystitis)
5. CT scan of the abdomen (neoplasm abscess, pancreatitis)
6. Serial electrocardiogram and cardiac enzymes (myocardial infarction)
7. Circulation time (CHF)
8. Breath test and *Helicobacter pylori* antibody test (peptic ulcer)
9. Serum gastrin (gastrinoma)
10. Stool for quantitative fat (malabsorption syndrome)
11. Lactose tolerance test

Case Presentation #56

A 55-year-old obese black mother of five complained of indigestion that she described as a fullness in the stomach and belching following meals. She denies abuse of alcohol or drugs but takes occasional aspirin for arthralgias.

Question #1. Utilizing the target method described above, what would be your differential diagnosis?

Her examination revealed mild tenderness in the right upper quadrant but was otherwise unremarkable. Stools were negative for occult blood, and ultrasonography was positive for gall stones.

Question #2. What is your diagnosis now?

(See Appendix B for the answers.)

INFERTILITY

Fertility depends on a healthy sperm reaching a freshly laid egg and impregnating it, and the fertilized egg digging into a healthy endometrium and being maintained in a healthy state until term. By visualizing the path the sperm must follow to reach the egg, one can identify many important causes of infertility. Male fertility, however, depends on a healthy pituitary gland and testicles, and female fertility depends on a healthy ovary and pituitary.

Thus, in the man, hypopituitarism, testicular atrophy (as in mumps), vas deferens obstruction (due to gonorrhea or tuberculosis), prostatitis and other prostatic disease, hypospadias, and other abnormalities of the urethra may cause infertility. Copulation may cause infertility; the causes of this disorder are discussed in the sections on frigidity and impotence (see pages 185 and 260).

In the female genital tract, the sperm may encounter antibodies, vaginitis, vaginal deformities, cervicitis, cervical

TABLE 41   Indigestion

	V Vascular	I Inflammatory	N Neoplasm	D Degenerative	I Intoxication Idiopathic	C Congenital	A Autoimmune Allergic	T Trauma	E Endocrine
Esophagus	Varices	Esophagitis	Esophageal carcinoma	Plummer–Vinson syndrome	Lye stricture	Hiatal hernia Diverticulitis Barrett esophagitis	Scleroderma		
Stomach		Gastritis Ulcer	Carcinoma	Atrophic gastritis Pernicious anemia	Aspirin Steroids Reserpine Alcohol Coffee syndrome	Cascade stomach		Gastrectomy	Zollinger–Ellison syndrome
Duodenum and Small Intestines	Abdominal angina	Duodenitis Ulcer	Polyp			Diverticuli	Scleroderma	Gastrectomy with afferent loop obstruction	Zollinger–Ellison syndrome
Gallbladder		Cholecystitis	Cholangiocarcinoma		Uremic ulcer				
Liver	CHF	Infectious hepatitis	Hepatoma			Stones from sickle cell anemia		Calculus	
Metastatic Carcinoma	Cirrhosis				Alcoholic cirrhosis				
Pancreas		Pancreatitis	Pancreatic carcinoma			Fibrocystic disease			Hyperparathyroidism
Kidney		Pyelonephritis			Uremia			Calculus	

carcinoma, endometritis, carcinoma of the endometrium, a retroverted uterus and other deformities, and obstruction of the tubes by a tubo-ovarian abscess or endometriosis. The ovary may not be able to develop an egg because of hypopituitarism or ovarian diseases, such as Stein–Leventhal polycystic ovaries, ovarian cysts, and tumors (especially hormone-secreting tumors of the ovary that prevent the variation in estrogen–progesterone concentration necessary during the cycle that allows maturation of the egg). There may be no ovaries present from birth (Turner syndrome), or there may be acquired ovarian failure (surgical removal or early menopause). Thyroid disorders (hyper- and hypothyroidism) are known to cause infertility. Adrenocortical tumors and hyperplasia may also cause infertility.

● Approach to the Diagnosis

The workup of infertility first involves doing a sperm count on the man. If that is normal and the examination of the woman discloses no gross abnormality, a temperature chart is kept by the patient or the Spinnbarkeit test is used to determine if ovulation occurs. Thyroid function studies and serum/prolactin, FSH, LH, estradiol, and progesterone levels may all be measured if ovulation is proved not to take place. Other tests such as tubal insufflation, hysterosalpingogram, and a trial of clomiphene will be useful in selected cases. Establishing the time of ovulation and ensuring copulation at that time often solve the problem. Cauterizing a chronic cervicitis may lead to fertility. Counseling about emotional problems may be necessary.

● Other Useful Tests

1. Gynecology consult
2. Sonogram (tubo-ovarian abscess)
3. Endometrial biopsy (polyps, neoplasm)
4. Laparoscopy (pelvic tumor, abscess)
5. CT scan of the brain (pituitary tumor)
6. Chromosomal analysis (Turner syndrome, etc.)

Case Presentation #57

A 23-year-old white woman and her husband have been trying to get pregnant for 2 years. Her periods are regular, but she has occasional vaginal discharge. The husband's sperm count is normal.

Question #1. Utilizing anatomy and physiology, what would be your list of possible causes of this woman's problem?

General physical and vaginal examinations are normal except for erythema and induration of the cervix.

Question #2. What is your diagnosis now?

(See Appendix B for the answers.)

INSOMNIA

It is customary to assume that the cause of the disorder is psychogenic and simply to prescribe a sleeping pill to anyone suffering from insomnia, hoping that it will go away by itself. Although this may be true in many cases, the conscientious clinician should rule out organic disease and investigate the hygiene and psyche of the patient before prescribing a medication that may launch a lifelong habit.

Anatomy is the key to a differential of the many organic causes. Visualizing the many organs of the body, one can discover most of the significant causes. Beginning with the **stomach** and the **esophagus**, one should recall indigestion from alcoholic gastritis, overeating, reflux esophagitis, or hiatal hernia. Cirrhosis of the **liver** may cause insomnia because of nocturnal delirium. **Renal** diseases may cause insomnia because of nocturia or because of the toxic effects of uremia. **Heart** diseases, particularly those associated with pulmonary edema or arrhythmias, may awaken the patient with paroxysmal nocturnal dyspnea or palpitations. In particular, aortic regurgitation awakens the patient because of the noise of his or her own heart. **Lung** diseases such as emphysema interfere with breathing, and both the cerebral anoxia and the fear of not being able to breathe cause insomnia. Upper airway obstruction from rhinitis, snoring, and epiglottitis causes insomnia. These conditions are grouped together under obstructive sleep apnea (page 00).

The **thyroid** may be the site of origin of insomnia, particularly in the thyroid storm of Graves disease. Anemia of any kind will cause insomnia if it is severe enough to cause cerebral anoxia. Skeletal deformities such as rheumatoid spondylitis may cause insomnia by forcing the patient to sleep in a chair. In the **nervous system**, the many neurologic disorders that can cause insomnia can be remembered by using **INSOMNIA** as a mnemonic.

I—Intoxication results from CNS stimulants such as amphetamines and caffeine. Although drugs and alcohol initially sedate the drinker, they produce a subsequent period of excitation.

N—Neuropsychiatric disorders include neurosis, manic–depressive psychosis, and schizophrenia. In the elderly, look for restless leg syndrome and periodic limb movement disorders.

S—Syphilis, seizure disorders, and senile dementia are included.

O—Opiate addiction may be responsible for insomnia.

M—Mental retardation and **malformations** such as hydrocephalus may be responsible for insomnia. The hyperactive child syndrome is just one example of a brain-damaged child with potential insomnia. Bedwetting is a cause in children.

N—Neoplasms of the brain may cause insomnia or somnolence. When the tumor leads to increased intracranial pressure, coma may eventually occur.

I—Inflammatory diseases include viral encephalitis, tuberculosis, cryptococcosis, and various parasites.

A—Arteriosclerosis includes diffuse and focal cerebrovascular insufficiency and sleep apnea.

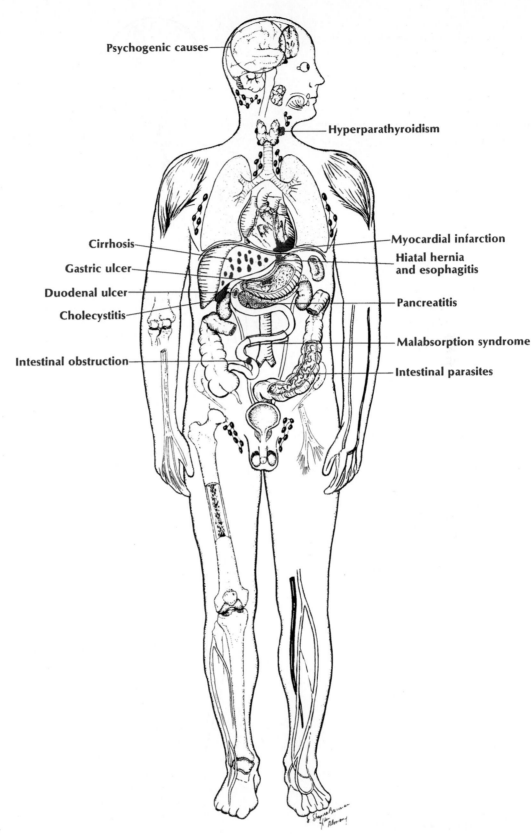

● **FIGURE 3** Indigestion.

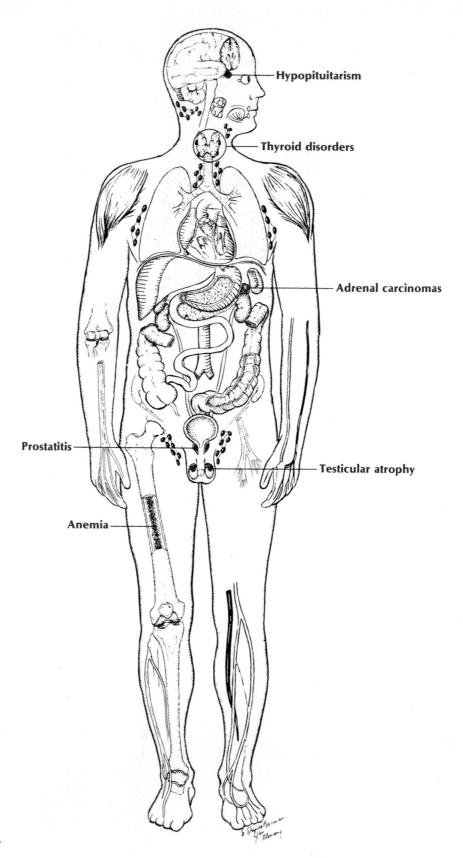

● **FIGURE 4** Infertility.

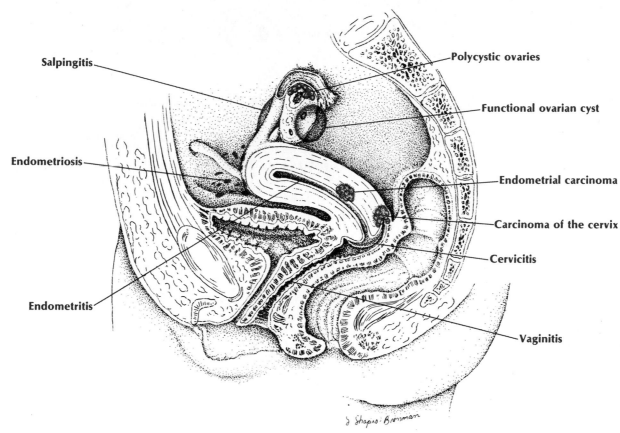

Salpingitis
Endometriosis
Endometritis
Polycystic ovaries
Functional ovarian cyst
Endometrial carcinoma
Carcinoma of the cervix
Cervicitis
Vaginitis

Shapiro-Brennman

● **FIGURE 5** Infertility.

Frequently the insomnia is related to some physiologic or environmental problem. A sagging mattress, a room that is too hot or too cold, an uncomfortable pillow (or too many pillows), and excessive noise or light all are environmental factors that may cause insomnia. Lack of exercise, mental exhaustion, muscular aches and pain from hard work or exercise, hunger, and too much sleep in the afternoon are some of the physiologic conditions that may cause insomnia.

● **Approach to the Diagnosis**

In the approach to the diagnosis, every physician should take the time to talk to the patient about possible reasons for fear or hostility. A nagging wife or mother-in-law, financial worries, a strict boss, or fear of losing a job are just a few examples of problems that can be handled with some sympathetic professional help. Caffeinated beverages including chocolate, coffee, tea, coke, Mountain Dew, etc. need to be eliminated. A good physical and neurologic examination may reveal an organic cause. The laboratory evaluation will be based on suspicion of one or more of the diseases mentioned above and will use the list of tests that follows this discussion. A skull x-ray, electroencephalogram, CT scan, and possibly a spinal tap are indicated if a neurologic disorder is strongly suspected.

● **Other Useful Tests**

1. Complete blood count (anemia)
2. Chemistry panel (chronic liver disease, renal disease)
3. Circulation time (CHF)

4. Arterial blood gases (chronic pulmonary disease)
5. Drug screen (drug abuse)
6. Venereal Disease Research Laboratory (VDRL) test (neurosyphilis)
7. Thyroid profile (hyperthyroidism)
8. MRI of the brain (brain tumor, senile dementia)
9. Polysomnography (e.g., sleep apnea)
10. Psychiatry consult

Case Presentation #58

A 46-year-old black man complained of insomnia, depression, and weight loss. He denies alcohol or drug abuse, although he has taken over-the-counter remedies to help him sleep. He has a history of smoking two packs of cigarettes a day for 20 years.

Question #1. What is your differential diagnosis at this point?

Physical examination reveals an enlarged nodular liver and 2+ pitting edema. On questioning a family member, you find out he has consumed significant amounts of alcohol for many years.

Question #2. What is your diagnosis now?

(See Appendix B for the answers.)

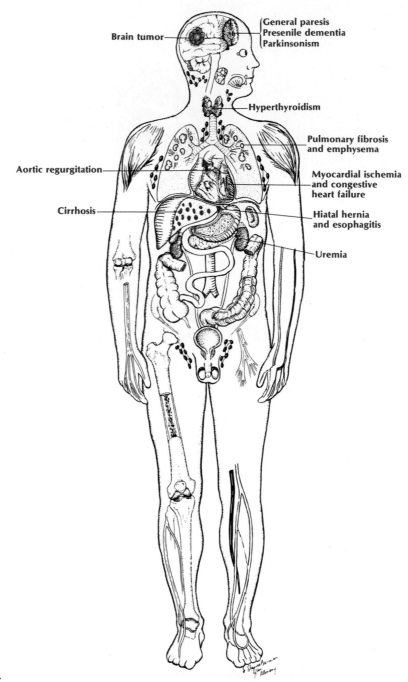

● **FIGURE 6** Insomnia.

INTRACRANIAL BRUIT

Intracranial bruits can be heard best over the orbits or mastoids. A list of possible causes can be developed by using the mnemonic **MINTS**.

M—Malformations should bring to mind arteriovenous malformations of the brain and persistent trigeminal artery.

I—Inflammatory lesions do not customarily cause intracranial bruits.

N—Neoplasm would bring to mind a cerebral angioma.

T—Trauma would suggest a traumatic caroticocavernous fistula.

S—Systemic disease such as anemia, thyrotoxicosis, and Paget disease may cause an intracranial bruit.

Bruit (page 92) may be transmitted to the orbit.

● Approach to the Diagnosis

If a systemic disease has been excluded by routine laboratory studies and a thyroid panel, serious investigation with an MRI or cerebral angiography should be considered. It is wise to consult a neurologist for guidance.

J

JAUNDICE

Jaundice is not to be confused with xanthochromia, in which the skin turns orange from carotene deposits but the sclerae remain normal in appearance. Carotenemia is often seen in hypothyroidism and diabetes mellitus, but jaundice is not usually a complication of these two conditions.

The causes of jaundice can best be established by applying **physiology** (Table 42). Jaundice develops from hyperbilirubinemia and may not be noticed until the bilirubin exceeds 3 or 4 mg/dL. Hyperbilirubinemia is due to an increased production of bilirubin, impaired transport of bilirubin to the liver for excretion, and decreased excretion of bilirubin.

1. Increased production: Bilirubin is produced by the release of hemoglobin from the red cells and its subsequent breakdown. Thus, the hemolytic anemias are the principal causes of this category of jaundice. These include hereditary spherocytosis, Cooley anemia, septicemia, autoimmune hemolytic anemia, and malaria. Neonatal jaundice is usually caused by hemolysis.
2. Impaired transport: Congestive heart failure (CHF) is the principal cause of this form of jaundice, but it must be advanced enough to cause cardiac cirrhosis.
3. Decreased excretion: This group of causes of jaundice is divided into conditions in which the liver is unable to transform unconjugated bilirubin to the conjugated form, such as Gilbert disease, infectious hepatitis, and cirrhosis; conditions in which the liver cannot transfer the conjugated bilirubin into the bile ducts, such as Dubin–Johnson syndrome; and conditions that obstruct the bile ducts, such as common duct stones, cholangitis, chlorpromazine toxicity, and carcinomas of the pancreas and ampulla of Vater. The cause of breast milk jaundice is unknown, but switching to formula usually alleviates the condition.

● Approach to the Diagnosis

The accurate diagnosis of jaundice is established by the association of other symptoms and the performance of liver function and special diagnostic procedures. For example, jaundice with fever, a prodromal phase of anorexia, malaise, and a tender liver suggests hepatitis. Jaundice with itching suggests xanthomatous or primary biliary cirrhosis. Jaundice and anemia suggest hemolytic anemia. Jaundice, back pain, and an abdominal mass suggest a carcinoma of the pancreas.

When liver functions show only an elevated indirect bilirubin level, Gilbert disease or hemolytic anemia is suggested. A normal urine urobilinogen will make Gilbert disease even more likely. Liver function analyses showing only elevated bilirubin and alkaline phosphatase levels suggest bile duct obstruction by a stone or tumor. Liver function results showing an impressive elevation of the bilirubin, serum aspartate aminotransferase, and serum alanine aminotransferase levels suggest hepatitis.

In cases in which obstruction versus parenchymal disease remains a dilemma after routine tests, several newer procedures have been developed that may help avoid an exploratory laparotomy. Endoscopic retrograde cholangiopancreatography (ERCP), cutaneous transhepatic cholangiography, and peritoneoscopy are very useful in these cases. Computed tomography (CT) scans and ultrasonography are also valuable. The old steroid whitewash is still useful. This is done by administering 20 mg of prednisone daily for 5 days and monitoring the bilirubin level. A positive test, indicating parenchymal diseases, is considered a drop of the bilirubin to one half its original value or more. Exploratory laparotomy may be necessary despite an extensive workup.

● Other Useful Tests

1. Complete blood count (CBC) (hemolytic anemia, infection)
2. Chemistry panel (hepatitis, e.g.)
3. Hepatitis panel (viral hepatitis)
4. Febrile agglutinins (*Salmonella*, brucellosis)
5. Monospot test (infectious mononucleosis)
6. Cytomegalic virus antibody titer (cytomegalic inclusion disease)
7. Leptospirosis antibody titer (leptospirosis)
8. Antinuclear antibody (ANA) analysis (lupoid hepatitis)
9. Serum iron and iron-binding capacity (Wilson disease)
10. Serum haptoglobins (hemolytic anemia)
11. Hemoglobin electrophoresis (hemolytic anemia)
12. Sickle cell prep (sickle cell anemia)
13. Blood smear for malarial parasites (malaria)
14. Gallbladder sonogram (cholelithiasis)
15. Peritoneoscopy and biopsy (neoplasm, cirrhosis)
16. Antimitochondrial antibodies (biliary cirrhosis)
17. Gastroenterology consult
18. Magnetic resonance cholangiopancreatography (common duct stone)
19. ERCP (common duct stone)

Case Presentation #59

A 26-year-old intern complained of loss of appetite, fever, and malaise for 1 week prior to admission. On the day of admission, he is noted to have icteric sclera.

Question #1. Utilizing your knowledge of physiology, what is your differential diagnosis?

He denies alcohol or intravenous drug abuse. He has not been exposed to anyone with hepatitis in the past 3 months. However, he did start taking ranitidine hydrochloride for heartburn a few days prior to the onset of symptoms. Physical examination revealed icteric sclera and slightly enlarged tender liver.

Question #2. What is your diagnosis now?

(See Appendix B for the answers.)

JAW PAIN

The key to formulating a list of causes of jaw pain is **anatomy.** Visualizing the area, one notes the skin, arteries, veins, nerves, salivary glands, teeth, bone, and joints. These structures should prompt the recall of the various causes of jaw pain as follows:

1. Skin: Cellulitis, herpes zoster, etc.
2. Arteries: Histamine cephalgia, migraine, etc.
3. Veins: Not usually a cause of jaw pain.
4. Nerves: Trigeminal neuralgia, glossopharyngeal neuralgia.
5. Teeth: Dental caries, alveolar abscess, impacted wisdom teeth, gingivitis, etc.
6. Bone: Osteomyelitis, fracture, bone tumors.
7. Salivary glands: Mumps, calculi, neoplasms.
8. Joints: Temporomandibular joint (TMJ) syndrome, rheumatoid arthritis (RA).

● Approach to the Diagnosis

Obviously, the history and physical examination will help to diagnose many causes of jaw pain. If trigger points can be found, suspect trigeminal neuralgia. A significant swelling would prompt the suspicion of cellulitis, mumps, or an alveolar abscess. Swollen gums should raise the question of gingivitis, periodontitis, or alveolar abscess. Malocclusion would suggest TMJ syndrome.

ACBC, arthritis panel, and x-rays of the teeth, jaw, and TMJ may disclose abnormalities. Referral to a dentist or

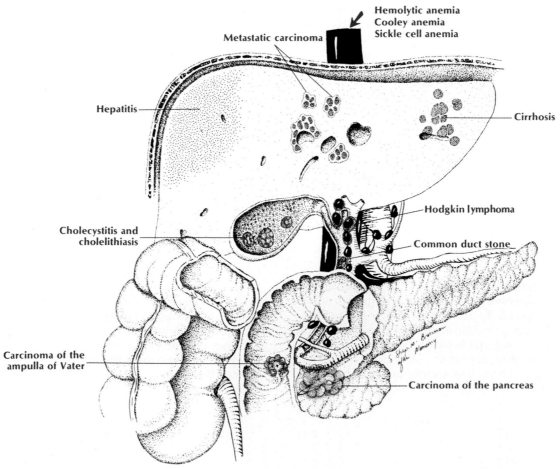

● FIGURE 1 Jaundice.

TABLE 42 Jaundice

	V Vascular	I Inflammatory	N Neoplasm	D Degenerative	I Intoxication	C Congenital	A Allergic and Autoimmune	T Trauma	E Endocrine
Increased Production of Bilirubin	Pulmonary infarction	Septicemia Malaria Oroya fever Mycoplasma infection	Leukemia Myeloid Metaplasia		α-methyldopa, quinine Primaquine Other drugs	Hereditary spherocytosis Cooley anemia	Lupus erythematosus Transfusion reaction	Valve prosthesis Intra-abdominal hemorrhage	
Impaired Transport of Bilirubin	Congestive heart failure								
Decreased Excretion Due to Decreased Conjugation	Budd–Chiari syndrome Pyelophlebitis	Viral hepatitis Leptospirosis Amebic abscess Yellow fever Infectious mononucleosis	Metastatic carcinoma	Idiopathic cirrhosis	Toxic hepatitis Wilson disease Alcoholic cirrhosis	Gilbert disease	Periarteritis nodosa sarcoid		Hyperthyroidism
Decreased Excretion Due to Decreased Transfer of Conjugated Bilirubin		Syphilis	Metastatic carcinoma			Dubin–Johnson syndrome			
Decreased Excretion Due to Obstruction of the Bile Ducts		Cholecystitis and cholangitis Chronic pancreatitis	Carcinoma of pancreas Carcinoma of ampulla or ducts Hodgkin lymphoma	Biliary cirrhosis	Toxic hepatitis Chlorpromazine	Biliary cirrhosis Congenital atresia of bile duct		Surgical ligation	

J

oral surgeon is indicated if the diagnosis is obscure after these studies are done. A magnetic resonance imaging (MRI) of the TMJ may need to be done to exclude the TMJ syndrome. If all tests are negative, a psychiatric consult may be in order.

JAW SWELLING

Applying **anatomy,** one can quickly ascertain that a lump in the jaw may come from the skin and subcutaneous tissues, glands, or bones.

1. Skin and subcutaneous tissue: This will remind one of lipomas, fibromas, and sebaceous cysts, although cellulitis and carbuncles may occur too. Other skin masses are discussed on page 381.
2. Parotid gland: Important lesions here are mumps, Mikulicz syndrome in Hodgkin lymphoma, Behçet disease of uveoparotid fever, and mixed tumors of the salivary gland. A stone in the Stensen duct may cause intermittent swelling of the parotid gland. Parotid gland swelling is also a component of Sjögren syndrome.
3. Jaw bone: These are best divided into etiologic groups using the mnemonic **MINT.**
   M—Malformations include congenital protrusions of the jaw, acquired protrusion from acromegaly, and thickening of the jaw in Paget disease.
   I—Inflammation suggests alveolar abscesses, osteomyelitis, actinomycosis, tuberculosis, or syphilis.
   N—Neoplasms include osteomas, adamantomas, sarcomas, myelomas, metastatic carcinomas, and odontomas.
   T—Trauma obviously can cause severe fracture dislocations, subperiosteal hematomas, and dislocation of the jaw. It is worthwhile to mention that hyperparathyroidism may cause cystic lesions of the jaw (generalized osteitis fibrosa cystica).

● Approach to the Diagnosis

The approach to the diagnosis is to obtain x-rays of the jaw and teeth; ascertain calcium, phosphorus, and alkaline phosphatase levels; and perform biopsy and excision when indicated. Sialography and bone scans may be useful in selected cases. It is wise to consult a dentist at the outset.

JOINT PAIN

Because most joints may be affected by the same etiologic processes, a general discussion of the differential diagnosis of joint pain will be undertaken, followed by a discussion of exceptions that apply to certain joints.

Anatomic and histologic breakdown of the joint is not of much value in the differential diagnosis. It is sufficient to say that extrinsic lesions around the joint, such as cellulitis, bursitis, and tendonitis, must be considered in the differential diagnosis. Nonarticular rheumatism or fibromyositis comes to mind here also. To develop a differential list of intrinsic conditions of the joints, the mnemonic **VINDICATE** is useful.

V—Vascular suggests hemophilia and scurvy as well as aseptic bone necrosis (Osgood–Schlatter disease and so forth).

I—Inflammatory suggests several infectious lesions, but gonorrhea, Lyme disease, *Staphylococcus, Streptococcus* organisms, tuberculosis, and syphilis are most likely. Although uncommon, viral infections such as rubella, herpes simplex, human immunodeficiency virus (HIV), and cytomegalovirus may cause arthritis.

N—Neoplastic disorders to be ruled out are osteogenic sarcoma and giant cell tumors.

D—Degenerative disorders bring to mind degenerative joint disease or osteoarthritis, which is so common that it is often the first condition to be considered in joint pain.

I—Intoxication suggests gout (uric acid) and pseudogout (calcium pyrophosphate). Drugs infrequently initiate joint disease, but the lupus syndrome of hydralazine (Apresoline) and procainamide and the "gout syndrome" of diuretics should be kept in mind.

C—Congenital and acquired malformations bring to mind the joint deformities of tabes dorsalis and syringomyelia and congenital dislocation of the hip. Alkaptonuria is also considered here.

A—Autoimmune indicates another commonly encountered group of diseases. RA is the most prevalent of these, but serum sickness, lupus erythematosus, rheumatic fever, Reiter syndrome, ulcerative colitis, regional ileitis, and psoriatic arthritis must be also considered. Do not forget polymyalgia rheumatica in elderly persons.

T—Trauma suggests numerous disorders. In addition to traumatic synovitis, one must consider tear or rupture of the collateral or cruciate ligaments, subluxation or laceration of the meniscus (semilunar cartilage), dislocation of the joint or patella, a sprain of the joint, and fracture of the bones of the joint.

E—Endocrine disorders that affect the joints include acromegaly, menopause, and diabetes mellitus (pseudogout).

Now it is useful to consider individual joints where special etiologies apply. The **TMJ** is often affected by malocclusion. The **cervical spine** is affected by cervical spondylosis, a condition where hypertrophic lipping of the vertebrae occurs in response to degeneration of the discs. Inflammation of the **sacroiliac joint** occurs most commonly in Marie–Strümpell disease, psoriatic arthritis, Reiter disease, and regional ileitis.

● Approach to the Diagnosis

The approach to the diagnosis of joint pain includes a careful history and examination for other signs such as swelling, redness, and hyperthermia of the joints. Joint pain that is sudden in onset should be considered septic arthritis until proven otherwise. If the joint pain is worse in the morning, consider RA. If multiple joints are involved, look for RA, lupus, and osteoarthritis. Multiple joint involvement with oral and/or genital ulcers suggests Behçet disease. Single joint involvement suggests gonorrhea, septic arthritis, tuberculosis, or gout, among other things. Small joints are

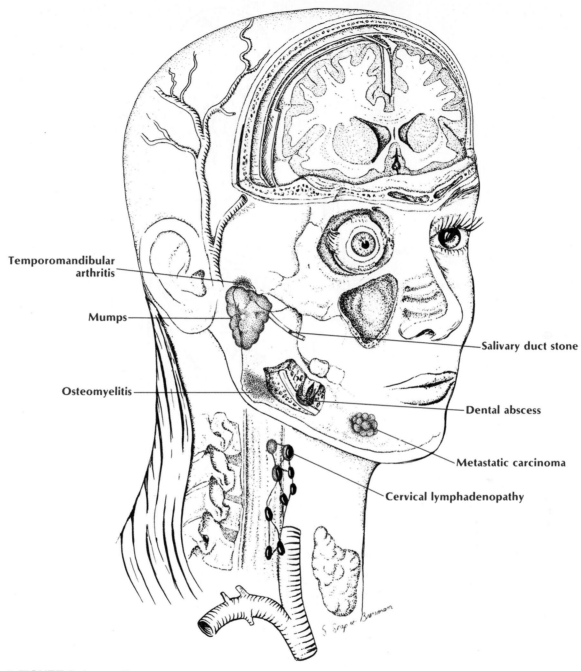

Temporomandibular arthritis

Mumps

Osteomyelitis

Salivary duct stone

Dental abscess

Metastatic carcinoma

Cervical lymphadenopathy

● **FIGURE 2** Jaw swelling.

involved more frequently in RA, Reiter syndrome, and lupus, although the large joints are more frequently involved in osteoarthritis, gonorrhea, tuberculosis, and other infections. Remember, however, that both osteoarthritis and gonorrhea may involve the small joints of the hands and feet. Rheumatic fever presents a migratory arthritis; this is a helpful differential point. When the knee joint is involved, the astute clinician will always examine for a torn or subluxated meniscus and loose cruciate or collateral ligaments. MRI or arthroscopy will pin down this diagnosis. Listed below are the most valuable diagnostic tests. Synovial fluid

analysis for uric acid and calcium pyrophosphate, the character of the mucin clot, a white cell count, and culture can be done in the office and may make the diagnosis almost immediately. This may eliminate the need for hospitalization. CT scans or MRIs may be diagnostic.

A therapeutic trial of aspirin or colchicine is useful in diagnosing rheumatic fever or gout, respectively. If the joint fluid examination is nonspecific and no systemic signs of infection are evident, the injection of steroids into the joint is reasonable while the physician waits for the results of more sophisticated diagnostic tests.

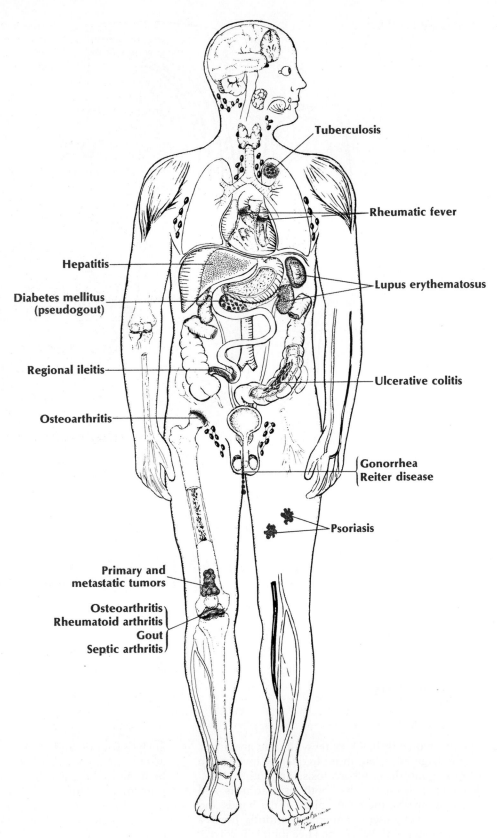

● **FIGURE 3** Joint pain.

● Other Useful Tests

1. CBC (sickle cell anemia, infectious arthritis)
2. Sedimentation rate (inflammatory joint disease)
3. RA test
4. ANA (collagen disease)
5. Chemistry panel (gout, diabetes, e.g.)
6. Coagulation profile (hemophilia)
7. Antistreptolysin O (ASO) titer (rheumatic fever)
8. Brucellin antibody titer (brucellosis)
9. Serologic test for Lyme disease
10. Sickle cell prep
11. X-ray of the joint
12. Bone scan (rheumatoid spondylitis)
13. Urine for homogentisic acid (ochronosis)
14. Rheumatology consult
15. Orthopedic consult
16. Cultures of the joint fluid for atypical mycobacteria of fungi
17. Human leukocyte antigen (HLA)-B27 (rheumatoid spondylitis)
18. Anti–cyclic citrullinated peptide (CCP) antibody titer (RA)
19. 1, 25 hydroxy vitamin D3
20. Serum Parvovirus B19 IgM

Case Presentation #60

A 52-year-old diabetic man presents with acute onset of pain and swelling in the left knee.

Question #1. Utilizing anatomy and histology, what would be the most likely causes of this man's problem?

There is no history of trauma or illicit sexual activity. The patient has not experienced fever or chills or other systemic symptomatology. Synovial fluid analysis is done.

Question #2. What is your differential diagnosis now?

(See Appendix B for the answers.)

JOINT SWELLING

The best approach to analysis of this symptom is **anatomic** and **histologic** (Table 43). However, if one remembers the biochemical causes of joint disease, gout, pseudogout, and ochronosis immediately come to mind.

Let us discuss the conditions to be considered in an anatomic and histologic breakdown of the joint. In the **skin,** an abscess or hematoma is a possibility. Subcutaneous lipoma and pretibial myxedema may involve the joint area as may edema, particularly in phlebitis. Around all joints are **bursae** that can become inflamed and swollen, especially when torn ligaments constantly rub against them.

Next let us consider the **ligaments** of the joint, especially those in the knee. Weak collateral ligaments will lead to recurrent swelling from fluid accumulation in the knee.

Ruptured anterior or posterior cruciate ligaments will also create intermittent pain and swelling. To diagnose this condition, bend the knee and pull the tibia and lower leg forward and backward like opening and closing a drawer. If the meniscus is ruptured, a distinct popping or locking of the joint will occur when the joint is flexed and then extended under pressure, especially with internal or external rotation of the lower leg.

The **synovium** is the site of most pathologic conditions of the knee. Rheumatic fever, RA, lupus erythematosus, and Reiter disease are classic collagen diseases affecting the synovium. The most common infectious diseases are gonorrhea and *Streptococcus* organisms, but tuberculosis and brucellosis should not be forgotten. Trauma to the synovium produces hemarthrosis, but it does not take much to cause hemarthrosis in hemophilia and occasionally in other coagulation disorders.

Moving on to the bone, osteomyelitis and syphilis must be considered: *Staphylococcus* and tuberculosis are common offenders. Aseptic bone necrosis (e.g., Osgood–Schlatter disease of the knee) is another condition of the bone that causes apparent joint swelling.

Idiopathic degeneration of the cartilage is a common cause of joint disease in the form of osteoarthritis. Ochronosis may lead to degeneration, but there is usually calcification of the cartilage on radiographs.

● Approach to the Diagnosis

The clinical picture will often help identify the cause of the joint swelling. If there is fever and migratory arthritis, one suspects rheumatic fever or Lyme disease. Fever with involvement of several joints would suggest RA, lupus erythematosus, or gonorrhea.

Fever and involvement of one joint primarily is found in septic arthritis and tuberculosis but may be found in gonorrhea. No fever and large joint involvement may be found in osteoarthritis, gout, and pseudogout. Osteoarthritis customarily affects the distal phalangeal joints, whereas RA affects the metacarpophalangeal joints. Psoriatic arthritis also affects the distal phalangeal joints primarily. Charcot joints are usually large.

The initial workup of joint swelling includes a CBC, sedimentation rate, urinalysis, chemistry panel, and x-rays of the involved joints. If a large joint is involved, joint fluid can be aspirated and analyzed. A culture should also be done.

If gonococcal arthritis is suspected, urethral or cervical smears and cultures will be helpful, but culture of the fluid on special medium is most important. If gout or pseudogout is suspected, it is important to examine the joint fluid for crystals under polarized light. If RA is suspected, an RA titer will often be positive. Lupus erythematosus can be confirmed by a positive ANA and anti–double-stranded DNA antibodies. Rheumatic fever can be confirmed by a positive ASO titer or streptozyme test. If the synovial fluid has a high white count, hospitalization and initiation of parenteral antibiotics are indicated without delay.

TABLE 43 Joint Swelling

	V Vascular	I Infection	N Neoplasm	D Degenerative	I Intoxication	C Congenital or Collagen	A Allergic Autoimmune	T Trauma	E Endocrine
Skin		Carbuncle						Hematoma	
Subcutaneous Tissue		Cellulitis	Lipoma						
Bursa		Bursitis							
Synovium		Gonococcal arthritis Tuberculous arthritis Streptococcal arthritis	Synovioma			Lupus Rheumatoid arthritis	Reiter disease Serum sickness	Hemarthrosis	
Ligaments of Joint								Ruptured ligament	
Joint Space				"Joint mice"				Hemarthrosis	
Cartilage				Degenerative osteoarthritis	Gout, pseudogout	Rheumatic fever		Torn meniscus	Intermittent hydrarthrosis
Bone	Aseptic bone necrosis	Staphylococcal osteomyelitis Tuberculous osteomyelitis				Ochronosis			
Blood Vessels	Sickle cell anemia	Phlebitis				Hemophilia			

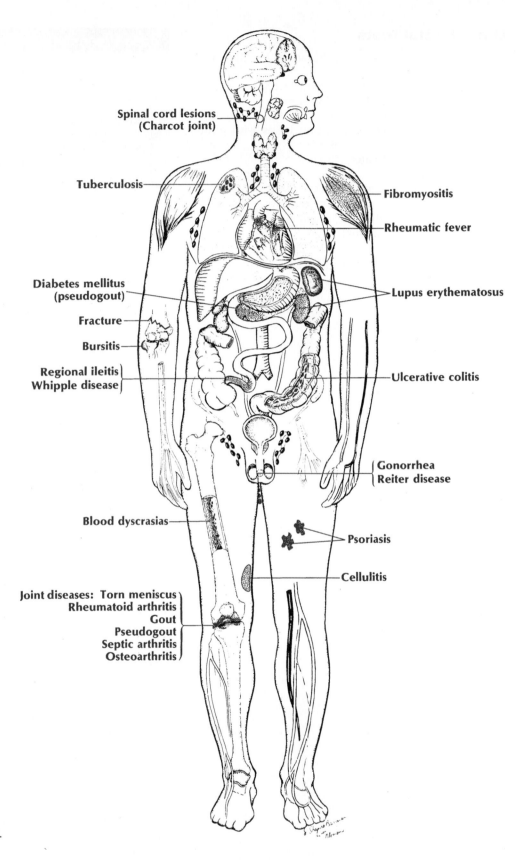

Spinal cord lesions
(Charcot joint)

Tuberculosis

Diabetes mellitus
(pseudogout)

Fracture

Bursitis

Regional ileitis
Whipple disease

Blood dyscrasias

Joint diseases: Torn meniscus
Rheumatoid arthritis
Gout
Pseudogout
Septic arthritis
Osteoarthritis

Fibromyositis

Rheumatic fever

Lupus erythematosus

Ulcerative colitis

Gonorrhea
Reiter disease

Psoriasis

Cellulitis

● FIGURE 4 Joint swelling.

J

● **Other Useful Tests**

1. Venereal Disease Research Laboratory (VDRL) test (Charcot joints)
2. Electrocardiogram (ECG) (rheumatic fever)
3. Tuberculin test (tuberculosis of the joint)
4. Blood cultures (septic arthritis)
5. Monospot test (infectious mononucleosis with joint involvement)
6. Lyme disease antibody titer
7. Sickle cell prep
8. Coagulation profile (hemophilia)
9. Cervical or urethral smears and cultures for gonococci
10. Febrile agglutinins (infectious arthritis)
11. MRI of joint (torn meniscus)
12. Synovial biopsy (RA)
13. Therapeutic trial of colchicine (gout)
14. Bone scan (osteomyelitis)

Case Presentation #61

A 26-year-old black woman presents to your office with fever, chills, and stiffness and pain in the joints of her hands and feet for the last 10 days.

Question #1. Utilizing your knowledge of anatomy and histology, what would be your list of possible causes?

On further questioning, she admits to a vaginal discharge for a couple of months and promiscuous sexual activity. Examination shows a maculopapular rash of the hands and feet.

Question #2. What is your diagnosis?

_____

(See Appendix B for the answers.)

K

KNEE PAIN

The main causes of knee pain can best be recalled by utilizing an etiologic mnemonic such as **VINDICATE**.

V—**Vascular:** This brings to mind aseptic bone necrosis (Osgood–Schlatter disease), thrombophlebitis, hemophilia, scurvy, and sickle cell anemia.

I—**Inflammatory** suggests septic arthritis of gonorrhea, streptococcus, Lyme disease, and rat bite fever, as well as tuberculosis and syphilis. Cellulitis may involve the subcutaneous tissue around the joint.

N—**Neoplasm** raises the possibility of osteogenic sarcoma and giant cell tumors.

D—**Degenerative disorders** prompt the recall of osteoarthritis.

I—**Intoxication** suggests gout, pseudogout, and drugs such as hydralazine that initiate a lupus syndrome and diuretics that induce gout.

C—**Congenital disorders** bring to mind alkaptonuria as a cause of joint pathology.

A—**Autoimmune disorders** include lupus erythematosus, rheumatic fever, rheumatoid arthritis, serum sickness, Reiter syndrome, and the arthritis associated with gastrointestinal disease such as granulomatous colitis.

T—**Trauma** brings to mind sprains, fractures, dislocations, torn collateral or cruciate ligaments, laceration of the meniscus, and hematomas. Iliotibial band syndrome, compartment syndrome, and patellofemoral syndrome are important to consider in athletes, particularly gymnasts and ballet artists.

E—**Endocrine disorders** causing joint pain include diabetes mellitus (pseudogout), hyperparathyroidism, and acromegaly.

● Approach to the Diagnosis

Many causes of joint pain can be isolated by a careful history and physical examination. A history of trauma would suggest a sprain, torn meniscus, or fracture. If there is fever, look for septic arthritis. Bilateral involvement of the knee joint is typical of osteoarthritis or rheumatoid arthritis, whereas unilateral involvement would suggest gout, pseudogout, septic arthritis, and hemophilia. Younger patients are more prone to a traumatic lesion such as sprain or torn meniscus, stress fractures, and Osgood–Schlatter disease. Older patients are more likely to have osteoarthritis or gout.

With the history of trauma, the first thing to do is anterior, posterior, lateral, and oblique x-rays of the joint. Stress fractures won't usually be seen on plain films. A magnetic resonance imaging (MRI) or arthroscopy may be necessary, but consult an orthopedic surgeon first.

Without a history of trauma, add a laboratory workup including complete blood count (CBC), sedimentation rate, antistreptolysin O titer, chemistry panel, arthritis panel, and blood cultures (if there is fever). Synovial fluid analysis and cultures may need to be done if there is sufficient joint fluid. A therapeutic trial of colchicine may be diagnostic of gout.

● Other Useful Tests

1. Antinuclear antibody (lupus erythematosus)
2. Coagulation profile (hemophilia)
3. Serologic test for Lyme disease
4. Bone scan (osteomyelitis)
5. Rheumatology consult
6. Orthopedic consult

KNEE SWELLING

Think of the anatomy of the knee in developing a differential diagnosis. Starting from the surface and penetrating deep in the knee, you have skin, subcutaneous tissue, Bursa, ligaments, synovium, cartilage, and bone. We should not forget the arteries and veins. Let's see what conditions each of these anatomic structures prompts us to recall.

Skin—Carbuncle, hematoma, and angioneurotic edema may cause swelling.

Subcutaneous tissue—Cellulitis, erythema nodosum, and lipoma may cause swelling.

Bursa—Inflammation of numerous bursa about the knee may cause swelling.

Ligaments—Torn or strained collateral ligaments and anterior or posterior cruciate ligaments may lead to instability of the joint and associated swelling.

Synovium—This is the site of infections such as streptococcus, gonorrhea, tuberculosis, and brucellosis. It is also the site of autoimmune disorders such as rheumatoid arthritis, lupus erythematosus, and rheumatic fever. Gout and pseudogout affect the synovium of the knee. Hemorrhage into the synovium is common in hemophilia and other coagulation disorders.

Cartilage—Trauma to the meniscus causes rupture and swelling. Degeneration of the cartilage in osteoarthritis produces significant swelling. Repeated trauma to the cartilage occurs in Charcot joints.

Bone—Osteomyelitis, bone tumors, aseptic bone necrosis (Osgood–Schlatter disease), and ochronosis are considered here.

Arteries—A popliteal aneurysm is brought to mind by remembering this structure.

Veins—Varices and thrombophlebitis may produce swelling around the knee.

● Approach to the Diagnosis

The history and physical are very important in ruling out some of the various possibilities. If the swelling is painless, Charcot joints should be considered. A history of fever suggests septic arthritis but is also common in rheumatic fever and rheumatoid arthritis. Unilateral swelling is most likely the result of trauma, gout, pseudogout, torn meniscus, or septic arthritis, whereas bilateral swelling is seen more commonly in rheumatoid arthritis, osteoarthritis, lupus erythematosus, and Reiter disease. The age of the patient will suggest the most likely possibilities. Knee swelling in a young individual would most likely be due to rheumatoid arthritis, rheumatic fever, gonorrhea, or lupus erythematosus, whereas knee swelling in elderly persons is more likely to be due to osteoarthritis, gout, or pseudogout.

The workup should begin with a CBC, urinalysis, sedimentation rate, arthritis panel, chemistry panel, and x-ray of the knees. If it can be determined that the swelling is due to synovial fluid, arthrocentesis should be done and the fluid analyzed for crystals, mucin clot, leukocyte count, and microorganism by smear and culture. An MRI or arthroscopy may be necessary, but an orthopedic surgeon or rheumatologist should be consulted before ordering these expensive tests.

● Other Useful Tests

1. Venereal disease research laboratory test (Charcot joints)
2. Blood cultures (septic arthritis)
3. Tuberculin test (tuberculosis)
4. Electrocardiogram (rheumatic fever)
5. Monospot test (infectious mononucleosis)
6. Coagulation profile (hemophilia)
7. Cervical or urethral smears and cultures (gonorrhea)
8. Lyme disease antibody titer
9. Synovial biopsy
10. Therapeutic trial (gout)
11. Bone scan (osteomyelitis, neoplasm)
12. Febrile agglutinins (brucellosis)

KYPHOSIS

The mnemonic **MINT** lends itself well to producing a list of possible causes of kyphosis.

M—**Malformation** includes mucopolysaccharidosis and Scheuermann disease. M also brings to mind **menopausal** osteoporosis.
I—**Inflammation** brings to mind tuberculosis and ankylosing spondylitis, and **idiopathic** prompts the recall of Paget disease (osteitis deformans) and osteoarthritis.
N—**Neoplasm** suggests metastatic neoplasm of the spine, which can cause kyphosis.
T—**Trauma** allows the recall of crush fractures of the vertebral bodies, especially in osteoporosis and osteomalacia.

This mnemonic fails to facilitate the recall of emphysema, which produces kyphosis also.

● Approach to the Diagnosis

The clinical picture will help establish the diagnosis in many cases. The large skull and bowing of the legs in Paget disease, the generalized abnormalities of the skeleton in mucopolysaccharidosis, and the barrel chest and shortness of breath seen in emphysema assure the identification of the cause. x-Ray of the thoracolumbar spine will be diagnostic in Paget disease, menopausal osteoporosis, ricket fractures, and Scheuermann disease.

If menopause is suspected, a serum follicle-stimulating hormone, luteinizing hormone, and estradiol will confirm the diagnosis. A human leukocyte antigen B27 antigen test should be ordered if ankylosing spondylitis is suspected. A bone scan will be useful in diagnosing ankylosing spondylitis, osteomyelitis, and metastatic carcinoma. A bone biopsy may be necessary when the diagnosis is in doubt.

LEG PAIN

Anatomic breakdown of the leg into its various anatomic components is the basis of a sound differential diagnosis (Table 44). Before that, however, one should determine if the pain is actually originating from the hip or if it is the result of knee joint disease. Diagnosis of these must be considered (see pages 226 and 274).

Beginning with the **skin**, consider herpes zoster and various dermatologic conditions. In the **subcutaneous tissue**, one encounters cellulitis and occasionally filariasis, which may produce a similar picture. Beneath this layer, the **muscle** and **fascia** suggest numerous causes of leg pain. There may be hematomas of the muscle, trichinosis or cysticercosis, nonarticular rheumatism, or fibromyositis. Muscle cramping from low sodium or other electrolyte disturbances must be considered.

The superficial and deep **veins** are the site of thrombophlebitis, a prominent cause of leg pain. The **arteries** may be involved by emboli (from auricular fibrillation, acute myocardial infarction, and subacute bacterial endocarditis), thrombosis (especially in Buerger disease and blood dyscrasias), and vasculitis (from arteriosclerosis and collagen diseases). Acute trauma to the artery or veins may cause pain. As usual, when one moves centrally along the arterial pathways additional causes of pain come to mind. Leriche syndrome and dissecting aneurysm must be considered. When superficial or deep infections of the leg spread to the lymphatics, lymphangitis is important in the differential.

The **nerves** may be involved locally, centrally, or systemically. Buerger disease, cellulitis, and osteomyelitis may involve the nerve locally. Neuromas may occasionally cause focal pain in the distribution of the nerve involved. More important are the central causes of nerve pain in the limbs. Probably herniated discs of the lumbar spine account for most of these cases, but Pott disease, lumbar spondylosis (osteoarthritis?), metastatic and primary tumors, multiple myeloma, fractures, spondylolisthesis, and osteomyelitis of the spine all may compress the cauda equina and cause pain in the lower limbs.

Pelvic tumors, endometriosis, and sciatic neuritis are, in a sense, "central" causes of leg pain, and all patients deserve a rectal and pelvic examination when the diagnosis is obscure. Pelvic inflammatory disease and obturator hernias may rarely involve the obturator nerve. Meralgia paresthetica from diabetes mellitus and other causes must be considered in thigh pain and in causalgia. Finally, the thalamic syndrome and diseases of the cervical spine must be considered. Dissecting the limb layer by layer, we finally reach the **bone**, which suggests osteomyelitis, bone tumors, Osgood–Schlatter disease, tuberculous osteomyelitis, and Paget disease. Joggers may experience shin splints, stress fractures, or compartment syndrome. Gymnasts, ballet dancers, and skiers experience patella–femoral problems. For leg pain originating in the joints, see page 274.

Systemic diseases that may involve the nerves causing pain in the legs include tabes dorsalis, periarteritis nodosa, diabetes mellitus, metabolic and nutritional neuropathies, and blood dyscrasias.

● Approach to the Diagnosis

The approach to the diagnosis of leg pain involves numerous ancillary examinations that one may not routinely do. Leg pain that is sudden in onset should be considered osteomyelitis until proven otherwise. Thus, arterial pulses must be checked all the way up. One should look for a positive Moses or Homans sign. Straight leg raising (SLR) and meticulous mapping of sensory changes are valuable. The SLR sign may be negative and the patient could still have a herniated disc higher up. Thus, a femoral stretch test is done[11] and when positive suggests a herniated disk at L2–3 or L3–4. Patients with pain in the hip should always be examined for greater trochanter bursitis, a common condition (page 274). Edema associated with phlebitis or atrophy associated with a herniated disc can be detected only with careful measurement of the calf and thigh. Deep vein thrombophlebitis can be diagnosed by ultrasonography or impedance plethysmography. Arterial circulation is best evaluated with an ultrasound flow study. Venography and arteriography may be necessary if plain x-ray films are unremarkable. One should almost always x-ray the spine, hips, knee joints, and, in difficult cases, the entire legs. Pain that is precipitated by walking suggests peripheral arteriosclerosis, but spinal stenosis is also possible.

● Other Useful Tests

1. Complete blood count (CBC) (infection)
2. Sedimentation rate (infection, arthritis)
3. Chemistry panel (gout, diabetes, etc.)
4. Arthritis panel
5. Serum protein electrophoresis (multiple myeloma)
6. Electromyogram (EMG) and nerve conduction velocity (NCV) (radiculopathy, neuropathy)
7. Computed tomography (CT) scan or magnetic resonance imaging (MRI) of the lumbar spine (herniated disc, etc.)
8. Orthopedic consult
9. Exploratory surgery
10. Lyme titer (Lyme disease)
11. Bone scan (osteomyelitis)
12. Ankle–brachial index (Leriche syndrome, arteriosclerosis)
13. Iodine 125-radioactive-labeled fibrinogen leg scanning (thrombophlebitis)
14. Arthrocentesis (gout, pseudogout, etc.)
15. MRI (stress fractures)

---

[1] Wiles P, Sweetnam R. *Essentials of orthopedics*. Boston: Little, Brown, 1965.

TABLE 44 Leg Pain

	V Vascular	I Inflammatory	N Neoplasm	D Degenerative	I Intoxication	C Congenital	A Autoimmune Allergic	T Trauma	E Endocrine
Skin	Embolism	Herpes zoster Carbuncle	Kaposi sarcoma				Pyoderma gangrenosum Periarteritis nodosa	Contusion Laceration	
Subcutaneous Tissue		Cellulitis Filariasis					Weber–Christian disease	Hematoma	
Muscle, Fascia, and Bursa		Tetanus Trichinosis Cysticercosis Epidemic myalgia			Low sodium from diuretic Black widow spider bite	McArdle syndrome Myositis ossificans	Dermatomyositis Fibrositis	Hematoma Laceration Rupture	Tetany
Veins and Capillaries	Thrombophlebitis Subacute bacterial endocarditis		Hemangioma	Scurvy		Varicose vein Buerger disease		Hemorrhage	
Arteries	Leriche syndrome Dissecting aneurysm Embolism	Subacute bacterial endocarditis		Arteriosclerosis			Periarteritis nodosa	Hemorrhage	
Lymphatics		Lymphangitis Filariasis	Hodgkin lymphoma Lymphangioma			Milroy disease			
Nerves	Ischemic neuropathy Buerger disease	Viral neuritis Tabes dorsalis	Pelvic tumor Neuroma Cord tumor Metastatic tumor			Obturator hernia Porphyria Blood dyscrasia		Fracture Hematoma Ruptured disc	Diabetic neuropathy
Bone	Aseptic necrosis	Osteomyelitis Relapsing polychondritis	Osteogenic sarcoma Metastatic carcinoma Multiple myeloma	Scurvy Paget disease	Radiation osteitis	Sickle cell anemia Osteogenesis imperfecta		Fracture Hematoma	Osteomalacia Polyosteotic fibrosa cystica Osteoporosis

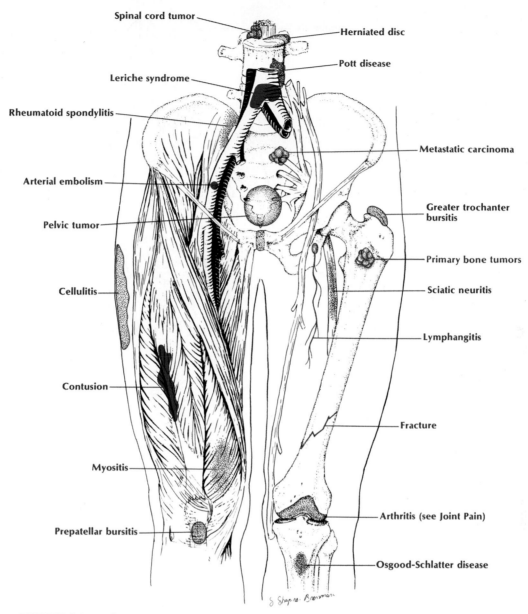

Spinal cord tumor
Herniated disc
Pott disease
Leriche syndrome
Metastatic carcinoma
Rheumatoid spondylitis
Greater trochanter bursitis
Arterial embolism
Pelvic tumor
Primary bone tumors
Cellulitis
Sciatic neuritis
Lymphangitis
Contusion
Fracture
Myositis
Arthritis (see Joint Pain)
Prepatellar bursitis
Osgood-Schlatter disease

● **FIGURE 1** Leg pain.

Case Presentation #62

A 36-year-old white female cashier developed acute pain in her right calf 2 hours before admission. She gives a history of taking birth control pills for several years.

Question #1. Considering the anatomy of the area, what would be your differential diagnosis?

Examination revealed that she had excellent peripheral pulses, but there was 2+ pitting edema of the right leg and a positive Homans sign.

Question #2. What is your diagnosis now?

(See Appendix B for the answers.)

LEUKOCYTOSIS

Numerous disorders cause leukocytosis. How can we recall all possibilities in the differential? The mnemonic **VINDICATE** would seem to be the answer.

V—Vascular would call to mind myocardial infarction, pulmonary infarction, cerebral vascular accident, and thrombophlebitis.

I—Inflammation should bring to mind bacterial infections anywhere in the body, but especially septicemia. Parasitic infections would cause an eosinophilia. Severe systemic fungal infections would also cause leukocytosis. Viral infections are not usually associated with leukocytosis but there are notable exceptions, such as infectious mononucleosis.

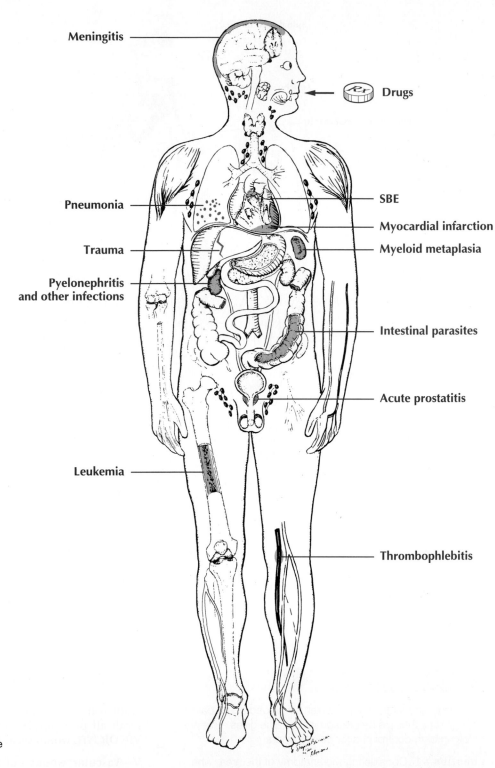

● **FIGURE 2** Leukocytosis (obscure causes).

N—Neoplasm would of course prompt the recall of acute and chronic leukemias and agnogenic myeloid metaplasia.

D—Degenerative disorders do not prompt the recall of any important disorder.

I—Intoxication would bring to mind various drugs that are associated with a leukocytosis, such as lithium, corticosteroids, and lead.

C—Congenital would bring to mind Down syndrome.

A—Allergic and **Autoimmune** would prompt the recall of anaphylactic shock, asthma, and other diffuse hypersensitivity reactions as well as polyarteritis nodosa and dermatomyositis.

T—Trauma reminds us that burns, fractures, massive hemorrhage, or contusions of various parts of the body cause a leukocytosis.

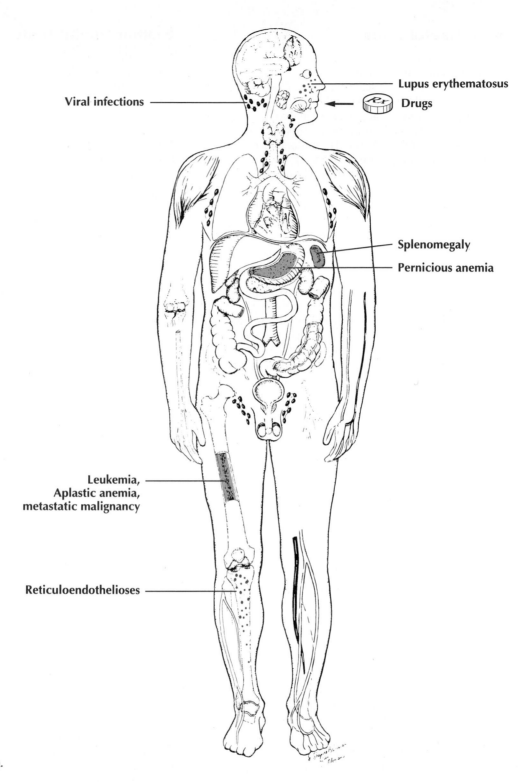

Viral infections

Lupus erythematosus

Drugs

Splenomegaly

Pernicious anemia

Leukemia,
Aplastic anemia,
metastatic malignancy

Reticuloendothelioses

● **FIGURE 3** Leukopenia.

E—Endocrine causes Cushing syndrome, and exogenous corticosteroids cause leukocytosis. Pregnancy thyroid storm and diabetic ketoacidosis are also associated with leukocytosis.

● Approach to the Diagnosis

Because infection is the most common and often the most life-threatening cause, the history and physical are of most importance in locating a source. All suspicious body fluids should be analyzed and cultured. Urinalysis, urine culture, blood cultures, and spinal fluid cultures are just a few. It is important to look at the blood smear and differential count. If the count is very high, a pathologist or hematologist should be called in without delay. An infectious disease specialist may be necessary.

● Other Useful Tests

1. CBC (leukemia)
2. Sedimentation rate (infection)
3. Chemistry panel (liver disease, kidney disease, infarction)
4. Antinuclear antibody (ANA) analysis (collagen disease)
5. Blood smear for malarial parasites (malaria)
6. Monospot test (infectious mononucleosis)
7. Antistreptolysin O (ASO) titer (rheumatic fever)
8. Bone marrow examination (leukemia)
9. Liver–spleen scan (neoplasm, myeloid metaplasia)
10. Bone scan (metastasis)

LEUKOPENIA

The mnemonic **VINDICATE** is most useful in developing a list of possible causes of leukopenia.

V—**Vascular** disorders are not usually associated with leukopenia.
I—**Inflammation** will help recall viral infections, typhoid fever, tularemia, brucellosis, and miliary tuberculosis, which are associated with leukopenia. Malaria and various rickettsial infections are also associated with leukopenia.
N—**Neoplasms and nutritional:** Neoplasms that invade the bone marrow may cause leukopenia. Aleukemic leukemia is also a cause of leukopenia. Nutritional disorders under this category include B_{12} and folate deficiencies.
D—**Degenerative** disorders are not usually associated with leukopenia.
I—**Intoxication and idiopathic** disorders will call to mind the leukopenia (agranulocytosis) of benzene, chemotherapy, sulfonamides, anticonvulsants, antibiotics, and many other drugs. It should also prompt the recall of aplastic anemia, myelofibrosis, and benign familial neutropenia.
C—**Congenital** should bring to mind the reticuloendothelioses such as Gaucher disease.
A—**Autoimmune** collagen vascular disorders such as lupus erythematosus and autoimmune neutropenia should be remembered by this classification.
T—**Trauma** mechanism is not usually a cause of leukopenia (with the exception of radiation).
E—**Endocrine** disorders are not usually associated with a leukopenia. Addison disease is a notable exception. Unfortunately, this method of recalling the possibilities would leave out the leukopenia that occurs with splenomegaly of many causes.

● Approach to the Diagnosis

The history may disclose the use of various drugs and exposure to radiation and other toxins. If there are associated anemia and thrombocytopenia, the possibility of aplastic anemia should be considered. An enlarged spleen suggests that hypersplenism is the cause. The initial laboratory workup includes a CBC, urinalysis, sedimentation rate, differential count, chemistry panel, febrile agglutinins, ANA, platelet count, serum B_{12} and folic acid levels, and serum protein electrophoresis. A bone marrow examination and hematology consult is next in line.

● Other Useful Tests

1. Donath–Landsteiner test (paroxysmal cold hemoglobinuria)
2. Liver–spleen scan (splenomegaly)
3. CT scan of the abdomen (splenomegaly, liver disease, neoplasm)
4. Bone scan (metastatic neoplasm)
5. Skeletal survey (metastatic neoplasm)
6. Lymph node biopsy (Hodgkin lymphoma, metastasis)

LIP SWELLING

The mnemonic **MAINTAIN** will help recall the principle causes of lip swelling.

M—This letter will help to recall the diffuse swelling of the lips in myxedema and cretinism.
A—**Allergy** should bring to mind angioneurotic edema, urticaria, and contact dermatitis.
I—**Inflammation** facilitates the recall of herpes simplex, syphilis, alveolar abscess, and cellulitis.
N—**Neoplasm** prompts the recall of carcinoma.
T—**Trauma** would suggest the swelling and contusions caused by trauma, especially in victims of abuse.
A—The second letter **A** stands for autoimmune disorders such as Crohn disease, which may cause granulomatous cheilitis.
I—The second letter **I** signifies insect bites or stings.
N—The second letter **N** should help to recall the deformity of the lips in facial nerve palsies.

● Approach to the Diagnosis

In many cases the cause will be obvious from the clinical picture. Obscure cases require x-rays of the teeth and jaw to exclude alveolar abscess, a venereal disease research laboratory test to exclude syphilis, and cultures to exclude abscess. A thyroid panel may be necessary to exclude myxedema. A therapeutic trial of antibiotics or antiviral therapy may be indicated. A referral to an oral surgeon or dermatologist will often help resolve the diagnostic dilemma.

LORDOSIS

This condition is often congenital and idiopathic, but it is seen in untreated bilateral congenital dislocation of the hips and muscular dystrophy. It is also seen due to the forward slipping of the fifth lumbar vertebra in spondylolisthesis.

An x-ray of the lumbar spine and hips will diagnose the cause in most cases. A muscle biopsy may be needed to diagnose muscular dystrophy.

LOW BACK PAIN

Nothing is more challenging to diagnose than a case of low back pain. That is why it is so important to have an extensive list of causes in mind before approaching the patient. **Anatomy** forms the basis for developing such a list (Table 45).

TABLE 45 Low Back Pain

	V Vascular	I Inflammatory	N Neoplasm	D Degenerative and Deficiency	I Intoxication Idiopathic	C Congenital and Acquired Anomaly	A Autoimmune Allergic	T Trauma	E Endocrine
Skin		Herpes zoster				Pilonidal cyst		Contusion Laceration	
Muscle, Fascia, and Ligaments		Fibromyositis Trichinosis				Herniation of subfascial fat Faulty posture		Contusion Tear Lumbosacral sprain	
Lumbosacral Spine		Tuberculosis Osteomyelitis	Hodgkin lymphoma Metastatic carcinoma Multiple myeloma	Osteomalacia Osteoporosis Osteoarthritis Lumbar spondylosis Spinal stenosis	Paget disease Alkaptonuria Gout	Herniated disc Spina bifida Spondylolisthesis Coccydynia Scoliosis, idiopathic Scoliosis from a short leg syndrome	Rheumatoid spondyitis	Herniated disc Fracture Sprung back Coccydynia	Osteitis fibrosa cystica
Spinal Cord and Cauda Equina	Atrioventricular anomaly	Epidural abscess Myelitis	Primary and metastatic tumors			Atrioventricular anomaly			
Aorta	Aortic aneurysm			Dissecting aneurysm					
Rectum	Hemorrhoid	Anal fissure Perirectal abscess	Carcinoma			Fistula			
Uterus, Tubes, and Ovaries		Endometritis Tubo-ovarian abscess	Fibroid Carcinoma Endometriosis Ovarian cyst			Retroversion or retroflexion			Dysmenorrhea
Bladder and Prostate		Cystitis Urethritis Prostatitis	Prostatic carcinoma					Ruptured urethra or bladder	

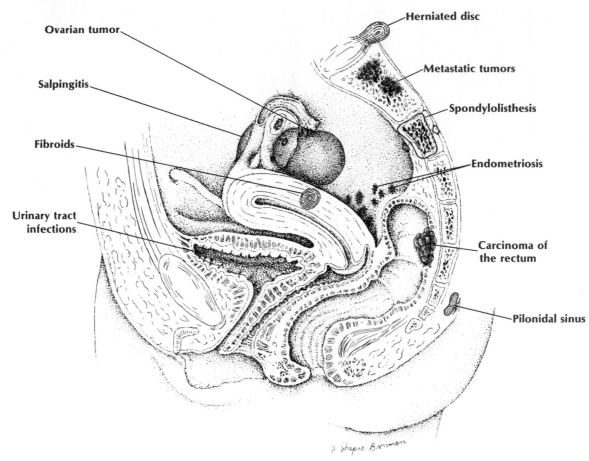

Ovarian tumor

Salpingitis

Fibroids

Urinary tract
infections

Herniated disc

Metastatic tumors

Spondylolisthesis

Endometriosis

Carcinoma of
the rectum

Pilonidal sinus

● **FIGURE 4** Low back pain.

Moving posteriorly from the skin inward, one encounters the muscle and fascial planes, the lumbosacral spine and its ligaments, the spinal cord and cauda equina, the abdominal aorta and its branches, the rectum, the prostate in the male, the uterus and pelvic organs in the female, and finally the bladder.

The **skin** may be involved by a pilonidal cyst, contusions and lacerations, or herpes zoster. The **muscle** and **fascia** are involved by fibromyositis, trichinosis, contusions, lacerations, strains, sprains, and herniation of fat through the subfascial plain. (The latter has been espoused as a common cause of lumbago.) A more important cause of muscle spasms and irritation is faulty posture. Slumping over a typewriter or computer, wearing the wrong shoes (e.g., very high heels), or having one leg shorter than the other may cause this.

The next layer is the **lumbosacral spine**. Vascular lesions are infrequent here, but inflammation caused by osteomyelitis and tuberculosis (Pott disease) is still seen in some countries. More common lesions of the spine inducing low back pain are metastatic carcinoma, herniated discs, rheumatoid spondylitis, or lumbar spondylosis (often erroneously labeled osteoarthritis). Osteoarthritis and other arthridites may involve the facets of the zygapophyseal joints, and produce back pain ("facet syndrome"). Advanced osteoarthritis leads to spinal stenosis,

especially in elderly persons. Multiple myeloma is not an uncommon cause and should be looked for in each case. Fractures are particularly frequent in association with this disease. Fractures are also seen with osteoporosis, osteitis fibrosa cystica, and osteomalacia. Paget disease, gout, and sprung back (in which the interspinous ligament is torn) are less common causes of low back pain originating in the spine. Congenital anomalies such as spondylolisthesis and scoliosis are important causes. In the **spinal cord** arteriovenous anomalies, myelitis, epidural abscesses, and primary tumors are important causes.

Moving deeper one encounters the aorta, and arteriosclerotic and dissecting aneurysms come to mind. Disease of the **rectum** may refer pain to the low back, particularly hemorrhoids, fissures, perirectal abscesses, and carcinomas. In the **prostate**, prostatitis and prostate carcinoma are frequent causes. Prostate carcinoma, however, produces low back pain most frequently by metastasis. The **bladder** and **urethra** are infrequent causes of low back pain, but a urinalysis and culture may be necessary to rule out infections.

To diagnose low back pain in women, the **uterus** and other **pelvic organs** must be examined. Dysmenorrhea (functional) is often the cause, but tubo-ovarian abscess, ovarian cysts, endometriosis, fibroids, retroversion or flexion of the uterus, and uterine carcinomas must be looked for.

● Approach to the Diagnosis

First, you must rule out malingering (page 274). Our next priority in a patient who presents with low back pain is to rule out anything serious such as a herniated disc or cauda equina tumor. A pelvic and rectal examination must be performed to exclude a pelvic tumor or prostate carcinoma. A careful neurologic examination must be done. If one is too busy to do that, referral to an orthopedic surgeon or neurologist is indicated. The neurologic examination should include an SLR test, femoral stretch test, careful sensory examination, and an assessment for asymmetric reflexes. It is wise to carefully measure the thighs and calves to reveal muscular atrophy. Also measure the leg length from the superior iliac spine to the medial malleolus. The

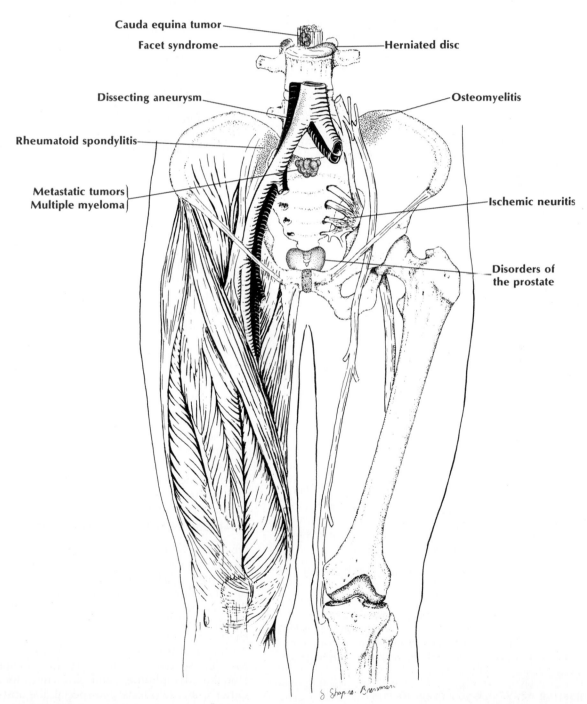

● **FIGURE 5** Low back pain.

L

author has found many cases of back pain are due to a short leg syndrome. Any findings to support a diagnosis of radiculopathy are a reasonable indication for a CT scan or MRI of the lumbar spine. However, it may be wise to have a neurologist or neurosurgeon examine the patient first because these tests are expensive.

If the patient has normal neurologic, pelvic, and rectal examinations, it is perfectly legitimate to manage the patient conservatively for a while without any testing other than clinical. Close follow-up is important in these cases, however. Should the pain persist despite rest and conservative treatment, a more thorough diagnostic workup is indicated regardless of the lack of objective findings. This will include plain films, MRI or CT scans, and an arthritis panel.

● Other Useful Tests

1. CBC
2. Urinalysis (pyelonephritis)
3. Urine for Bence–Jones protein (multiple myeloma)
4. Protein electrophoresis (multiple myeloma)
5. Chemistry panel (metastatic carcinoma)
6. Prostate-specific antigen (prostatic carcinoma)
7. Urine culture and colony count (pyelonephritis)
8. Intravenous pyelogram (renal calculus, carcinoma)
9. Aortogram (abdominal aneurysm)
10. Nerve blocks (radiculopathy)
11. Lidocaine infiltration of trigger points
12. Bone scan (rheumatoid spondylitis)
13. Human leukocyte antigen-B27 antigen (rheumatoid spondylitis)
14. EMG and NCV (radiculopathy)
15. Myelogram (herniated disc, neoplasm)
16. Plain films of the lumbar spine
17. Sedimentation rate (polymyalgia rheumatica)
18. Bone densitometry (osteoporosis)
19. Plain films to measure leg length (short leg syndrome)

Case Presentation #63

A 34-year-old oil refinery worker complained of increasing low back pain radiating into both lower extremities. He denies paresthesias or increase of the pain on coughing or sneezing, but the pain is relieved by lying down. The pain is aggravated by lifting, bending, and stooping. His grandfather had similar back pain beginning in his 30s.

Question #1. Utilizing anatomy, what is your differential diagnosis at this point?

Neurologic examination revealed good sensation, power, and symmetrical reflexes in the lower extremities. The SLR and femoral stretch tests were negative bilaterally. Rectal examination was normal. X-rays of the lumbar spine revealed calcification of the intervertebral discs and degenerative changes.

Question #2. What is your diagnosis now?

LYMPHADENOPATHY, GENERALIZED

Many of the conditions that cause splenomegaly also cause generalized lymphadenopathy. They are best recalled with the use of the mnemonic **MINT**.

M—Malformations include sickle cell anemia and other congenital hemolytic anemias, the reticuloendothelioses (Niemann–Pick disease, Hand–Schüller–Christian disease, and Gaucher disease), and lymphangiomas.

I—Inflammatory disorders constitute the largest group of lymphadenopathies. Breaking them down into subgroups according to the size of the organism further assists the recall.

1. **Viral illnesses** include infectious mononucleosis, acquired immunodeficiency syndrome (AIDS), lymphogranuloma venereum, German measles, chickenpox, and viral upper respiratory illnesses. There are many other conditions in this category.
2. **Rickettsial diseases** include typhus and Rocky Mountain spotted fever.
3. **Bacterial diseases** include typhoid, plague, tuberculosis, skin infections, tularemia, meningococcemia, and brucellosis.
4. **Spirochetes** include syphilis and *Borrelia vincentii*.
5. **Parasites** include malaria, filariasis, and trypanosomiasis.
6. **Fungi** include histoplasmosis, disseminated coccidioidomycosis, and blastomycosis.

N—Neoplasms: Dissemination of almost every malignancy may cause generalized lymphadenopathy. The most likely ones to present with generalized lymphadenopathy, however, are lymphatic leukemia, monocytic leukemia, Hodgkin lymphoma, and lymphosarcoma. Myelophthisic anemia must be considered too.

T—Toxic disorders that cause generalized lymphadenopathy are numerous. Dilantin toxicity may mimic Hodgkin lymphoma. Drug allergies from sulfonamides, hydralazine, and iodides are just a few of the others.

In addition to the conditions listed above, **systemic diseases** that may cause lymphadenopathy include the autoimmune disorders such as lupus erythematosus (50% of the cases with lupus erythematosus are associated with lymphadenopathy), dermatomyositis, sarcoidosis, and Still disease.

● Approach to the Diagnosis

Obviously, it is tempting simply to do a lymph node biopsy, but certain other procedures should be done first. If the patient is febrile, febrile agglutinins, monospot test, blood cultures, and cultures of any other suspicious body fluid should be made. A fluorescent treponemal antibody absorption (FTA-ABS) test should be done as well as a chest x-ray and tuberculin test to rule out tuberculosis. A blood count usually shows leukemia, but a bone marrow biopsy may be necessary to diagnose leukemia, Hodgkin lymphoma, and the reticuloendothelioses. Other x-rays, skin tests, and special diagnostic procedures may be necessary.

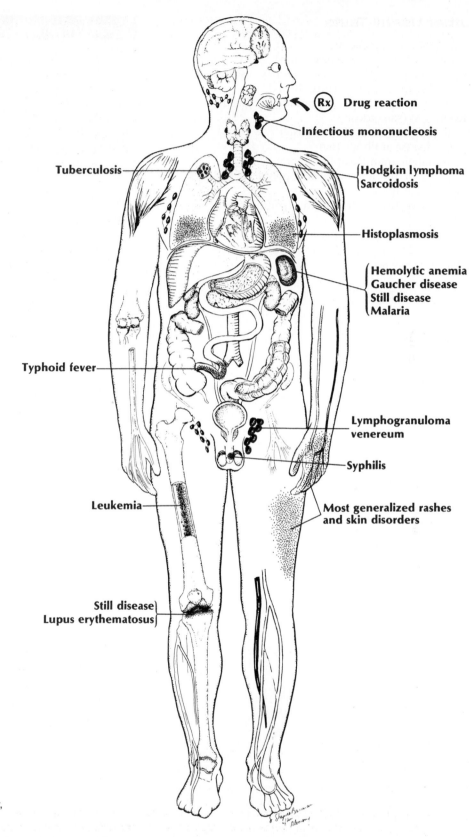

Rx Drug reaction

Infectious mononucleosis

Tuberculosis

Hodgkin lymphoma
Sarcoidosis

Histoplasmosis

Hemolytic anemia
Gaucher disease
Still disease
Malaria

Typhoid fever

Lymphogranuloma
venereum

Syphilis

Most generalized rashes
and skin disorders

Leukemia

Still disease
Lupus erythematosus

● **FIGURE 6** Lymphadenopathy,
generalized.

● Other Useful Tests

1. CBC (infection, leukemia)
2. Sedimentation rate (inflammation)
3. Chemistry panel (liver disease, kidney disease)
4. Brucellin antibody titer (brucellosis)
5. X-ray of the long bones (metastatic neoplasm)
6. Kveim test (sarcoidosis)
7. Brucellergen skin test (brucellosis)
8. Lyme disease antibody titer
9. Lymphangiogram (lymphosarcoma)
10. CT scan of the abdomen and pelvis (Hodgkin lymphoma, lymphoma)
11. CT scan of the mediastinum (lymphoma, metastatic neoplasm)
12. ANA analysis (collagen disease)
13. Skin tests for fungi (e.g., histoplasmosis)
14. HIV antibody test

Case Presentation #64

A 38-year-old black woman was admitted with a 6-week history of mild generalized abdominal pain and low-grade fever. Physical examination revealed generalized lymphadenopathy, abdominal distention with diffuse tenderness, and rebound throughout. A fluid level could be found on percussion.

Question #1. Utilizing your knowledge of anatomy and bacteriology, what are the most likely causes of this woman's problem?

A peritoneal tap revealed numerous lymphocytes in the fluid.

Question #2. What is your diagnosis now?

(See Appendix B for the answers.)

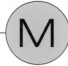

MEMORY LOSS AND DEMENTIA

Memory loss is a real symptom and sign, but organic brain syndrome should be dropped from usage because it is a wastebasket term. Unless the memory loss is functional ("supratentorial"), the cerebrum is the principal anatomic site of diseases that produce memory loss. Applying the mnemonic **VINDICATE** to this area provides a method for the prompt recall of causes.

V—Vascular disease includes cerebral arteriosclerosis, thrombi, emboli, and hemorrhages.

I—Inflammatory disorders include syphilis, chronic encephalitis (inclusion body encephalitis and Jacob–Creutzfeldt disease), and cerebral abscess.

N—Neoplasms include primary and metastatic neoplasms of the brain and meninges.

D—Degenerative and deficiency diseases suggest senile and presenile dementia, Pick disease, Wernicke encephalopathy, and pellagra. Pernicious anemia may be associated with dementia.

I—Intoxication brings to mind alcoholism, bromism, lead poisoning, and a host of other toxic or drug-induced encephalopathies. **I** may also stand for **idiopathic** and suggest normal-pressure hydrocephalus.

C—Congenital disorders include the encephalopathies, Tay–Sachs disease, cerebral palsy, Down syndrome, Wilson disease, and Huntington chorea. Congenital hydrocephalus and many other causes must be considered. Porphyria is often forgotten in the differential.

A—Autoimmune disease suggests lupus erythematosus and multiple sclerosis, although severe dementia is uncommon in the latter.

T—Trauma should prompt the recall of concussion and epidural, subdural, and intracerebral hematomas. Heat stroke may cause temporary memory loss. The dissociative reaction of psychoneurosis may be precipitated by trauma.

E—Endocrine disorders with memory loss are myxedema, insulinoma with chronic hypoglycemia, and hypoparathyroidism. If a pituitary tumor invades the hypothalamus, there may be memory loss. Addison disease and aldosteronism may affect memory by the associated disturbance in potassium balance.

● Approach to the Diagnosis

Once again, the presence or absence of other neurologic signs and symptoms is important. A mini-mental status exam is done. If one does not have the skills or the time for a complete neurologic examination, immediate referral is indicated. Next, a careful drug history is done. Withdrawal

of all drugs may clear the dementia. An electroencephalogram (EEG), skull x-ray film, computed tomography (CT) scan, or magnetic resonance imaging (MRI), spinal tap (if there is no papilledema), and psychometric tests are basic to any workup. If the CT scan or MRI shows dilated ventricles, a spinal fluid nuclear flow study is indicated to exclude normal-pressure hydrocephalus. In the absence of other neurologic signs and negative spinal fluid analysis for syphilis and other chronic encephalopathies, one should do an endocrine workup and look for systemic diseases such as porphyria. Drug screens for lead intoxication and bromism should also be performed.

● Other Useful Tests

1. Complete blood count (CBC) (pernicious anemia)
2. Chemistry panel (uremia, liver disease, electrolyte disorder)
3. Serum B_{12} (pernicious anemia)
4. Urine thiamine afterload (Wernicke encephalopathy)
5. Drug screen (drug or alcohol abuse)
6. Neurology consult
7. Human immunodeficiency virus antibody titer (acquired immunodeficiency syndrome)
8. Schilling test (pernicious anemia)
9. Free thyroxine (FT_4), sensitive thyroid-stimulating hormone (hypothyroidism)
10. Fluorescent treponemal antibody absorption (FTA-ABS) test (neurosyphilis)

Case Presentation #65

A 62-year-old blue-eyed white man complained of increasing forgetfulness. He would occasionally leave a faucet running and when he drove to town he would have to ask directions to get back home. He also suffered indigestion and occasional shortness of breath after walking half a block.

Question #1. Utilizing the mnemonic **VINDICATE**, what would be your differential diagnosis?

Neurologic examination revealed that he was oriented in time and place but could not name the current president. He has slightly diminished vibratory sense in the lower extremities but no other focal neurologic signs. His hemoglobin was 13.2 g/100 mL.

Question #2. What is your diagnosis?

(See Appendix B for the answers.)

M

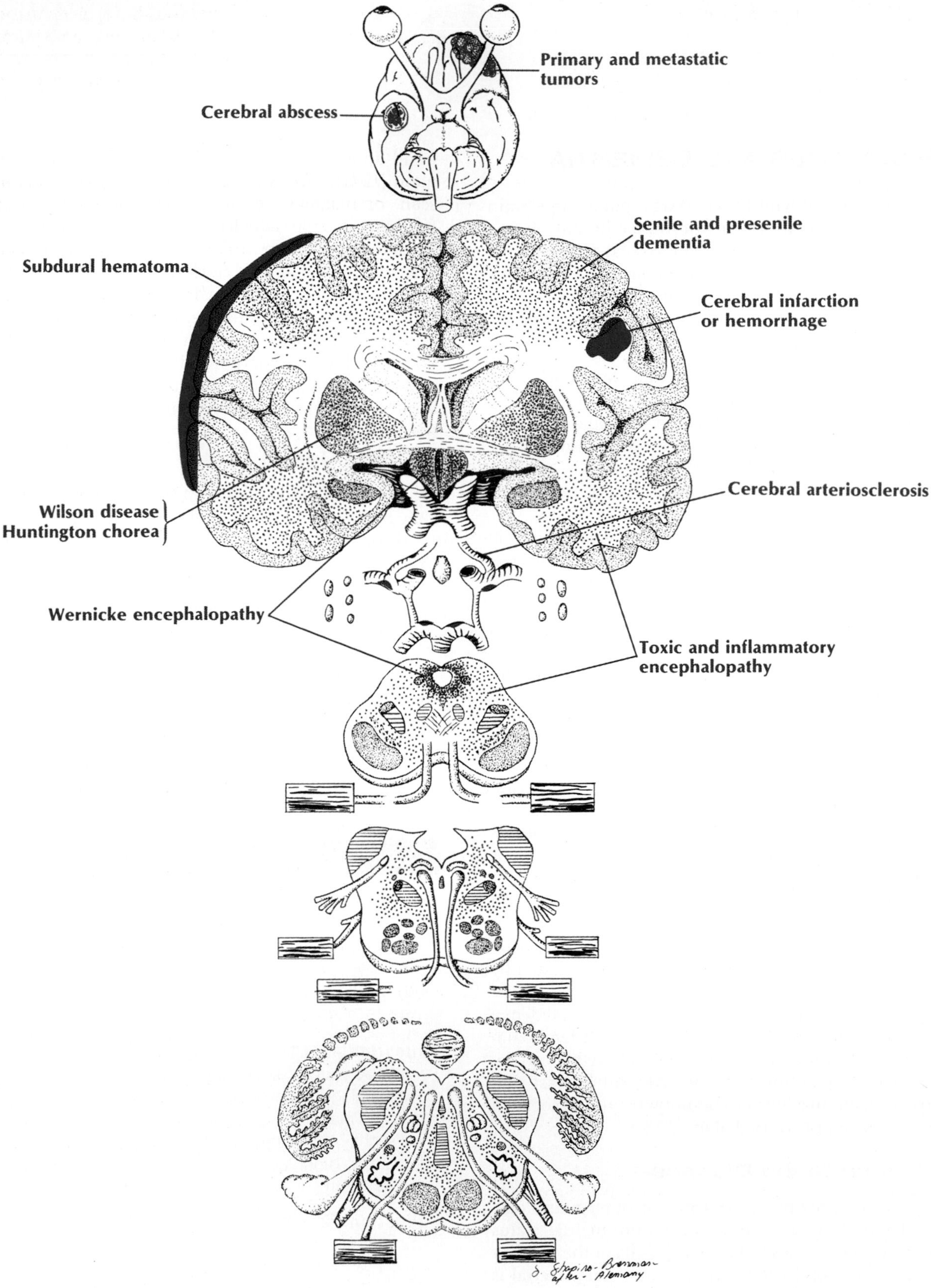

Primary and metastatic tumors

Cerebral abscess

Senile and presenile dementia

Subdural hematoma

Cerebral infarction or hemorrhage

Cerebral arteriosclerosis

Wilson disease
Huntington chorea

Wernicke encephalopathy

Toxic and inflammatory encephalopathy

● **FIGURE 1** Memory loss and dementia.

MENSTRUAL CRAMPS

Visualizing the **anatomy** of the female reproductive system will give an appropriate differential diagnosis:

Cervix: Cervical stenosis (congenital or acquired), cervical polyp, cervicitis
Uterus: Fibroids, retroverted uterus, adenomyosis
Fallopian tubes: Pelvic inflammatory disease (PID), ectopic pregnancy, endometriosis
Ovary: Ovarian neoplasm (especially functional tumors), ectopic pregnancy, endometriosis, and PID
Physiologic analysis would bring to mind the endocrinologic causes of menstrual cramps such as thyroid or pituitary disorders. Finally, do not forget psychogenic causes in the differential diagnosis.

● Approach to the Diagnosis

A thorough pelvic and rectal examination must be performed to rule out secondary causes such as ovarian cyst, uterine fibroids, and ectopic pregnancy. A sonogram and pregnancy test should be performed if there is an adnexal mass, as well as a smear and culture for gonococcus and Chlamydia. A gynecologist should be consulted. If test results are negative, the patient may be tried on oral contraceptives. Diuretics may be used to treat pelvic congestion. Resistant cases may need laparoscopy and ultimately a dilatation and curettage. A psychiatric consult may be necessary.

METEORISM

This is the accumulation of gas in the intestines causing distention. The mnemonic **VINDICATE** lends itself well to facilitate the recall of most of the possible causes.

V—Vascular would prompt the recall of mesenteric thrombosis or embolism. Aortic aneurysms may precipitate bouts of meteorism by causing mesenteric vascular insufficiency.
I—Inflammatory conditions cause meteorism, most notably peritonitis and pancreatitis. However, lobar pneumonia, typhoid, fever, and dysentery should not be forgotten.
N—Neurologic conditions such as transverse myelitis, spinal cord trauma, and anterior spinal artery occlusion may cause meteorism. Conversion hysteria may present with pseudopregnancy and phantom tumors.
D—Degenerative conditions of the intestinal tract or nervous system do not usually cause distention until late in their course.
I—Intoxication should bring to mind the many parasympatholytic drugs (i.e., Pro-Banthine) that cause paralytic ileus.
C—Congenital conditions that may cause this symptom are Hirschsprung disease and malrotation.
A—Allergy would suggest food allergies such as sensitivity to chocolate, peanuts, etc. **Autoimmune** conditions such as granulomatous colitis and ulcerative colitis may produce meteorism.

T—Trauma to the spinal cord has already been mentioned, but penetrating wounds, contusions, and intraperitoneal bleeding may cause meteorism.
E—Endocrine disorders such as myxedema may cause gaseous distention of the bowel.

● Approach to the Diagnosis

A flat plate of the abdomen, chest x-ray, and routine laboratory tests including a CBC, sedimentation rate, chemistry panel, serum amylase and lipase, and stool for occult blood, ovum, and parasites may be indicated depending on the clinical picture. A general surgeon or gastroenterologist may need to be consulted in the acute cases. CT scans, ultrasonography, or contrast radiography may be necessary before the diagnosis can be certain. An exploratory laparotomy is occasionally the only way to pin down the diagnosis.

● Other Useful Tests

1. Quantitative stool fat (malabsorption syndrome)
2. Thyroid panel (myxedema)
3. MRI of the thoracolumbar spine (spinal cord trauma, transverse myelitis)
4. Peritoneal taps (intraperitoneal hemorrhage, peritonitis)

MISCELLANEOUS SITES OF BLEEDING

Bleeding from the ear: This is not usually a serious condition. **Anatomy** is again applied to formulate a diagnosis. The blood may be from the external or middle ear, and usually is caused by diseases of the skin or drum. Trauma is the most significant cause and is usually related to self-inflicted lacerations from digging at wax with hairpins or pencils, for example, which may occasionally rupture the eardrum. Children are prone to lodge foreign bodies in their ears. Skull fractures of the posterior fossa may present with bleeding from the ear. External otitis and otitis media may cause a bloody discharge, but this is not common. If the drum is ruptured by infection, there is usually bleeding from the ear. Carcinomas of the skin of the external canal may cause a bloody discharge, and cholesteatomas will cause bleeding when they ulcerate through the tympanic membrane. Coagulation disorders rarely present with bleeding from the ear, in contrast to epistaxis and bleeding from the gums.

Bleeding from the gums: No anatomic breakdown is necessary here. The causes may be divided into local and systemic categories but, by using the word **VINDICATE**, one can cover all the etiologic categories adequately.

V—Vascular would suggest the hemorrhagic disorders, especially hemophilia, thrombocytopenia, heparin and warfarin (Coumadin) therapy, and fibrinogenopenia, as in disseminated intravascular coagulopathy. In children, idiopathic thrombocytopenic purpura may present with bleeding gums and petechiae following an upper respiratory infection.
I—Inflammatory includes acute gingivitis, dental abscesses, pyorrhea, actinomycosis, or syphilis.

M

N—**Neoplasms** suggest both local neoplasms (e.g., odontoma, papillomas, and epulis) and systemic neoplasms (Hodgkin lymphoma and leukemia).

D—**Degenerative** disorders include aplastic anemia and deficiencies such as scurvy and vitamin K deficiencies.

I—**Intoxication** recalls mercury, phosphorus, and diphenylhydantoin intoxication, in which the gums are usually severely hypertrophied as well.

C—**Congenital** conditions, other than congenital blood dyscrasias (e.g., sickle cell anemia), include erythema bullosum.

A—**Autoimmune** suggests thrombocytopenic purpura, Henoch purpura, and lupus erythematosus.

T—**Trauma** indicates bleeding from vigorous brushing or picking with a toothpick.

E—**Endocrine** disorders are not likely to cause bleeding except secondarily, as in diabetes-induced pyorrhea or the alveolar bone degeneration or dysplasia (osteotic) of hyperparathyroidism.

Gingivitis as part of a diffuse stomatitis may be seen in pemphigus, Stevens–Johnson syndrome, Vincent stomatitis (spirilla and bacilli fusiformis), and various other bacterial forms. The job of the clinician is to exclude the systemic causes and then refer the patient to a periodontist for evaluation and treatment of the local causes.

Bleeding from the breast, hemorrhagic discharge: Suspect a neoplasm, such as a ductal carcinoma (Paget disease), fibroadenosis, and ductal papillomas, unless proven otherwise. With a magnifying glass, one may be able to tell which of the 20 or so ducts is bleeding, but expressing one small segment at a time, working spirally, is also helpful.

MONOPLEGIA

Monoplegia is the paralysis of one extremity. Following the nerve impulse from the cerebral cortex down through the spinal cord, nerve roots, brachial and lumbosacral plexus, peripheral nerve, myoneural junction, and muscles allows us to recall the most significant causes of monoplegia.

Cerebral cortex: Monoplegia may result from a parasagittal tumor or abscess and anterior cerebral artery embolism or thrombosis. Occasionally an occlusion of the middle cerebral artery or its branches may cause monoplegia of the upper extremity, but there are almost always neurologic signs in the lower extremities in these cases.

Spinal cord: Early space-occupying lesions of the spinal cord and amyotrophic lateral sclerosis may present with monoplegia. It is unlikely for multiple sclerosis or transverse myelitis to present this way.

Nerve roots: Poliomyelitis, progressive muscular atrophy, and herniated discs may present with monoplegia. Early cauda equina tumors may present with monoplegia as well.

Brachial plexus: This would bring to mind brachial plexus neuropathy, thoracic outlet syndrome, and Pancoast tumors.

Sciatic plexus: This would suggest sciatic neuritis or injury.

Peripheral nerve: Trauma or entrapment of the peripheral nerves may present as a monoplegia. Charcot–Marie tooth disease may begin in one extremity.

Myoneural junction: Myasthenia gravis or Eaton–Lambert syndrome may occasionally present as weakness in one extremity.

Muscle: It is unusual for the various forms of muscular dystrophy and dermatomyositis to present with monoplegia.

● Approach to the Diagnosis

The neurologic examination will help determine the site of the lesion and thus the likely etiology. If there are hyperactive reflexes in the involved extremity, the lesion is probably in the upper spinal cord or cerebral cortex. If there is associated facial palsy or other cranial nerve signs, the lesion is probably in the brain or brainstem.

Hypoactive reflexes in the involved extremity indicate a lesion in the nerve roots, nerve plexus, or peripheral nerves. However, acute cerebral thrombosis, hemorrhage, or embolism may present with hypoactive reflexes in the involved extremity. Before proceeding with an expensive workup, a neurologist needs to be consulted.

Monoplegia of the upper extremities with hyperactive reflexes would indicate the need for an MRI or CT scan of the brain or cervical spinal cord. Monoplegia of the lower extremities with hyperactive reflexes would suggest the need for an MRI of the thoracic spine. However, a CT scan or MRI of the brain may still be required to rule out a parasagittal lesion.

Monoplegia with hypoactive reflexes may require an MRI or CT scan of the spine, electromyogram (EMG), and nerve conduction velocity (NCV) studies. Blood lead levels, glucose tolerance tests, and other studies indicated in a neuropathy workup (page 331) may be required. Muscle biopsy and acetylcholine receptor antibody titers may be necessary.

MOUTH PIGMENTATION

A key to remembering the cause of a mouth pigmentation is found in the mnemonic **MINTS**.

M—**Malformation** would bring to mind familial intestinal polyposis (Peutz–Jegher syndrome) and Fabry disease. Small red spots of the mouth and tongue suggest hereditary telangiectasia.

I—**Inflammation** would suggest the pigmentation of the buccal mucosa seen in pulmonary tuberculosis of the adrenal gland leading to Addison disease.

N—**Neoplasm** suggests the pigmentation seen in metastatic malignant melanoma and carcinomatosis.

T—**Toxic** helps recall the toxic substances that cause mouth pigmentation such as silver, bismuth, contraceptives, tranquilizers, antimalarials, lead, arsenic, and mercury.

S—**Systemic** diseases associated with mouth pigmentation include Addison disease, hemochromatosis, and porphyria.

● Approach to the Diagnosis

If lead or arsenic poisoning is suspected, hair analysis may be done. If Addison disease is suspected, serum cortisol or a 24-hour urine 17-hydroxysteroids and 17-ketosteroids should be done. A gastrointestinal (GI) series, small bowel follow-through, and barium enema may be done to rule out Peutz–Jegher syndrome. Alternatively, a colonoscopy can be done. Urine porphobilinogen and porphyrins will help diagnose porphyria.

● Other Useful Tests

1. Rapid adrenocorticotropic hormone tests (Addison disease)
2. Urine melanin (malignant malenoma)

MURMURS

The first consideration on hearing a heart murmur is to determine whether the murmur is functional or organic. Certainly, the low-grade systolic murmurs tend to be functional; if the murmur changes or disappears on position, inspiration, or exercise it is likely to be functional. A diastolic murmur, however, is invariably organic. Perhaps the most significant question to ask is, "Are the heart sounds normal?" This is a decisive factor in many cases. If the heart sounds are normal, organic disease is unlikely. After the murmur is determined to be organic, one needs to have a working differential diagnosis in mind to proceed efficiently. **VINDICATE** provides a mnemonic for this purpose.

V—**Vascular** suggests myocardial infarction, ball–valve thrombi, mural thrombus, and congestive heart failure (CHF). Hypertensive cardiovascular disease may lead to cardiac dilatation and murmurs.
I—**Inflammatory** recalls acute and subacute bacterial endocarditis (SBE), viral myocarditis, and the myocarditis of trichinosis and Chagas disease. Intravenous drug use is a major cause of SBE today. Syphilis is also a prominent cause of aortic insufficiency.
N—**Neoplasm** includes atrial myxomas, the most significant disorder to remember here, but leukemic infiltration of the heart and all the neoplasms associated with anemia might be considered.
D—**Degenerative** disease recalls atherosclerotic heart disease, muscular dystrophy, and Friedreich ataxia. Atherosclerotic heart disease should be emphasized because it frequently causes aortic murmurs. Medionecrosis may lead to murmurs when a dissecting aneurysm begins. This may be associated with Marfan syndrome.
I—**Intoxication** reminds one that there may be no murmur in alcoholic myocardiopathy until failure develops, but it is a condition to consider nevertheless.
I—**Idiopathic disorders** include mitral valve prolapse although in some cases, this is hereditary.
C—**Congenital** heart disease is a well-known cause of murmurs.

A—**Autoimmune** disease includes rheumatic fever, the best known of these disorders, although it is now a less frequent consideration in murmurs. Libman–Sacks mitral valvular disease occurs in lupus erythematosus.
T—**Traumatic** disorders recall a ventricular or aortic aneurysm and occasionally a coronary arteriovenous fistula or valvular insufficiency that may result from a stab wound.
E—**Endocrinopathies** indicate hyperthyroidism and hypothyroidism, particularly because the associated CHF may lead to cardiac dilatation and murmurs. Hyperthyroidism produces murmurs in some cases because of the rushing blood and rapid rate, causing many eddy currents.

● Approach to the Diagnosis

A chest x-ray with anterior oblique films during a barium swallow along with an electrocardiogram (ECG), sedimentation rate, blood serology thyroid profile, and CBC are basic in the workup of a murmur. Echocardiography will need to be done in most cases. If there is a fever or if there is recent onset of the murmur, blood cultures, an antistreptolysin-O (ASO) titer, and a C-reactive protein (CRP) test should be done. An antinuclear antibody (ANA) test, ECG, and phonocardiogram are frequently done. Referral to a cardiologist is wise if the cause is obscure or if one is unable to spend the time for a careful workup. Angiocardiography and cardiac catheterization are the only sure ways to determine the location of the valvular disease, and, in many cases, the exact cause.

MUSCULAR ATROPHY

This symptom is developed using both **anatomy** and **physiology**. Atrophy of any muscle may develop in seven ways:

1. Lack of use of the muscle
2. Malnutrition or increased body metabolism
3. Primary muscle disease
4. Myoneural junction disease
5. Peripheral nerve disease
6. Nerve root disease
7. Spinal cord disease

When recalling the differential diagnosis of muscular atrophy, think of these seven factors and the causes will unfold.

1. **Lack of use of the muscle:** In focal or generalized bone or joint disease there is diminished use of the extremity or part involved, so the muscles atrophy. "Disuse" atrophy may also occur in compensation neurosis, hysteria, depression, and in many central nervous system diseases in which motivation is gone.
2. **Malnutrition or body hypermetabolism:** Starvation causes diffuse muscular wasting. Diffuse muscular wasting also occurs in anything that speeds up body metabolism, including hyperthyroidism, metastatic carcinoma and other diffuse neoplasms, chronic inflammatory conditions such as rheumatoid arthritis (RA) and collagen disease, and chronic fever of any cause.

M

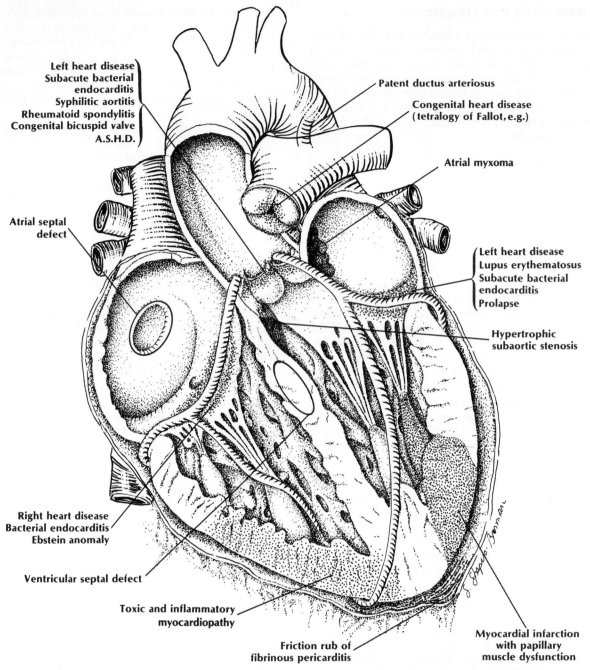

Left heart disease
Subacute bacterial
endocarditis
Syphilitic aortitis
Rheumatoid spondylitis
Congenital bicuspid valve
A.S.H.D.

Atrial septal
defect

Right heart disease
Bacterial endocarditis
Ebstein anomaly

Ventricular septal defect

Toxic and inflammatory
myocardiopathy

Patent ductus arteriosus

Congenital heart disease
(tetralogy of Fallot, e.g.)

Atrial myxoma

Left heart disease
Lupus erythematosus
Subacute bacterial
endocarditis
Prolapse

Hypertrophic
subaortic stenosis

Myocardial infarction
with papillary
muscle dysfunction

Friction rub of
fibrinous pericarditis

● **FIGURE 2** Murmurs.

3. **Primary muscle disease:** Muscular dystrophy, dermato-myositis, trichinosis, and McArdle syndrome should be considered here.

4. **Myoneural junction:** This category makes one think of myasthenia gravis.

5. **Peripheral nerve disease:** Diabetic neuropathy and the neuropathy from lead, arsenic, and other toxins should be considered here. Periarteritis nodosa and trauma to the nerve may give an asymmetric neuritis. Hereditary neuropathies such as Charcot–Marie–Tooth disease and Dejerine–Sottas hereditary hypertrophic neuritis are also

considered here. Porphyria is another cause to recall in this category.

6. **Nerve root disease:** Spinal column disorders that compress the root include fractures, herniated disks, spondylolisthesis, tuberculosis, metastatic tumors, and multiple myelomas.

7. **Spinal cord disease:** The degenerative diseases such as amyotrophic lateral sclerosis, progressive muscular atrophy, and syringomyelia must be considered here. In addition, poliomyelitis, transverse myelitis of various areas, anterior spinal artery occlusion, infectious polyneuritis, and spinal cord tumors must be recalled.

● Approach to the Diagnosis

Focal atrophy of a muscle often means a damaged peripheral nerve or root. If there are visible fasciculations, a lesion of the spinal cord or root is most likely. Electromyography will determine which portion of the nerve is affected. It will also be helpful in diagnosing muscle disease. Muscle biopsy is valuable in ruling out trichinosis, dermatomyositis, or muscular dystrophy. If there are fasciculations, a spine x-ray, spinal tap, and myelography or MRI may be necessary to establish the diagnosis. Sedimentation rate, CRP, RA titer, ANA, and tuberculin tests may be necessary.

● Other Useful Tests

1. Serum protein electrophoresis (collagen disease, multiple myeloma)
2. Muscle enzyme tests (muscular dystrophy, dermatomyositis)
3. 24-hour urine creatine and creatinine levels (muscular dystrophy)
4. Acetylcholine receptor antibody titer (myasthenia gravis)
5. Thyroid function tests (hypothyroid myopathy)
6. Glucose tolerance test (diabetic neuropathy)

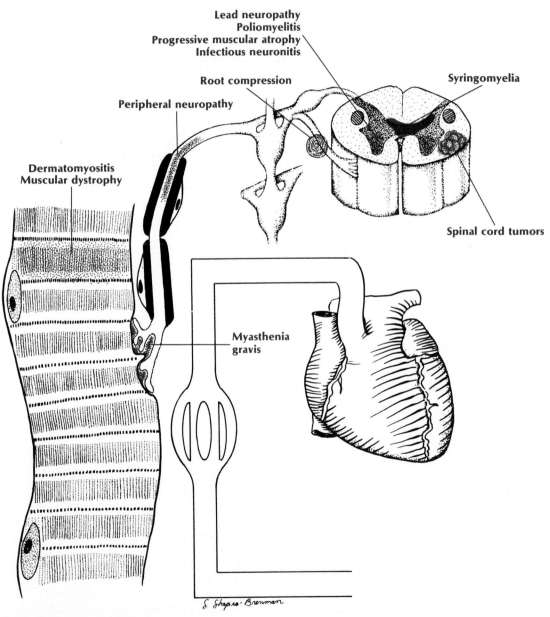

● **FIGURE 3** Muscular atrophy.

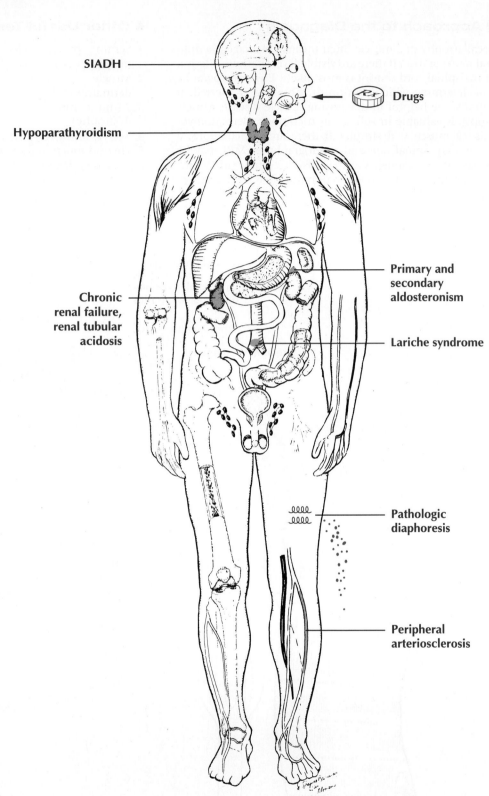

SIADH

Drugs

Hypoparathyroidism

Primary and secondary aldosteronism

Chronic renal failure, renal tubular acidosis

Lariche syndrome

Pathologic diaphoresis

Peripheral arteriosclerosis

● **FIGURE 4** Muscular cramps.

Case Presentation #66

A 40-year-old white male factory worker complained of back pain and weakness of his right leg ever since an injury at work 8 months ago. He has not been back to work. There is no loss of bladder control.

Question #1. Based on your knowledge of neuroanatomy, what would be your differential diagnosis?

Your examination shows diffuse atrophy of the muscles of the right leg along with diffuse hypesthesia and hypalgesia. However, the reflexes are equal and active in both lower extremities, and there are no pathologic reflexes.

Question #2. What is your diagnosis now?

(See Appendix B for the answers.)

MUSCULAR CRAMPS

To develop a list of possible causes of muscular cramps, think of **anatomy** and **physiology**. Anatomically a muscle bundle is supplied by arteries, veins, and nerves. Considering the arteries will prompt the recall of arteriosclerosis, emboli, Leriche syndrome, and other conditions that interfere with the blood supply to the muscles. This is manifested by the familiar intermittent claudication. Considering the veins will call to mind varicose veins as a frequent cause of muscle cramps. Turning our attention to the nerve supply will help recall the various neurologic conditions that are associated with muscle cramps. Multiple sclerosis, amyotrophic lateral sclerosis, spinal cord injury, and any upper motor neuron lesion may be the cause of muscular cramps. Finally, the muscle itself may be involved by myositis, myotonic dystrophy, traumatic hemorrhage (i.e., charley horse), and "professional" cramps from the overuse of certain muscle groups.

Next, applying physiology to the analysis of possible causes of muscular cramps, we should easily remember the various fluid and electrolyte disorders that may be implicated. Hypocalcemia and hypomagnesemia due to hypoparathyroidism, rickets, malabsorption syndrome, chronic renal failure, and renal tubular acidosis are a prominent cause of muscular cramps. Hyponatremia from pathologic diaphoresis, diuretics, dilutional hyponatremia, inappropriate antidiuretic hormone secretion, and chronic renal failure are also associated with muscle cramps. Finally, hypokalemia or alkalosis due to primary and secondary hyperaldosteronism, intestinal obstruction, milk–alkali syndrome, and hyperventilation may be the cause.

A few additional disorders that may not be recalled by the above methods are lead poisoning, certain drugs such

M

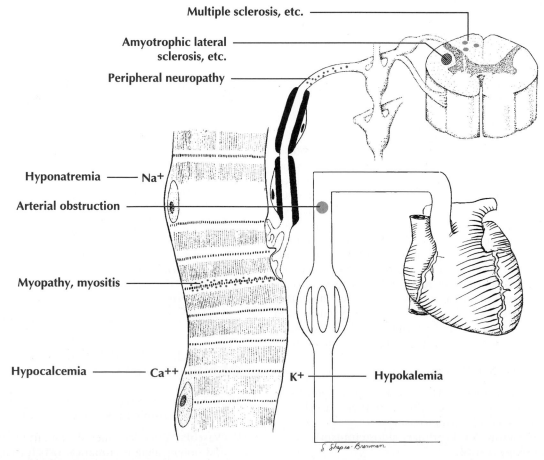

● **FIGURE 5** Muscular cramps.

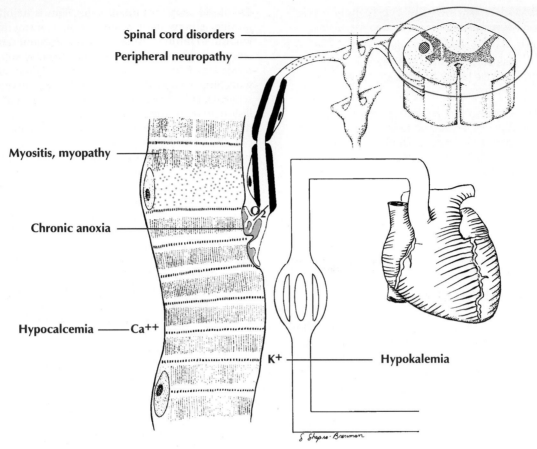

● **FIGURE 6** Musculoskeletal pain, generalized.

as phenytoin and rifampin, hysteria, fever, pregnancy, and strychnine poisoning.

● **Approach to the Diagnosis**

Clinically, one should look for absent or diminished pulses in the extremity involved, Chvostek and Trousseau signs of tetany, and neurologic signs of an upper motor neuron lesion. An occupational history may disclose that the patient is a miner or ironworker or is exposed to excessive heat on the job. Occupations such as painters, writers, seamstresses, and compositors suggest the so-called professional cramps. Adson signs are positive in thoracic outlet syndrome. Cramps in the legs produced by walking a certain distance suggest peripheral arteriosclerosis and Leriche syndrome. This is also a sign of spinal stenosis. The initial laboratory workup involves a CBC, urinalysis, chemistry panel, and electrolytes. If a vascular cause is suspected, ultrasonography and perhaps venography or angiography may be indicated.

● **Other Useful Tests**

1. Parathyroid hormone (PTH) assay (hypoparathyroidism)
2. 24-hour urine calcium level (hypoparathyroidism)
3. Plasma renin level (aldosteronism)
4. Urine aldosterone level (primary aldosteronism)
5. Endocrinology consult
6. Neurology consult

Case Presentation #67

A 67-year-old white man complained of cramps in both legs on walking one block. He also suffered chronic low back pain for the past year.

Question #1. Utilizing your knowledge of anatomy and physiology, what is your differential diagnosis?

Further history reveals that he is on medication for hypertension. Physical examination reveals good pulses in all four extremities. Neurologic examination aside from limited range of motion of his lumbar spine is unremarkable.

Question #2. What is your diagnosis now?

(See Appendix B for the answers.)

MUSCULOSKELETAL PAIN, GENERALIZED

The mnemonic **VINDICATE** is extremely useful in developing a list of possible causes of musculoskeletal pain.

V—Vascular disorders include periarteritis nodosa, SBE, and polymyalgia rheumatica, which also could be classified under collagen disorders.

I—**Infectious** diseases include brucellosis, poliomyelitis, influenza, leptospirosis, measles, dengue fever, epidemic myalgia, trichinosis, cysticercosis, malaria, and toxoplasmosis. Almost any febrile illness may begin with generalized myalgia.

N—**Neoplastic** diseases that may cause generalized myalgia are those that are associated with fever such as Hodgkin lymphoma and leukemia.

D—**Deficiency** disorders associated with myalgia are rickets and osteomalacia.

I—**Intoxication** with lead, alcohol, lithium, and drugs such as vincristine, amphotericin B, cimetidine, and amphetamines may cause generalized myalgia.

C—**Congenital** disorders such as McArdle syndrome (type V glycogen storage disease), porphyria, and myoglobinuria may cause generalized myalgia.

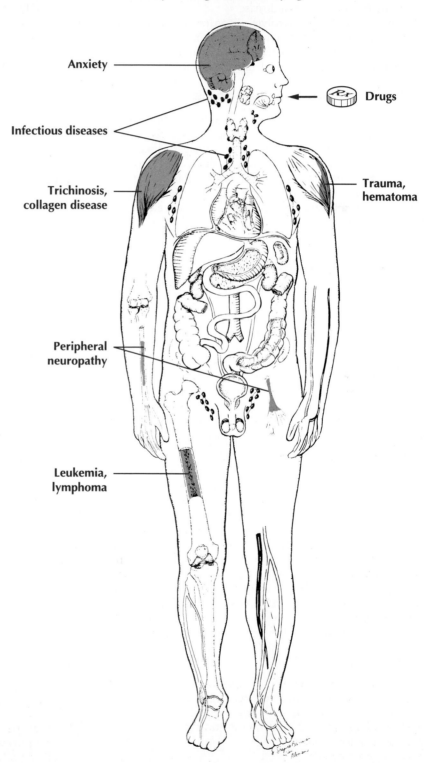

● **FIGURE 7** Musculoskeletal pain, generalized.

A—Autoimmune disorders include periarteritis nodosa, lupus erythematosus, rheumatic fever, Guillain–Barré syndrome, and dermatomyositis.

T—Trauma causing muscular hemorrhages or injury is usually associated with focal myalgia and cramps, but after prolonged exercise, there may be generalized myalgia. Prolonged anxiety and tension may cause myalgia by the same mechanism. However, it is unlikely that the entity fibromyalgia is a disease.

E—Endocrine and electrolyte disorders bring to mind hypothyroidism, hypoparathyroidism, prolonged corticosteroid therapy, hyperaldosteronism, hyponatremia, hypokalemia, and hypocalcemia (see page 246).

● Approach to the Diagnosis

On history and physical examination one may find the history of the use of alcohol and/or drugs, signs of fever, paralysis, or psychiatric symptomatology. Collagen disease will show certain telltale symptoms and signs. The laboratory workup includes a CBC, urinalysis, sedimentation rate, ANA test, chemistry panel, and electrolytes. Febrile agglutinins, ASO titers, *Trichinella* antibody titer, and protein electrophoresis may be indicated. It may be wise to consult a neurologist, endocrinologist, or infectious disease specialist.

● Other Useful Tests

1. NCV (neuropathy, radiculopathy)
2. EMG (myopathy, radiculopathy)
3. Muscle biopsy (collagen disease, myopathy)
4. Spinal tap (Guillain–Barré syndrome, neurosyphilis, multiple sclerosis)
5. RA test
6. 24-hour urine calcium, sodium, or potassium level (endocrine disorder, electrolyte disorder)
7. Urine aldosterone (primary aldosteronism)
8. Serum PTH assay (hypoparathyroidism)
9. Urine porphyrin and porphobilinogen levels (porphyria)
10. Urine myoglobin (muscle injury)

Case Presentation #68

A 70-year-old white woman complained of early morning pain and stiffness in the shoulders, hips, and proximal extremities for the past month. She has lost 15 lb and was fatigued all the time.

Question #1. Utilizing the mnemonic VINDICATE, what would be your differential diagnosis?

Physical examination revealed diffuse tenderness of the proximal muscles and joints but no focal neurologic signs. The sedimentation rate was 70 mm. Other laboratory tests were unremarkable.

Question #2. What is your diagnosis now?

(See Appendix B for the answers.)

MYOCLONUS

The differential diagnosis of this sign is similar to that of tremors (see page 420), but a few additional possibilities should be kept in mind. Idiopathic myoclonus epilepsy, petit mal epilepsy (with the *petit mal* triad), *grand mal* epilepsy, and hysteria are the important ones to remember. Congenital hypsarrhythmia may present with salaam seizures. Decerebrate states are associated with myoclonic jerks in which there are flexion of the arms and extension of the legs. Phenothiazine and other tranquilizers may cause myoclonus. L-Dopa will cause oculogyric crisis and smacking of lips. The workup of these conditions includes a skull x-ray, EEG (preferably sleep), possibly a CT scan, and, if there is no evidence of increased intracranial pressure, a spinal tap. It is recommended that the patient be referred to a neurologist for this workup.

N

NAIL CHANGES

There are various types of nail changes, such as thickening (onychogryposis), thinning, deformity, and separation from the nail bed (onycholysis). Whenever a peculiarity of the nail exists, the mnemonic **VINDICATE** will help to recall all the causes.

V—Vascular disease includes the anoxic disorders that cause clubbing (see page 97), iron deficiency anemia that causes spoon nails or koilonychia, Raynaud disease, vasculitis (periarteritis nodosa), and peripheral arteriosclerosis, which causes dystrophy or onychogryposis of the nails.

I—Inflammatory diseases that involve the nail bring to mind fungus infections causing onychia (nail bed inflammation), paronychia, syphilis (which can cause almost any nail change), subacute bacterial endocarditis (SBE), and trichinosis, which causes splinter hemorrhages of the nail.

N—Neoplasms do not usually cause nail changes, with the exception of clubbing and pallor from secondary anemia. Chondromas, melanomas, and angiomas are a few neoplasms that do. Intestinal polyposis may cause nail atrophy. The **N**, however, can be used to recall **neurologic** disorders such as peripheral neuropathy (dystrophy or onychogryposis), syringomyelia, and multiple sclerosis.

D—suggests **deficiency** diseases such as avitaminosis (B$_2$ and D).

I—Intoxication includes arsenic (white lines and transverse ridges across the nails) and radiodermatitis.

C—Congenital disorders include psoriasis, congenital ectodermal defects, absence of nails (onychia), micronychia, and macronychia.

A—Autoimmune disorders suggest scleroderma, periarteritis nodosa, eczema, and lupus.

T—Trauma causes the familiar subungual hematoma that turns the nail to turn dark red or black.

E—Endocrine disorders are probably some of the most important causes of nail changes. Hypothyroidism produces nail dystrophy, brittleness, and onycholysis; similar changes, plus spooning of the nails, occur in hyperthyroidism. In hypopituitarism, these may be dystrophy, loss of the subcuticular moons, and spooning. Thickening and transverse grooving of the nails may be seen in hypoparathyroidism.

● Approach to the Diagnosis

The diagnosis of nail abnormalities begins by correlating the nail changes with other findings (e.g., neurologic and endocrinologic). Laboratory workup depends on the particular disease or diseases suggested by the nail changes (see Appendix A).

● Other Useful Tests

1. Complete blood count (CBC) (iron deficiency anemia)
2. Sedimentation rate (chronic infectious disease)
3. Blood cultures (SBE)
4. Trichinella antibody titer (trichinosis)
5. Free thyroxine (FT$_4$) and sensitive thyroid-stimulating hormone levels (hyperthyroidism, hypothyroidism)
6. Serum parathyroid hormone (PTH) (hypoparathyroidism)
7. Serum growth hormone, luteinizing hormone, follicle-stimulating hormone (hypopituitarism)
8. Computed tomography (CT) scan of the brain (pituitary tumor)
9. Chest x-ray (neoplasm, tuberculosis, bronchiectasis)
10. Arterial blood gas (pulmonary disease, heart disease)
11. Hair analysis for arsenic (arsenic poisoning)
12. Antinuclear antibody (ANA) analysis (collagen disease)
13. Glucose tolerance test (diabetic arteriolar sclerosis)

NASAL DISCHARGE

With nasal discharge (rhinorrhea and postnasal drip), **anatomy** is the key. In visualizing the structure from outside in, one encounters the external nares, the choana with the turbinates, the maxillary, ethmoid, frontal and sphenoid sinuses, and the nasopharynx with the openings of the eustachian tubes surrounded by the adenoids. In addition, the inferior meatus provides the opening for the nasolacrimal ducts. The etiologies of a nonbloody discharge of the nose are almost invariably inflammatory (infectious or allergic), but a fracture of the sinuses or cribriform plate may cause a cerebrospinal fluid (CSF) rhinorrhea. As in nonbloody discharges elsewhere, it is incumbent on the diagnostician to keep the possibility of neoplasm, foreign body, and other causes of obstruction in mind, because these may set the stage for infection.

Nasal conditions causing acute nonbloody rhinorrhea include the common cold (due to any one of at least 60 viruses), viral influenza, pertussis, measles, and allergic rhinitis (hay fever). The discharge is at first clear; however, after a few hours of obstruction, secondary bacterial infection may set in and the discharge often becomes purulent. Chronic rhinitis is usually allergic, bacterial, or fungal (as in mucormycosis), but it can be on an autoimmune basis (Wegener granulomatosis). Toxins in the environment (e.g., smoke) may cause serous rhinorrhea. Too frequent use of nasal sprays and cocaine should always be considered. Chronic rhinitis may also be idiopathic (vasomotor rhinitis).

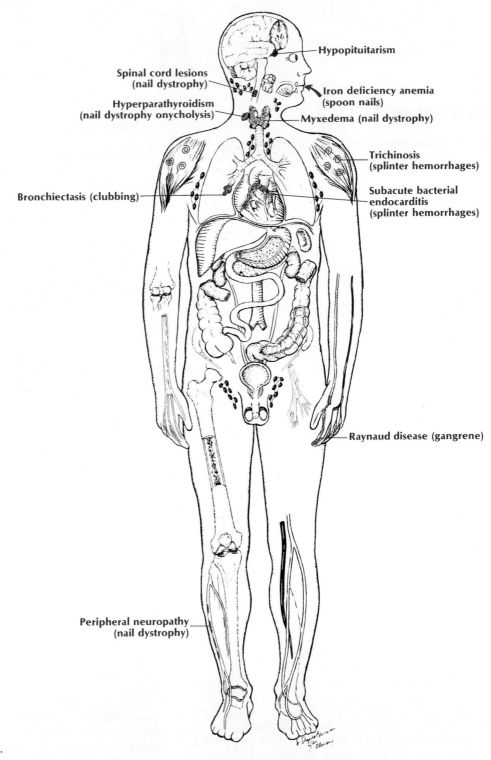

Hypopituitarism

Spinal cord lesions
(nail dystrophy)

Iron deficiency anemia
(spoon nails)

Hyperparathyroidism
(nail dystrophy onycholysis)

Myxedema (nail dystrophy)

Trichinosis
(splinter hemorrhages)

Bronchiectasis (clubbing)

Subacute bacterial
endocarditis
(splinter hemorrhages)

Raynaud disease (gangrene)

Peripheral neuropathy
(nail dystrophy)

● **FIGURE 1** Nail changes.

The **sinuses** may be inflamed in the same conditions that involve the nose. However, concern about whether a discharge is coming from the sinuses arises when the discharge becomes purulent, when there is associated pain over the sinus, or when the discharge becomes chronic. In chronic sinusitis the discharge may frequently be a postnasal drip.

The **nasopharynx** is also involved by the same viral, bacterial, and fungal conditions as the rest of the nasal passages, but, in addition, diphtheria may begin here. If the **adenoids** become large enough, they may obstruct the nasal canals and produce a secondary bacterial rhinitis with discharge.

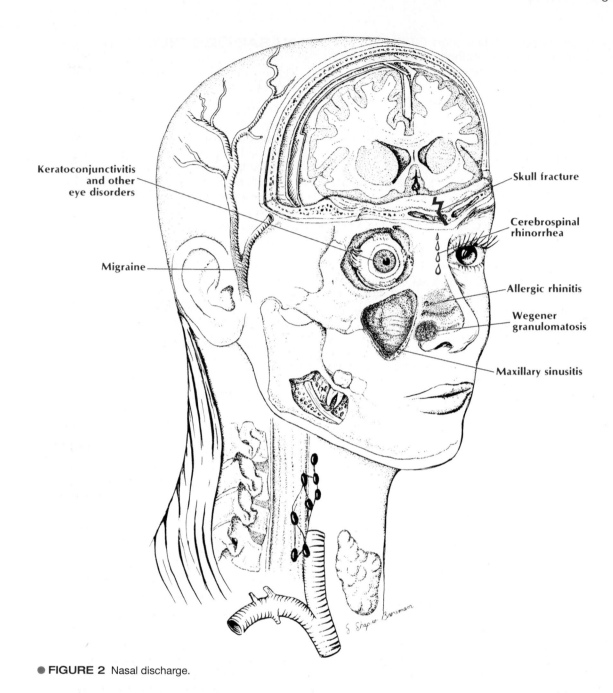

● **FIGURE 2** Nasal discharge.

Because the **nasolacrimal ducts** open into the inferior meatus, any eye condition that may cause excessive tearing may also produce rhinorrhea. The unilateral rhinorrhea of histamine headaches is partially related to this mechanism, as is trigeminal neuralgia.

● Approach to the Diagnosis

The diagnosis of nonbloody rhinorrhea is not usually difficult in acute cases because it is frequently due to the common cold or allergic rhinitis (in which case the history will be helpful). However, the first thing to do is eliminate nasal sprays. When rhinorrhea persists, a smear for eosinophils and appropriate skin testing are useful if the discharge is nonpurulent; Gram stain, culture for bacteria and fungi, and x-rays of the sinuses will be valuable if the discharge is purulent. Cerebrospinal rhinorrhea is a possibility. Idiopathic vasomotor rhinitis can be diagnosed by the response to Atrovent (topical anticholinergic agents). A CT scan is the preferred method to diagnose sinusitis.

● Other Useful Tests

1. CBC (infection)
2. Sedimentation rate (infection)
3. Tuberculin test

4. Venereal disease research laboratory (VDRL) test
5. Fluorescent treponemal antibody absorption (FTA-ABS) test (more definitive test for syphilis)
6. ANA analysis (collagen disease)
7. Antineutrophil cytoplasmic antigen (ANCA) antibodies for Wegener granulomatosis
8. Fungal culture (mucormycosis)
9. Nasopharyngoscopy (neoplasm, granuloma)
10. CT scan of brain and sinuses (neoplasm, sinus abscess)
11. Biopsy
12. Radioimmunosorbent assay study of CSF (cerebrospinal rhinorrhea)
13. Viral antigen testing (influenza)

NASAL MASS OR SWELLING

Although anatomy may assist somewhat in developing the differential here, it is probably an unnecessary exercise because the mnemonic **MINT** will bring to mind virtually all the etiologies.

M—**Malformation** reminds one of the broad nose of cretinism, Down syndrome, gargoylism, myxedema, and acromegaly.
I—**Inflammation** suggests carbuncles, cellulitis, syphilis, acne rosacea with rhinophyma, Wegener midline granuloma, and granulomas from tuberculosis, aspergillosis, rhinosporidiosis, mucormycosis, and other chronic infections.
N—**Neoplasms** suggest carcinomas of the external nares, squamous cell carcinoma of the nasal mucosa (such as Schmincke tumors), and nasal polyps secondary to allergic rhinitis.
T—**Trauma** reminds one of fractures, dislocations, and contusions, although these diagnoses are usually obvious.

● Approach to the Diagnosis

The diagnosis is not difficult except in the case of granulomas and carcinomas, when skillful biopsy and culture are necessary. In Wegener midline granuloma, a search for alveolitis and glomerulonephritis will help to determine the diagnosis. Serum for ANCA antibodies is often diagnostic.

● Other Useful Tests

1. CBC (infection)
2. Nasal smear and culture
3. Tuberculin test (tuberculosis)
4. Acid-fast bacillus smear and culture (tuberculosis)
5. VDRL test (syphilis)
6. Fungal smear and culture (mucormycosis)
7. X-ray of skull and sinuses (granuloma, neoplasm)
8. CT scan of brain and sinuses (sinusitis, neoplasm, granuloma)
9. Nasal smear for eosinophils (nasal polyps)
10. Nasopharyngoscopy (polyps, carcinoma)
11. Serum immunoglobulin E (IgE) level (allergic rhinitis)
12. Radioallergosorbent test (RAST) (allergic rhinitis)
13. Allergy skin testing (nasal polyps)

NASAL OBSTRUCTION

The mnemonic **MINTS** will be very helpful in recalling the various causes of nasal obstruction.

M—**Malformation** prompts the recall of deviated nasal septum and congenital atesia.
I—**Inflammation** brings to mind nasal obstruction due to viral, bacterial, and allergic rhinitis and sinusitis. It should also help to recall the obstruction caused by mucormycosis in diabetes. Inflamed swollen adenoids cause acute and chronic obstruction.
N—**Neoplasm** reminds one of nasal polyps, fibromas, osteomas, teratomas, and advanced carcinomas.
T—**Trauma** prompts the recall of hematomas of the septum, fracture, and displacement of the nasal bones. T should also suggest toxic swelling of the membranes due to rhinitis medicamentosus.
S—**Systemic** causes facilitate the recall of Wegener granulomatosis.

● Approach to the Diagnosis

If there is fever, one must suspect an upper respiratory infection or acute sinusitis and rhinitis. It is extremely important to ask about chronic use of topical nasal decongestants to rule out rhinitis medicamentosa. If allergic rhinitis is suspected, a nasal smear for eosinophils and serum IgE antibodies can be done. If there is a purulent discharge, smear and cultures for bacteria should be done. Wegener granulomatosis is diagnosed by an ANA, ANCA, or biopsy. In difficult cases, an otolaryngologist should be consulted.

● Other Useful Tests

1. X-rays of the nose and sinuses (sinusitis, deviated septum, polyps)
2. CT scan of the sinuses (sinusitis, polyps)
3. Nasopharyngoscopy (adenoids, polyps, neoplasm)
4. Allergy skin tests (allergic rhinitis)
5. Viral antigen testing (influenza)

NAUSEA AND VOMITING

These two should be considered together, because nausea is just a *forme fruste* of vomiting. A patient with acute nausea and vomiting and diarrhea almost always has viral or bacterial gastroenteritis although acute appendicitis, cholecystitis, and pancreatitis must be kept in mind. It is the chronic cases of nausea and vomiting that present a diagnostic dilemma. This symptom lends itself well to **anatomic** analysis, particularly by the target method illustrated on page 312. The focus should be on the gastrointestinal (GI) tract. Starting from the top and working to the bottom, and at the same time cross-indexing this with etiologies (Table 46), one can review the most important causes of vomiting.

In the **nasopharynx**, one encounters tonsillitis and foreign bodies. In the **esophagus**, achalasia, esophageal diverticulum, reflux esophagitis, and carcinoma are important,

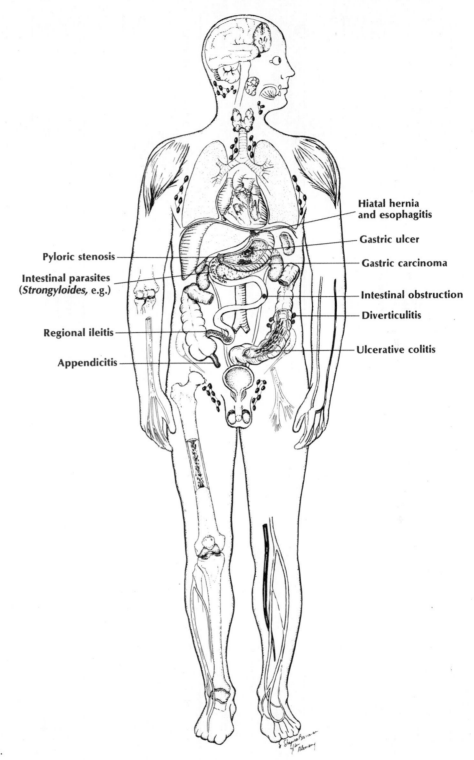

Hiatal hernia
and esophagitis

Gastric ulcer

Gastric carcinoma

Intestinal obstruction

Diverticulitis

Ulcerative colitis

Pyloric stenosis

Intestinal parasites
(*Strongyloides,* e.g.)

Regional ileitis

Appendicitis

● **FIGURE 3** Nausea and vomiting.

although they are more likely to produce dysphagia (see page 128). In the **stomach**, gastritis, gastric ulcers, and gastric carcinoma are important causes of vomiting. A polyp, carcinoma, or ulcer at the pylorus is most likely to produce vomiting because of gastric outlet obstruction. In children, one must not forget pyloric stenosis. In the **duodenum**,

one must consider not only ulcers and duodenitis but also the afferent loop obstructions that occur after Billroth II surgery and the "dumping syndrome" in Billroth I and II surgery. Bile gastritis is also a cause. Intestinal obstruction from a variety of causes (e.g., volvulus, intussusception, malrotation, bezoar, carcinoma, and regional ileitis) must

TABLE 46   Nausea and Vomiting

	V Vascular	I Inflammatory	N Neoplasm	D Degenerative and Deficiency	I Intoxication	C Congenital and Collagen	A Autoimmune Allergic	T Trauma	E Endocrine
Pharynx		Tonsillitis Diphtheria		Plummer–Vinson syndrome			Vincent angina	Foreign body	
Esophagus	Aortic aneurysm	Esophagitis Chagas disease	Carcinoma		Lye stricture	Achalasia scleroderma		Foreign body	
Stomach		Gastritis Ulcers	Carcinoma	Pernicious Anemia	Aspirin Reserpine	Pyloric stenosis Cascade stomach			Gastrinoma Hyperparathyroidism
Duodenum		Ulcers Duodenitis Strongyloides				Duodenal atresia or stenosis			Gastrinoma
Jejunum and Ileum	Mesenteric thrombosis	Tinea solium and other parasites (e.g., Salmonella, Shigella)	Carcinoid Sarcoma	Pellagra Malabsorption syndrome	Botulism	Whipple disease Meckel diverticulum	Regional enteritis	Ruptured viscus	Vasoactive intestinal peptide syndrome
Appendix		Appendicitis	Carcinoid					Rupture Fecalith	
Colon	Mesenteric thrombosis	Amebic colitis Staphylococcal colitis	Carcinoma			Malrotation Diverticulum	Ulcerative colitis Granulomatous colitis	Ruptured viscus	
Gallbladder		Cholecystitis	Cholangioma					Stone	
Pancreas		Pancreatitis	Pancreatic cyst and carcinoma			Mucoviscidosis			
Kidneys	Renal artery thrombosis	Pyelonephritis	Carcinoma with obstruction		Drug neuropathy	Polycystic kidney	Glomerulonephritis	Rupture Stone Obstruction	
Pelvic Organs	Torsion of ovary or cyst	Pelvic inflammatory disease	Ectopic pregnancy					Induced abortion	
Blood	Chronic anemia		Leukemia Multiple myeloma	Iron deficiency anemia	Uremia				

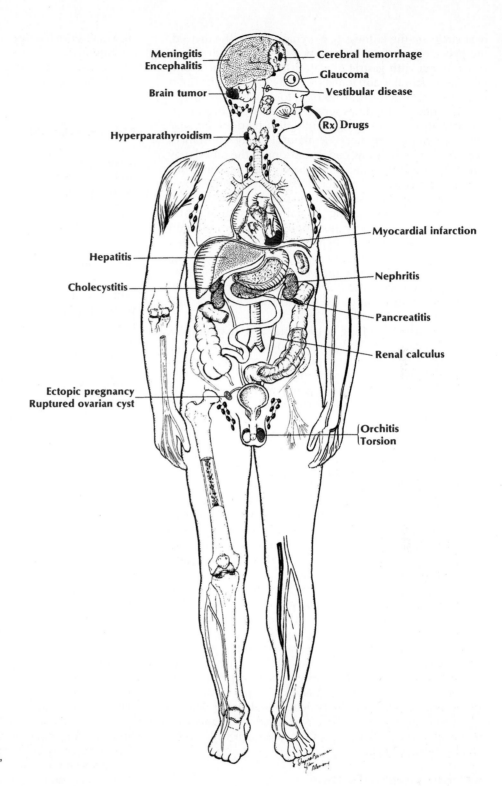

● **FIGURE 4** Nausea and vomiting, systemic causes.

be considered in the jejunum and ileum. Parasites such as *Strongyloides, Ascaris,* and *Taenia solium* must also be considered in this part of the GI tract.

An obstructed Meckel **diverticulum** or **appendix** may present with vomiting. In the large bowel, ulcerative colitis, amebiasis, and neoplasms should be considered. Mesenteric thrombosis can cause vomiting regardless of

which portion of the intestine it involves. Acute viral or bacterial enteritis is associated with nausea and vomiting, but almost invariably there is diarrhea in botulism, salmonellosis, and shigellosis.

In the next circle in the target one encounters cholecystitis and cholelithiasis, pancreatitis, gastrinomas, pancreatic cysts, peritonitis, and myocardial infarction. In the next circle are the kidneys (e.g., renal stones), the thyroid, the pelvic organs (e.g., ectopic pregnancy), and the lungs (pneumonia with gastric dilatation). The next circle contains the vestibular apparatus (Ménière disease), the brain (e.g., tumor), and the testicles (e.g., torsion and orchitis).

The target method has served us well, but a biochemical evaluation of vomiting should also be done because many foreign substances or natural body substances occurring in high or low concentrations in the blood may affect the vomiting centers or cause a paralytic ileus. Thus uremia, increased ammonia and nitrogen breakdown products in hepatic disease, and hypokalemia and hyperkalemia may cause vomiting. Alterations in sodium, chloride, and CO_2 may also cause vomiting. More important is hypercalcemia due to hyperparathyroidism or other causes. Almost any drug can cause nausea and vomiting. When intractable nausea and vomiting develops following the flu, consider Reye syndrome. Vitamin A intoxication may cause increased intracranial pressure and vomiting in children.

In summary, vomiting is best analyzed anatomically. Physiologically, the symptoms of vomiting should suggest obstruction, either functional or mechanical. When all studies (see page 314) are normal, consider a neuropsychiatric disorder. Remember migraine may cause vomiting without headache, especially in children.

● Approach to the Diagnosis

First ask if the patient is on any drugs. Almost any drugs can cause nausea and vomiting, especially digoxin, nonsteroidal anti-inflammatory drugs, aspirin, iron preparations, and narcotics. Also ask if the patient is alcoholic. The association of other symptoms and signs is essential in pinpointing the diagnosis of vomiting. For example, vomiting with tinnitus and vertigo suggests Ménière disease, whereas vomiting with hematemesis suggests gastritis, esophageal varices, and gastric ulcers. Vomiting with significant abdominal pain will most likely be due to appendicitis, cholecystitis, pancreatitis, or intestinal obstruction. The laboratory workup should include a flat plate of the abdomen, upper GI series, esophagram, cholecystogram, gastric analysis, serum electrolytes, and amylase and lipase levels. Stools for occult blood, ova, and parasites are usually indicated. Gastroscopy and esophagoscopy are often indicated in the acute case, but an exploratory laparotomy should not be delayed if the patient's condition is deteriorating and pancreatitis has been excluded. In infants with duodenal atresia, a flat plate of the abdomen will show a "double bubble" sign.

● Other Useful Tests

1. CBC (anemia, infection)
2. Chemistry panel (liver disease, uremia)
3. Serial electrocardiograms and cardiac enzymes (myocardial infarction)
4. Pregnancy test (ectopic pregnancy)
5. Arterial blood gases (pulmonary embolism)
6. Lung scan (pulmonary embolism)
7. Gallbladder sonogram (gallstones)
8. Small-bowel series (neoplasm, diverticulum, regional enteritis)
9. CT scan of the abdomen (neoplasm, abscess)
10. Laparoscopy (neoplasm of pancreas or liver)
11. Angiogram (mesenteric thrombosis)

NECK MASS

Anatomy is the most important basic science used in developing the differential diagnosis in the case of a neck mass. **Histology** is then applied to each anatomic structure to further develop the list. As with any mass, a neck mass may be due to the proliferation of tissues in any of the anatomic structures, a displacement or malposition of tissues or anatomic structures, or the presence of fluid, air, bleeding, or other substances foreign to the neck.

Visualize the anatomy of the neck and think of the skin, thyroid, lymph nodes, trachea, esophagus, jugular veins, carotid arteries, brachial plexus, cervical spine, and muscles. Thus, taking **thyroid** enlargement, hypertrophy and cystic formation (endemic goiter), hyperplasia (Graves disease), neoplasm (adenomas and carcinomas), thyroiditis (subacute or Hashimoto), cyst (colloid type), and hemorrhage come to mind. Thyroglossal duct cysts also occur.

Lymph nodes may be enlarged by many inflammatory diseases, but when they present as an isolated mass they are usually infiltrated with Hodgkin lymphoma or a metastatic carcinoma from the thyroid, lungs, breast, or stomach. Tuberculosis, actinomycosis, and other chronic inflammatory diseases may present this way. **Tracheal** enlargement is rarely a problem in differential diagnosis, but bronchial cleft cysts may present as a mass. Pulsion diverticula are the main masses of **esophageal** origin, but carcinoma of the esophagus may involve the upper third on rare occasions. There is rarely a problem distinguishing **jugular veins** from a mass of other origin. **Carotid or subclavian artery** aneurysms are distinguished by their pulsatile nature; occasionally, an aortic aneurysm may be felt in the neck. When there is severe atherosclerotic disease of the carotids, one or both may be felt as a "lead pipe" in the neck. Neurofibromas of the **brachial plexus** are rare but must be considered. Any neoplasm that metastasizes to the **cervical spine** may spread into the neck; a plasmacytoma is likely to do this in multiple myeloma. A cervical rib may occasionally be felt in the neck. Finally, a large scalenus anterior muscle may be felt as a mass in the neck.

Neoplasms of the skin present here, as elsewhere (e.g., lipoma). Abnormal accumulations of fluid, air, or other substances in colloid cysts and bronchial cleft cysts have already been mentioned, but what about carbuncles, sebaceous cysts, and angioneurotic edema? Cystic hygromas present from birth contain a serous or mucoid material and may be huge. Finally, subcutaneous emphysema must not be forgotten. These conditions are illustrated in Table 47.

● Approach to the Diagnosis

The clinical picture will help to determine the diagnosis in many cases. For example, a neck mass with hemoptysis suggests carcinoma of the lung with metastasis to the lymph

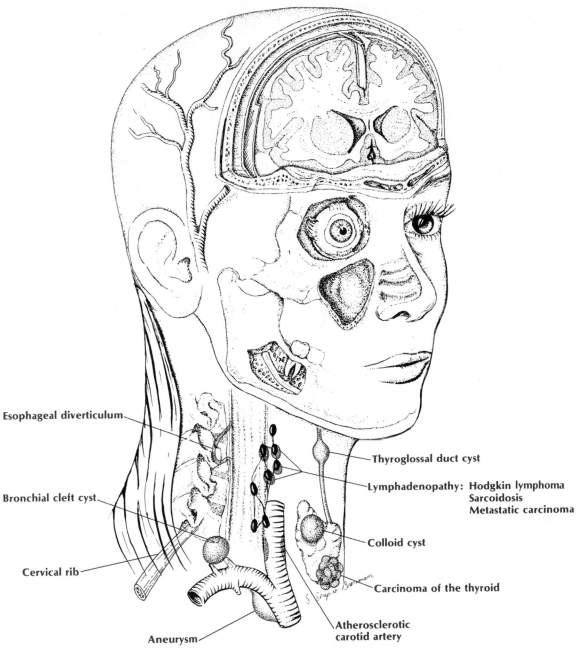

Esophageal diverticulum

Thyroglossal duct cyst

Lymphadenopathy: **Hodgkin lymphoma**
Sarcoidosis
Metastatic carcinoma

Bronchial cleft cyst

Colloid cyst

Cervical rib

Carcinoma of the thyroid

Aneurysm

Atherosclerotic
carotid artery

● **FIGURE 5** Neck mass.

node. A diffuse, tender, and enlarged thyroid suggests subacute thyroiditis. If the mass increases in size after swallowing food or liquid, an esophageal diverticulum is likely. A thyroglossal duct cyst moves on protruding the tongue.

The workup will depend on the type of lesion suspected. If the mass is suspected to be an enlarged lymph node, exploration and biopsy may be appropriate. An esophageal diverticulum can be ruled out by a barium swallow or esophagoscopy. A thyroid profile will show an increased T_4 in subacute thyroiditis. A radioiodine uptake and scan may be indicated to diagnose other thyroid masses. A thyroid cyst may be suspected by ultrasonography or CT scan, but it is confirmed by fine needle aspiration. If the mass

is connected to the cervical spine, a CT scan or magnetic resonance imaging (MRI) of the cervical spine should be ordered. One can now see that the diagnostic workup can be developed by visualizing the anatomy of the area.

● **Other Useful Tests**

1. CBC
2. Sedimentation rate (inflammation)
3. Chest x-ray (neoplasm, tuberculosis, fungal disease)
4. X-ray of cervical spine (neoplasm)
5. Tuberculin test (tuberculosis)
6. Serum protein electrophoresis (multiple myeloma)

TABLE 47 Neck Mass

	V Vascular	I Inflammatory	N Neoplasm	D Degenerative	I Intoxication	C Congenital	A Allergic and Autoimmune	T Trauma	E Endocrine
Skin		Subcutaneous emphysema	Lipoma Angioma Carcinoma			Cystic hygroma	Angioneurotic edema	Contusion Fractured rib	
Thyroid		Cyst (colloid type) Thyroiditis	Adenoma Carcinoma	Endemic goiter					Graves disease Thyroid carcinoma
Lymph Nodes		Tuberculosis Actinomycosis Lymphadenitis	Hodgkin lymphoma Metastatic carcinoma				Sarcoidosis		
Trachea		Bronchial cleft cyst							
Esophagus			Carcinoma of esophagus			Diverticulum of esophagus		Surgical esophageal bypass	
Jugular Veins	Thrombosis Varicocele Obstruction		Hemangioma					Hemorrhage	
Carotid Arteries	Aneurysms			Atherosclerotic disease				Contusion	
Brachial Plexus			Neurofibroma						
Cervical Spine		Tuberculosis	Multiple myeloma Metastatic carcinoma			Cervical rib		Fracture Sprain Contusion	
Muscles of Neck		Myositis	Rhabdomyosarcoma			Scalenus anticus			

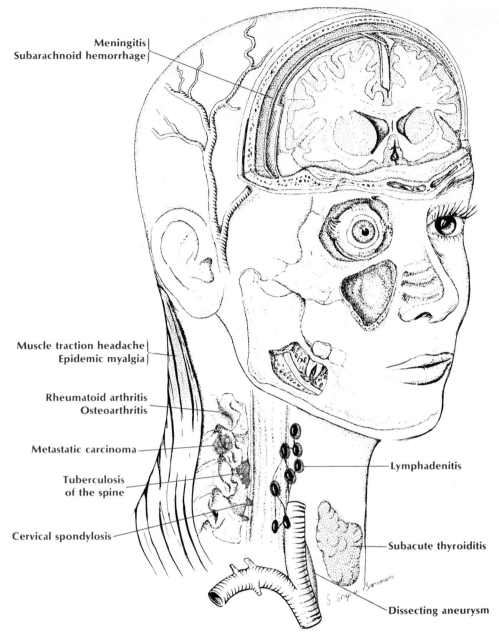

Meningitis
Subarachnoid hemorrhage

Muscle traction headache
Epidemic myalgia

Rheumatoid arthritis
Osteoarthritis

Metastatic carcinoma

Tuberculosis
of the spine

Cervical spondylosis

Lymphadenitis

Subacute thyroiditis

Dissecting aneurysm

● **FIGURE 6** Neck pain.

7. Bone scan (osteomyelitis, neoplasm)
8. Bronchoscopy (neoplasm of the lung)
9. CT scan of the mediastinum (neoplasm, superior vena cava syndrome)
10. CT scan of the neck (thyroid malignancies)

NECK PAIN

The analysis of the cause of neck pain is similar to that of headache. First, the anatomic components are distinguished, then the various etiologies are applied to each (Table 48). Moving from the skin to the spinal cord layer by layer, we encounter the fascia, muscles, arteries, veins, brachial and cervical plexus, and lymph nodes. Next are the esophagus, trachea, and thyroid gland. Finally, there is the cervical spine encircling the spinal cord and meninges and designed to allow uninfringed exit of the cervical nerve roots.

Taking each of these structures and applying the etiologic categories of **MINT**, we can arrive at a respectable differential diagnosis of neck pain. Inflammation and trauma are the principal causes. The **skin** may be involved by herpes zoster, cellulitis, contusions, and lacerations. An infected bronchial cleft cyst may occasionally be the offender. In the **muscle** and **fascia**, one encounters fibromyositis, dermatomyositis, and trichinosis as well as traumatic contusions and pulled or torn ligaments (strains). Remember Ludwig's angina, which is a painful swelling under the chin caused by the spread of a dental abscess to the neck! The muscles

TABLE 48	Neck Pain			
	M **Malformation**	**I** **Inflammation**	**N** **Neoplasm**	**T** **Trauma**
Skin		Herpes zoster Cellulitis Carbuncle		Contusion Laceration
Muscle and Fascia		Epidemic myalgia Trichinosis		
Arteries	Dissecting aneurysm Subarachnoid hemorrhage from cerebral aneurysm	Temporal arteritis		Hemorrhage
Veins		Thrombophlebitis		Hemorrhage
Lymph Nodes		Lymphadenitis	Hodgkin lymphoma	
		Tuberculosis	Metastatic carcinoma	
Nerves	Cervical rib Scalenus anticus syndrome	Brachial plexus neuritis	Pancoast tumor	Contusion Laceration Compression
Thyroid		Subacute thyroiditis Riedel struma	Metastatic thyroid carcinoma	Ruptured colloid cyst
Esophagus	Congenital diverticulum	Esophagitis	Carcinoma	Pulsion diverticulum
Cervical Spine	Platybasia	Rheumatoid arthritis Tuberculosis Osteoarthritis	Metastatic carcinoma Spinal cord tumor	Fracture Herniated disc

may be involved by tension headache, poor posture, and occasionally by epidemic myalgia. Meningitis causes nuchal rigidity and neck pain. Torticollis causes painful spasms, but the jerking of the neck makes the condition obvious.

The **arteries** of the neck are infrequently tender or painful as are most aneurysms (aside from dissecting aneurysms) unless they compress adjacent structures. Arteritis is unusual here, but a common carotid thrombosis may be tender and painful. Referred pain from angina pectoris is not uncommon.

As with the arteries, it is rare for the **jugular veins** and smaller veins of the neck to cause pain by thrombosis or rupture; however, it occasionally happens in superior vena cava obstruction. In contrast, the **lymph nodes** are a frequent site of neck pain. They are usually enlarged and tender in association with pharyngitis, otitis media, sinusitis, dental abscesses, and mediastinitis.

The **brachial plexus** may be involved by a primary neuritis or by compression from a scalenus anticus syndrome, a Pancoast tumor, the clavical (costoclavicular) syndrome, or a cervical rib. More often, the roots are compressed by diseases of the **spine**, such as a herniated disk, fracture, cervical spondylosis, tuberculous or nontuberculous osteomyelitis, and primary or metastatic tumors of the spine and spinal cord. In the case of the **spinal cord**, one should

also remember the meninges as a cause of neck pain in meningitis, arachnoiditis, and subarachnoid hemorrhage. Rheumatoid arthritis of the spine will cause neck pain without compression.

The esophagus is not usually a cause of neck pain, but pain may be referred to the neck from a hiatal hernia or subdiaphragmatic abscess. Pulsion diverticula of the esophagus may also compress adjacent structures and cause painful symptoms. Like the esophagus, the **trachea** is an infrequent source of neck pain, but occasionally acute laryngotracheitis will be the source of severe pain. Finally, **subacute thyroiditis** and inflammatory or obstructive lesions of the salivary glands may be the offenders in neck pain, even though the patient complains of a sore throat.

● Approach to the Diagnosis

The patient who presents with neck pain most commonly has a cervical sprain or muscle contraction headache. However, we must rule out more serious pathology such as meningitis, subarachnoid hemorrhage, herniated disks, and neoplasms before we send the patient home with a collar and a bag of pills. This means checking for nuchal rigidity, doing a thorough neurologic examination, and checking for a thyroid or lymph node mass. If the neurologic examination is abnormal, referral to a neurologist or a neurosurgeon is indicated before ordering expensive diagnostic tests.

If the neurologic examination is normal and there are no neck masses or other significant findings, conservative treatment may be initiated without ordering expensive diagnostic tests. However, most physicians consider it wise to at least do plain films of the cervical spine. Careful and close follow-up is necessary so that something serious is not missed in these cases. When the pain persists despite adequate medical therapy, an MRI of the cervical spine should be done as well as an electromyogram. Again, it is wise to consult a neurologist first. Always keep in mind that the pain may be referred from the heart, lungs, esophagus, or gallbladder. Act accordingly.

● Other Useful Tests

1. CBC
2. Sedimentation rate (subacute thyroiditis)
3. FT$_4$, thyrotropin (subacute thyroiditis)
4. Chest x-ray (neoplasm, mediastinal tumor)
5. Exercise tolerance test (coronary insufficiency)
6. Arthritis panel
7. Chemistry panel (bone metastasis)
8. Serum protein electrophoresis (multiple myeloma)
9. Upper GI series and esophagram (reflux esophagitis and hiatal hernia)
10. Gallbladder sonogram (cholecystitis)
11. MRI of the cervical spine (herniated disk)
12. Cervical myelogram (tumor, herniated disk)
13. Bone scan (osteomyelitis, metastasis, small fractures)

Case Presentation #69

A 45-year-old Filipino female nurse complained of pain in the neck that began after turning a patient over in bed. Two weeks prior to admission, the pain began radiating down her right arm.

Question #1. Utilizing your knowledge of anatomy, what is your differential diagnosis?

Neurologic examination revealed loss of sensation to touch, pain in the right thumb, and diminished right biceps reflex.

Question #2. What is your diagnosis now?

(See Appendix B for the answers.)

NIGHTMARES

The mnemonic **PINT** will help to recall the causes of nightmares.

P—Psychiatric causes include anxiety, neurosis, and the various psychoses.
I—Inflammation prompts the recall of nightmares associated with systemic infections, and **intoxication** brings to mind the nightmares due to alcohol and drugs such as the benzodiazepines.

N—Neurologic disorders prompt the recall of epilepsy.
T—Trauma facilitates the recall of head injury as a common cause of nightmares.

● Approach to the Diagnosis

If an infectious disease is suspected, a CBC, sedimentation rate, and chemistry panel should be done. Alcohol- or drug-induced nightmares may be diagnosed by the history and a drug screen. The history should also be useful in cases of head injury, especially when questioning the family or closely associated persons. If epilepsy is suspected, a wake-and-sleep electroencephalogram should be ordered; a trial of anticonvulsants may be necessary to rule out epilepsy. It may be useful to order a psychiatric consult early in the evaluation.

NOCTURIA

The differential diagnosis of nocturia is similar to that of polyuria. A pathophysiologic analysis of the symptoms would indicate that the patient is producing excessive urine at night, there is an obstruction to the output of urine so that the bladder cannot be emptied fully on one voiding, or there is an irritative focus in the urinary tract stimulating the patient to urinate more frequently.

1. **Excessive urine production at night:** This category includes all the causes of polyuria: diabetes insipidus, diabetes mellitus, hyperthyroidism, diuretic drugs, nephrogenic diabetes insipidus, and chronic nephritis. In addition, the one condition that produces excessive urine output almost exclusively at night—congestive heart failure—must be considered. In heart failure, edema accumulates in the extremities during the day while the patient is in the upright position and is returned to the circulation and poured out through the kidneys at night while the patient is in the recumbent position.
2. **Obstructive uropathy:** Bladder neck obstruction by a calculus, enlarged or inflamed prostate, median bar hypertrophy, or urethral stricture is a condition to consider here. Neurogenic bladder from poliomyelitis, multiple sclerosis, and other spinal cord diseases must also be considered.
3. **Irritative focus in the urinary tract:** Nocturia may result from inflammation of the bladder, prostate, urethra, and kidney on this basis. Occasionally a bladder tumor or prostate carcinoma may be the irritative focus. Inflammation of the vagina, fallopian tubes, and rectum are also occasionally responsible.

● Approach to the Diagnosis

The workup of nocturia is essentially the same as the workup of polyuria and urinary frequency (see page 345). Obviously, the search for obstruction and infection are most important. Venous pressure, circulation time, and pulmonary function studies to rule out congestive heart failure should be done if the urinary tract is clean.

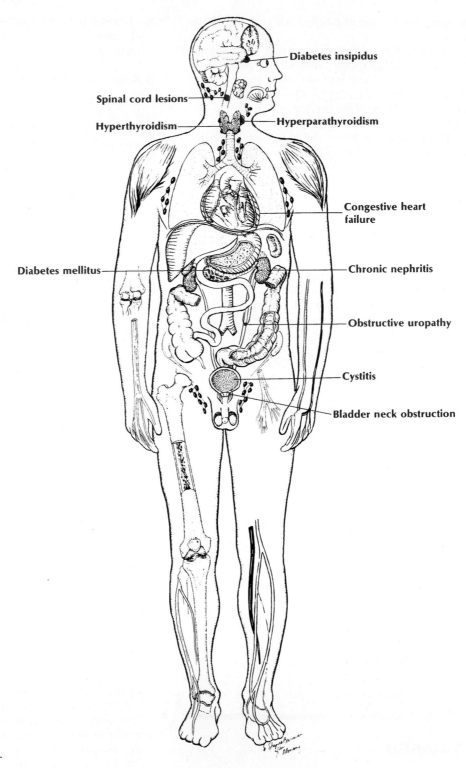

Diabetes insipidus

Spinal cord lesions

Hyperthyroidism

Hyperparathyroidism

Congestive heart failure

Chronic nephritis

Diabetes mellitus

Obstructive uropathy

Cystitis

Bladder neck obstruction

● **FIGURE 7** Nocturia.

NOSE, REGURGITATION OF FOOD THROUGH

Here again the mnemonic **MINT** will facilitate the recall of the many possibilities.

M—Malformation brings to mind cleft palate and a congenital short soft palate.

I—Inflammation prompts the recall of disorders that destroy the palate such as syphilis, leprosy, and tuberculosis.

N—Neurologic disorders that paralyze the palate include poliomyelitis, Guillain–Barré syndrome, pseudobulbar palsy, brainstem tumors, and myasthenia gravis.

T—Trauma should make one suspect palatal fenestration from gunshot wounds or surgery, posttonsillectomy weakness, and trauma to the brain stem.

● Approach to the Diagnosis

Cleft palate and many other conditions will be diagnosed by a careful nose and throat examination; all that is necessary is a referral to an otolaryngologist. If the local examination is negative, a referral to a neurologist is probably in order. Myasthenia gravis is diagnosed by a Tension test or acetylcholine receptor antibody titers; an MRI of the brain will diagnose tumors, multiple sclerosis, and other causes of pseudobulbar palsy; and a spinal fluid analysis is necessary to diagnose Guillain–Barré syndrome and poliomyelitis.

NUCHAL RIGIDITY

Finding nuchal rigidity on examination has almost invariably prompted the diagnosis of meningitis and lumbar puncture, but the astute clinician will want to consider other possibilities to avoid a potentially hazardous procedure. **Anatomy** is the key. Visualize the structures of the neck and the many causes come quickly to mind.

Cellulitis of the back of the neck or a carbuncle may be the cause in the **skin**. The **muscles** of the neck may be rigid from parkinsonism or pyramidal tract disease. Diseases of

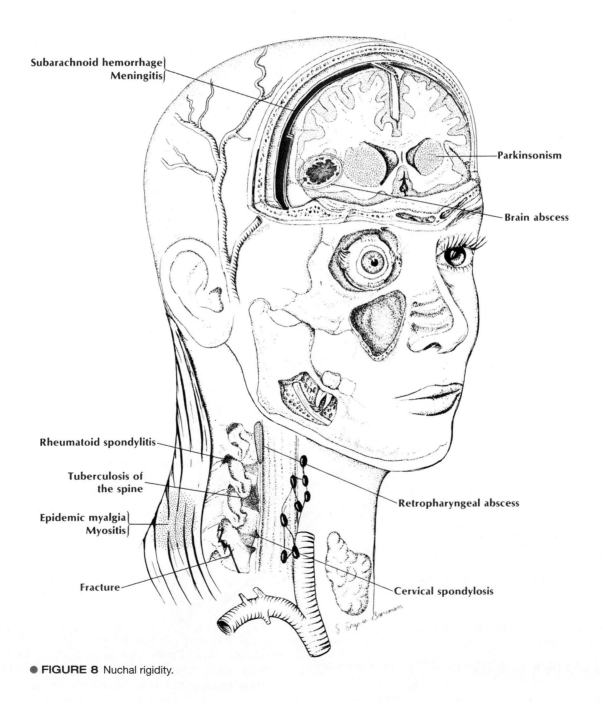

● **FIGURE 8** Nuchal rigidity.

the **spine** such as cervical spondylosis, rheumatoid spondylitis, and tuberculosis may cause nuchal rigidity. An acute fracture of the cervical spine should be considered if no history can be obtained. The respiratory tree recalls retropharyngeal abscess, mediastinal emphysema, and endotracheal intubation. Finally, the spinal cord and meninges may be involved by meningitis, epidural abscess, subarachnoid hemorrhage, and primary and metastatic tumors, resulting in nuchal rigidity.

● Approach to the Diagnosis

The workup of nuchal rigidity requires a good history, but if one is unobtainable, no spinal tap should be performed until the cervical spine is x-rayed and the eyegrounds are examined. Even with a good history, a spinal tap should be withheld if there is papilledema: A neurosurgeon should be consulted immediately under these circumstances. In a patient with fever, nuchal rigidity, no papilledema, and no focal neurologic signs (particularly a dilated pupil), a spinal tap can be performed for diagnosis and immediate therapy. It is preferable, however, to have CT scan results in hand first. Meningitis or a subarachnoid hemorrhage is frequently found in these circumstances. CT scans and x-rays of the cervical spine and skull will still be indicated in cases where the diagnosis remains obscure.

NYSTAGMUS

Why not consider the differential diagnosis of nystagmus under vertigo, because **anatomic pathophysiology** is the key to the differential in both? The reason is that there are two forms of nystagmus (ocular and cerebellar) that do not necessarily occur with vertigo. In addition to these two categories, nystagmus that usually occurs with vertigo is divided into nystagmus of middle ear diseases, nystagmus of inner ear diseases, nystagmus due to auditory nerve involvement, and nystagmus due to brain stem and cerebral diseases.

1. **Ocular nystagmus:** This is a pendular to-and-fro nystagmus with no fast component, which is usually due to congenital visual defects but which may be due to working in poor lighting (miner's nystagmus). It is really an effort of the eye to find a better visual image. Infants with spasmus nutans have this type of nystagmus.
2. **Middle ear disorders:** Nystagmus may result from otitis media, which causes associated inflammation of the labyrinth.
3. **Inner ear diseases:** Labyrinthitis may be viral, postinfectious, traumatic, or toxic (e.g., from salicylates, quinine, streptomycin, or gentamycin). A cholesteatoma also causes nystagmus, as does Ménière disease.
4. **Auditory nerve:** Acoustic neuromas, internal auditory artery occlusions, or aneurysms and basilar meningitis

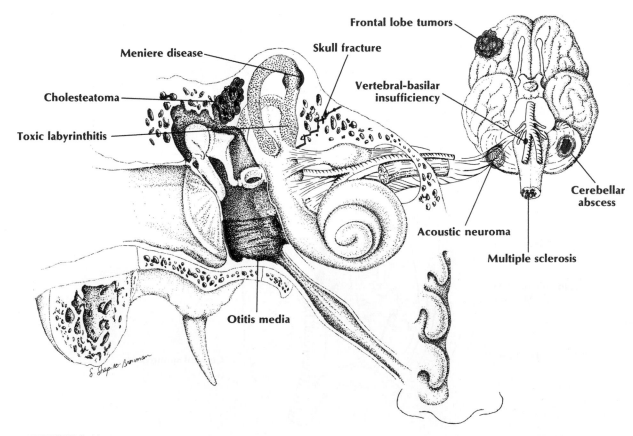

● **FIGURE 9** Nystagmus.

may be considered in this category. Diabetic neuritis is another cause.

5. **Brain stem:** Transient ischemic attack (TIA) from basilar artery insufficiency, multiple sclerosis, gliomas, syphilis, and tuberculosis are the major conditions to consider here. Thrombi, emboli, and hemorrhages in the branches of the basilar artery are important too. With TIA the possibility of migraine and emboli from SBE or atrial fibrillation should be investigated. Dissemination encephalomyelitis and other forms of encephalitis should not be overlooked. Degenerative diseases such as syringobulbia and olivopontocerebellar atrophy are possibilities.

6. **Cerebellum:** In addition to the causes of nystagmus mentioned under brain stem, the physician should consider cerebellar tumors, abscesses, posterior fossa subdural hematomas, and diphenylhydantoin toxicity, as well as Friedreich ataxia and other forms of hereditary cerebellar ataxia. Alcoholic cerebellar degeneration is a significant cause of nystagmus. Acute cerebellar ataxia of children cannot be forgotten. Platybasia may compress the cerebellum and cause nystagmus. Cerebellar degeneration associated with carcinoma of the lung is often misdiagnosed.

7. **Cerebrum:** Curiously enough, frontal lobe tumors may cause nystagmus. Head injuries, encephalitis, chronic subdural hematomas, occipital meningiomas, and the aura of an epileptic seizure may also cause nystagmus.

● Approach to the Diagnosis

The workup here is similar to that of vertigo. Nystagmus without other signs of central nervous system disease is usually ocular or peripheral in the middle or inner ear. Vertigo is almost invariably present in nystagmus of aural origin. Nystagmus with long tract signs such as hemiplegia or hemianesthesia is invariably brain stem in origin. Purely cerebellar nystagmus is not easily fatigued and is associated with dyskinesia and dyssynergia of the extremities as well as ataxia. There are no long tract or cranial nerve signs. Nystagmus with vertigo, nausea, vomiting, tinnitus, and deafness suggests Ménière disease.

Confirmation of the diagnosis is made by audiograms, caloric tests, skull x-rays (with special views of the mastoids and petrous bones), angiography, CT scans, and myelography. MRI scans are useful, especially in diagnosing brain stem lesions and multiple sclerosis. They also provide a better view of the internal auditory canal. A spinal tap will help in the diagnosis of multiple sclerosis and neurolues as well as acoustic neuromas.

OBESITY

The differential diagnosis of obesity, like that of weight loss, is best developed using **physiology** because most cases of obesity are caused by an absolute increased intake of calories or a relative increased intake of calories over output of energy. Fluid retention may also be associated with weight gain.

Increased intake of calories: This type of obesity is due to an increased appetite. Under this heading are idiopathic obesity, psychogenic obesity, hypothalamic obesity (due to pituitary tumors and other lesions affecting the hypothalamus), islet cell adenomas and carcinomas (causing hypoglycemia and, consequently, a big appetite), early stages of diabetes mellitus when functional hypoglycemia is common, Cushing syndrome and exogenous corticosteroids (which increase appetite), and alcoholism, which stimulates the appetite but which also adds calories in the alcohol (up to 250 calories per cocktail). Polycystic ovary syndrome causes increased appetite, but the hirsutism is a dead giveaway.

Decreased output of energy: Under this heading should be listed hypothyroidism and possibly hypogonadism (such as Klinefelter syndrome), where the motivation to work or exercise may be impaired. Mild pituitary insufficiency (as in Sheehan or Fröhlich syndrome) may also cause obesity by this mechanism. A primary growth hormone deficiency in adults may cause obesity. This type of obesity may be occupational (e.g., white-collar workers) or environmental (i.e., watching television all day).

"Obesity" due to fluid retention: This increase is in reality an increase in weight from fluid retention. Inappropriate antidiuretic hormone syndromes such as those that occur in carcinoma of the lung, hypothalamic lesions, and drugs are the most important obscure causes. Congestive heart failure, nephrosis, cirrhosis, beriberi, and myxedema rank as significant among the obvious causes.

Miscellaneous causes: Heredity is a cause of obesity, but the physiologic mechanism is uncertain. Several drugs may cause obesity including corticosteroids, tricyclic antidepressants, selective serotonin reuptake inhibitors, oral contraceptives, and estrogen.

● Approach to the Diagnosis

It would be ridiculous to do a complete endocrine workup on every case of obesity, but thyroid function studies may be worthwhile. Patients who fail to lose weight on a strict diet may require hospitalization with observation. If they still fail to lose weight, a complete endocrine workup would seem to be indicated.

● Other Useful Tests

1. 48-hour fast with glucose monitoring (insulinoma)
2. Plasma insulin (insulinoma)
3. C-peptide (insulinoma)
4. Serum cortisol (Cushing syndrome)
5. Dexamethasone suppression test (Cushing syndrome)
6. Pelvic sonogram (polycystic ovary)
7. Chromosomal analysis (Klinefelter syndrome)
8. Psychiatry consult

Case Presentation #70

A 14-year-old boy is brought to your office by his mother because of obesity. She complains that at times he has a ravenous appetite.

Question #1. Utilizing your knowledge of physiology, what is your differential diagnosis?

Your examination reveals mild hypertension, acne, and purple abdominal striae.

Question #2. What is your diagnosis now?

(See Appendix B for your answers.)

ORAL OR LINGUAL MASS

Most of these lesions are tumors, but because some are caused by other etiologies, it is well to use the mnemonic **MINT** to review the possibilities.

M—Malformations include dermoid cysts, ranula, Wharton duct cysts or stones, mucous cysts, and thyroglossal cysts.

I—Inflammation should suggest peritonsillar abscesses, tonsillitis, sialadenitis, Ludwig angina, and actinomycosis. Alveolar abscesses and granulomas may present as a mass inside the mouth.

N—Neoplasms are most commonly squamous cell carcinomas and are usually ulcerated. Angiomas, lipomas, papillomas, and sarcomas also occur.

T—Trauma suggests subperiosteal and submucosal hematomas and fractures–dislocations.

● Approach to the Diagnosis

Most of these lesions are referred to the oral surgeon for diagnosis and treatment, so an elaborate discussion of the workup is unnecessary in a text of this scope.

Obviously, cultures should be made in cases of suspected infectious granulomas, whereas biopsy or excision is the main diagnostic tool for neoplasms.

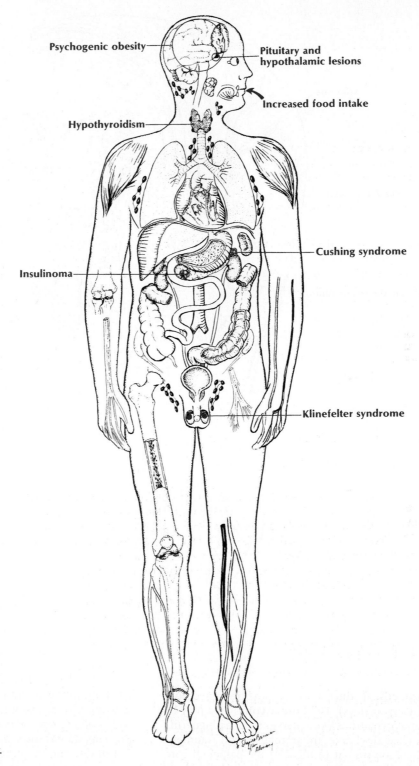

● **FIGURE 1** Obesity.

ORBITAL DISCHARGE

A clear or purulent discharge from the eye is usually due to allergy or infection, but a few notable exceptions exist. In addition to using **anatomy** to formulate the list of diagnostic possibilities, it is well to apply the mnemonic **MINT** to the various anatomic components. Beginning with the **eyelids**, one should recall the following:

M—Malformations like a chalazion, ectropion, and entropion

I—Inflammatory conditions like blepharitis, a hordeolum (stye), and allergic or infectious conjunctivitis

N—Neoplasms such as squamous cell carcinoma and angioma

T—Traumatic conditions, especially foreign bodies

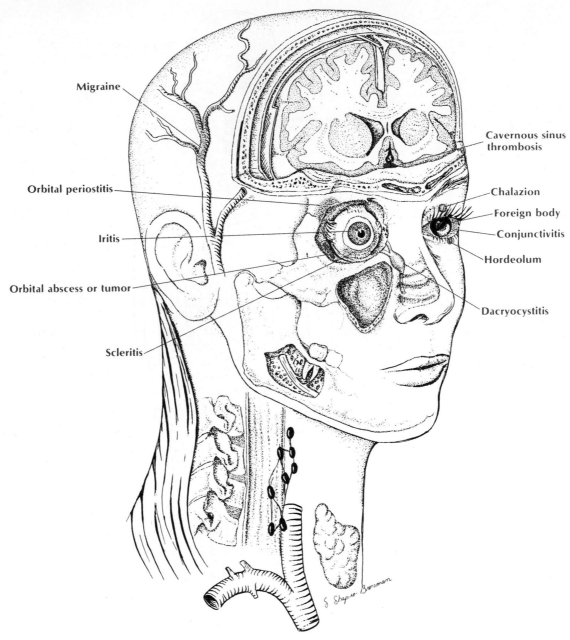

● **FIGURE 2** Orbital discharge.

The **nasolacrimal duct** may become inflamed and obstructed (dacryocystitis). The **bulbar conjuctiva** may be involved by malformations like a pterygium or a pinguecula and cause a clear discharge. Inflammatory and traumatic conditions here are similar to those of the palpebral conjunctiva. It is well to mention toxic causes of a nonbloody discharge, such as irritation from tobacco smoke, cold, and irritating gases; chronic alcoholism, arsenic poisoning, and iodism may cause a clear discharge.

Separating the **eyeball** into its various components, one recalls the **cornea** and immediately one should think of a foreign body of the cornea or of a laceration, a keratitis, and malformations like keratoconus. Next, the **iris** suggests iritis as a cause of discharge, but by using the mnemonic one will

not forget albinism as a cause of excessive tearing. In addition, the iris angle should remind one of acute glaucoma, which often presents with lacrimation as well as with pain. The **lens** should suggest refractive errors as a major cause of a clear discharge and predisposition to infection of the lids. Finally, the **sclera** is the site of episcleritis and scleritis, which are frequently associated with a nonbloody discharge.

Turning to the **lacrimal gland**, one should remember mumps of this gland and other infections. The **vascular supply** to the eye should suggest the tearful discharge of histamine cephalalgia and obstruction of the venous drainage by a cavernous sinus thrombosis. Paralysis of the **muscles** of the eye, especially the facial nerve, creates a discharge by excessive exposure to dust and air.

● Approach to the Diagnosis

Anatomy has served us well in developing a differential, although the cause of a discharge from the eye is often easy to establish. Foreign bodies, trauma, toxins, and conjunctivitis are the conditions most commonly responsible. This is why in the approach to the diagnosis one will first examine the eye carefully under magnification and use fluorescein to rule out a foreign body or laceration. Then, a careful history of exposure to toxins (e.g., industrial) is in order. Finally, if the discharge is unilateral, a smear and culture of specific bacteria are valuable before treatment. If it is bilateral, allergy should be considered, as well as refractive errors. Tonometry should be performed. Referral to an ophthalmologist may be appropriate at any one of these stages (when in doubt, refer it out).

● Other Useful Tests

1. Complete blood count and differential
2. Sedimentation rate
3. Urinalysis
4. Smear and culture of discharge
5. Venereal disease research laboratory test
6. Tuberculin test
7. Antinuclear antibody test (uveitis)
8. Smear for eosinophils (allergic conjunctivitis)
9. Tonometry (glaucoma)
10. Refraction
11. Thyroid function test (Graves disease)
12. Visual fields
13. X-ray of skull
14. X-ray of sinuses (acute sinusitis)
15. Sonogram
16. Computed tomography scan (orbital tumor)
17. Biopsy
18. Exploratory surgery
19. Mumps skin test
20. Histamine test (histamine cephalalgia)

ORBITAL MASS

Because most orbital masses cause exophthalmos, the differential diagnosis of the two is very similar (for illustration, see section on exophthalmos, page 158). The best method to use to arrive at the causes is to visualize the **anatomy** of the orbit and then to think of the mnemonic **MINT**.

1. **Subcutaneous tissue:** Subcutaneous tissue proliferation in the orbit occurs in hyperthyroidism. There may be an orbital cellulitis or orbital hemorrhage into the subcutaneous tissue. Wegener granulomatosis, orbital cysts, sarcomas, and metastatic carcinomas may occur here.
2. **Eyeballs:** An orbital echinococcal cyst may occur. Tumors, infections, and trauma to the eyeball may occasionally spread to the orbit.
3. **Veins:** These are distended in cavernous sinus thrombosis, carotid–cavernous fistulas, and hemangiomas.
4. **Arteries:** Aneurysms of the ophthalmic artery are rare, but they may cause an orbital mass.
5. **Lacrimal gland:** Tumors and inflammation of this gland (e.g., in Boeck sarcoid) should be remembered.
6. **Sinuses:** Inflammatory lesions and tumors of the sinuses may spread to the orbit.
7. **Bone:** Sphenoid ridge meningiomas, metastatic carcinomas, tuberculous, syphilitic orbital periostitis, and Hodgkin lymphoma may involve the bones of the orbit. Orbital fractures and hematomas may result from trauma.

The workup of these lesions is similar to the workup for exophthalmos (see page 158).

P

PALLOR OF THE FACE, NAILS, OR CONJUNCTIVA

Pallor is almost invariably caused by anemia and is best analyzed with the application of **pathophysiology**. Anemia may be caused by decreased production of blood, increased destruction of blood, or loss of blood. **Decreased production** results from poor nutrition particularly, poor absorption or intake of B_{12} (pernicious anemia), iron (iron deficiency anemia), and folic acid (malabsorption syndrome). It may also result from suppressed bone marrow (aplastic anemia) or infiltrated bone marrow (leukemia or metastatic carcinoma). **Increased destruction** is caused by hemolysis from intrinsic defects in the red cells (e.g., sickle cell anemia and thalassemia) or extrinsic defects in the circulation (autoimmune hemolytic anemia of many disorders). **Blood loss** may result from peptic ulcers and carcinomas of the gastrointestinal (GI) tract, excessive menstruation or metrorrhagia from tumors of the uterus, or dysfunctional uterine bleeding. These are the principal causes of anemia, but the reader will be able to think of several more. What is important here is to have a systematic method to recall them.

If anemia is ruled out, the less frequent causes of pallor should be considered. Shock, congestive heart failure (CHF), and arteriosclerosis cause pallor by poor circulation of blood to the skin. Patients who have hypertension may be pale from reflex vasomotor spasms of the arterioles supplying the skin. Aortic regurgitation and stenosis, as well as mitral stenosis, cause pallor for the same reasons, but the malar flush of mitral stenosis may negate this. The reason that tuberculosis, rheumatoid arthritis, carcinomatosis, and glomerulonephritis cause pallor even when their victims are not anemic or hypertensive is not known.

● Approach to the Diagnosis

The approach to the diagnosis of pallor is obviously to check for anemia first and then to examine for the other chronic disorders. Chest x-ray, electrocardiogram (ECG), sedimentation rate, and a check for rheumatoid factor are all appropriate in specific cases.

● Other Useful Tests

1. Complete blood count (CBC) (anemia)
2. Sedimentation rate (chronic infection)
3. Chemistry panel (anemia of liver and kidney disease)
4. Serum B_{12} level (pernicious anemia)
5. Serum folic acid level (folic acid deficiency)
6. Serum iron and ferritin levels (iron deficiency anemia)
7. Stool for occult blood (GI bleeding)
8. Stool for ova and parasites (anemia due to parasite infestation)
9. Serum haptoglobins (hemolytic anemia)
10. Antinuclear antibody (ANA) analysis (collagen disease)
11. Bone marrow examination (aplastic anemia)

PALPITATIONS

Because anxiety is the common cause of palpitations, there is a tremendous temptation to jump to this conclusion as the cause in an otherwise healthy-looking individual. If we use the mnemonic **VINDICATE**, we may avoid a misdiagnosis in many cases.

V—**Vascular** causes help to recall aortic aneurysms, arteriovenous fistulas, anemia, postural hypotension, migraine, and cardiac disorders such as aortic regurgitation, aortic stenosis, tricuspid insufficiency, mitral valve prolapse, CHF, and various arrhythmias (see page 85).
I—**Inflammation** reminds us of fever, pericarditis, subacute bacterial endocarditis, and rheumatic fever.
N—**Neoplasms** are not usually associated with palpitations.
D—**Deficiency** of thiamine can lead to beriberi heart disease resulting in palpitations.
I—**Intoxication** prompts us to recall that alcohol, tobacco, coffee, soft drinks, and tea can cause palpitations. It should also remind us that palpitations are common side effects of many drugs, including digitalis, aminophylline, sympathomimetics, ganglionic blocking agents, nitrates, and other drugs.
C—**Congenital** disorders that may cause palpitations include patent ductus, ventricular septal defect, and hiatal hernia. Disorders of the conduction system such as Wolff–Parkinson–White syndrome should be considered here.
A—**Anxiety** is a common cause of palpitations.
T—**Trauma** causes palpitations by inducing the release of epinephrine, but there is no diagnostic dilemma in these cases.
E—**Endocrine** disorders that cause palpitations include thyrotoxicosis, pheochromocytoma, menopausal syndrome, and hypoglycemia.

● Approach to the Diagnosis

Valvular heart disease, anemia, and febrile disorders will usually be revealed on physical examination. It is important to inquire about drug, alcohol, and tobacco use. Caffeine is a frequent offender. It is helpful to eliminate any suspicious medications if possible. A drug screen may be useful in many cases. The initial diagnostic workup should include a CBC, chemistry profile, thyroid profile, sedimentation rate, antistreptolysin O (ASO) titer, ECG, and chest x-ray. If these have normal findings, 24-hour Holter monitoring or continuous loop event recording of the ECG should be undertaken.

P

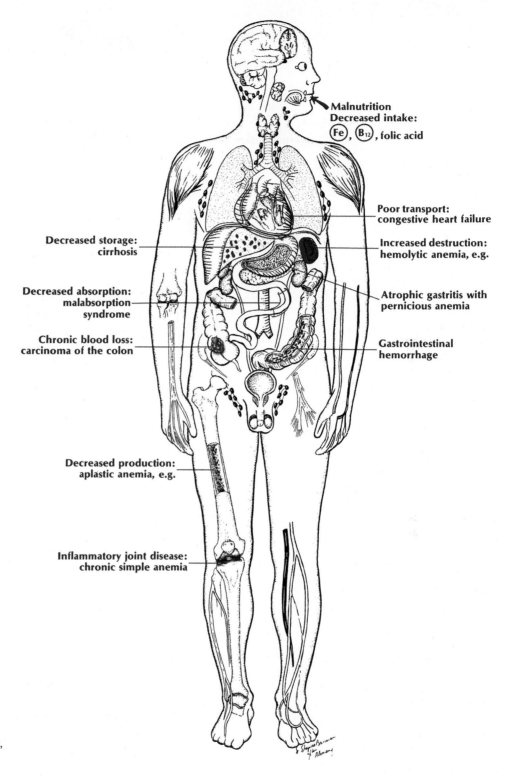

Malnutrition
Decreased intake:
(Fe), (B₁₂), folic acid

Poor transport:
congestive heart failure

Increased destruction:
hemolytic anemia, e.g.

Decreased storage:
cirrhosis

Atrophic gastritis with
pernicious anemia

Decreased absorption:
malabsorption
syndrome

Chronic blood loss:
carcinoma of the colon

Gastrointestinal
hemorrhage

Decreased production:
aplastic anemia, e.g.

Inflammatory joint disease:
chronic simple anemia

● **FIGURE 1** Pallor of the face, nails,
or conjunctiva.

● Other Useful Tests

1. 24-hour urine catecholamine or vanillylmandelic acid (pheochromocytoma)
2. Arm-to-tongue circulation time (CHF)
3. Echocardiography (CHF, valvular heart disease)
4. Exercise tolerance test (coronary insufficiency)
5. Upper GI series and esophagram (hiatal hernia)
6. 24-hour blood pressure monitoring (pheochromocytoma)
7. Psychometric testing (hysteria)
8. Serum estradiol, follicle-stimulating hormone (FSH) and luteinizing hormone (LH) (menopause)

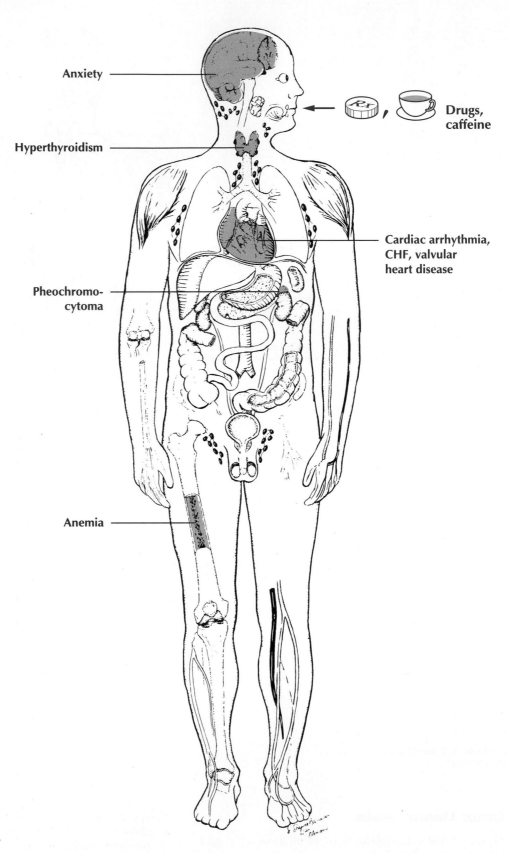

Anxiety

Hyperthyroidism

Pheochromo-
cytoma

Anemia

Drugs,
caffeine

Cardiac arrhythmia,
CHF, valvular
heart disease

● **FIGURE 2** Palpitation.

> ## Case Presentation #71
>
> A 62-year-old physician complained of frequently awakening at night with palpitations. It would take him at least an hour to go back to sleep. He also had to urinate at least twice at night but denied daytime frequency of urination. He denied the use of alcohol, tobacco, or drugs but usually has a cup of coffee in the morning and a coke at lunch.
>
> **Question #1.** Utilizing your knowledge of physiology and the mnemonic **VINDICATE**, what is your differential diagnosis?
>
> Physical examination was unremarkable. His blood pressure was 110/70 mm Hg, and his pulse was 66 bpm. Results of laboratory studies and an exercise tolerance test were normal.
>
> **Question #2.** What is your diagnosis now?
>
> _____
>
> *(See Appendix B for the answers.)*

PAPILLEDEMA

No anatomic analysis of this condition is necessary because most cases of papilledema are caused by intracranial pathology. Three notable extracranial conditions are optic neuritis, hypertension, and pseudotumor cerebri. The polycythemia and right heart failure of chronic pulmonary emphysema may combine to produce papilledema, but this is uncommon. Analysis of the intracranial causes of papilledema is performed using the mnemonic **VINDICATE**.

V—Vascular lesions are aneurysms and arteriovenous malformations that cause subarachnoid hemorrhages. Severe hypertension may lead to an intracerebral hemorrhage or hypertensive encephalopathy, thus causing papilledema. Cerebral thrombosis and emboli rarely lead to papilledema.

I—Infection is not a common cause of papilledema unless a space-occupying lesion is produced or the condition persists. Thus, a brain abscess is often associated with papilledema, whereas acute bacterial meningitis is not. Chronic cryptococcal meningitis, syphilitic meningitis, and tuberculous meningitis, in contrast, are often associated with some degree of papilledema. Viral encephalitis may occasionally be associated with papilledema. Cavernous sinus thrombosis and septic thrombosis of the other venous sinuses may produce papilledema.

N—Neoplasms, primary and metastatic, are the most common cause of papilledema.

D—Degenerative diseases are rarely the cause.

I—Intoxication brings to mind lead encephalopathy, but other toxins and drugs rarely cause papilledema.

C—Congenital malformations that cause papilledema include the aneurysms and arteriovenous malformations already mentioned plus the various types of hydrocephalus, skull deformities (oxycephaly), hemophilia (because of intracranial hemorrhages), and, occasionally, Schilder disease and other congenital encephalopathies.

A—Autoimmune disorders recall lupus cerebritis and periarteritis nodosa (when associated with severe hypertension).

T—Trauma does not usually produce papilledema in the early stages of concussions or epidural or subdural hematomas, but in chronic subdural hematomas, it is the rule.

E—Endocrine disorders bring to mind the papilledema of malignant pheochromocytomas (with hypertension) and the fact that pseudotumor cerebri occurs in obese, amenorrheic, and emotionally disturbed women.

● Approach to the Diagnosis

The approach to the diagnosis of papilledema in someone without hypertension or hypertensive retinopathy must include a thorough neurologic examination and a computed tomography (CT) scan. If focal signs are present or the CT scan shows positive findings, referral to a neurosurgeon is indicated. He or she can decide if a magnetic resonance imaging (MRI) is indicated. A spinal tap is contraindicated. If there are no focal signs, it may be worthwhile to differentiate papilledema from optic neuritis by having an ophthalmologist perform a visual field examination. This may also be helpful in differentiating pseudotumor cerebri because there may be bilateral visual defects in the inferior nasal quadrants. Papilledema from increased intracranial pressure will show only an enlarged blind spot (unless there is a tumor of the optic tracts, radiations, or occipital cortex), whereas optic neuritis will show scotomata peripheral to the blind spot (disk). Appendix A will be useful for confirming the diagnosis of a specific disease.

● Other Useful Tests

1. CBC (polycythemia)
2. Sedimentation rate (cerebral abscess, infection)
3. Urinalysis (renal disease associated with hypertension)
4. ANA analysis (collagen disease)
5. Blood lead level
6. Visual evoked potentials (optic neuritis)
7. Pulmonary function tests (emphysema)
8. Blood volume (polycythemia vera)
9. 24-hour blood pressure monitoring (hypertension)
10. Spinal tap when imaging study is negative (pseudotumor cerebri)

PARESTHESIAS, DYSESTHESIAS, AND NUMBNESS

Anatomically, tingling and numbness or other abnormal sensations in the extremities result from involvement of the peripheral nerve, the nerve plexus (brachial or sciatic), the nerve root, the spinal cord, or the brain. When each of these is cross-indexed with the etiologies suggested by the mnemonic **VINDICATE**, most of the causes can be developed (Table 49). Only the most important conditions are mentioned in this discussion.

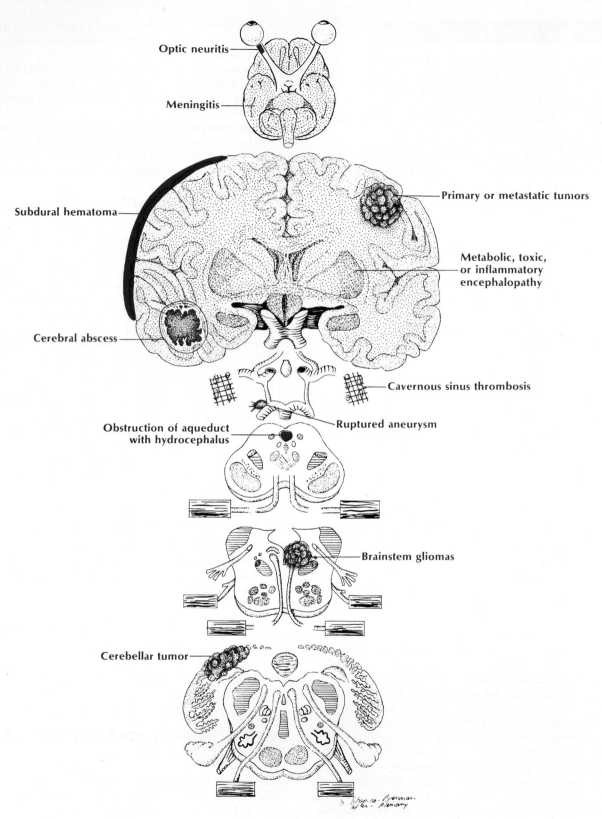

● **FIGURE 3** Papilledema.

TABLE 49 Paresthesias, Dysesthesias, and Numbness

	V Vascular	I Inflammatory	N Neoplasm	D Degenerative	I Intoxication	C Congenital	A Autoimmune Allergic	T Trauma	E Endocrine
Peripheral Nerve	Causalgia Raynaud disease Buerger disease Arteriosclerosis Ischemic neuritis			Pellagra Beriberi Nutritional neuropathy	Alcoholic neuropathy Isoniazid toxicity Lead and arseric neuropathy	Porphyria	Infectious neuronitis Periarteritis nodosa	Trauma Hematoma Laceration Neuroma Frostbite	Tetany of hypoparathyroidism Aldosteronism
Nerve Plexus	Leriche syndrome		Pancoast tumor			Scalenus anticus Cervical rib	Infectious neuronitis	Contusion Laceration Fracture	Diabetic neuropathy
Nerve Root		Tabes dorsalis Tuberculosis	Metastatic and primary tumors of the cord and spine (multiple myeloma)	Herniated disk Cervical and lumbar spondylosis		Spondylolisthesis		Fracture Herniated disk	
Spinal Cord	Anterior spinal artery occlusion Aortic aneurysm	Poliomyelitis Epidural abscess Tuberculosis Syphilis	Metastatic and primary tumors of the cord and spine	Spondylosis Disk disease Pernicious anemia	Transverse myelitis from radiation	Spina bifida Myelocele Syringomyelia	Guillain–Barré syndrome Multiple sclerosis	Fracture Herniated disk Hematoma	
Brain	Cerebral embolus, thrombus, hemorrhage Carotid or basilar artery insufficiency Migraine	Neurosyphilis Encephalitis Brain abscess	Brain tumor	Senile dementia Presenile dementia	Alcoholism Bromism Encephalopathy Opiates, barbiturates, etc.	Atrioventricular anomalies Aneurysm Epilepsy Cerebral palsy	Lupus cerebritis Multiple sclerosis	Depressed fracture Subdural hematoma	Pituitary tumor Acromegaly

Peripheral nerve: Peripheral neuropathies from alcohol, diabetes, and other causes are important in this category, but one should not forget vascular diseases that may cause paresthesias, such as peripheral arteriosclerosis, Raynaud syndrome, and Buerger disease. In addition, metabolic disorders such as tetany and uremia should be considered. Chronic acute inflammatory demyelinating polyneuropathy (Guillain–Barré syndrome) is brought to mind here. Excessive intake of vitamin B$_6$ (Pyridoxine) may cause a peripheral neuropathy. Finally, nerve entrapments such as carpal tunnel syndrome need to be checked. Tingling of the third and fourth toes would suggest Morton neuroma.

Nerve plexus: The brachial plexus may be involved by the scalenus anticus syndrome, a cervical rib, or Pancoast tumor. The sciatic plexus may be compressed by pelvic tumors.

Nerve root: Herniated disks, spondylosis, tabes dorsalis, and infiltration of the spine by tuberculosis, metastatic tumor, and multiple myeloma need to be remembered here. Don't forget Polio and postpolio syndrome.

Spinal cord: Spinal cord tumors, pernicious anemia, and tabes dorsalis are the most important conditions to recall here. Be alert to a myelopathy associated with acute onset of numbness around the waist and lower extremities that may occur in scuba divers.

Brain: Transient ischemic attacks, emboli, and migraines are vascular diseases to remember in addition to the diseases that affect the spinal cord. The aura of epilepsy is also important. One would not want to miss brain tumors, abscesses, and toxic encephalopathy because these are potentially treatable.

● Approach to the Diagnosis

This would be the same as the workup of weakness in one or more extremities. If the condition is in the hand, one would check for Tinel and Adson signs and x-ray the cervical spine for a cervical rib or disk degeneration. The next steps are nerve conduction studies and electromyogram (EMG). Objective signs of radiculopathy are a clear indication for an MRI or cervical myelography, preferably combined with a CT scan. MRI may reveal tiny disk herniations. With associated pain in certain roots, diagnostic nerve blocks may be indicated. If there is coldness in the hand, a stellate ganglion block may be helpful.

If the condition is in the lower extremity, a careful examination of the arterial pulses, particularly the femoral, is performed. If these are abnormal, ultrasonography, a flow study, or femoral angiography may be indicated. X-rays of the spine to rule out a herniated disk or tumor of the spine are done routinely. One must not forget a pelvic examination in a female. If other neurologic signs are present, an MRI or CT scan may be necessary. When a disk herniation is still likely, myelography should be ordered. EMG has the same usefulness here as in the upper extremity. When a cerebral lesion is suspected, a CT scan, MRI, and four-vessel angiography should be considered.

● Other Useful Tests

1. CBC (anemia)
2. Chemistry panel (hypoparathyroidism, electrolyte disturbance, uremia)
3. Fluorescent treponemal antibody absorption (FTA-ABS) test (neurosyphilis)
4. Serum B$_{12}$ and folic acid levels (pernicious anemia)
5. Schilling test (pernicious anemia)
6. Blood lead level (lead neuropathy)
7. ANA analysis (collagen disease)
8. Glucose tolerance test (diabetic neuropathy)
9. Urine porphobilinogen (porphyria)
10. Hair analysis for arsenic
11. Somatosensory evoked potentials (multiple sclerosis)
12. Spinal tap (neurosyphilis, multiple sclerosis)
13. Anticentromere antibody (scleroderma)
14. Muscle biopsy (periarteritis nodosa)

Case Presentation #72

A 25-year-old white male intern complained of intermittent numbness and tingling for several months of the lower extremities and, to a lesser extent, the upper extremities. He had occasional weakness in his left arm and hand but was told on an insurance examination that that was due to a scalenus anticus syndrome. He denies alcohol or substance abuse.

Question #1. Utilizing your knowledge of neuroanatomy, what is your differential diagnosis?

Further history reveals that he had an episode of optic neuritis at age 17. His neurologic examination reveals hyperactive reflexes of the left upper and lower extremities but is otherwise unremarkable.

Question #2. What is your diagnosis now?

(See Appendix B for the answers.)

PELVIC MASS

A mass in the pelvis is usually (but not always) a neoplasm. Is there a quick way to recall all the various causes while examining the pelvis? **Anatomy** is the key. Apply the mnemonic **MINT** to develop a list of the many possibilities (Table 50).

Anatomically, there are three major groups of structures: the urinary tract, the female genital tract, and the lower intestinal tract. Breaking these down into their components, there are the bladder and ureters; the vagina, cervix, uterus, fallopian tubes, and ovaries; and the rectum and sigmoid colon. In addition to these structures, the diseases of the aorta and iliac vessels, spine, and surrounding muscles and fascia must be considered. Other structures fill the pelvis from above. The small intestines, the omentum, and the appendix may be felt; even the kidney may drop into the pelvis.

P

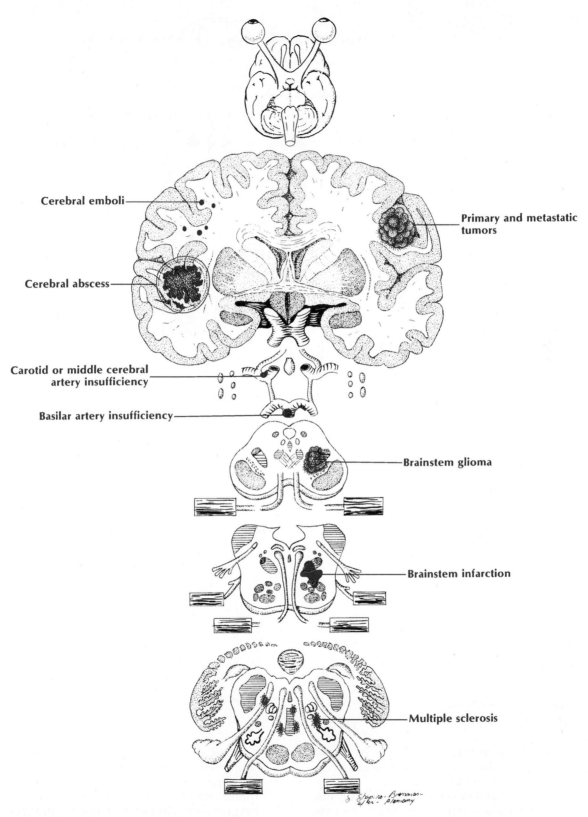

Cerebral emboli

Primary and metastatic tumors

Cerebral abscess

Carotid or middle cerebral artery insufficiency

Basilar artery insufficiency

Brainstem glioma

Brainstem infarction

Multiple sclerosis

● **FIGURE 4** Paresthesias, dysethesias, and numbness.

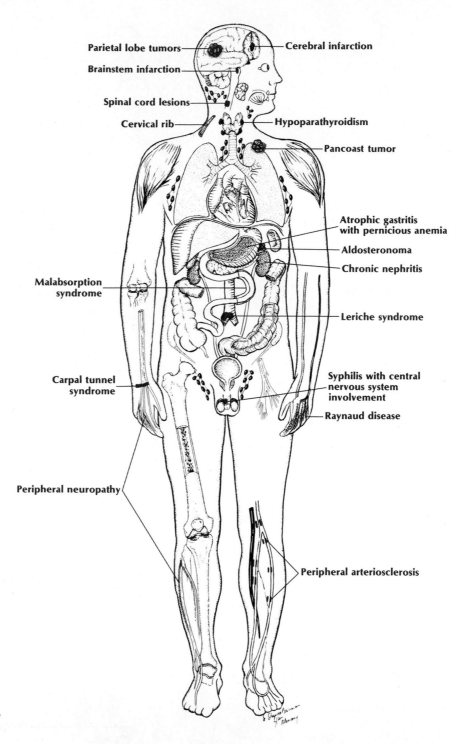

Parietal lobe tumors
Brainstem infarction
Spinal cord lesions
Cervical rib
Cerebral infarction
Hypoparathyroidism
Pancoast tumor
Atrophic gastritis with pernicious anemia
Aldosteronoma
Chronic nephritis
Malabsorption syndrome
Leriche syndrome
Carpal tunnel syndrome
Syphilis with central nervous system involvement
Raynaud disease
Peripheral neuropathy
Peripheral arteriosclerosis

● **FIGURE 5** Paresthesias, dysethesias, and numbness.

1. **Bladder:** Prominent conditions that must be considered here are stones, diverticula, Hunner ulcer, and carcinomas. A distended bladder is deceptive.

2. **Urethra:** A cystocele and urethrocele are felt easily during a pelvic examination, but if they are not, have the patient strain or stand up.

3. **Ureters:** A ureteral calculus or ureterocele may be felt.

4. **Vagina:** Vaginal carcinomas, prolapsed cervix or procidentia, rectocele, and Bartholin cysts may be felt. A foreign body (e.g., a pessary) should be considered.

5. **Cervix:** Carcinoma or polyps are the main considerations here, because an inflamed cervix does not usually cause a mass.

6. **Uterus:** Fibroids are the most likely tumor to be felt, but pregnancy, chronic endometritis, choriocarcinoma, and endometrial carcinomas all present as a mass. A retroverted uterus may masquerade as a mass in the cul-de-sac.

7. **Fallopian tubes:** Tubo-ovarian abscesses and endometriosis of these structures account for most cases. Ectopic pregnancy is always possible.

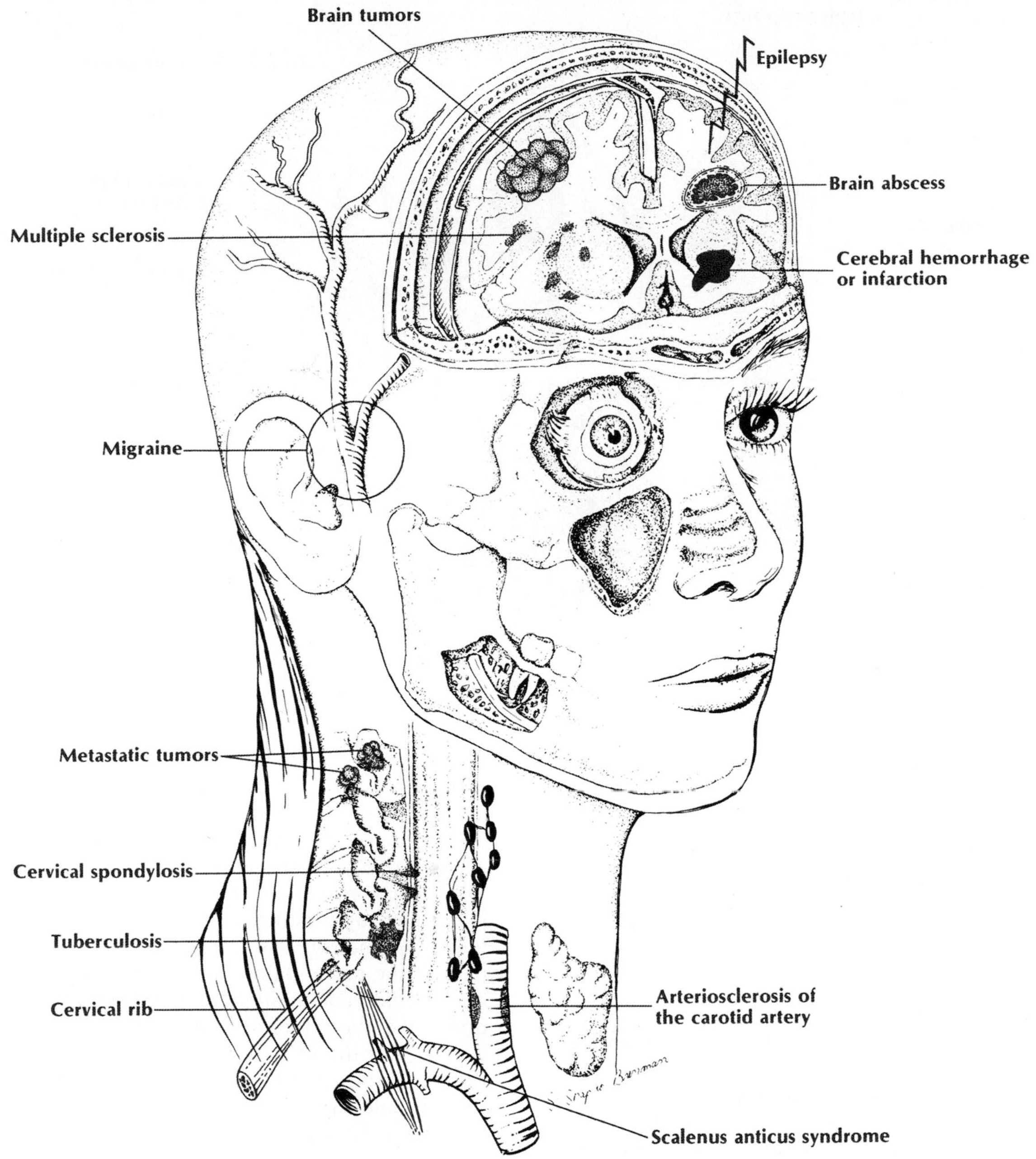

● **FIGURE 6** Paresthesias, dysethesias, and numbness.

8. **Ovary:** Ovarian cysts and carcinomas must be considered as well as endometriosis.
9. **Rectum:** Carcinoma, abscesses, diverticula, and prolapse are good possibilities here. Feces may masquerade as a mass.
10. **Sigmoid colon:** Again, the disorders mentioned in the section on the rectum (see page 372) must be considered. Granulomatous or ulcerative colitis may present as a mass.
11. **Arteries:** It is unusual for an aortic or iliac aneurysm to be felt here, but they should be kept in mind.
12. **Spine:** Deformities of the spine (e.g., lordosis), tuberculosis (Pott disease), and metastatic or primary malignancies of the spine (e.g., myeloma) may present as a pelvic mass.

13. **Miscellaneous:** A pelvic kidney may be felt. An inflamed segment of ileum (regional ileitis) or the appendix should be considered, as should omental cysts and adhesions.

● **Approach to the Diagnosis**

The association with other symptoms is the key to the clinical diagnosis. A painless mass is likely to be a neoplasm, whereas a tender mass with fever suggests pelvic inflammatory disease (PID) or a diverticular abscess. Obviously, an ectopic pregnancy should be associated with tender breasts, frequency of urination, and morning sickness. The next logical step is ultrasonography and a gynecologic consult.

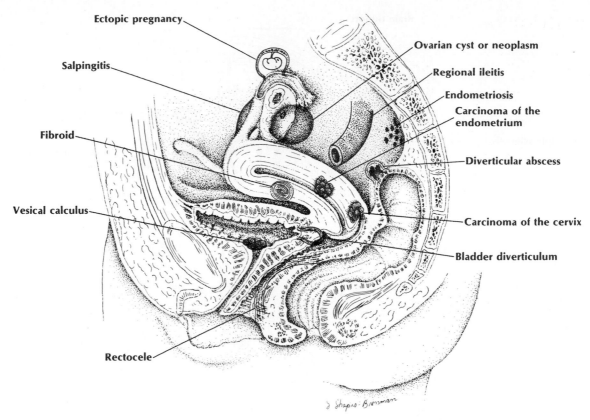

Ectopic pregnancy

Salpingitis

Fibroid

Vesical calculus

Rectocele

Ovarian cyst or neoplasm

Regional ileitis

Endometriosis

Carcinoma of the endometrium

Diverticular abscess

Carcinoma of the cervix

Bladder diverticulum

● **FIGURE 7** Pelvic mass.

Laboratory tests include urinalysis and culture, pregnancy test, stool for blood and parasites, and vaginal cultures. A proctoscopy and barium enema may be useful. Colonoscopy, culdoscopy, peritoneoscopy, and cystoscopy may all need to be done before an exploratory laparotomy is performed.

● Other Useful Tests

1. Sedimentation rate (PID)
2. Tuberculin test (tuberculosis of the fallopian tubes)
3. Catheterization for residual urine
4. Culdocentesis (ruptured ectopic pregnancy)
5. Laparoscopy (ectopic pregnancy, neoplasm)
6. CT scan of the pelvis (neoplasm, stone, diverticulum, abscess)
7. Aortogram (aortic aneurysm)
8. Exploratory laparotomy
9. Urology consult
10. Gynecology consult
11. CA 125 (ovarian carcinoma)
12. Therapeutic trial of oral contraceptives (ovarian cysts)

PELVIC PAIN

Visualizing the anatomy of the pelvic area is the key to forming a list of the causes of pelvic pain. Starting at the skin and working inward, we have the muscles and fascia, bladder, peritoneum, uterus, ovaries, fallopian tubes, intestines, rectum, and spine. The skin helps to recall herpes zoster, the muscle and fascia suggest contusion and hernia,

and the peritoneum would remind one of peritonitis and endometriosis. The uterus, ovary, and tubes would prompt consideration of PID, dysmenorrhea, pelvic congestion, and ectopic pregnancy. Ovarian tumors can also cause pelvic pain by twisting on their pedicle. A pedunculated uterine fibroid can also twist on its pedicle causing severe pain. If the pelvic pain is related to the menstrual cycle, one should recall mittelschmerz. Considering the intestines, one should recall appendicitis and diverticulitis. Considering the rectum should prompt recall of hemorrhoids, fissures, and rectal abscess. Finally, thinking of the spine should suggest rheumatoid spondylitis, osteomyelitis, herniated disk, and other conditions.

● Approach to the Diagnosis

A good pelvic and rectal examination is essential. These will often disclose a mass or other pathology to explain the pain. If there is a vaginal discharge, a smear and culture for gonococcus and *Chlamydia* need to be done. A pregnancy test will help rule out an ectopic pregnancy, but ultrasonography is most useful.

A gynecology consult should be obtained when there is any doubt. In acute cases, the gynecologist may proceed with an exploratory laparotomy immediately.

● Other Useful Tests

1. CBC (PID, ruptured ectopic pregnancy)
2. Chemistry panel
3. Urinalysis (cystitis, pyelonephritis)

TABLE 50	**Pelvic Mass**			
Anatomy	**M** **Malformation**	**I** **Inflammation**	**N** **Neoplasms**	**T** **Trauma**
Bladder	Obstruction with diverticulum Calculi	Hunner ulcer	Carcinoma Polyp	Rupture of the bladder
Urethra	Urethrocele Cystocele			
Ureters	Double ureter Calculus Ureterocele		Papilloma	
Vagina	Prolapsed cervix Rectocele	Bartholinitis fistula with rectum or bladder	Carcinoma	Foreign body Tear
Cervix		Cervicitis (rarely)	Carcinoma Polyp	
Uterus	Bicornuate uterus Retroversion	Endometritis	Endometrial carcinoma Choriocarcinoma Fibroid	Rupture during pregnancy
Fallopian Tubes	Ectopic pregnancy Endometriosis	Salpingitis	Carcinoma (rarely)	
Ovary	Benign congenital ovarian cyst (e.g., Morgagni)	Oophoritis	Cystadenoma Cystadenocarcinoma Follicular and granulosa cell cyst	
Rectum	Prolapse Rectocele	Inflamed hemorrhoid Rectal abscess Fistula	Rectal carcinoma	
Sigmoid	Diverticulum	Diverticulitis Granulomatous colitis Ulcerative colitis	Carcinoma of polyp	Foreign body
Arteries	Aneurysm			
Spine	Lordosis Scoliosis	Rheumatoid arthritis Spondylosis Tuberculosis	Metastatic carcinoma Myeloma Hodgkin lymphoma	Fracture Ruptured disk
Miscellaneous	Pelvic kidney Omental cyst and adhesions	Appendicitis Regional ileitis	Pelvic metastasis from stomach, etc.	Blood clot in cul-de-sac Surgical abscess

4. Urine culture (cystitis, urinary tract infection [UTI])
5. Pregnancy test (ectopic pregnancy)
6. CT scan of abdomen and pelvis (only if pregnancy has been ruled out) (neoplasm, abscess)
7. Culdocentesis (PID, neoplasm, ectopic pregnancy)
8. Laparoscopy (PID, neoplasm, ectopic pregnancy)
9. Peritoneal tap (peritonitis, ruptured ectopic pregnancy)

PENILE PAIN

Perhaps no other pain will bring a patient to the doctor more quickly in this age of sexual candor. Most cases will be caused by **inflammation**, so a mnemonic of etiologies is, for the most part, superfluous. Utilization of **anatomy** is valuable, however. Let us begin, then, with the **head of the penis** and proceed upward to the prostate, the bladder, and the kidney.

The **head of the penis** may be inflamed by a painful chancroid ulcer or lymphogranuloma venereum, but one must remember that a chancre (syphilitic ulcer) is not painful. Herpes progenitalis, in contrast, is extremely painful. Balanitis is usually caused by a nonspecific infection, but one should caution the uncircumcised patient about proper cleaning of the area and rule out Reiter disease. (Look for conjunctivitis and joint symptoms.) Trauma to the head of the penis should be obvious, but some patients may be too shy to mention its origin without careful questioning. Carcinoma of the penis rarely causes pain, but like all carcinomas, it will often be painful when it is secondarily infected.

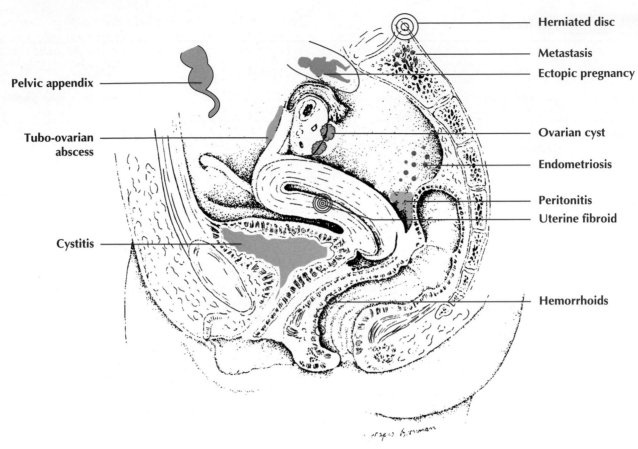

Pelvic appendix

Tubo-ovarian
abscess

Cystitis

Herniated disc

Metastasis

Ectopic pregnancy

Ovarian cyst

Endometriosis

Peritonitis

Uterine fibroid

Hemorrhoids

● **FIGURE 8** Pelvic pain.

Next, let us consider the **urethra**. Inflammation here is probably the most common cause of penile pain. It is almost invariably associated with a discharge, and the smear will usually disclose the typical gram-negative intracellular diplococci of gonorrhea. The clinician is reminded that nonspecific urethritis is more frequently encountered each year and that *Chlamydia* and mima polymorpha are common causes. Reiter disease must also be considered. Passage of a stone through the urethra causes pain in the penis.

The **shaft** of the penis is one of the few areas in which a vascular lesion may account for penile pain. Thrombosis of the corpus cavernosum is often encountered in blood dyscrasias (particularly leukemia), and the resulting permanent erection may be enviable and even humorous to the observer but not to the patient. Peyronie disease will cause a painful erection.

Moving to the **prostate**, one hardly needs to be reminded that both acute and chronic prostatitis are frequent causes of penile pain. In contrast, carcinoma and hypertrophy of the prostate are rarely associated with pain unless there is associated infection.

The **bladder** is another common source of penile pain, but because there is often an associated urethritis, it is uncertain whether pure cystitis causes penile pain by itself except on urination. Bladder stones cause pain in the penis, especially on urination. Carcinoma of the bladder will not usually cause penile pain unless it is complicated by infection. Hunner ulcer, in contrast, causes great pain in the

penis at times. Occasionally, ureteral and renal stones will cause penile pain, but pyelonephritis is very unlikely to do so. Referred pain from the rectum caused by hemorrhoids and fissures is common.

● Approach to the Diagnosis

Finding any lesion of the penis should prompt a smear and culture of the exudate or scrapings. A dark field examination will often be indicated by the history of sexual contact. Any urethral discharge must also be examined after a Gram stain and cultured for gonococci and *Chlamydia*. Prostatic massage may be necessary to get adequate urethral material. Next, a urinalysis is done and a fresh drop is examined under high power for motile bacteria signifying cystitis or pyelonephritis. A urine culture and colony count will be wise in any case. If the diagnosis is still obscure, it is wise to consult a urologist before proceeding with an intravenous pyelogram (IVP) or other expensive tests.

● Other Useful Tests

1. Cystoscopy (stricture, tumor, stone)
2. Retrograde pyelography (tumor, stone, malformation)
3. CBC (infection)
4. Chemistry panel (hypercalcemia, hyperuricemia)
5. Strain urine for stone
6. CT scan of the abdomen and pelvis (tumors, stones, malformation)

PENILE SORES

To recall the possible causes of penile sores, think of the smallest microorganism up to the largest.

Virus: This brings to mind genital herpes (herpes simplex virus 2 [HSV2]). Genital warts are included here but are rarely difficult to diagnose.

Bacteria: This should facilitate the recall of chancroid (caused by *Haemophilus ducreyi*; *Bacillus*) and lymphogranuloma venereum and granuloma inguinale (caused by *Calymmatobacterium Granulomatous*). Abscess and balanitis should also be recalled here.

Spirochete: This suggests chancre, the first stage of syphilis.

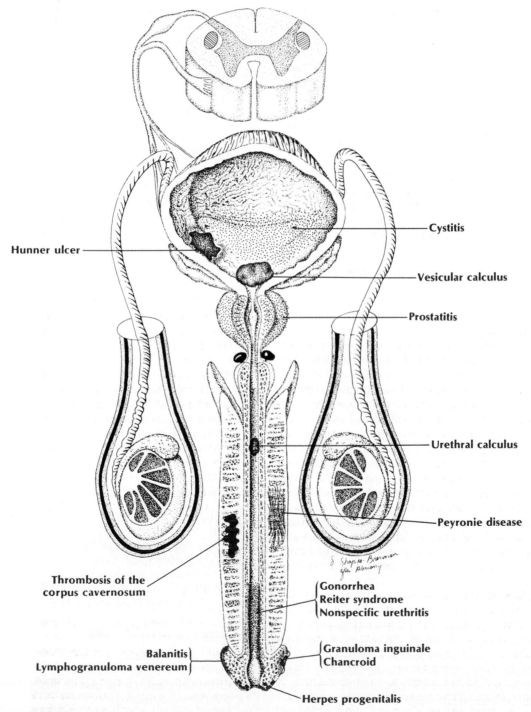

● **FIGURE 9** Penile pain.

The above classification would not help recall an epithelioma or laceration and other lesions caused by trauma.

● Approach to the Diagnosis

Something that is often neglected today is the tracking down of contacts, which can assist in the diagnosis. A painless lesion suggests chancre, whereas a painful lesion is typical of chancroid, herpes simplex, or balanitis. The presence of inguinal lymphadenopathy should alert the clinician to lymphogranuloma venereum, chancre, and epithelioma.

A smear and culture should be done if balanitis or chancroid is the clinical diagnosis. A dark field examination is done to confirm the diagnosis of chancre. The finding of intracellular Donovan bodies will confirm the diagnosis of granuloma inguinale. A Tzanck test and rapid immunofluorescent antibody study will assist in the diagnosis of genital herpes but is not usually necessary. Serologic tests or a Giemsa stain of scrapings of the primary lesion may be examined for inclusion bodies in cases of lymphogranuloma venereum. A biopsy is necessary to diagnose an epithelioma.

PERIORBITAL AND FACIAL EDEMA

The mechanism for periorbital and facial edema is similar to that for edema of the extremities. Thus, increased back-pressure of the veins will cause periorbital edema in right heart failure, constrictive pericarditis, advanced pulmonary emphysema, and thrombosis or extrinsic obstruction of the superior vena cava (as in mediastinal tumors). High blood pressure from acute glomerulonephritis and malignant hypertension will cause periorbital and facial edema. Low serum albumin will lead to periorbital and facial edema in nephrosis and cirrhosis. Mucoprotein in the subcutaneous tissue will cause periorbital edema in hypothyroidism.

Other causes for periorbital edema are not associated as frequently with edema in the extremities. Allergic or inflammatory dilatation of the capillaries around the eyelids will cause periorbital edema in dermatomyositis and trichinosis. A thrombosed cavernous sinus will also cause periorbital edema, but this is similar to thrombophlebitis of an extremity. Local causes for periorbital edema include orbital cellulitis, urticaria, angioneurotic edema, contusions, and other orbital trauma. Angiotensin-converting enzyme inhibitors and angiotensin receptor blockers may cause angioneurotic edema. The workup for periorbital edema is similar to that for edema of the extremities (see page 149).

PHOTOPHOBIA

Sensitivity to light may be due to local eye disease or systemic disease, but in both cases it is usually due to inflammation, with three exceptions: albinism because there is poor pigmentation of the iris and choroid, allowing more light to get in; migraine, where the explanation is still not available; and eye strain from astigmatism and, in particular, hyperopia.

Local eye disease: Following the path of light from the conjunctiva to the retina, one may easily recall the causes of photophobia. Conjunctivitis (chemical, allergic, and infectious), keratitis, foreign bodies of the cornea, iritis, retinitis, chorioretinitis, and optic neuritis may all be associated with photophobia.

Systemic disease: All the febrile states, especially those associated with conjunctival infection, cause photophobia. Measles, meningitis, encephalitis, hay fever, influenza, the common cold, and trichinosis are just a few. Certain toxins can cause photophobia, notably iodine, bromide, and atropine derivatives. Simply staying in the dark will cause photophobia. Hysteria and simple fear or annoyance with crowds will also cause this condition.

● Approach to the Diagnosis

The approach to the diagnosis of photophobia is the same as that of blurred vision (see page 76).

POLYCYTHEMIA

Pathophysiology will help to form a list of diagnostic possibilities in a case of polycythemia. First, it is important to exclude those cases of polycythemia that are due to a reduced plasma volume such as dehydration, diarrhea, and Gaisböck syndrome in which the actual red cell mass is normal. Next, separate those cases of polycythemia that are caused by an outside stimulus to the bone marrow. This involves two groups: those with anoxia as the stimulus and those with the hormone erythropoietin as the stimulus. The anoxic group includes pulmonary emphysema, alveolar hypoventilation, and cyanotic congenital heart disease. The group with erythropoietin as the stimulus includes pheochromocytoma, Cushing disease, hydronephrosis, renal cell carcinoma, renal cyst, cerebellar hemangioblastoma, and hematoma. Finally, we are left with the form of polycythemia that has no outside stimulus for red cell production: polycythemia vera. This is most likely a neoplastic disorder, and, in fact, it has been termed a "myeloproliferative" syndrome. In this disorder, there is also leukocytosis and thrombocytosis, which are distinguishing features.

● Approach to the Diagnosis

Blood volume studies, serum and urine osmolality studies, and electrolyte assessment will help differentiate relative or spurious forms of polycythemia. Arterial blood gas analysis will distinguish those cases associated with anoxia such as pulmonary emphysema and cyanotic heart disease. Determining the blood erythropoietin will help to differentiate cases of erythropoietin as the stimulus.

● Other Useful Tests

1. CBC (polycythemia)
2. Platelet count (polycythemia vera)
3. Chemistry panel (renal disease, heart disease)
4. IVP (hypernephroma)
5. CT scan of the abdomen (hypernephroma)

P

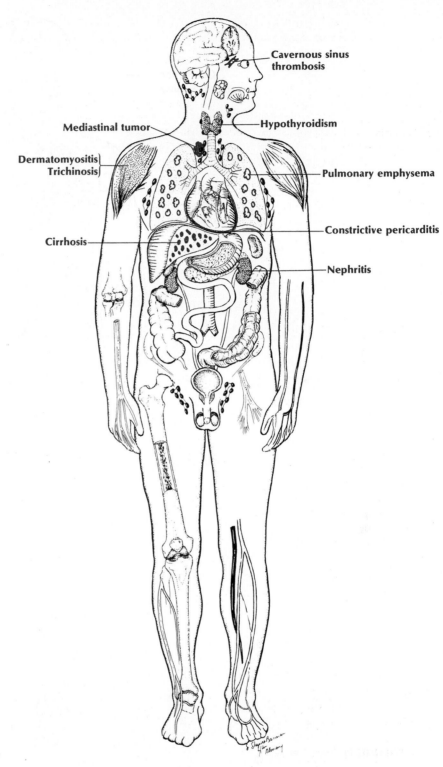

Labels on figure:
- Cavernous sinus thrombosis
- Hypothyroidism
- Mediastinal tumor
- Dermatomyositis
- Trichinosis
- Pulmonary emphysema
- Constrictive pericarditis
- Cirrhosis
- Nephritis

● **FIGURE 10** Periorbital and facial edema.

6. Chest x-ray (pulmonary emphysema)
7. Pulmonary function studies (pulmonary fibrosis or emphysema)
8. Cardiac catheterization (congenital heart disease)
9. Pulmonary consult
10. Hematology consult
11. Bone marrow examination (myeloproliferative disorder)

POLYDIPSIA

Excessive thirst is best analyzed by the application of **physiology**. Increased desire for water may be due to a **decreased intake**, as in prolonged abstinence, vomiting of pyloric stenosis and intestinal obstruction, and diarrhea of any cause. **Poor transport** of fluid in hemorrhagic or

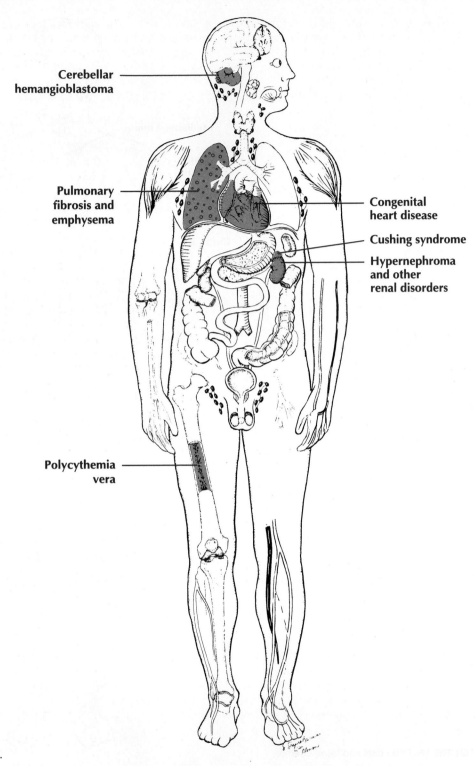

- **FIGURE 11** Polycythemia.

vasomotor shock and CHF may be the cause. Anything that decreases the effective circulatory volume, such as hypoalbuminemia, may cause retention of salt and consequent thirst through the rennin–angiotensin–aldosterone mechanism. **Increased output** of water may be responsible for polydipsia. The increased output may result from a solute diuresis in diabetes mellitus and hypercalcemic states (e.g., hyperparathyroidism); an increased glomerular filtration rate in hyperthyroidism; inability of the kidney to respond to antidiuretic hormone (ADH) in chronic glomerulonephritis, aldosteronism, and renal diabetes insipidus; or a lack of ADH in diabetes insipidus. **Increased output** of salt and water in excessive sweating of work or fever will lead to thirst. This mechanism is an additional factor in hyperthyroidism and diabetes mellitus where diaphoresis is common.

A neurosis may be responsible for polydipsia in neurogenic diabetes insipidus. Drugs such as lithium and demeclocycline hydrochloride (Declomycin) can damage the distal tubule and cause renal diabetes insipidus. Drugs such as belladonna alkaloids, amitriptyline hydrochloride, parasympatholytic drugs, and gallic acid may cause a dry mouth and an excessive thirst. Alcohol may cause excessive thirst by inhibiting ADH.

● Approach to the Diagnosis

The approach to the diagnosis of polydipsia involves establishing the presence or absence of other symptoms such as polyuria, polyphagia, weakness, and weight loss. Polydipsia with polyuria and excessive appetite (polyphagia) should suggest diabetes mellitus or hyperthyroidism, whereas polydipsia with polyuria alone should suggest a form of diabetes insipidus (pituitary, renal, or psychogenic). The laboratory workup involves checking intake and output, blood sugars, electrolytes, and a thyroid profile.

● Other Useful Tests

1. Urinalysis (renal or pituitary diabetes insipidus)
2. Serum and urine osmolality (diabetes insipidus)
3. Serum parathyroid hormone (PTH) level (hyperparathyroidism)
4. Serum ADH level (diabetes insipidus)
5. 24-hour urine calcium (hyperparathyroidism)
6. Serum growth hormone, LH, and FSH levels (pituitary tumor)
7. Hickey–Hare test (diabetes insipidus)
8. Pitressin test (renal diabetes insipidus)
9. CT scan or MRI of the brain (pituitary tumor)
10. Microscopic examination of the urinary sediment (chronic renal disease)

Case Presentation #73

A 44-year-old white male YMCA Summer Camp supervisor complained of a 1-week history of excessive thirst, polyuria, and weight loss. He denied fever, chills, or palpitations.

Question #1. Utilizing your knowledge of physiology, what would be on your list of possible causes?

Further history reveals that he has a ravenous appetite. Physical examination was unremarkable, but he had a sweet odor to his breath. Urinalysis revealed 4+ glucose and was strongly positive for acetone.

Question #2. What is your diagnosis now?

(See Appendix B for the answers.)

POLYPHAGIA

The causes of increased appetite are similar to those of obesity and can be recalled with the help of **physiology**.

The appetite may be based on a psychic desire for food, a lack of food or a particular vitamin, impaired intake of food, an increased metabolism of the body (and consequently an increased need for food), increased uptake of food by the cell, and inability of the cell to absorb food, causing "cell starvation."

1. **Psychic desire for food:** This occurs in many chronic anxiety and depressed states and is frequently associated with obesity.
2. **Lack of food or a particular ingredient in food:** Starvation and avitaminosis can cause polyphagia.
3. **Impaired uptake of food:** Rapid mobility of food in gastric hypersecretion and intestinal bypass as well as preempting of food by intestinal worms may cause polyphagia on this basis.
4. **Increased body metabolism:** Hyperthyroidism, rapid growth of adolescence, and gigantism are included in this category.
5. **Increased uptake of food by the cell:** Any condition associated with hyperinsulinism (functional hypoglycemia and **insulinomas**) is recalled in this category.
6. **"Cell starvation":** Here diabetes mellitus and acromegaly are associated with diabetes where the cell cannot absorb glucose.

● Approach to the Diagnosis

Association with other symptoms is the key to a definitive diagnosis of polyphagia. Thus, polyphagia and obesity suggest an islet cell adenoma. Polyphagia with polyuria, polydipsia, weakness, and weight loss suggest hyperthyroidism or diabetes mellitus.

The laboratory workup should include thyroid function studies, a skull x-ray for pituitary size, glucose tolerance tests, and, possibly, a 48-hour fast with frequent blood sugar determinations. An MRI of the pituitary is the best way to reveal microadenomas.

Case Presentation #74

A 28-year-old white man complained of a ravenous appetite for several months.

Question #1. Utilizing your knowledge of physiology, what would be your differential diagnosis?

Further history reveals that the patient had experienced episodes of weakness, palpitations, and sweating during the same period of time. He had recently gained 25 lb.

Question #2. What is your diagnosis now?

(See Appendix B for the answers.)

POLYURIA

Polyuria is an absolute increase in the urine output in a 24-hour period. The average individual excretes 1,500 mL of urine a day. Many physiologic conditions increase the

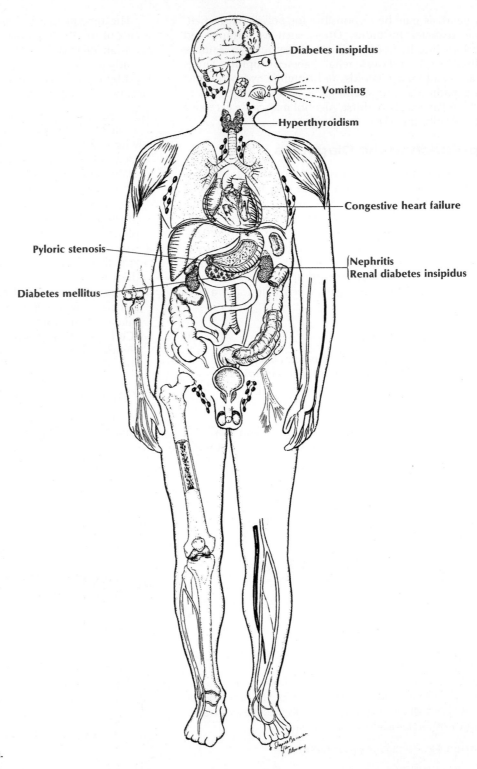

● **FIGURE 12** Polydipsia.

output of urine (stress, exercise, and warm weather associated with copious drinking). From a pathophysiologic standpoint, polyuria results from one of four mechanisms: (a) increased intake of fluids, (b) increased glomerular filtration rate, (c) increased output of solutes such as sodium chloride and glucose, and (d) inability of the kidney to reabsorb water in the distal tubule.

1. **Increased intake of fluid:** As already mentioned, increased intake can occur under stress and nervous tension. It becomes pathologic in psychogenic diabetes insipidus when 6 to 10 L of fluid may be ingested each day.
2. **Increased glomerular filtration rate:** This is a factor in the polyuria of hyperthyroidism and fever of any cause.

P

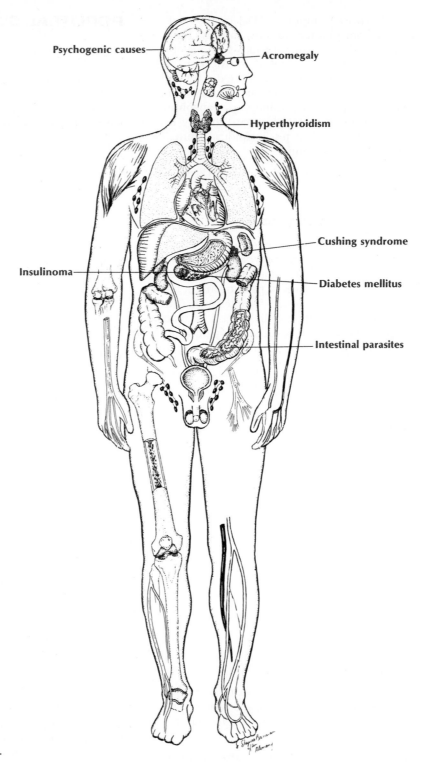

Psychogenic causes

Acromegaly

Hyperthyroidism

Cushing syndrome

Insulinoma

Diabetes mellitus

Intestinal parasites

● **FIGURE 13** Polyphagia.

3. **Increased output of solutes:** Uncontrolled diabetes mellitus (where the solute is glucose) and hyperthyroidism (where the solute may be glucose or urea) are examples of this type of polyuria. Hyperparathyroidism is another important cause (increased calcium output). Diuretics are a significant cause of this type of polyuria because they increase the amount of solute arriving at the distal tubule and hold onto the water that would otherwise be absorbed.

4. **Decreased reabsorption of water in the distal tubule:** This, the most common cause of polyuria, is divided into two groups: Conditions in which there is inadequate or blocked output of ADH and conditions in which the distal tubule and collecting ducts are unable to respond

to the ADH. Decreased output of ADH occurs in diabetes insipidus from pituitary tumors, infarcts, Hand–Schüller–Christian disease, and sarcoidosis among other causes. It also results from alcohol intoxication and hypothalamus lesions. The inability of the distal tubule to respond to ADH occurs in aldosteronism, chronic glomerulonephritis, polycystic kidneys, pyelonephritis, lithium and demeclocycline (Declomycin) therapy, and idiopathic nephrogenic diabetes insipidus. Diuretics operate somewhat in this manner.

Cases of myxedema with polyuria have been reported, but the mechanism is unclear.

● Approach to the Diagnosis

The diagnosis of polyuria depends largely on the association of other symptoms. Polyuria, polyphagia, and polydipsia suggest diabetes mellitus and hyperthyroidism. Polyuria with only polydipsia suggests psychogenic or idiopathic diabetes insipidus; the Hickey–Hare test will differentiate the two. Polyuria with polydipsia and weakness but with no significant weight loss suggests hypercalcemia and possible hyperparathyroidism. Chronic nephritis will be diagnosed by examination of the urine sediment and a specific gravity that remains at 1.010. Nephrogenic diabetes insipidus can be differentiated from neurogenic diabetes insipidus by the inability of the kidney to respond to a pitressin injection.

● Other Useful Tests

1. Thyroid profile (hyperthyroidism)
2. Glucose tolerance test (diabetes mellitus)
3. 24-hour intake and output (diabetes insipidus)
4. Addis count (chronic nephritis)
5. Serum ADH assay (diabetes insipidus)
6. Serum and urine osmolality (pituitary diabetes insipidus, nephrogenic diabetes insipidus)
7. Spot urine sodium (diabetes insipidus)
8. CT scan of the brain (diabetes insipidus)
9. PTH assay (hyperparathyroidism)
10. Endocrine consult

Case Presentation #75

A 38-year-old white woman presents to your office with a history of weakness, fatigue, depression, and frequency of urination over the past year. She denies fever, dysuria, or significant weight loss.

Question #1. Utilizing your knowledge of pathophysiology, what is your differential diagnosis?

Further history reveals that she had an episode of right flank pain and hematuria 6 months ago.

Question #2. What is your diagnosis now?

(See Appendix B for the answers.)

POPLITEAL SWELLING

The key to recalling the causes of a popliteal swelling is **anatomy**. Each structure in the popliteal space may be involved by one or two conditions that cause a mass or swelling. In visualizing the anatomy, one encounters the skin, subcutaneous tissues, muscles, bursae, veins, arteries, lymphatics, nerves, and bones.

1. **Skin:** The skin may be involved by urticaria, sebaceous cysts, carbuncles, lipomas, hemangiomas, and various other skin masses.
2. **Subcutaneous tissue:** Lipomas, sarcomas, and cellulitis are the main lesions encountered.
3. **Muscle:** Contusions of the gastrocnemius and semimembranous muscles may cause a mass in the popliteal fossa.
4. **Bursae:** Popliteal cysts (Baker cysts) may result from filling of the bursa between the gastrocnemius and semimembranous muscles with a gelatinous or serous substance.
5. **Veins:** The veins may enlarge from a varicocele or thrombophlebitis.
6. **Artery:** An aneurysm of the popliteal artery may result from atherosclerosis or a gunshot wound. When there is a loud bruit over the artery and distention of the veins, an arteriovenous fistula should be considered.
7. **Lymphatics:** Enlarged popliteal nodes may result from infections in the distal portion of the extremity, tuberculous adenopathy, or metastatic malignancy.
8. **Nerves:** Traumatic neuromas or neurofibromas may involve the nerves here.
9. **Bone:** Exostosis arising from the epiphyseal cartilage of the femur is a well-defined tumor of children or young adults. Medullary giant cell tumors, fibrosarcomas of the periosteum, and osteomyelitis may present as a mass in this area also. Fractures and periosteal hematomas should present no problem in diagnosis.

● Approach to the Diagnosis

Initial workup includes a CBC, sedimentation rate, and an x-ray of the knee. If these have negative findings, it may be wise to consult an orthopedic surgeon before any other tests are done. If a Baker cyst is suspected, aspiration will help make the diagnosis. Before doing this, it is wise to rule out a varicocele by watching for the disappearance of the mass on elevation of the leg. Ultrasonography can also assist in this differentiation. Ultrasonography will also be helpful in ruling out an aortic aneurysm. If there is joint swelling or other signs of joint involvement, an MRI should be performed. If the mass seems fixed to the bone, a bone scan or CT scan of the bone and joint is ordered.

● Other Useful Tests

1. CBC
2. Sedimentation rate (abscess)
3. Tuberculin test
4. Arthritis profile (gout, lupus, rheumatoid arthritis)

P

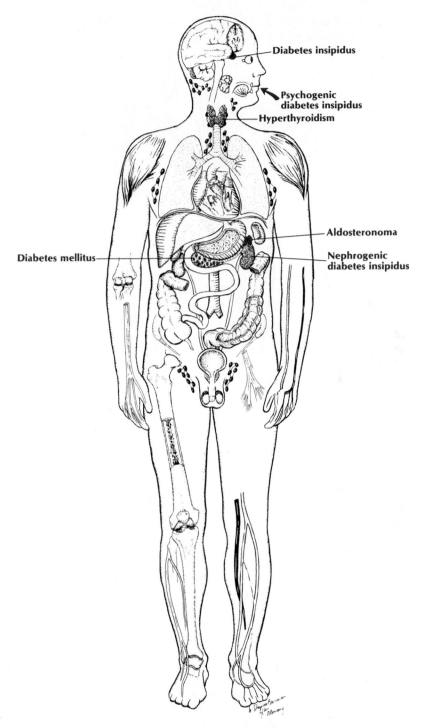

Diabetes insipidus

Psychogenic
diabetes insipidus

Hyperthyroidism

Aldosteronoma

Nephrogenic
diabetes insipidus

Diabetes mellitus

● **FIGURE 14** Polyuria.

5. Synovial fluid analysis (septic arthritis, rheumatoid arthritis, lupus)
6. Arthroscopy (torn meniscus)
7. Lymphangiogram (lymph node mass)
8. Exploratory surgery and biopsy
9. Arteriogram (Baker cyst, aneurysm)

PRIAPISM

This unfortunate condition may be humorous to everyone but the one who is "blessed" with it. The common causes are few, and the mnemonic **MINT** is an easy method for recall of these.

M—Malformation suggests phimosis and other deformities of the penis.

I—Inflammation and **intoxication** suggest posterior urethritis, prostatitis, and cystitis, as well as aphrodisiac drugs such as sildenafil citrate, alcohol, cannabis, indica, camphor, and damiana.

N—Neoplasms suggest two common causes of priapism—chronic lymphatic or myeloid leukemia and nasal polyps. The **N** also suggests **neurologic** disorders

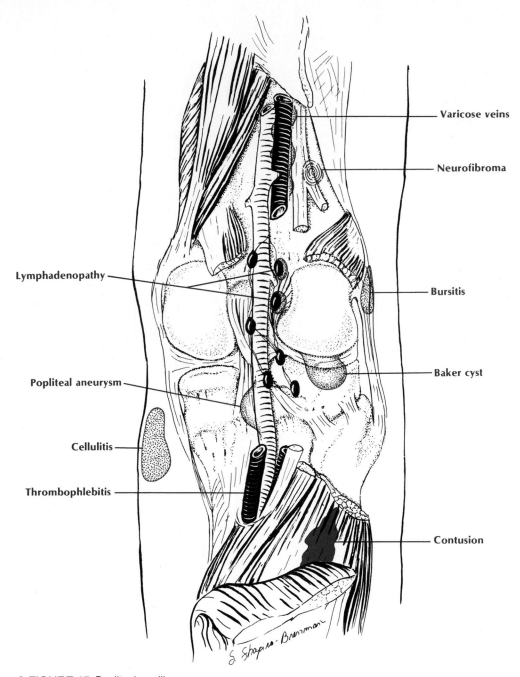

● **FIGURE 15** Popliteal swelling.

such as neurosyphilis, multiple sclerosis, and diabetic neuropathy.

T—**Trauma** recalls not only direct trauma to the penis producing a local hematoma but also trauma to the spinal cord with fractures or contusion.

● Approach to the Diagnosis

The diagnosis of priapism usually depends on the association of other symptoms and signs (e.g., boggy prostate), but a blood smear or bone marrow examination may be necessary to exclude leukemia. A careful history of the patient's sexual activities to rule out too frequent masturbation or sexual excesses may be indicated.

● Other Useful Tests

1. CBC (leukemia, sickle cell anemia)
2. Coagulation studies (blood dyscrasias)
3. Prostatic massage and examination of the discharge (prostatitis)
4. Urine culture (cystitis, pyelonephritis)
5. Serum protein electrophoresis (macroglobulinemia)

P

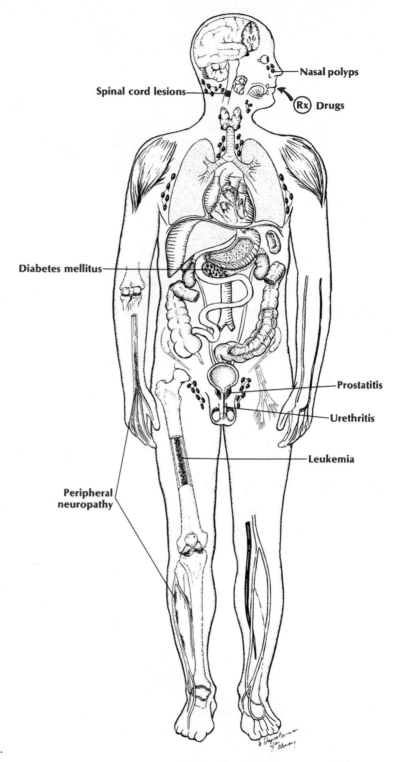

Nasal polyps

Spinal cord lesions

(Rx) Drugs

Diabetes mellitus

Prostatitis

Urethritis

Leukemia

Peripheral
neuropathy

● **FIGURE 16** Priapism.

6. MRI of the brain (tumor, cerebrovascular accident, multiple sclerosis)
7. MRI of spinal cord (multiple sclerosis, space-occupying lesion)
8. Spinal tap (multiple sclerosis, neurosyphilis)
9. Neurology consult
10. Urology consult

PROSTATIC MASS OR ENLARGEMENT

Generally, when the physician examines the prostate in a routine physical, there are only two conditions that he or she is looking for—benign prostatic hypertrophy and prostate carcinoma. The former presents a diffuse enlargement,

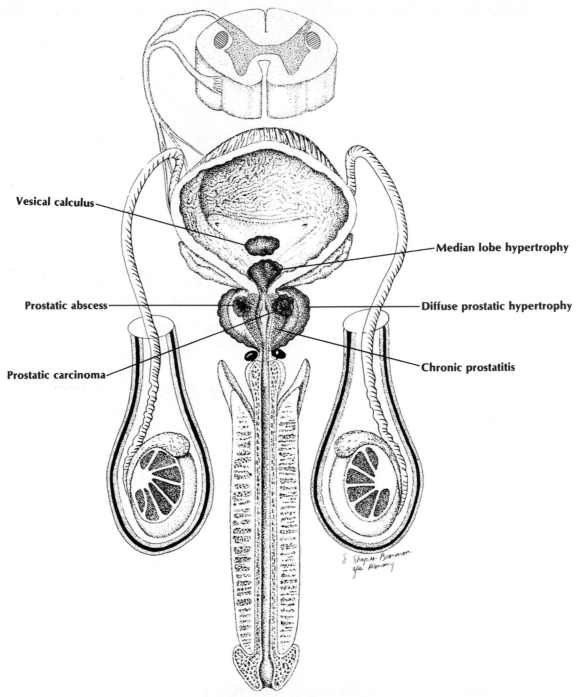

● **FIGURE 17** Prostatic mass or enlargement.

soft in consistency, and the prostate varies in size from a plum to an orange. Prostate carcinomas, in contrast, present as a stony, hard nodule in the lateral superior or inferior areas in the early stages or as a diffuse, hard, nodular enlargement in the more advanced stages. The approach is different for the patient presenting with a urethral discharge or difficulty voiding, because then one must include **acute** and **chronic prostatitis** and **prostatic abscess** in the differential.

In brief, that is the differential diagnosis of an enlarged prostate. The only trick that might be useful in remembering it is to keep in mind the ages 20, 40, 60, and 80. In general, 20-year-old men usually have acute prostatitis from gonorrhea or other bacteria. The 40-year-old men usually have chronic prostatitis from previous gonorrhea or from nonspecific prostatitis. The 60-year-old men generally have prostatic hypertrophy, and the 80-year-old men most likely have prostatic carcinoma. However, it is important to remember that any one of these diseases may appear at the ages of 40, 60, and 80.

● Approach to the Diagnosis

The main consideration in diagnosing a prostatic mass is to rule out carcinoma. It is therefore wise to draw blood for prostate-specific antigen (PSA) before proceeding in anyone who is suspected of having prostate cancer. If the mass is located in the posterior lobes, there is further support for the diagnosis. Ultrasonography can be done for further localization before proceeding with a biopsy. Obviously, if the PSA test is positive, referral to a urologist is mandatory, although false positives can occur in this test. A large, boggy prostate suggests a prostatic abscess or prostatitis. If there is no urethral discharge, one can elicit a discharge by prostatic massage. However, this should not be done if the patient has fever and significant tenderness of the prostate. It is better to proceed with antibiotic therapy and reexamine the patient after the fever has subsided. A smear and culture of the discharge is made. If upon examining the discharge under high-power microscopy, four or more white blood cells (WBCs) per high-power field are found, the diagnosis of prostatitis can be made. If benign prostatic hypertrophy is suspected, cystoscopy and retrograde pyelography can be done.

● Other Useful Tests

1. CBC
2. Sedimentation rate (infection)
3. Chemistry panel (uremia)
4. Urinalysis (cystitis, UTI)
5. Cystogram (prostatic hypertrophy)
6. Skeletal survey (metastatic carcinoma)
7. Bone scan (metastatic carcinoma)
8. Acid phosphatase level (metastatic carcinoma)
9. CT scan of pelvic lymph nodes (metastasis)
10. Lymphoscintigraphy (node metastasis)
11. Cystoscopy (bladder neck obstruction)

PROTEINURIA

There are many causes of proteinuria. The mnemonic **VINDICATE** is a helpful way of developing a list of possibilities.

V—Vascular category should call to mind CHF, hypertension, and renal vein thrombosis.

I—Inflammation: An important cause of proteinuria is UTI. In addition to the common bacterial infection, one should not forget tuberculosis, schistosomiasis, viral hepatitis, syphilis, and malaria.

N—Neoplasm category includes Wilms tumor, renal cell carcinoma, papilloma of the renal pelvis and bladder, and multiple myeloma.

D—Degenerative disorders are not a common cause of proteinuria.

I—Intoxication category includes toxic reactions to gold, mercury, gentamycin, penicillamine, captopril, and anticonvulsants. There are many other drugs that cause

proteinuria. **Idiopathic** prompts the recall of orthostatic proteinuria. Also remember primary amyloidosis.

C—Congenital causes should bring to mind polycystic kidneys, Alport syndrome, Fabry disease, horseshoe kidney, and other congenital anomalies.

A—Allergic and **autoimmune** should call to mind acute glomerulonephritis, collagen diseases, Wegener granulomatosis, Henoch–Schönlein purpura, amyloidosis, sarcoidosis, and chronic interstitial nephritis.

T—Trauma: The kidneys are involved in various forms of trauma causing proteinuria, but usually there is associated hematuria. Stones should also be included in this category because they cause trauma, inducing proteinuria and hematuria.

E—Endocrine disorders include diabetic nephrosis, myxedema, and Graves disease.

● Approach to the Diagnosis

The first step is to determine whether the proteinuria is caused by infection. A urinalysis for WBCs and examination of a fresh drop of unspun urine under the microscope for the bacteria are the fastest ways of determining this. The urine can also be cultured. Next, determine if there are red cells in the urine. This would indicate a more serious cause for the proteinuria such as collagen disease, stone, glomerulonephritis, or neoplasm, and prompts the need for an IVP, cystoscopy, and urology consult.

● Other Useful Tests

1. CBC (pyelonephritis, infectious disease)
2. Sedimentation rate (infectious disease)
3. 24-hour urine protein (nephrosis)
4. Chemistry panel (uremia, liver disease)
5. Urine for Bence–Jones protein (multiple myeloma)
6. Serum protein electrophoresis (multiple myeloma, collagen disease)
7. ANA analysis (collagen disease)
8. Addis count (glomerulonephritis)
9. ASO titer (acute glomerulonephritis)
10. CT scan of the abdomen and pelvis (neoplasm, malformation)
11. Retrograde pyelography (neoplasm, hydronephrosis)
12. Nephrology consult
13. Renal biopsy (glomerulonephritis)
14. Renal angiogram (renal artery stenosis, renal vein thrombosis)

PRURITUS

The differential diagnosis of pruritus is best developed by **anatomy**. Local conditions such as bites and parasitic infestations (e.g., scabies, hookworms, and schistosomiasis) usually reveal an obvious lesion. Generalized skin conditions such as dermatitis herpetiformis, atopic dermatitis, and exfoliative dermatitis are also more likely to show obvious skin manifestations and severe itching. These conditions are to be distinguished from cutaneous syphilis, where there is no itching at all, and psoriasis and pemphigus, where the

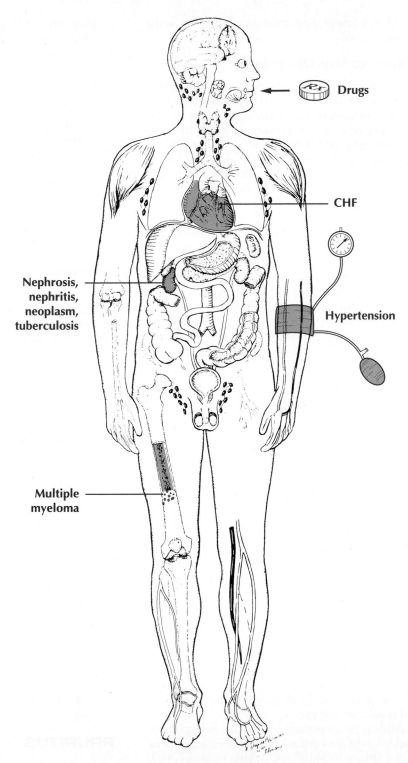

● **FIGURE 18** Proteinuria.

itching is minimal. Numerous other skin conditions cause pruritus, but we are more concerned with the systemic causes because they are more difficult to diagnose.

Jaundice, particularly obstructive jaundice, is associated with marked pruritus. Primary biliary cirrhosis may begin with pruritus without jaundice because the liver must turn more than 30 g of bile salts (the cause of the itching) a day to only 1 g of bilirubin. Thus, although there may be

enough function left to turn over the bilirubin, there is not enough to turn over the bile salts.

Diabetes mellitus may cause pruritus, particularly vulvar, where it predisposes to moniliasis. Renal disease may also cause pruritus, presumably because of the retention of toxic waste products. Pruritis during the first trimester of pregnancy called pruritis gravidarum may be due to retention of bile salts. Finally, leukemia and Hodgkin lymphoma

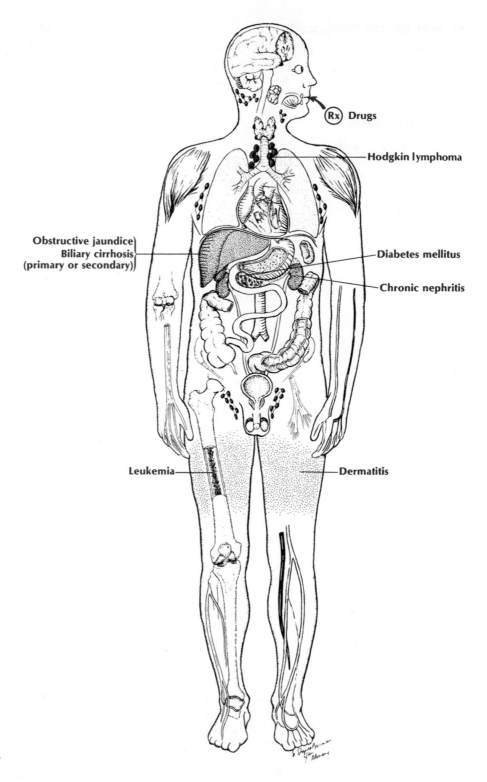

(Rx) **Drugs**

Hodgkin lymphoma

Obstructive jaundice)
Biliary cirrhosis
(primary or secondary))

Diabetes mellitus

Chronic nephritis

Leukemia

Dermatitis

● **FIGURE 19** Pruritus.

are systemic causes of pruritus. Of course, psychoneurosis and malingering must be considered.

In addition to systemic conditions mentioned above, one should search for local conditions in the anus and rectum (pruritus ani), especially hemorrhoids (internal ones may not be obvious), anal fissure, anal abscess or fistula,

and anal moniliasis or pinworms. Condyloma acuminatum may contribute to pruritus.

Any vaginal discharge may cause pruritus vulvae. Thus, *Trichomonas* and *Candida* organisms should be looked for. One should also consider lack of estrogen leading to atrophic vaginitis and dermatitis.

● Approach to the Diagnosis

It should be obvious that the clinical approach to pruritus without an obvious dermatologic manifestation is to order appropriate tests. See below to rule out the above systemic disorders.

● Other Useful Tests

1. CBC (leukemia, polycythemia)
2. Chemistry panel (liver disease, uremia)
3. Thyroid profile (hyperthyroidism)
4. Glucose tolerance test (diabetes mellitus)
5. Protein electrophoresis (lymphoma, myeloma)
6. CT scan of abdomen (malignancy)
7. Skin biopsy
8. Dermatology consult
9. Antimitochondrial antibody titer (primary biliary cirrhosis)

PTOSIS

A drooping eyelid may result from direct involvement of the levator palpebrae superioris muscle (end organ) or from involvement of the sympathetic or oculomotor nerve pathways from the muscle to the central nervous system. Consequently, visualizing **neuroanatomy** is the key to a differential diagnosis.

1. **End organ** (levator palpebrae superioris muscle): The end organ can be involved in congenital ptosis (defective development of the muscle), injury to the tendon of the muscle, neoplasms of the eye or orbit, or dermatomyositis.
2. **Sympathetic pathway:** If the sympathetic pathways are involved there is almost invariably an associated miosis and enophthalmos (Horner syndrome). The lesion may be along the intracranial pathways of the postganglionic fibers around the carotid artery in internal carotid aneurysms, thrombosis, and migraine. Orbital cellulitis or tumors may rarely affect the sympathetic nerve pathways here. The lesion may be in the stellate ganglion and its connections in cervical rib, scalenus anticus syndrome, Pancoast tumors, cervical Hodgkin lymphoma, and brachial plexus injuries. The lesion may be in the spinal cord or nerve roots in spinal cord tumors, syringomyelia, syphilis, thoracic spondylosis, metastatic carcinoma, myeloma, or tuberculosis of the spinal column. Finally, the lesion may be in the brain stem in gliomas, posterior inferior cerebellar artery occlusions, syringobulbia, and encephalitis.
3. **Oculomotor nerve pathways:** When the ptosis is due to involvement in this pathway, there are usually other extraocular muscle palsies as well. The levator muscle may be affected by myotonic dystrophy. The myoneural junction may be affected by myasthenia gravis. The oculomotor nerve may be involved by orbital tumors or cellulitis by compression from herniation of the uncus in cerebral tumors or subdural hematomas, by cavernous sinus thrombosis or carotid aneurysms, and

occasionally by syphilitic or tuberculous meningitis or pituitary and suprasellar tumors. Diabetic neuropathy may cause ptosis due to oculomotor nerve involvement. In the brain stem, the nuclei or supranuclear connections of the oculomotor nerve may be involved by syphilis (e.g., general paresis), gliomas, pinealomas, basilar artery occlusions, encephalitis, botulism, and progressive muscular atrophy.

● Approach to the Diagnosis

As always, the diagnosis is usually established by the presence or absence of other neurologic signs and symptoms. Bilateral partial ptosis suggests myotonic dystrophy, a congenital origin, or progressive muscular dystrophy. Unilateral ptosis without miosis or extraocular muscle palsy suggests injury to the levator palpebrae superioris muscle or myasthenia gravis. A Tensilon test should always be considered. When all the components of Horner syndrome are present, x-rays of the skull, cervical and thoracic spine, and chest should be done. A spinal tap and arteriography should be considered.

If oculomotor involvement is certain, a glucose tolerance test, skull x-rays, serologic tests for syphilis, spinal tap (if no contraindications), CT scans, and, possibly, arteriography are indicated. The need for other tests depends on the presence of other neurologic signs. An ophthalmologist and neurologist should probably be consulted in all cases of unilateral ptosis.

● Other Useful Tests

1. CBC (orbital cellulitis)
2. ANA analysis (collagen disease)
3. Acetylcholine receptor antibody titer (myasthenia gravis)
4. MRI of the brain (brain tumor or other space-occupying lesion)
5. Cerebral angiogram (cerebral aneurysm)
6. Response to intravenous thiamine (Wernicke encephalopathy)
7. 24-hour urine creatinine and creatine (muscular dystrophy)
8. CT scan of mediastinum (mediastinal tumor, aneurysm)
9. Chest x-ray (malignancy)
10. Lymph node biopsy (lymphoma)

PTYALISM

The mnemonic **MINT** will facilitate the recall of the most important causes of ptyalism.

M—Malformation would prompt the recall of congenital esophageal atresia.
I—Inflammation ought to suggest herpes simplex, aphthous stomatitis, and peritonsillar abscess. Syphilis and tuberculosis rarely cause ptyalism.
N—Neurologic disorders that cause ptyalism include bulbar palsy (as in amyotrophic lateral sclerosis and

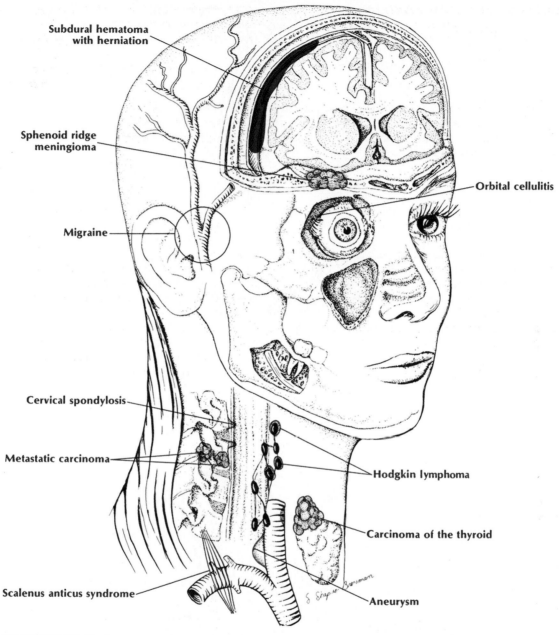

Subdural hematoma
with herniation

Sphenoid ridge
meningioma

Migraine

Orbital cellulitis

Cervical spondylosis

Metastatic carcinoma

Hodgkin lymphoma

Carcinoma of the thyroid

Scalenus anticus syndrome

Aneurysm

● **FIGURE 20** Ptosis.

poliomyelitis) and pseudobulbar palsy (as in multiple sclerosis and brain stem gliomas). They should also suggest myasthenia gravis, Parkinsonism, and ptyalism associated with dementia.

T—**Toxic disorders** that cause ptyalism include iodine medications, mercury poisoning, pilocarpine, and other parasympathomimetic drugs.

● **Approach to the Diagnosis**

The most important thing to do is look for ulcerations or other abnormalities of the mouth and oropharynx. Dental cares and gingivitis may cause ptyalism as may an ill-fitted dental plate. If local conditions can be excluded, a thorough neurologic examination should be done to rule out bulbar and pseudobulbar palsy. A Tensilon test or serum

acetylcholine receptor antibody titer can be done to exclude myasthenia gravis. The busy physician will want to consult a neurologist to do this. Although a CT scan or MRI may be needed, a neurologic consult is more cost-effective. Do not hesitate to consult a dentist or oral surgeon if the diagnosis is in doubt.

PULSATILE MASS

Simply by thinking of the location of the pulsatile mass, one can identify the cause or causes of a pulsatile mass.

Orbit: This is most likely an arteriovenous fistula related to trauma or the spontaneous rupture of an aneurysm into the cavernous sinus.

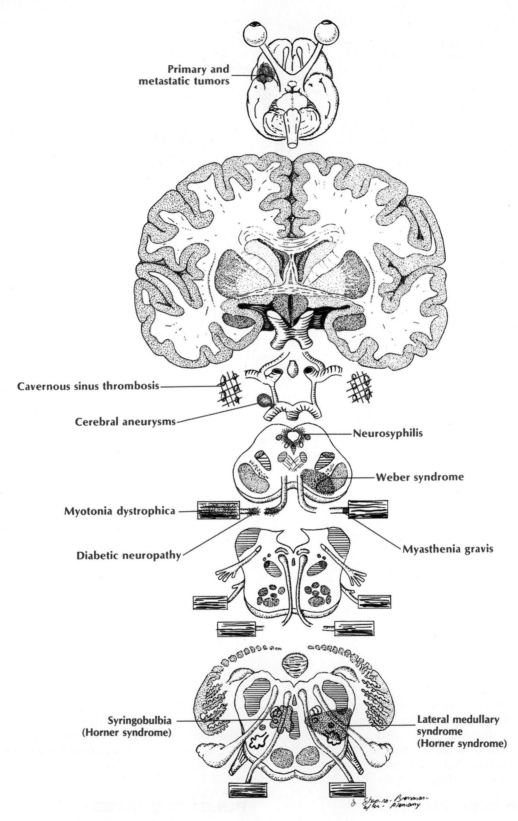

● **FIGURE 21** Ptosis.

Neck: A carotid, innominate, or brachial artery aneurysm is the most likely cause here, but pulsations may be felt in the neck from aortic regurgitation as well.

Chest: An aneurysm of the thoracic aorta is the most likely cause here, but an enlarged heart or cardiac aneurysm may give a noticeable heave on inspection.

Abdomen: Tricuspid regurgitation may cause pulsations of the liver in the right upper quadrant, but the associated ascites and dependent edema should make the diagnosis obvious. A pulsating abdominal aorta is usually an atherosclerotic aneurysm, but it may be an abnormal finding in asthenic individuals. It is also possible that the pulsating mass is a tumor over a normal abdominal aorta.

Extremities: A pulsating mass in the axilla, groin, or popliteal fossa is usually an aneurysm, but osteosarcoma can produce a pulsating mass along with eggshell cracking.

● Approach to the Diagnosis

Ultrasonography will usually confirm the diagnosis of these lesions, but a CT scan or angiography may be necessary, particularly when surgical intervention is planned. A cardiovascular surgeon should be consulted before ordering these expensive tests.

PULSE RHYTHM ABNORMALITIES

Visualizing the conduction system of the heart from its beginning in the sinus node to its ends in the ventricular muscle, one can develop a list of the causes of pulse irregularities.

Sinus node: Pulse irregularities associated with this node include sinus arrhythmia and sick sinus syndrome.

Atrium: Paroxysmal atrial tachycardia, atrial premature contractions, atrial flutter, and fibrillation are brought to mind when we focus on the atrium.

Arterioventricular (A-V) node: A-V nodal rhythm and nodal tachycardia are suggested by this anatomic structure.

Bundle of Hiss: This structure prompts the recall of first-, second-, and third-degree heart block.

Ventricular muscle: This tissue facilitates the recall of premature ventricular contractions, ventricular tachycardia, and ventricular fibrillation.

Simply visualizing the cardiac conduction system will not help to recall the slow pulse of vasovagal syncope or parasympathomimetic drugs. Furthermore, a method of recalling the various causes of these cardiac arrhythmias is still needed. These are considered on pages 85 through 86.

● Approach to the Diagnosis

It is wise to get a cardiology consult at the outset. Routine workup includes a CBC, sedimentation rate, thyroid panel, chemistry panel, ECG, and chest x-rays. If rheumatic fever is suspected, an ASO titer or streptozyme test will be ordered. Echocardiography, Hiss bundle studies, and 24-hour

Holter monitoring may be necessary. If a valvular lesion or coronary artery disease is suspected, cardiac catheterization and angiocardiography will be necessary.

PYURIA

Pyuria is included here although it is not a symptom or a definitive finding on physical examination. Examination of the urine, however, is so frequently a part of every physical examination that the causes of pyuria should be available for immediate recall for all primary care physicians.

As in other cases of purulent discharge, inflammation is the cause of pyuria in most cases, thus an etiologic mnemonic would seem unnecessary. However, the mnemonic **MINT** must be considered at the outset so that one recalls the malformations, neoplasms, and traumatic foreign bodies that may cause an obstruction or provide a fruitful soil for bacterial growth. Unlike a non-bloody discharge elsewhere, pyuria is rarely associated with inflammation of a noninfectious nature; more than that, it is almost invariably due to bacteria. What is more, the bacteria are usually gram-negative bacilli, particularly *Escherichia coli*, *Enterobacter*, *Proteus*, or *Pseudomonas* organisms.

With this in mind, let us visualize the **anatomy** of the genitourinary tree and develop a system for ready recall of the diagnostic possibilities. The **urethra** brings to mind all the various causes of urethritis (see page 425). The **prostate** reminds one of prostatitis and prostatic abscess. The **bladder** suggests cystitis, stricture, Hunner ulcers, calculi, and papillomas that may initiate infection. Some urologists may recall finding a vesicovaginal fistula or rectovesical fistula in patients who have had previous abdominal surgery; a fistula may also form in regional ileitis. The **ureters** suggest the numerous congenital anomalies (e.g., stricture, congenital band, and aberrant vessel) that may cause obstruction and infection. The **renal pelvis** and **kidney** recall pyelitis and pyelonephritis, as well as renal carcinoma, calculi, and congenital anomalies, all of which may contribute to infection.

The rare causes of pyuria must be considered. Tuberculosis of the kidney should be mentioned, because when routine cultures are negative, this is one of the conditions to look for. Even actinomycosis can cause pyuria, thus a culture on Sabouraud media may be warranted. Although *Bilharzia haematobium* parasites usually cause hematuria, pyuria is occasionally the initial finding. An interstitial nephritis of toxic or autoimmune origin may occasionally cause a "shower" of eosinophils into the urine. Finally, there is probably not a surgeon alive who has not been fooled by the pyuria of an acute appendicitis, salpingitis, or diverticulitis.

● Approach to the Diagnosis

How does one track down the cause of pyuria? First, it must be determined that the cloudy urine is really pyuria. Amorphous phosphates and other inert material will disappear on treating the urine with dilute acetic acid. Then, just

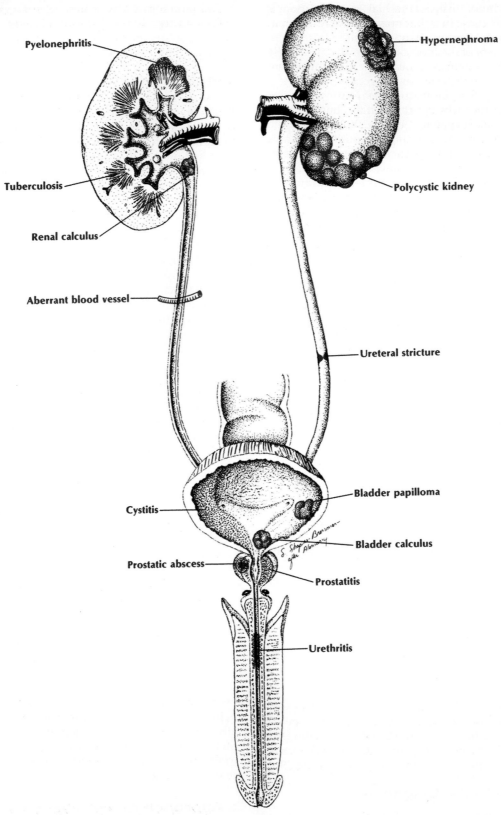

Pyelonephritis

Tuberculosis

Renal calculus

Aberrant blood vessel

Hypernephroma

Polycystic kidney

Ureteral stricture

Cystitis

Bladder papilloma

Bladder calculus

Prostatic abscess

Prostatitis

Urethritis

● **FIGURE 22** Pyuria.

as for other nonbloody discharges, one must do a smear and culture for the offending organism; an examination of the urine, especially the unspun specimen, is axiomatic. If one finds clumps of leukocytes, renal gitter cells, or WBC casts, the infection almost certainly comes from the kidney. Motile bacteria in an unspun specimen examined under high-power microscopy and a colony count of over 100,000 per mL signify infection. A three-glass test may be helpful in localizing the site of origin of the pyuria. Anaerobic cultures and cultures for *Chlamydia* may be needed. Look for eosinophils on a Wright stain of the urine if toxic nephritis is suspected.

Vaginal examination and culture may disclose a source for the infection. In the male, one episode of pyuria should be sufficient indication for an IVP; a female should have one after her second episode, especially if no cause can be found on physical examination. Cystoscopy and a voiding cystogram are often indicated at this time.

● Other Useful Tests

1. CBC (pyelonephritis)
2. Sedimentation rate (pyelonephritis)
3. Chemistry panel (diabetes mellitus, nephritis)
4. ANA analysis (collagen disease)
5. Retrograde pyelography (tumor, malformation, obstructive uropathy)
6. Urine for acid-fast bacillus smear and culture and guinea pig inoculation (tuberculosis)
7. Sonogram (diverticulum, pelvic mass, cyst, abscess)
8. CT scan of abdomen and pelvis (tumor, malformation, obstructive uropathy, extrinsic mass)

R

RASH, GENERAL

The best way to recall the causes of a general rash while still examining the patient is to think of the mnemonic **DERMATITIS**.

D—Deficiency diseases include pellagra, scurvy, and vitamin A deficiency.

E—Endocrine diseases recall the acne and plethora of Cushing disease, the pretibial myxedema of hyperthyroidism, and the necrobiosis lipoidica diabeticorum of diabetes mellitus. Xanthoma diabeticorum should also be mentioned. Carcinoid tumors may cause a general erythema and cyanosis.

R—Reticuloendotheliosis suggests Niemann–Pick disease, Hand–Schöller–Christian disease, and Gaucher disease, as well as Letterer–Siwe disease.

M—Malignancies suggest the rash of leukemia, Hodgkin lymphoma, and metastatic carcinoma. In addition, certain malignancies induce skin conditions such as herpes zoster (lymphomas), dermatitis herpetiformis, dermatomyositis (gastrointestinal [GI] malignancy), or acanthosis nigricans (abdominal malignancy). Multiple small metastases to the skin may suggest a rash. Neurofibromatosis is a cause of multiple skin fibromas. Dysplastic nevi syndrome is a hereditary condition associated with numerous moles of the scalp, trunk, and buttocks. Malignant transformation to melanomas is not uncommon.

A—Allergic and **autoimmune** diseases include angioneurotic edema, urticaria, allergic dermatitis, erythema nodosum and multiforme, and other skin lesions of rheumatic fever, dermatomyositis, scleroderma, lupus erythematosus, periarteritis nodosa, and pemphigus. Allergies to many foods and inhalants may cause a skin reaction. Thrombocytopenia purpura and allergic purpura belong in this category.

T—Toxic disorders include drug eruptions from sulfa, penicillin, and a host of other drugs. Serum sickness should be recalled here. Iodides, boric acid, and many toxins in the environment may be responsible.

I—Infectious diseases are perhaps the largest category to consider. They are best classified by the size of the organism working from the smallest on up.

Figures on pages 364, 365, 366, 368, and 369 from Sauer GC. *Manual of Skin Diseases*, 4th ed. Philadelphia: JB Lippincott, 1980, with permission.

1. **Viruses** include the exanthema of measles, infectious mononucleosis, rubella, smallpox, chickenpox, human immunodeficiency virus (HIV), herpes zoster, viral hepatitis, and various Coxsackie and echoviruses.
2. **Rickettsiae** include Rocky Mountain spotted fever and typhus.

3. **Bacteria** include typhoid, meningococcemia, miliary tuberculosis (usually a focal lesion), Haverhill fever, brucellosis, leprosy, and subacute bacterial endocarditis (SBE).
4. **Spirochetes** include syphilis, which may present any form of a rash, but the lesions are usually small, indurated macules on the trunk, palm, and, to a lesser degree, the extremities. Rat-bite fever and *Borrelia recurrentis* may also cause a rash.
5. **Parasites** suggest New World leishmaniasis, hookworm, toxoplasmosis, and trichinosis.
6. **Fungi** suggest histoplasmosis, which is more likely to produce a general rash than coccidioidomycosis, blastomycosis, and spirotrichosis, although all are associated on occasion with rash. Tinea versicolor is also responsible for a diffuse rash, but most of the other fungi cause a local rash.

T—Trauma suggests sunburn and other types of burns, such as radiation.

I—Idiopathic disorders account for a number of diseases. In this category one should remember psoriasis, lichen planus, epidermolysis bullosum, ichthyosis, porphyria, neurodermatitis or eczema, the adenoma sebaceum of tuberous sclerosis, and keratosis pilaris. Pityriasis rosea may be due to a virus, but this is not established yet.

S—Sweat gland and **sebaceous** gland disorders include miliaria (prickly heat) of the sweat glands and milia, folliculitis, and carbuncles and furuncles involving the base of the hair follicle and sebaceous glands. Acne rosacea and acne vulgaris can also be recalled here.

The diagnosis of a rash depends on a good history and a description of the type of rash and its distribution.

● Description (only the most typical are listed)

1. **Macular rash:** Typhoid, syphilis, pityriasis rosea, variola (in early stages), rubella (first stages), and tinea versicolor fall into this group.
2. **Papular rash:** Measles, German measles, HIV, miliaria, scabies, drug eruptions, lichen planus, urticaria papulosa, warts, lupus erythematosus, erythema multiforme, rat-bite fever, and infectious mononucleosis generally present this way. Rocky Mountain spotted fever may have a maculopapular rash prior to the purpuric rash. Reticuloendotheliosis may also present this way.
3. **Purpural rash:** Meningococcemia, thrombocytopenic purpura from any cause, Henoch–Schönlein purpura, Letterer–Siwe disease, trichinosis, leukemia, SBE, and Rocky Mountain spotted fever and other rickettsiae are in this category.

4. **Vesicles:** Contact or allergic dermatitis, miliaria, eczema, variola and varicella, dermatophytosis, tinea circinata, herpes zoster, poison ivy, scabies (one stage), and some drug allergies present this way. Impetigo may start as a vesicle but usually quickly becomes bullous.

5. **Bullae:** Pemphigus, impetigo contagiosa, hereditary syphilis, herpes zoster, dermatitis herpetiformis, and epidermolysis bullosa are considered here.

6. **Scales:** Psoriasis, parapsoriasis, and lichen planus are the most typical causes of this lesion, but most dermatoses may get to this stage after chronic itching. Scarlet fever

R

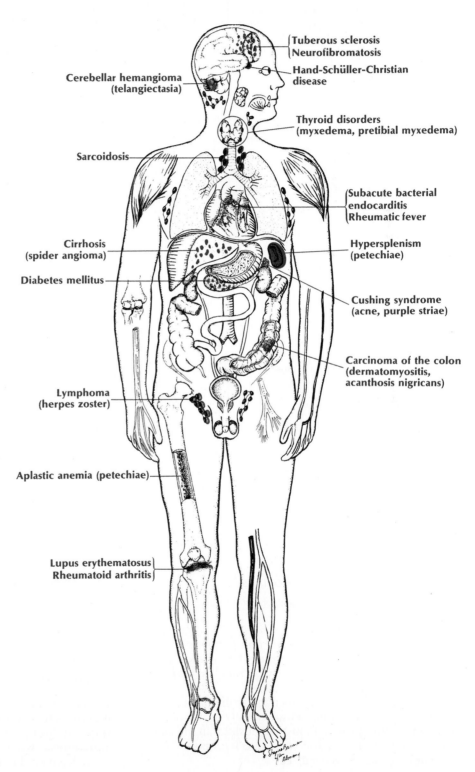

● **FIGURE 1** Rash, systemic causes.

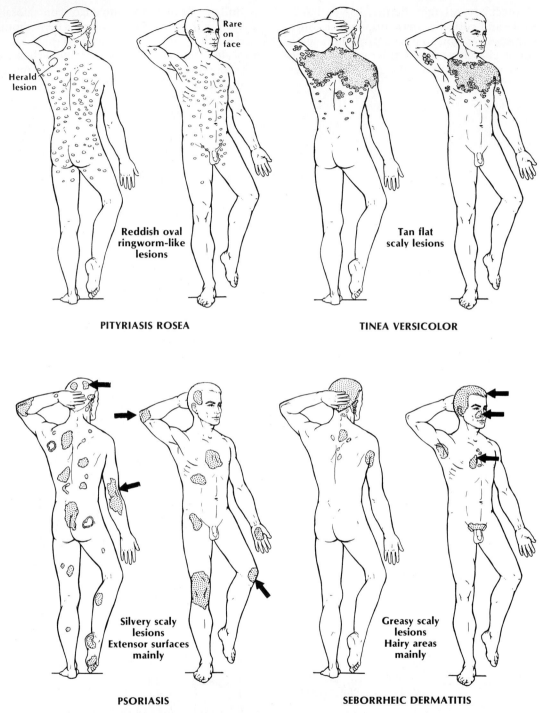

PITYRIASIS ROSEA

Herald lesion

Rare on face

Reddish oval ringworm-like lesions

TINEA VERSICOLOR

Tan flat scaly lesions

PSORIASIS

Silvery scaly lesions
Extensor surfaces mainly

SEBORRHEIC DERMATITIS

Greasy scaly lesions
Hairy areas mainly

● **FIGURE 2** Rash, general.

has a definite desquamative phase, and pityriasis rosea will demonstrate scaling on scratching. Tinea versicolor, the dermatophytoses, and exfoliative dermatitis must be considered here.

7. **Pustules:** Furunculosis and impetigo are the most typical types of this lesion but they are usually focal rashes. Smallpox (variola) will demonstrate pustules in the late stages, and chickenpox may do the same. It is unusual for pustular lesions to be generalized.

8. **Nodules:** Erythema nodosum, erythema induratum, and Weber–Christian disease fall into this category.

● **Distribution**

1. **Trunk:** Pityriasis rosea, drug eruptions, herpes zoster, dermatitis herpetiformis, chickenpox, seborrheic dermatitis, and tinea versicolor occur typically on the trunk.

2. **Extremities:** Smallpox and Rocky Mountain spotted fever often begin on the extremities and work centripetally.

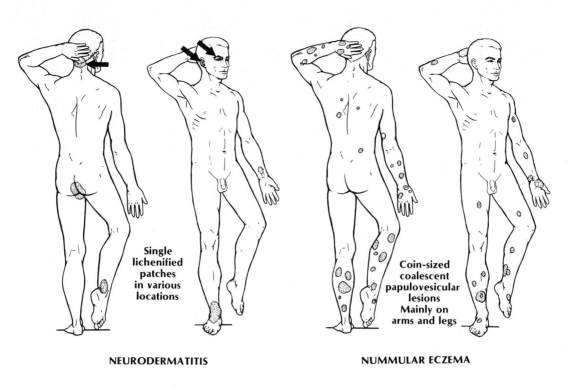

NEURODERMATITIS

Single lichenified patches in various locations

NUMMULAR ECZEMA

Coin-sized coalescent papulovesicular lesions Mainly on arms and legs

R

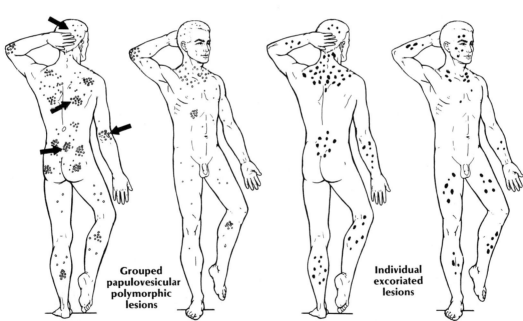

DERMATITIS HERPETIFORMIS

Grouped papulovesicular polymorphic lesions

NEUROTIC EXCORIATIONS

Individual excoriated lesions

● **FIGURE 3** Rash, general.

3. **Palms of the hands:** Four conditions typically occur here: Rocky Mountain spotted fever, penicillin allergy, syphilis, and erythema multiforme. Contact dermatitis, keratoderma, climacterium, warts, keratoderma palmaris, dyshidrosis, and psoriasis may also occur here. Hand, foot, and mouth disease is associated with a vesicular rash of the hands, feet, and mouth and is caused by a coxsackie virus.

4. **Feet:** Tinea pedis, warts, purpuras, psoriasis, keratoderma plantaris, syphilis, penicillin allergy, Rocky Mountain spotted fever, acrodynia, varicose ulcers, diabetic ulcers, and ischemic ulcers may occur here more often than elsewhere. Contact dermatitis from leather is important to consider here.

5. **Face:** Acne vulgaris and rosacea, impetigo, seborrheic dermatitis, milia, lupus erythematosus, lupus vulgaris,

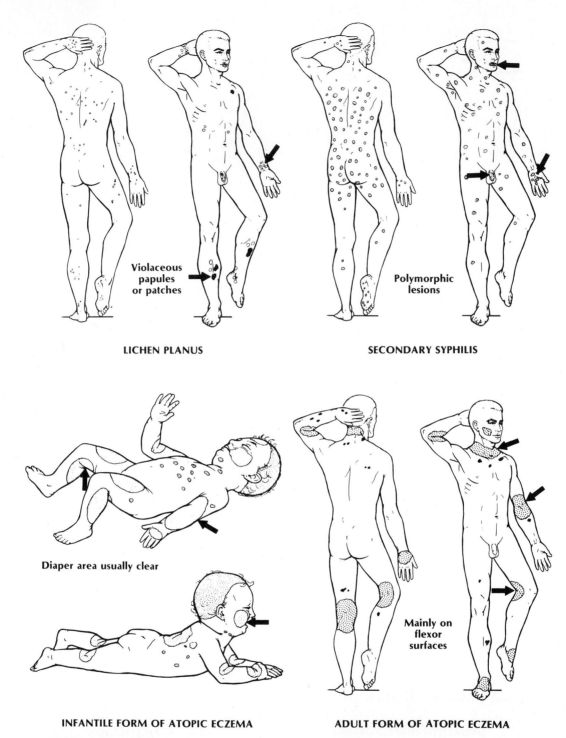

LICHEN PLANUS

Violaceous papules or patches

SECONDARY SYPHILIS

Polymorphic lesions

INFANTILE FORM OF ATOPIC ECZEMA

Diaper area usually clear

ADULT FORM OF ATOPIC ECZEMA

Mainly on flexor surfaces

● **FIGURE 4** Rash, general.

basal cell and squamous cell carcinomas, eczema, contact dermatitis, and erythema multiforme have a predilection for the face.

6. **Groins and thighs:** Scabies, pediculosis, intertrigo, tinea cruris, moniliasis, and Weber–Christian disease occur here.
7. **Antecubital and popliteal spaces:** Eczema occurs here.
8. **Extensor surfaces of elbow and knees:** Psoriasis and epidermolysis bullosa should be considered.
9. **Shins:** Erythema nodosum occurs here.

The description and distribution of all the dermatologic conditions would take volumes. Only the most common or important ones have been considered here.

● **Approach to the Diagnosis**

The association of other symptoms and signs is extremely helpful in differential diagnosis. For example, a rash with bloody diarrhea might suggest Crohn disease or ulcerative colitis. A rash with joint pain would suggest lupus or gonorrhea. A rash with lymphadenopathy should suggest syphilis or Kaposi sarcoma. Any condition with pus should be cultured. If a fungus is suspected, a Wood lamp examination and a fresh potassium hydroxide (KOH) preparation should be done. Skin biopsy is useful and is necessary in some cases. A dermatologist should be consulted if there is any question about a malignancy, if the condition persists, or if the symptoms are systemic. It is foolish to persist in treatment without a definitive diagnosis for more than 2 or 3 weeks when one may be dealing with something serious.

● Other Useful Tests

1. Complete blood count (CBC) (chronic infectious disease)
2. Sedimentation rate (infectious disease)
3. Chemistry panel (collagen disease)
4. Platelet count (thrombocytopenia)
5. Blood cultures (SBE)
6. Venereal disease research laboratory (VDRL) test (secondary syphilis)
7. Antinuclear antibody (ANA) analysis (collagen disease)
8. Allergy skin testing (allergic dermatitis)
9. Chest x-ray, barium enema, GI series, long bone survey (survey for malignancy and various forms of colitis)
10. HIV antibody titer (acquired immunodeficiency syndrome [AIDS])
11. Well–Felix reaction (*Rickettsia disease*)
12. Serology for Rocky Mountain spotted fever
13. Coagulation profile (disseminated intravascular coagulation [DIC])
14. Serum immunoglobulin E (IgE) level (allergy)
15. Serum for viral studies (viral disease)
16. Streptozyme test (rheumatic fever)
17. Anticentromere antibody (scleroderma)

Case Presentation #76

A 26-year-old white man presents with an erythematous macular rash on his trunk and proximal extremities for the past week. There is no fever, chills, or other constitutional symptoms. There is no pruritis associated with the rash.

Question #1. What is your differential diagnosis?

On further questioning, he denies a urethral discharge or genital ulcer. He has not been exposed to any drugs. However, he recalls a large oval red patch that appeared in the epigastrium a few days before the generalized rash.

Question #2. What is your diagnosis now?

(See Appendix B for the answers.)

RASH, LOCAL

The differential diagnosis of a local rash is best approached with the mnemonic **VINDICATE**.

V—**Vascular** lesions suggest livedo reticularis, acrocyanosis, gangrene of Raynaud syndrome, necrotic areas of periarteritis nodosa, and petechiae from emboli. Varicose and ischemic ulcers may also be considered here.

I—**Inflammatory** lesions include boils, carbuncles, folliculitis, hydradenitis suppurativa, abscesses, and erysipelas. Dermatophytosis, chancre, chancroid, and yaws, pinta, and tularemia are important. Scabies, insect bites, anthrax, tuberculosis, or actinomycotic sinus fall into this category. The bull's-eye lesion of a brown recluse spider bite deserves special mention here. The fistulous tracts of regional ileitis may belong here. Warts and moluscum contagiosa also need mentioning here.

N—**Neoplasms** of the skin include fibromas, melanomas, lipomas, basal cell and squamous cell carcinomas, and metastatic carcinoma. Kaposi sarcoma and mycosis fungoides must also be considered.

D—**Degenerative** lesions such as senile keratosis are considered here. Kraurosis vulvae may be recalled here.

I—**Intoxication** includes acid or alkaline burns of the skin. Fixed-drug eruptions should not be forgotten.

C—**Congenital** lesions include epidermolysis bullosa, eczema, neurofibromatosis, and lipomas.

A—**Allergic** and **autoimmune** diseases suggest pyoderma gangrenosum (ulcerative colitis), necrotic lesions of periarteritis nodosa, and subcutaneous fat necrosis of Weber–Christian disease. Seventeen percent of health care workers are allergic to latex.

T—**Trauma** suggests burns, contusions, lacerations, and hemorrhages.

E—**Endocrine** diseases immediately recall pretibial myxedema, necrobiosis lipoidica diabeticorum, diabetic ulcers, the flushed face of Cushing syndrome, and carcinoid.

● Approach to the Diagnosis

The approach to the diagnosis is similar to that of the general rash (see page 366).

RECTAL BLEEDING

This discussion considers the causes of bright red or maroon stools. (The causes of melena or black stools are the same as the causes of hematemesis; the differential diagnosis is given on page 208.) Bright-red blood may occasionally result from an upper GI lesion if there is associated diarrhea.

A list of the causes of rectal bleeding of fresh blood is best developed with the use of the mnemonic **VINDICATE**.

V—**Vascular** conditions prompt the recall of hemorrhoids, but one cannot forget mesenteric infarctions.

I—**Inflammation** suggests perirectal abscess, anal fissure or ulcer, amebic colitis, or condyloma latum and acuminatum.

N—**Neoplasms** call to mind polyps and carcinomas of the rectum and anus.

D—**Degenerative** disorders do not suggest anything in particular.

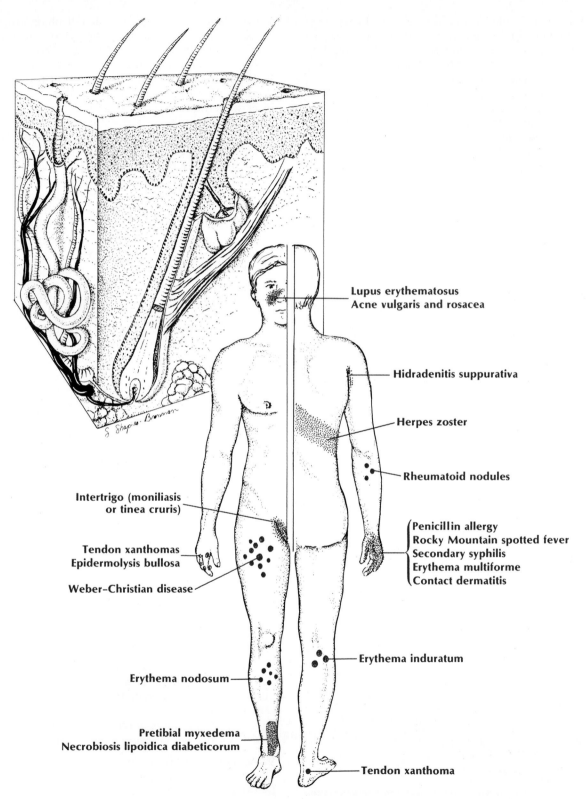

S. Shapira-Brosman

● **FIGURE 5** Rash, local.

I—Intoxication suggests pseudomembranous colitis complicating gentamicin, clindamycin, and other antibiotic therapy. Jejunal ulcers from potassium chloride tablets should be considered here.

C—Congenital and **acquired** anomalies suggest fistula in ano, bleeding Meckel diverticulum, and bleeding colonic diverticula, among other congenital conditions. Intussusception would fall into this category also.

R

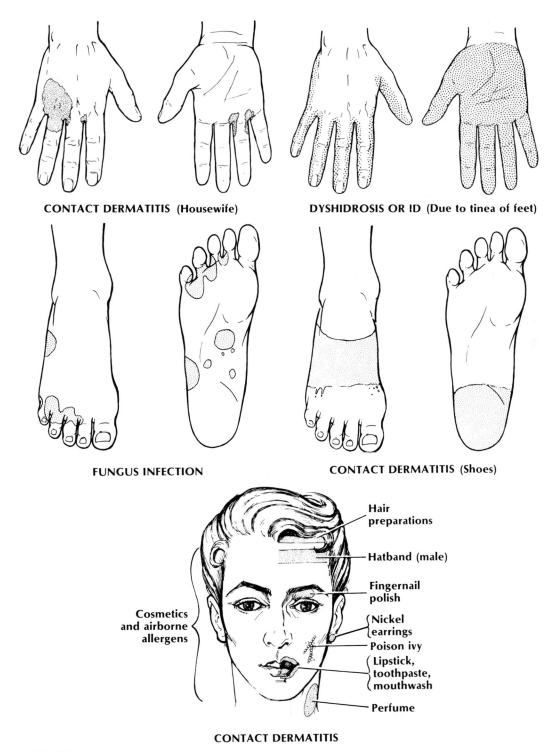

CONTACT DERMATITIS (Housewife)

DYSHIDROSIS OR ID (Due to tinea of feet)

FUNGUS INFECTION

CONTACT DERMATITIS (Shoes)

Hair
preparations

Hatband (male)

Fingernail
polish

Nickel
earrings

Poison ivy

Lipstick,
toothpaste,
mouthwash

Perfume

Cosmetics
and airborne
allergens

CONTACT DERMATITIS

● **FIGURE 6** Rash, local.

A—Autoimmune diseases recall granulomatous colitis and ulcerative colitis.

T—Trauma suggests the bleeding from any foreign body inserted into the rectum, including the male organ.

E—Endocrine disorders do not suggest anything other than the Zollinger–Ellison syndrome, which, because it causes ulceration of the jejunum, may be associated with maroon stools.

In disorders of the upper colon and small intestines, the blood is older and thus a maroon color is likely. In addition, the blood is mixed with the stool and may indeed

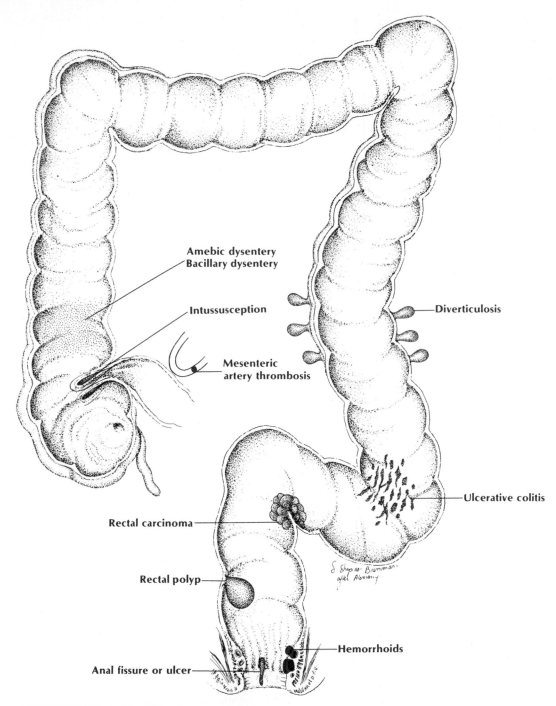

Ambic dysentery
Bacillary dysentery

Intussusception

Diverticulosis

Mesenteric
artery thrombosis

Ulcerative colitis

Rectal carcinoma

Rectal polyp

Hemorrhoids

Anal fissure or ulcer

● **FIGURE 7** Rectal bleeding.

be so well mixed that it will not be discovered without a test for occult blood. Other features are more prominent in bacillary dysentery and salmonellosis.

● **Approach to the Diagnosis**

Armed with a more comprehensive list of causes of rectal bleeding, the clinician is ready to eliminate some of them as he or she asks appropriate questions during the history and performs the examination with all the causes in mind. The diagnosis may be pinned down by the presence or absence of other symptoms and signs. The principal diagnostic procedures are stool cultures, stool examination for ova and parasites, proctoscopy, barium enema, and colonoscopy. Radioactive bleeding scans may be necessary if these studies are negative.

● **Other Useful Tests**

1. CBC (infection)
2. Urinalysis (systemic disease)

3. Sedimentation rate (infection, granulomatous, or ulcerative colitis)
4. Chemistry panel (liver disease)
5. Frei test (lymphogranuloma venereum)
6. Rectal biopsy (colitis, neoplasm)
7. Carcinoembryonic antigen (CEA) (colorectal cancer)
8. Small-bowel series (neoplasm)
9. CT scan of the abdomen
10. Angiogram (mesenteric thrombosis)
11. Exploratory laparotomy

Case Presentation #77

A 72-year-old white woman presents to your office with the chief complaint of blood in her stool for several weeks. She also has noted intermittent constipation and diarrhea during that time. She denies painful bowel movements.

Question #1. Utilizing the mnemonic **VINDICATE**, what is your differential diagnosis?

General physical examination was unremarkable. Rectal examination failed to reveal the cause of her rectal bleeding, but the stool was positive for occult blood. A barium enema revealed a napkin ring constriction in the sigmoid colon.

Question #2. What is your diagnosis now?

(See Appendix B for the answers.)

RECTAL DISCHARGE

Rectal discharges are usually bloody, but the two notable exceptions to this are a **ruptured perirectal abscess** and an **anal fistula** (really the end result of the former). Use the mnemonic **MINT**, and a few other conditions that might otherwise be overlooked come to mind.

M—**Malformation** that creates a nonbloody rectal discharge is loss of sphincter control, often due to rectal surgery or a deep midline episiotomy, but perhaps even more frequently due to neurologic disturbances such as spinal cord injury or stroke (really fecal incontinence). A **pilonidal sinus**, although not specifically related to the rectum, may suggest that the patient has a rectal discharge.

I—**Inflammation**, in addition to those disorders already mentioned, recalls an anal fissure or ulcer that not only causes purulent material to weep on its own but also often permits fecal material to leak onto the underclothes of the patient. The fistulous tracts from regional ileitis and lymphogranuloma venereum must be considered here. Condyloma latum and acuminatum, although not causing a discharge themselves, may prevent complete closure of the anal canal and permit fecal material to leak.

N—**Neoplasms** of the rectum and anus and even thrombosed hemorrhoids can behave in a similar manner.

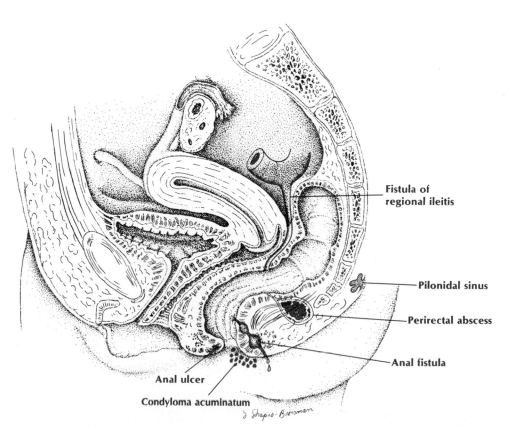

Fistula of regional ileitis

Pilonidal sinus

Perirectal abscess

Anal fistula

Anal ulcer

Condyloma acuminatum

● **FIGURE 8** Rectal discharge.

T—**Trauma** is mentioned merely to remind one again of episiotomies and rectal surgery that may create poor control and allow chronic escape of feces, especially the liquid form.

● Approach to the Diagnosis

Smear and culture of the discharge are axiomatic. Visualization of the lesion with the anoscope or sigmoidoscope is usually necessary. A Frei test should be done if lymphogranuloma venereum is suspected.

● Other Useful Tests

1. CBC (inflammation, abscess)
2. Sedimentation rate (abscess)
3. VDRL test
4. Frei test (lymphogranuloma venereum)
5. Barium enema (ulcerative colitis)
6. Cystogram (fistulous tract)
7. Stool for ova and parasites (amebiasis)
8. Proctology consult
9. Computed tomography (CT) scan of pelvis (neoplasm, fistulous tract, abscess)
10. Indium scan (abscess)
11. Exploratory surgery
12. Biopsy of lesion
13. HIV antibody titer

RECTAL MASS

Of course, the physician is looking for a rectal carcinoma when performing a routine rectal examination, but what else might be found? Use the mnemonic **VINDICATE** to have a list of possibilities clearly in mind before the examination.

V—**Vascular** disorders suggest internal and external hemorrhoids.

I—**Inflammation** includes submucous and perirectal abscesses.

N—**Neoplasms** most often manifest as rectal polyps and carcinomas. Other conditions to be remembered include the Blummer shelf of metastatic carcinoma from many sites into the pouch of Douglas, prostatic hypertrophy, and carcinomas.

D—**Degenerative** conditions are not associated with a rectal mass.

I—**Intoxication** signifies a fecal impaction, particularly from a hunk of barium after a barium enema.

C—**Congenital** and acquired anomalies should remind one of diverticula that may become abscessed and create a mass in the cul-de-sac. They may also recall a pelvic appendix and rectal prolapse.

A—**Autoimmune** conditions include regional ileitis, which may lodge in the cul-de-sac and create a fistula with the rectum.

T—**Trauma** signifies a ruptured bladder.

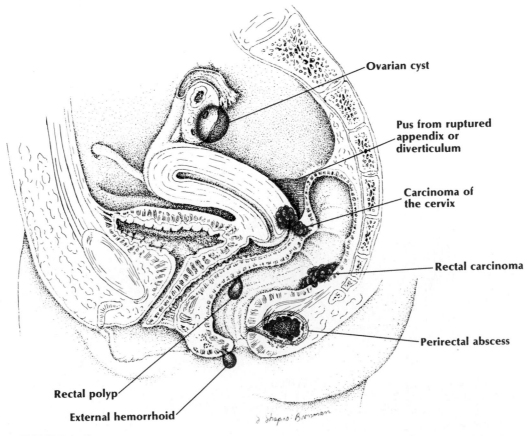

Ovarian cyst

Pus from ruptured appendix or diverticulum

Carcinoma of the cervix

Rectal carcinoma

Perirectal abscess

Rectal polyp

External hemorrhoid

● **FIGURE 9** Rectal mass.

E—**Endocrine** causes recall the various ovarian tumors and ruptured ectopic pregnancy that will produce a mass in the cul-de-sac.

There are, therefore, numerous disorders to keep in mind when examining the rectum.

● Approach to the Diagnosis

Anoscopy, sigmoidoscopy, and a barium enema are the most significant tools in the proctologist's armamentarium. Biopsy or excision of polyps is routine. When one polyp is found, a barium enema or colonoscopy is always done to look for others.

● Other Useful Tests

1. CBC (abscess)
2. Sedimentation rate (rectal abscess)
3. Stool for occult blood (carcinoma)
4. Incision and drainage (I & D) and culture of exudate (abscess)
5. Sonogram (ectopic pregnancy, peritoneal metastasis, tubo-ovarian abscess)
6. CT scan of the pelvis (metastasis)
7. CEA (colonic neoplasm)

RECTAL PAIN

Practically the whole specialty of proctology is devoted to taking care of patients with rectal pain. To develop the differential diagnosis it is useful first to divide the conditions into **extrinsic** and **intrinsic**. To recall the **extrinsic** causes, one simply visualizes the structures around the rectum. Noting the tubes and ovaries, one considers salpingitis, ovarian cysts, and ectopic pregnancy. Visualize the coccyx, and coccydynia is brought to mind. Just as important a cause of rectal pain is prostatitis or prostatic abscess. A pelvic appendix or ruptured diverticulum may inflame the rectum extrinsically.

Intrinsic causes are developed by the mnemonic **VINDICATE**.

V—**Vascular** conditions suggest hemorrhoids.
I—**Inflammation** suggests proctitis, anal ulcers, and perirectal abscess.
N—**Neoplasms** are not usually painful until the advanced stage of disease.
D—**Degenerative** disorders are suggested, but there are no degenerative diseases causing rectal pain.
I—**Intoxication** includes overuse of suppositories and phenylephrine HCl (Preparation H). An idiopathic condition to be considered here is proctalgia fugax.
C—**Congenital** and acquired malformations suggest fistula in ano, infected pilonidal cyst, diverticulum, and intussusception.
A—**Autoimmune** diseases suggest ulcerative proctitis and granulomatous colitis.
T—**Trauma** should bring to mind fecal impactions and foreign bodies or introduction of the male organ into the rectum.
E—**Endocrine** disorders suggest nothing other than the ovarian cysts and ectopic pregnancy already mentioned.

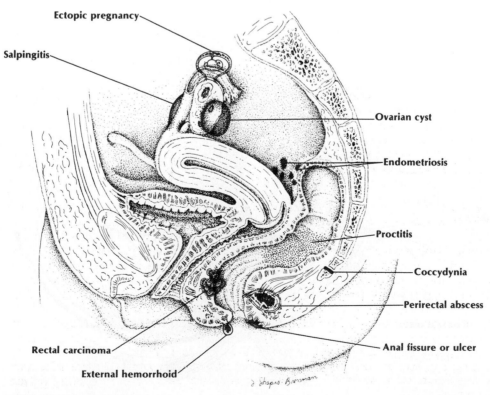

● **FIGURE 10** Rectal pain.

● Approach to the Diagnosis

The cause of rectal pain is usually obvious on examination with an anoscope or proctoscope. Careful palpation may be necessary to discover a perirectal abscess, coccydynia, or an ectopic pregnancy. Anal fissures may be missed unless all quadrants of the anus are examined with the slit anoscope. Lateral anal fissures (3 o'clock or 9 o'clock) suggest syphilis, tuberculosis, or other serious underlying causes.

● Other Useful Tests

1. Proctology consult
2. Sigmoidoscopy (rectal carcinoma)
3. Stool culture (proctitis)
4. Barium enema (Crohn disease, ulcerative colitis)
5. Frei test (lymphogranuloma venereum)
6. Prostatic massage and examination of the exudate (proctitis)
7. Urine culture and colony count
8. X-ray of lumbar spine (cauda equina syndrome, coccydynia)
9. HIV antibody titer (AIDS)
10. Gallium scan (perirectal abscess)
11. Pregnancy test
12. Pelvic sonogram (ectopic pregnancy)
13. Sedimentation rate (pelvic inflammatory disease [PID])

RED EYE

Most textbooks consider the causes of red eye to be conjunctivitis, iritis, or glaucoma, but it may be the result of taking the night plane from Los Angeles to New York. If these are all the causes you can remember, you will be sadly mistaken in some cases. Most of the causes can be quickly recalled by simply considering the **anatomy** of the eye, because trauma or inflammation is the usual cause.

Beginning with the **eyelids**, one recalls blepharitis and hordeolum. The **conjunctiva** suggests conjunctivitis. The **cornea** may be involved by a foreign body or keratitis; corneal ulcers should also be looked for. Proceeding to deeper layers, the physician should consider iritis, scleritis, or injury to these structures. Finally, between the cornea and iris is the **canal of Schlemm**, which recalls glaucoma. The **vascular supply** suggests a cavernous sinus thrombosis.

Another method that will bring to mind even more of the possibilities is to use the mnemonic **FOREIGN**. The word and the first letter signify foreign bodies. The **O** suggests otolaryngologic conditions such as upper respiratory infections. The **R** brings to mind refractive errors and astigmatism. The **E** suggests the exanthema and the conjunctivitis of measles. It will also help recall episcleritis and scleritis. **I** should signify iritis, conjunctivitis, and other

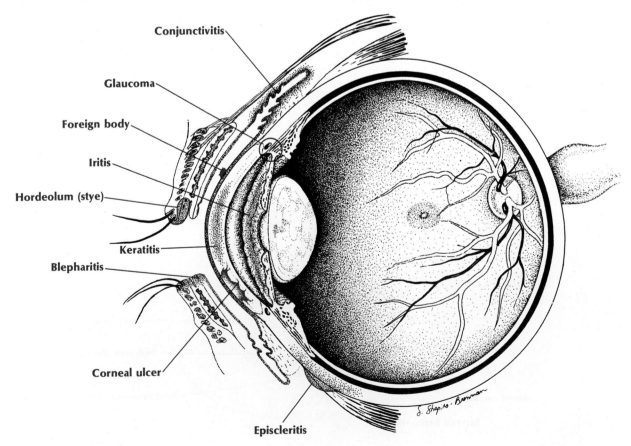

Conjunctivitis
Glaucoma
Foreign body
Iritis
Hordeolum (stye)
Keratitis
Blepharitis
Corneal ulcer
Episcleritis

● **FIGURE 11** Red eye.

inflammatory lesions. The **G** suggests glaucoma. Finally, the **N** should indicate neoplasms of the orbit.

● Approach to the Diagnosis

Pinning down the diagnosis of a red eye is usually not difficult because most causes will be evident to the naked eye. Even when conjunctivitis is likely, always check the visual acuity in the affected eye to rule out a more serious condition. However, a careful search for a foreign body with a magnifying glass and for a corneal abrasion using fluorescein will be necessary in some cases. The association of other signs and symptoms will be invaluable. A child with red eyes and cervical lymphadenopathy may have Kawasaki disease. Diffuse erythema of the eye usually indicates trauma, conjunctivitis, or scleritis, whereas circumcorneal injection suggests iritis or glaucoma. Episcleritis is a focal erythema that fails to blanch with one drop of phenylephrine 2.5%. A dilated pupil suggests glaucoma, whereas a constricted or distorted pupil suggests iritis. A slit lamp will differentiate keratitis and obscure foreign bodies. Tonometry is useful in differentiating glaucoma from other conditions. Acute closed angle glaucoma is associated with nausea, vomiting, and halos and is a medical emergency. A smear and culture will help differentiate infectious conjunctivitis from allergic conjunctivitis, but the latter is usually bilateral whereas the former is usually unilateral. An ophthalmologist should be consulted immediately if there is any doubt about the diagnosis.

● Other Useful Tests

1. Rheumatoid arthritis (RA) test (RA)
2. Human leukocyte antigen (HLA) B27 (rheumatoid spondylitis)
3. Colonoscopy (ulcerative colitis, Crohn disease)
4. Chest x-ray (sarcoidosis)

Case Presentation #78

A 17-year-old black boy presents to the emergency room with redness of his left eye. He denies a history of trauma or foreign body. His left pupil is slightly constricted but reacts to light and accommodation. Your initial examination fails to reveal a foreign body.

Question #1. Utilizing your knowledge of anatomy, what is your differential diagnosis at this point?

Further questioning reveals that he has had intermittent bloody diarrhea for several months.

Question #2. What is your diagnosis now?

(See Appendix B for the answers.)

RESTLESS LEG SYNDROME

The mnemonic **PINT** will facilitate the recall of causes of this peculiar disorder that presents with creeping, crawling, or other types of dysesthesias in the lower extremities.

P—Pregnancy may be associated with restless leg syndrome.
I—Many cases of restless leg syndrome are **idiopathic**.
N—Neurologic disorders associated with restless leg syndrome include uremic or diabetic neuropathy, Parkinson disease, and multiple sclerosis.
T—Toxic causes of this disorder include barbiturates, benzodiazepines, caffeine, and tricyclic antidepressants.

Unfortunately, the above list fails to include anemia, another significant cause.

● Approach to the Diagnosis

The workup of restless leg syndrome includes a CBC, chemistry panel, glucose tolerance test, urine drug screen, and nerve conduction velocity studies. If multiple sclerosis is suspected, a magnetic resonance imaging (MRI) of the brain or spinal cord can be done. A spinal tap may reveal an elevated gamma globulin or myelin basic protein. A neurologist should be consulted before ordering these expensive diagnostic tests.

RISUS SARDONICUS

This a fixed grin due to mild but sustained contraction of the facial muscle. It is almost invariably due to a wound infection with tetanus but may also give the appearance of a fixed grin.

● Approach to the Diagnosis

Careful examination of the trunk and extremities for a wound infection is extremely important. If the patient is not stripped down, the clinician can miss a tetanus infection caused by dirty needles in drug addicts. A history of mental illness should alert one to attempted suicide with strychnine. A urine drug screen is useful in ruling out narcotic addiction. Scleroderma can usually be excluded by an ANA and anticentromere antibody titer, but a skin biopsy may be necessary.

S

SCALP TENDERNESS

The cause of scalp tenderness can best be recalled utilizing the mnemonic **MINT**.

M—**Mental** disorders such as pseudoneurosis can be associated with diffuse scalp tenderness.

I—**Inflammation** would bring to mind herpes zoster, pediculosis, tinea capitis, cellulitis, an infected sebaceous cyst, and impetigo.

N—**Neurologic** disorders associated with a tender scalp include temporal arteritis, occipital nerve entrapment, trigeminal neuralgia, and neoplasms that involve the cranium and meninges (i.e., meningioma).

T—**Trauma** would suggest scalp contusions, fractures, and hematomas.

● Approach to the Diagnosis

Most skin conditions should be easily diagnosed by inspection. A Wood lamp inspection would assist in the diagnosis of tinea capitis. A potassium hydroxide (KOH) preparation of scraping may be necessary. Skin biopsy will diagnose other skin disorders. A sedimentation rate and biopsy of the superficial temporal artery will diagnose temporal arteritis. If occipital nerve entrapment is suspected, a nerve block should be done to confirm the diagnosis. X-rays of the skull and a magnetic resonance imaging (MRI) may be necessary, but a neurologist should be consulted before ordering expensive diagnostic tests.

SCOLIOSIS

The many causes of this deformity of the spine can be recalled by applying the mnemonic **MINTS**.

M—**Malformation** prompts the recall of osteogenesis imperfecta, congenital hemivertebra, Marfan syndrome, and arthrogryposis. It should also suggest a short leg syndrome.

I—**Inflammation** suggests tuberculosis and fungal disease of the spine. The **I** should also remind one of **idiopathic scoliosis**, responsible for 80% of the cases.

N—**Neurologic** disorders that may cause scoliosis include syringomyelia, poliomyelitis, muscular dystrophy, and Friedreich ataxia.

T—**Trauma** should facilitate the recall of thoracolumbar sprain, compression, fracture, and herniated disk. It should also remind one of **thoracoplasty** and other surgical causes.

S—**Systemic** diseases associated with scoliosis include Paget disease, pulmonary fibrosis, and Ehlers–Danlos syndrome.

Unfortunately, rickets and osteoporosis will not be recalled with this mnemonic.

● Approach to the Diagnosis

To diagnose scoliosis, have the patient bend over, and there will be asymmetry in the height of the scapulae (Adam test). Most causes of scoliosis will require only an x-ray of the spine to clarify the diagnosis. An orthopedic consult should be obtained before any further workup. Be sure to measure the leg length. If there are objective neurologic signs, a neurologist should be consulted. A bone scan, MRI, or computed tomography (CT) scan may be necessary in difficult diagnostic problems.

● Other Useful Tests

1. Complete blood count (CBC) (osteomyelitis)
2. Sedimentation rate (osteomyelitis, tuberculosis)
3. Arthritis panel (rheumatoid spondylitis)
4. Human leukocyte antigen (HLA) B-27 (rheumatoid spondylitis)
5. Pulmonary function tests (pulmonary fibrosis)
6. Bone survey (Paget disease)
7. Electromyogram (EMG) (muscular dystrophy)

SENSORY LOSS

Anatomy is the key to developing a list of possible causes of sensory loss. Tracing the nerve endings in the face or extremities to the brain we have the peripheral nerves, nerve plexus, nerve roots, spinal cord, brain stem, and cerebrum. Now cross-index these structures with the various etiologies (vascular, inflammatory, neoplastic, etc.), and you have an excellent list of possibilities.

1. Peripheral nerve—This structure should prompt the recall of carpal tunnel syndrome, ulnar entrapment in the hand or elbow, and diffuse peripheral neuropathy (diabetes, nutritional disorders, etc.).
2. Nerve plexus—This structure should suggest brachial plexus neuritis, sciatic neuritis, brachial plexus compression by a Pancoast tumor or thoracic outlet syndrome, or lumbosacral plexus compression by a pelvic tumor.
3. Nerve roots—This would facilitate the recall of space-occupying lesions of the spinal cord (e.g., tumor, abscess) and fractures of the spine compressing the root. It would also help to recall tabes dorsalis, herniated disk disease, osteoarthritis, cervical spondylosis, spinal stenosis, and spondylolisthesis. Guillain–Barré syndrome affects the nerve causing sensory loss.
4. Spinal cord—Lesions in the spinal cord that cause sensory loss include space-occupying lesions, syringomyelia,

pernicious anemia, multiple sclerosis, and Friedreich ataxia, acute traumatic or viral transverse myelitis, and anterior spinal artery occlusion may also cause sensory loss.

5. Brain stem—This should prompt the recall of brain stem tumors, abscess and hematomas, multiple sclerosis, syringobulbia, encephalomyelitis, basilar artery, thrombosis, posterior inferior cerebellar artery occlusion, and neurosyphilis. Do not forget the thalamic syndrome.

6. Cerebrum—Space-occupying lesions of the cerebrum, cerebral hemorrhage, thrombosis, or embolism should be considered here. Encephalitis, toxic encephalopathy, and multiple sclerosis are less likely to cause significant sensory loss if the lesions are confined to the cerebral cortex.

● Approach to the Diagnosis

The neurologic examination will help to determine the location of the lesion. Peripheral neuropathy presents with diffuse distal loss of sensation to all modalities. Nerve root involvement will present with sensory loss in a radicular distribution; spinal cord involvement will be associated with a sensory level. Sensory loss to pain and temperature on one side of the face and the opposite side of the body is typical of posterior inferior cerebellar artery occlusion. If there is only loss of vibratory and position sense, look for pernicious anemia or a cerebral tumor.

The workup for peripheral neuropathy and entrapment syndromes will include nerve conduction velocity (NCV) tests and EMGs. An MRI and CT scan can be done if brain and spinal cord pathology is suspected, but a neurologist should be consulted first. If a cerebrovascular disease is suspected, Doppler ultrasound and magnetic resonance angiography (MRA) may be necessary as well. Ultimately, four-vessel cerebral angiography may be indicated.

● Other Useful Tests

1. CBC (pernicious anemia)
2. Chemistry panel (e.g., diabetic neuropathy)
3. Fluorescent treponemal antibody absorption (FTA–ABS) test (neurosyphilis)
4. Serum B_{12} (pernicious anemia)
5. Blood lead level (lead neuropathy)
6. Spinal tap (neurosyphilis, multiple sclerosis, Guillain–Barré syndrome)
7. Urine porphobilinogen (porphyria)
8. Antinuclear antibody (ANA) (collagen disorders)

SHOULDER PAIN

The differential diagnosis of shoulder pain, like other forms of pain, is best established by **anatomy**, working from the outside in (Table 51). Beginning with the **skin**, one immediately thinks of cellulitis and herpes zoster. The **muscles** and **tendons** come next, and epidemic myalgia and the myalgias secondary to many infectious diseases lead the list. However, **trichinosis**, **dermatomyositis**, **fibromyositis**, and **trauma** must always be considered. Proceeding to

the blood vessels, keep in mind thrombophlebitis, Buerger disease, vascular occlusion from periarteritis nodosa, and other forms of vasculitis.

Inflammation of the **bursae** is probably the most common cause of shoulder pain. This should be considered traumatic because in most cases the torn ligamentum teres rubs the bursa and causes the inflammation. Interestingly enough, aside from gout, the bursae are rarely involved in other conditions. Biceps tendonitis needs to be considered here as well. The **shoulder joint** itself is also a frequent site of pain. Osteoarthritis, rheumatoid arthritis, gout, lupus, and various bacteria all may involve this joint, but dislocation of the shoulder, fractures, and frozen shoulder should be considered. Inflammation of the acromioclavicular joint is usually traumatic in origin. If the **bone** is the site of pain, there is usually a fracture involved. Osteomyelitis and metastatic tumors, however, ought to be ruled out.

Neurologic causes are not the last to be considered just because anatomically they come last. The **brachial plexus** may be compressed by a cervical rib, a large scalenus anticus or pectoralis muscle, or the clavicle (costoclavicular syndrome). When the **cervical sympathetics** are irritated or disrupted, a shoulder–hand syndrome develops. The **cervical spine** is the site or origin of shoulder pain in cervical spondylosis, spinal cord tumors, tuberculosis and syphilitic osteomyelitis, ruptured disks, or fractured vertebrae.

It would be a grave error to omit the **systemic causes** of shoulder pain. Thus, coronary insufficiency, cholecystitis, Pancoast tumors, pleurisy, and subdiaphragmatic abscesses should be ruled out.

● Approach to the Diagnosis

The approach to ruling out various causes is most often clinical, provided x-rays of the shoulder and cervical spine have negative findings. If a torn rotator cuff is strongly suspected, an MRI or arthrogram should be done. In the classical case of subacromial bursitis (recently called impingement syndrome), in which passive movement is much less restricted than active movement and a point of maximum tenderness can easily be located, lidocaine and steroid injections into the bursa (at the point of maximum tenderness) may be done without x-rays. Cervical root blocks, stellate ganglion blocks for shoulder–hand syndrome, and aspiration and injection of the shoulder joint with lidocaine and steroids may also be useful in establishing the cause. Adson maneuvers will help to establish the diagnosis of scalenus anticus syndrome, but the clinician must bear in mind that there are many false positives for this test and the job is not finished until tests for pectoralis minor and costoclavicular compression are done. The history will help to diagnose systemic causes, but checking for dermatomal hyperalgesia or hypalgesia and other sensory changes will be most helpful in diagnosing disease of the cervical spine. Remember that a negative cervical spine x-ray does not rule out a herniated disk. If the pain is increased by pressure on the top of the head or by coughing and sneezing, then a herniated disk must be ruled out by an MRI.

TABLE 51 Shoulder Pain

	V Vascular	I Inflammatory	N Neoplasm	D Degenerative and Deficiency	I Intoxication Idiopathic	C Congenital	A Autoimmune Allergic	T Trauma	E Endocrine
Skin		Herpes zoster			Fibromyositis		Dermatomyositis	Contusion Ruptured tendon	
Muscle and Tendons		Epidemic myalgia Trichinosis Tendonitis biceps				Hemophilia Quadrilateral space syndrome	Vasculitis		
Blood Vessels	Arterial thrombosis Buerger disease Dissecting aneurysm	Phlebitis			Gout				Pseudogout
Bursae		Bursitis			Gouty arthritis Frozen shoulder		Rheumatoid arthritis Rheumatic fever Lupus	Shoulder dislocation Shoulder separation Torn ligament	
Shoulder Joint		Purulent arthritis		Osteoarthritis				Fracture	
Bone	Aseptic bone necrosis	Osteomyelitis	Primary and metastatic tumors		Shoulder–hand syndrome	Cervical ribs Scalenus anticus syndrome		Traumatic neuroma	
Brachial Plexus and Sympathetics		Neuritis	Lymphoma		Cervical spondylosis	Klippel–Feil syndrome		Ruptured disk Fracture	
Cervical Spine		Osteomyelitis Tuberculosis Syphilis	Cord tumor (primary and metastatic)	Osteoarthritis					
Systemic Causes	Coronary insufficiency Aortic aneurysm	Cholecystitis Pleurisy Subdiaphragmatic abscess	Pancoast tumor						

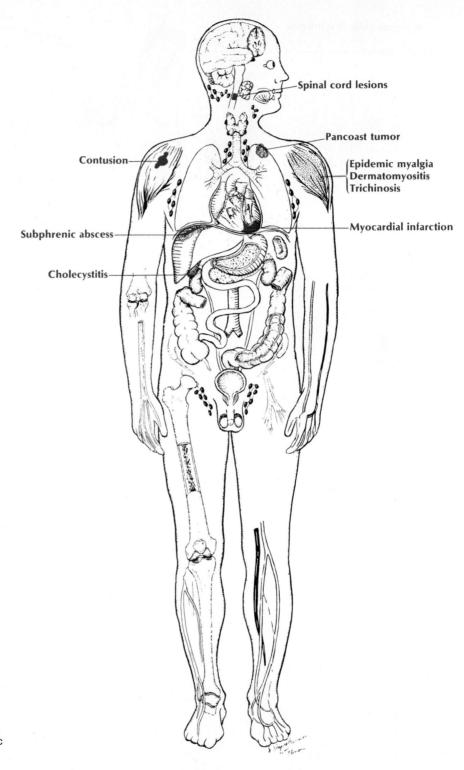

Spinal cord lesions

Pancoast tumor

Contusion

Epidemic myalgia
Dermatomyositis
Trichinosis

Subphrenic abscess

Myocardial infarction

Cholecystitis

S

● **FIGURE 1** Shoulder pain, systemic causes.

● Other Useful Tests

1. CBC
2. Sedimentation rate (collagen disease, infection)
3. Chemistry panel (gout, pseudogout)
4. Arthritis panel
5. ANA analysis (collagen disease)

6. Exercise tolerance test (coronary insufficiency)
7. Nerve blocks (radiculopathy)
8. EMG (radiculopathy)
9. Bone scan (small fractures, osteomyelitis)
10. Arteriogram (thoracic outlet syndrome)
11. Chest x-ray (Pancoast tumor)

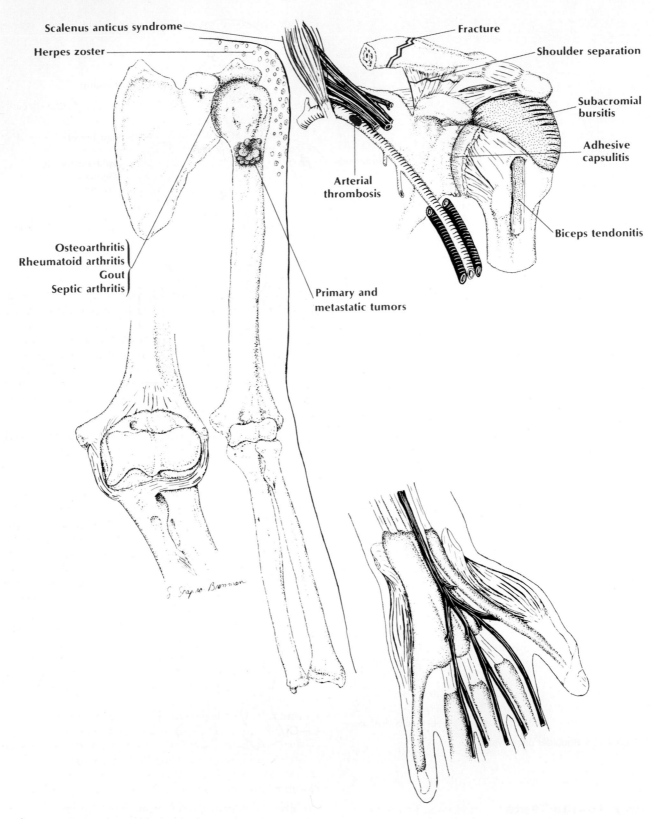

● **FIGURE 2** Shoulder pain, local causes.

Case Presentation #79

A 52-year-old white man complained of increasing stiffness and pain in his left shoulder for the past year. Physical examination revealed diffuse tenderness of the shoulder joint and limited abduction, extension, and rotation of the shoulder joint on both active and passive motion.

Question #1. Utilizing your knowledge of anatomy, what are the diagnostic possibilities at this point?

Further questioning revealed that he had a myocardial infarction 1 year ago.

Question #2. What is your diagnosis now?

(See Appendix B for the answers.)

SKIN DISCHARGE

The differential diagnosis of a weeping skin lesion is covered in the section on rash (see page 362), but certain conditions should be mentioned here. In all nonbloody discharges, infection (usually bacterial) is the most prominent etiology; *Staphylococcus* and *Streptococcus* organisms are the most common offenders in the skin. In working up from the smallest organism to the largest, however, one will not forget the weeping blisters of herpes zoster and simplex, smallpox, and chickenpox; the ulcers and bullae of syphilis; the draining sinuses and ulcers of actinomycosis, sporotrichosis, and other cutaneous mycosis; and the weeping ulcers of cutaneous leishmaniasis and amebiasis cutis. There are many more—but decidedly rare—infections in all these categories. By recalling the anatomy of the skin, the infected hair follicles and sebaceous cysts (furunculosis and carbuncles), infected apocrine glands (hidradenitis suppurativa), and inflamed sweat glands (milariasis) come to mind. Finally, using the mnemonic **VITAMIN** one will recall the following:

V—Vascular conditions of the skin (e.g., postphlebitic ulcers) that cause a discharge

I—Inflammatory conditions of a noninfectious nature (e.g., erythema multiforme, pyoderma gangrenosum, and pemphigus) that produce weeping. Specific infections are listed above.

T—Traumatic conditions such as third-degree burns

A—Autoimmune and **allergic** disorders associated with weeping vesicles and ulcers, such as periarteritis nodosa and contact dermatitis

M—Malformations such as bronchial clefts and urachal sinus tracts

I—Intoxicating lesions such as a vesicular or bullous drug eruption

N—Neoplasms such as basal cell carcinoma and mycosis fungoides that produce weeping ulcers

● Approach to the Diagnosis

Smear and culture of the lesion are most important, although a skin biopsy is sometimes necessary. Serologic tests or cultures on special media are necessary to diagnose fungi and parasites.

● Other Useful Tests

1. CBC (systemic infection)
2. Sedimentation rate (systemic infection, collagen disease)
3. Tuberculin test
4. Venereal disease research laboratory (VDRL) test (primary or secondary syphilis)
5. X-ray of area involved (abscess, osteomyelitis)
6. ANA analysis (collagen disease)
7. Skin test and serology for fungi
8. Biopsy
9. Muscle biopsy (collagen disease, trichinosis)

SKIN MASS

Masses of the skin may be better termed nodules if they are larger than 0.5 cm and are not just neoplastic in origin. The term **VINDICATE** serves as a useful mnemonic to recall the important skin masses. When the physician is considering the cause of a mass in any part of the body, he or she must include a possible skin mass in the differential. Therefore, although I have limited the discussion of skin lesions in other sections, the reader should turn to this section if the mass is thought to originate in the skin.

V—Vascular lesions include cavernous hemangiomas, varicose veins, hemorrhages from scurvy or coagulation disorders, and emboli from subacute bacterial endocarditis (SBE) (Osler nodules).

I—Inflammatory masses include caruncles, furuncles, warts, condyloma latum and acuminatum, molluscum contagiosum, tuberculomas, gummas, and granulomas from coccidioidomycosis, sporotrichosis, and other fungi.

N—Neoplasms constitute the largest group of skin masses. The important ones to remember are basal and squamous cell carcinomas, melanomas, nevi, sarcomas, metastatic nodules, Kaposi sarcomas, lipomas, neurofibromatosis, dermoid cysts, leiomyomas, lymphangiomas, and mycosis fungoides. Leukemic infiltration and Hodgkin disease may cause skin nodules or plaques.

D—Degenerative diseases do not produce any skin masses worthy of mention but do predispose to pressure sores. Heberden nodes of osteoarthritis should be considered here.

I—Intoxication suggests the lesions of bromism.

C—Cystic lesions of the skin include sebaceous cysts, epithelial cysts, and dermoid cysts. Congenital lesions such as eosinophilic granulomas of the skin, tuberous sclerosis, and neurofibromatosis should not be overlooked.

A—Autoimmune disease includes the aneurysms of periarteritis nodosa, rheumatoid and rheumatic nodules, localized lupus or amyloidosis, and Weber–Christian disease.

T—Trauma induces contusions and edema of the skin.

E—Endocrine and metabolic diseases that cause skin masses are diabetes mellitus (abscesses, necrobiosis lipoidica diabeticorum), hyperthyroidism (pretibial myxedema, acromegaly [tufting of the distal phalanges]), gout (tophaceous deposits), hyperlipemia and hypercholesterolemia with multiple xanthomas, and calcinosis in hypercalcemic states.

● Approach to the Diagnosis

A biopsy or excision is the best approach to the diagnosis. If a systemic disease is suspected because of a lesion, appropriate studies for these are listed below.

● Other Useful Tests

1. CBC (abscess)
2. Sedimentation rate (infection)
3. Incision and drainage (I & D) and culture of exudate
4. Tuberculin test
5. Skin tests and serology for fungi
6. Kveim test (sarcoidosis)
7. ANA analysis (collagen diseases)
8. Frei test (lymphogranuloma venereum)
9. Muscle biopsy (collagen disease)

SKIN PIGMENTATION AND OTHER PIGMENTARY CHANGES

To recall the causes of a diffuse pigmentation of the skin, one might simply visualize various organs of the body where a cause may originate. The **adrenal gland** brings to mind Addison disease, the **liver** suggests hemochromatosis, the **thyroid** suggests hyperthyroidism, the **uterus** suggests pregnancy (more likely to cause chloasma), and the **ovaries** suggest the chloasma of menopause and melasma of chronic birth control use. The liver is also the cause of jaundice (see page 271). The skin itself is the site of melanotic carcinoma, which in occasional cases causes a deeply pigmented skin, and tinea versicolor, which produces a patchy yellow-brown pigmented area over the trunk. Any dermatitis that takes a long time to heal may cause a patchy pigmentation. Cushing syndrome and ectopic adrenocorticotropic hormone (ACTH) production by a malignancy (especially a carcinoma of the lung) should be ruled out.

Other causes of patchy pigmentation are the *café au lait* spots of neurofibromatosis, stasis dermatitis from chronic thrombophlebitis and varicose veins, the pigmentation of the dorsal surfaces of the hands and face in pellagra, carcinoid syndrome, porphyria, and Gaucher disease. Ochronosis produces a bluish black or bluish brown pigment of the sclera, ears, skin, and nails. Vitiligo (idiopathic type) suggests a patchy pigmentation but is really a depigmentation. Acanthosis nigricans characterized by pigmented lesions of the skin flexures, neck, and nipples is often associated with malignancies.

● Approach to the Diagnosis

The workup for diffuse pigmentation involves ruling out hemochromatosis, hepatobiliary disease, and Addison disease with appropriate tests for these disorders (see Appendix A) and using the expertise of a dermatologist in the cases of patchy pigmentation.

● Other Useful Tests

1. Wood lamp (tinea versicolor)
2. Serum electrolytes (Addison disease)
3. Serum cortisol (Addison disease)
4. Serum iron and iron-binding capacity (hemochromatosis)
5. Urine porphyrins and porphobilinogen (porphyria)
6. Urine melanin (melanoma)
7. Urine for homogentisic acid (ochronosis)
8. Free thyroxine (FT_4) level (hyperthyroidism)
9. Serum follicle-stimulating hormone (FSH) and luteinizing hormone (LH) levels (menopause)
10. Skin biopsy
11. Serum ACTH (ectopic ACTH production)

SKIN THICKENING

Diffuse thickening of the skin is typical of myxedema, whereas thickening of the skin of the hands and face is also found in scleroderma and hereditary osteoar thropathy. Thickening of the skin of the lower legs is found in lymphedema and carcinoid syndrome. If the thickening is primarily localized to the face, consider the possibility of Chagas disease and porphyria cutanea tarda.

● Approach to the Diagnosis

If myxedema is suspected, a thyroid-stimulating hormone (TSH) test and FT_4 test can be ordered. If scleroderma is suspected, order an ANA, anticentromere antibody titer or a skin biopsy. Urine for porphyrins will help to identify porphyria. Carcinoid syndrome can be identified by a urine test for 5-hydroxyindole acetic acid (HIAA).

SKIN ULCERS

The differential diagnosis of skin ulcers may be approached with **anatomy** as the basic science, particularly if the ulcer is on one of the legs. Beginning with the skin itself and applying the mnemonic **MINT**, one can recall the following:

M—**Malformations** suggest sickle cell anemia.
I—**Infection** suggests syphilis, chancroid, lymphogranuloma, actinomycosis, tularemia, and other infections.
N—**Neoplasms** suggest basal cell and squamous cell carcinomas.
T—**Trauma** suggests third-degree burns, unsutured lacerations, and pressure sores (bedsores).

Now visualize the structure beneath the skin. The **arteries** suggest arteriosclerosis and diabetic ulcers; the **veins** prompt the recall of varicose ulcers or postphlebitic ulcers; the **nerves** suggest trophic ulcers of tabes dorsalis, syringomyelia, and peripheral neuropathy; and the **bone** suggests osteomyelitis (e.g., staphylococcal, tuberculosis) that penetrates the skin.

S

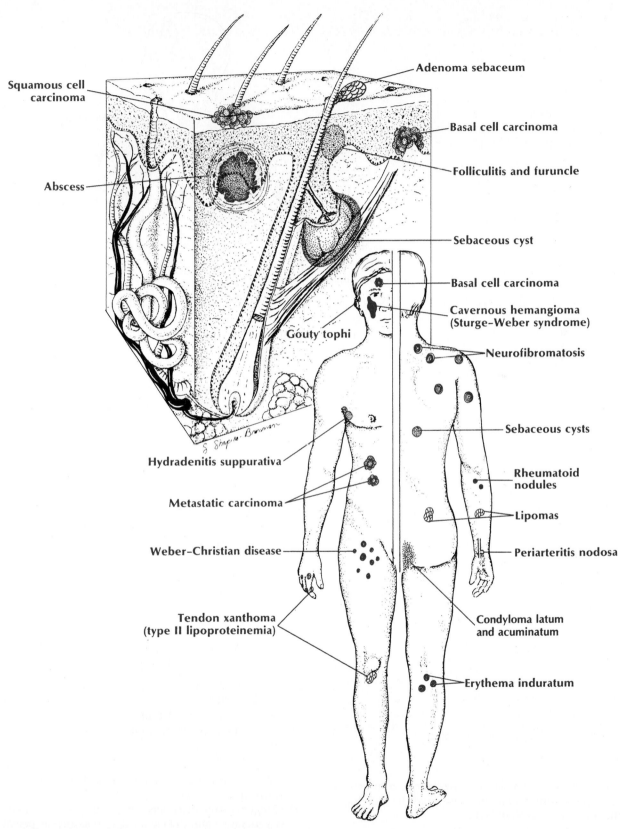

● FIGURE 3 Skin mass.

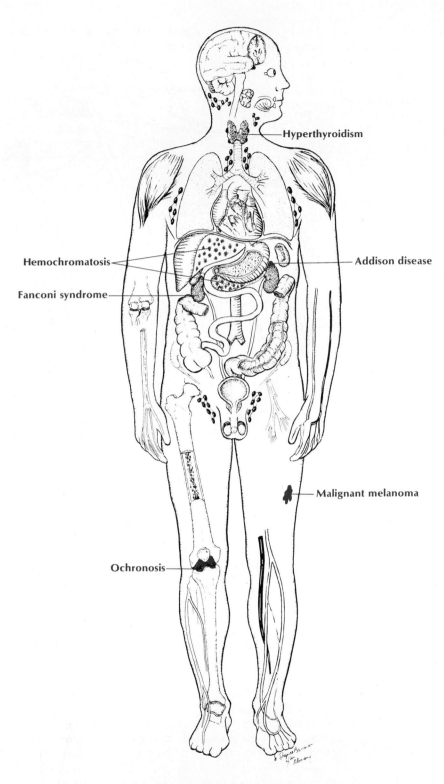

● **FIGURE 4** Skin pigmentation and other pigmentary changes.

In contrast to the method described above, a somewhat more complete differential diagnosis may be developed with the mnemonic **VINDICATE**.

V—Vascular disorders suggest peripheral arteriosclerosis, diabetic ulcers, and varicose ulcers.

I—Infections suggest syphilis, chancroid, yaws, and tularemia.

N—Neoplasm suggests carcinomas, sarcomas, and mycosis fungoides.

D—Degenerative disorders suggest ulcers associated with degenerative and deficiency diseases, such as peripheral neuropathy, syringomyelia, muscle atrophy, and peroneal muscular atrophy.

I—Intoxication suggests the ulcer of chronic dermatitis.

C—Congenital recalls the ulcers of sickle cell anemias.

A—**Autoimmune** brings to mind the ulcers of periarteritis nodosa, pyoderma gangrenosum (associated with ulcerative colitis and Crohn disease), and Stevens–Johnson syndrome.

T—**Trauma** identifies ulcers of burns and radiation secondary to unhealed lacerations and decubitus ulcers.

E—**Endocrine** disorders suggest diabetic ulcers.

I—**Infections** can be further elucidated by working from the smallest organism to the largest.

Beginning with **viruses**, herpes simplex, and lymphogranuloma is suggested. **Bacteria** remind one of tuberculosis, tularemia, leprosy, and cutaneous diphtheria. **Spirochetes** suggest syphilis and yaws. **Parasites** identify leishmaniasis and amebiasis cutis. The rest are **fungal** and include actinomycosis, blastomycosis, sporotrichosis, and cryptococcosis.

● Approach to the Diagnosis

The approach to the diagnosis of a skin ulcer involves an assessment of the vascular supply to the area, a neurologic examination, and a good history (especially important is venereal disease). The laboratory can support the diagnosis with a smear and culture, skin tests for tuberculosis and fungi, and serologic tests.

An x-ray of the bone may reveal the cause. A biopsy may be necessary. Radiographic and laboratory survey of other organs may be necessary if a systemic disease (e.g., collagen disease or ulcerative colitis) is suspected.

SLEEP APNEA

The differential diagnosis of sleep apnea may be arrived at by utilizing both **physiology** and **anatomy**. Normal sleep requires an unobstructed pathway from the nasopharynx to the lung and an intact central nervous system that responds to anoxia and the accumulation of CO_2 in the blood. It follows that sleep apnea may result from an obstructed airway (obstructive sleep apnea) or central suppression of respiration (central sleep apnea).

Obstructive sleep apnea: Think of the things that may obstruct the airway and many causes will come to mind. A deviated nasal septum, chronic infective or allergic rhinitis and sinusitis, tonsillitis and enlarged tonsils, obesity causing an enlarged soft palate or tongue, hypothyroidism, or acromegaly causing an enlarged tongue and nasal polyps must be considered. A small chin, deep overbite, or short neck may be the cause. Pickwickian syndrome may cause obstructive sleep apnea because of the associated obesity.

Central sleep apnea: Conditions that contribute to chronic anoxia such as congestive heart failure (CHF), Pickwickian syndrome, arteriovenous (AV) malformations (e.g., septal defects), and pulmonary fibrosis may be associated with this disorder. Conditions that cause chronic CO_2 retention such as pulmonary emphysema may also be causes. Finally, diseases of the central nervous system that depress the respiratory center may be involved. These include poliomyelitis, chronic drug or alcohol use, residual damage from viral encephalitis, brain stem tumors, and multiple sclerosis.

● Approach to the Diagnosis

A thorough examination of the upper respiratory system is essential: It may be wise to get an otolaryngologist to do this. A CBC to rule out anemia and arterial blood gases to rule out anoxia and hypercarbia may be helpful. Spirometry, chest x-ray, echocardiogram (ECG), and arm-to-tongue circulation time will help to rule out pulmonary and cardiovascular disorders. Ultimately, overnight polysomnography will be required to secure the diagnosis. A pulmonologist or otolaryngologist ought to be consulted before ordering this expensive test.

SLEEPWALKING

The differential diagnosis of this disorder is relatively simple, so we need not use a mnemonic or one of the basic sciences to develop a differential. It should be distinguished from night terrors which occur in stage 3 and 4 of non-REM (rapid eye movement) sleep. If sleepwalking and night terrors only occur occasionally, it is normal and of no pathologic significance. If they are frequent and associated with other signs of an emotional disorder such as bedwetting, temper tantrums, and anxiety, it is probably due to a psychologic or social problem and the patient needs to be referred to a psychiatrist. However, before doing so it is well to do a wake-and-sleep electroencephalogram (EEG) to exclude epilepsy. It may be necessary to do the EEG with nasopharyngeal electrodes inserted.

SMOOTH TONGUE AND OTHER CHANGES

There was a time when the first thing a physician did was to look at the tongue. The art of examining the tongue is all but lost, although more than 30 diseases can be diagnosed by looking at the tongue. Recalling these diseases may be best accomplished with the mnemonic **VINDICATE**. No attempt to cover all of them will be made, but the important ones are considered here.

V—**Vascular** diseases that may be diagnosed by looking at the tongue include the cyanosis of CHF, lung diseases, and polycythemia. The sublingual veins are also distended in these conditions.

I—**Inflammatory** diseases that cause tongue changes are streptococcal pharyngitis (strawberry tongue), tuberculosis (ulcers or furring of the tongue), chronic gastritis (coated gray), measles (furry tongue), appendicitis and peritonitis (moist and furry to dry and brown), typhoid (dense white fur), poliomyelitis (atrophy), syphilis (smooth or fissured tongue), herpes (ulcers), and moniliasis (white patches to white fur).

N—**Neoplasms** suggest carcinoma of the tongue (ulceration), leukoplakia (white plaques), diffuse lymphoma (small vesicles and a large tongue), fibroma (pediculated lesion on tongue), hemangioma (port-wine stain), and lingual warts.

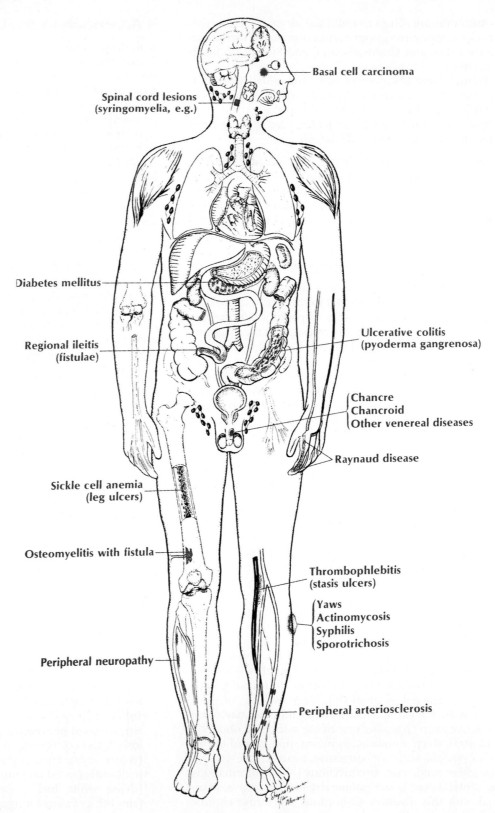

- Basal cell carcinoma

Spinal cord lesions
(syringomyelia, e.g.)

Diabetes mellitus

Regional ileitis
(fistulae)

Ulcerative colitis
(pyoderma gangrenosa)

Chancre
Chancroid
Other venereal diseases

Raynaud disease

Sickle cell anemia
(leg ulcers)

Osteomyelitis with fistula

Thrombophlebitis
(stasis ulcers)

Yaws
Actinomycosis
Syphilis
Sporotrichosis

Peripheral neuropathy

Peripheral arteriosclerosis

● **FIGURE 5** Skin ulcers.

D—Deficiency diseases include pernicious anemia (smooth tongue), iron deficiency anemia (smooth tongue), vitamin A deficiency, sprue, pellagra, and riboflavin deficiency (red and smooth tongue).

I—Intoxication suggests bromism (tremulous tongue with excessive salivation), alcoholism (tremulous, white furry tongue), mercury poisoning (ulcers), and lead poisoning (atrophy).

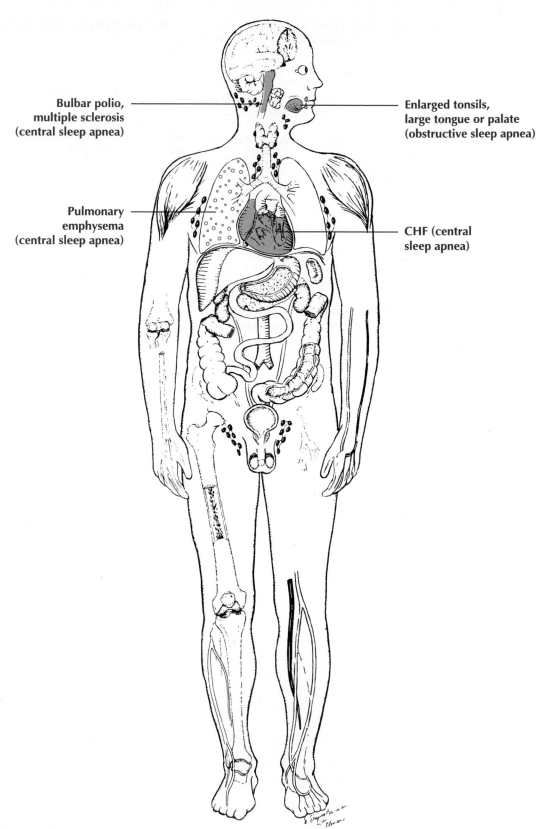

Bulbar polio,
multiple sclerosis
(central sleep apnea)

Enlarged tonsils,
large tongue or palate
(obstructive sleep apnea)

Pulmonary
emphysema
(central sleep apnea)

CHF (central
sleep apnea)

S

● **FIGURE 6** Sleep apnea.

C—**Congenital** disorders include Down syndrome (large, coarsely papillate tongue), geographic tongue, and cerebral palsy.

A—**Autoimmune** diseases include amyloidosis (swollen tongue), erythema multiforme (swollen tongue with ulcers and blisters), angioneurotic edema, and multiple sclerosis (tremulous tongue with fibrillary twitching).

T—**Trauma** to the tongue is important to look for in cases of undiagnosed epilepsy.

E—**Endocrine** disorders include acromegaly (swollen tongue), myxedema (large tongue), lingual thyroid, and thyroglossal cysts.

● Approach to the Diagnosis

The approach to the diagnosis will depend largely on the clinical picture. A smooth tongue with pallor of the nails and conjunctiva suggests pernicious anemia or iron deficiency anemia. A swollen tongue with cardiovascular abnormalities suggests amyloidosis. A swollen tongue and protruding jaw suggest acromegaly, whereas a swollen tongue and nonpitting edema prompt a diagnosis of myxedema. A dry, furry tongue suggests dehydration.

● Other Useful Tests

1. CBC (pernicious anemia or iron deficiency anemia)
2. Serum B_{12} (pernicious anemia)
3. Serum iron and ferritin levels (iron deficiency anemia)
4. Thyroid profile (myxedema)
5. Antistreptolysin O (ASO) titer (strawberry tongue of streptococcal infection)
6. Tongue biopsy (amyloidosis and focal lesions of the tongue)

SNEEZING

Allergic rhinitis (hay fever) is the most common cause of this condition, and perhaps any patient with sneezing as the chief complaint needs to have this excluded first. Other conditions, however, may present with sneezing, and the clinician needs to be able to recall these while examining the patient. The mnemonic **MINT** forms a good method for recalling these conditions.

M—**Malformations** include a deviated septum, a cleft palate that allows food to enter the nose, and large tonsils and adenoids.

I—**Inflammation** suggests pertussis, acute viral influenza, the common cold, chronic rhinitis, measles, and other upper respiratory infections. The **I** also suggests **immunologic** disorders; allergic rhinitis and bronchial asthma head the list.

N—**Neoplasms** suggest nasal polyps and carcinomas of the nasopharynx.

T—**Toxic** disorders suggest reactions to substances such as pepper, tear gas, phosphine, chlorine, and iodine compounds.

● Approach to the Diagnosis

The workup of sneezing involves a careful ear, nose, and throat (ENT) examination to exclude the presence of foreign bodies, polyps, and malformations. The typical mucoid bluish mucosa of allergic rhinitis may be spotted. A nasal smear for eosinophils or serum immunoglobulin E (IgE) level will clinch the diagnosis of allergic rhinitis, and skin testing or a radioallergosorbent test (RAST) can be performed, although a good allergy history may be more important.

SORE THROAT

Breaking down the oropharynx, nasopharynx, and larynx into anatomic components is not very valuable in developing a differential diagnosis of sore throat. What is useful is to use the mnemonic **VINDICATE** to establish the etiologies. Further analyzing the differential (because so many causes of sore throat are infectious), one may recall the inflammatory etiologies in a systematic fashion by starting with the smallest organism and working to the largest. Let us begin with **VINDICATE**.

V—**Vascular** disorders remind one of blood dyscrasias such as leukemia, agranulocytosis of numerous causes, and Hodgkin lymphoma.

I—**Inflammatory diseases** include the most common causes of sore throat, streptococcal or viral pharyngitis, but one must also consider the less frequent infectious diseases here. Beginning with the smallest organism and moving to the largest, one thinks of viral pharyngitis, particularly herpangina (due to Coxsackie virus), acquired immunodeficiency syndrome (AIDS), cytomegalic virus, pharyngoconjunctival fever (due to eight or more viruses), and infectious mononucleosis. Viral influenza may begin with a sore throat. Moving to a larger organism, one should remember that Eaton agent (*Mycoplasma*) pneumonia might be associated with pharyngitis. Next, **bacterial causes** such as group A hemolytic *Streptococcus* (with or without scarlet fever), diphtheria, *Listeria monocytogenes*, and meningococcemia should be considered. Gonorrhea is increasingly a cause of sore throat. Tuberculosis should also be mentioned, although it is rare in contemporary affluent societies. Consider among bacterial causes sinusitis, tonsillar or peritonsillar abscess (quinsy), and retropharyngeal abscess: *Staphylococcus* organisms may cause these, but they rarely cause the common sore throat. Moving to the next largest organisms, the spirochetes, think of syphilis and Vincent angina. Toxoplasmosis may present with a sore throat. Finally, remember the fungi, including thrush (moniliasis) and actinomycosis.

N—**Neoplasm** and carcinomas may include Hodgkin lymphoma and leukemia. The Schmincke tumor is of particular interest here.

D—**Degenerative diseases** are an unlikely cause of sore throat, just as they are unlikely to cause pain anywhere.

I—**Intoxication** brings to mind chronic alcoholism and smoker's throat. Agranulocytosis may also be included in this category, because it is so often drug induced.

C—**Congenital diseases** are an infrequent cause of sore throat, but a hiatal hernia with reflux esophagitis may cause recurrent sore throat, because there may be reflux of gastric juice all the way to the posterior pharynx in the recumbent position. An elongated uvula may also be responsible.

A—**Allergic diseases** include angioneurotic edema of the pharynx or uvula and allergic rhinitis; otherwise, this category is a rare cause of sore throat.

T—**Trauma** brings to mind foreign bodies such as chicken bones and tonsilloliths.

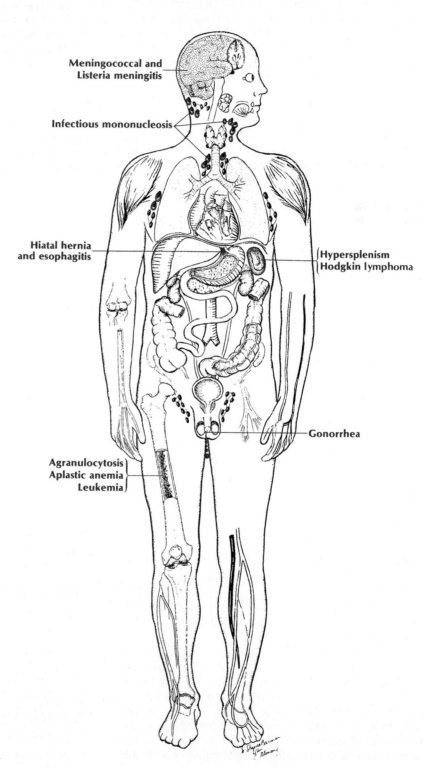

● **FIGURE 7** Sore throat, systemic causes.

E—**Endocrine** causes of sore throat should remind one of subacute thyroiditis; although the pain is really in the neck, the patient will report a "sore throat."

● Approach to the Diagnosis

Most cases of sore throat have a viral etiology. The absence of rhinorrhea and cough make strep pharyngitis more likely. In diagnosing the cause of sore throat, it has been traditional to do a throat culture and possibly a CBC and differential and to start the patient on penicillin until the culture comes back. Now Abbott Laboratories (Abbott Park, IL) has developed a rapid *Streptococcus* agglutination test on a throat swab. In resistant cases, repeated cultures (especially for diphtheria, gonorrhea, and *Listeria* organisms) and a monospot test will be useful. Because the titer for infectious mononucleosis may not be high initially, the differential test (Paul–Bunnell) or a repeated monospot test 1 to 3 weeks later may be necessary. Remember that subacute thyroiditis may present as a sore throat. Viral antigen testing is now available for influenza.

Case Presentation #80

A 16-year-old black girl presents to your office with a sore throat. Examination reveals exudative tonsillitis and enlarged anterior cervical lymph nodes.

Question #1. Utilizing the mnemonic **VINDICATE**, what would be your differential diagnosis at this point?
   The patient is given a course of penicillin, but 1 week later she returns to the office with no improvement. In addition to the previous findings, there is now splenomegaly and posterior cervical lymphadenopathy.

Question #2. What is your differential diagnosis now?

(See Appendix B for the answers.)

SPASTICITY

This is hypertonicity of the muscle and is almost invariably due to a lesion along the pyramidal tract from the spinal cord to the brain. Knowledge of neuroanatomy is extremely useful in developing a differential diagnosis.

Spinal cord: This prompts the recall of space-occupying lesions of the spinal cord, amyotrophic lateral sclerosis, Friedreich ataxia, transverse myelitis, neurosyphilis, multiple sclerosis, and anterior spinal artery occlusion. Advanced syringomyelia may also be a cause.
Brain stem: Common causes of spasticity originating here include brain stem tumors, hemorrhage, basilar artery thrombosis, multiple sclerosis, bulbar amyotrophic lateral sclerosis, encephalomyelitis, and neurosyphilis.
Cerebral hemispheres: Once again, space-occupying lesions are important to recall but hemorrhage, embolism, and thrombosis are also prominent causes. In children it is wise to consider cerebral palsy, encephalitis,

and Schilder disease. There are many degenerative disorders of the cerebrum that eventually develop spasticity, but the diagnosis will be well established by that time. Multiple sclerosis that predominantly involves the cerebral cortex also is unlikely to cause spasticity until late in the course of the disease.
Miscellaneous: The Stiffman syndrome is associated with stiffness of the muscles of the neck, trunk, and extremities. The location of the lesion is unknown.

● Approach to the Diagnosis

After the level of the lesion is established, an MRI or CT scan of that area can be ordered. A neurologist should be consulted first. A spinal tap will be useful in establishing the diagnosis of multiple sclerosis, encephalitis, and neurosyphilis if a space-occupying lesion has been ruled out.

● Other Useful Tests

1. MRA (cerebrovascular disease)
2. Visual evoked potential (VEP) and brainstem evoked potential (BSEP) (multiple sclerosis)
3. Carotid duplex scans (carotid stenosis or occlusion)
4. Four-vessel cerebral angiography (cerebrovascular disease)
5. CBC, serum B_{12} (pernicious anemia)

SPINE DEFORMITIES

Deformities of the spine are of four types: scoliosis (lateral curvature of the spine), lordosis (lumbar concavity of the spine), kyphosis (thoracic convexity of the spine or "hunchback"), and kyphoscoliosis (curvature with a "hunchback"). The differential diagnosis of all of these is essentially the same and may be best recalled by the mnemonic **VINDICATE**.

V—**Vascular** disorders suggest a large aortic aneurysm that may damage the vertebrae by compression, but this category is used with the prime purpose of recalling the spinal deformities associated with various congenital heart diseases (e.g., tetralogy of Fallot).
I—**Inflammatory** disorders recall osteomyelitis and tuberculosis of the spine; one should also remember infectious diseases of the nervous system such as poliomyelitis.
N—**Neoplasms** include metastatic tumors, myeloma, Hodgkin lymphoma, and primary tumors of the spinal cord.
D—**Degenerative** and **deficiency** diseases include degenerative disk disease, osteoarthritis, and spondylosis along the spine. In this category should be mentioned the kyphosis associated with pulmonary emphysema and fibrosis. Vitamin D deficiency will cause kyphoscoliosis.
I—**Intoxication** includes kyphosis associated with pneumoconiosis and osteoporosis from menopause or long-term corticosteroid therapy.
C—**Congenital** disorders are perhaps the largest category, including congenital scoliosis, kyphoscoliosis, Hurler disease, hemivertebra, muscular dystrophy, Friedreich ataxia, achondroplasia, and spondylolisthesis.

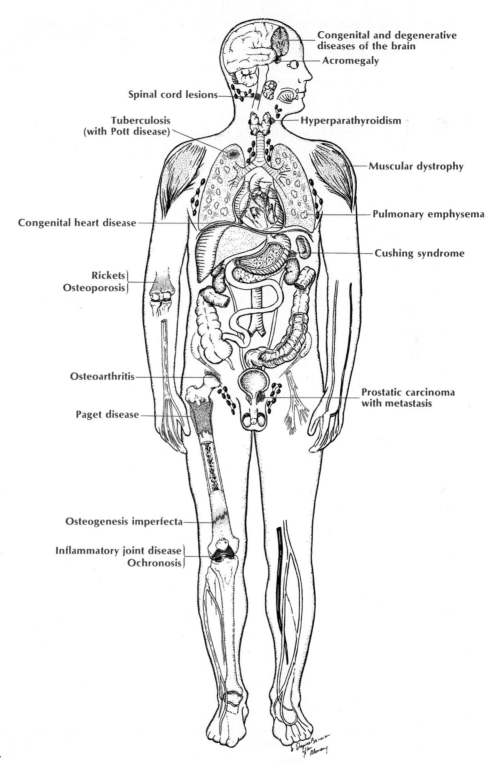

Congenital and degenerative
diseases of the brain
Acromegaly
Spinal cord lesions
Tuberculosis
(with Pott disease)
Hyperparathyroidism
Muscular dystrophy
Congenital heart disease
Pulmonary emphysema
Cushing syndrome
Rickets
Osteoporosis
Osteoarthritis
Paget disease
Prostatic carcinoma
with metastasis
Osteogenesis imperfecta
Inflammatory joint disease
Ochronosis

● **FIGURE 8** Spine deformities.

A—Autoimmune disease suggests rheumatoid spondylitis with the characteristic "poker spine."

T—Trauma indicates fractures, ruptured disks, and spinal cord injuries, all of which may leave a residual deformity of the spine.

E—Endocrine diseases remind one of the kyphosis associated with menopausal osteoporosis and osteomalacia of hyperparathyroidism. Acromegaly may also cause a kyphosis from osteoarthritis and osteoporosis.

● Approach to the Diagnosis

Obviously, a good family history and a thorough physical and neurologic examination are essential. The busy physician who does not have the time to perform a neurologic examination should refer the patient to a neurologist or orthopedist. A spine x-ray will often reveal the lesion, but a bone scan or CT scan and bone biopsy may be necessary. The bone scan has become especially useful in diagnosing early rheumatoid spondylitis.

● Other Useful Tests

1. CBC (osteomyelitis)
2. Chemistry panel (Paget disease)
3. Tuberculin test (tuberculosis of the spine)
4. Urine for mucopolysaccharides (Hurler disease)
5. HLA-B27 typing (rheumatoid spondylitis)
6. Urine creatinine and creatine levels (muscular dystrophy)
7. Serum protein electrophoresis (multiple myeloma)
8. Serum growth hormone assay (acromegaly)
9. Pulmonary function tests (emphysema)
10. Urine for homogentisic acid (ochronosis)

SPLENOMEGALY

The patient is lying on the table and has a palpable mass in the left upper quadrant. The mass has a hard, smooth surface with a notch on the edge and descends on inspiration. The patient has an enlarged spleen. What can be done about it? What is causing it?

The key word is **histology**. Think about the histologic components: parenchyma, supporting tissue, arteries, veins, and a capsule. What is parenchyma? It is nothing more than the components of the blood: red cells, white cells, lymph tissue, and platelets. Now it is possible to form a differential. Increased numbers of red cells recall polycythemia; increased numbers of white cells recall leukemia and infection. Increased lymph tissue suggests Hodgkin lymphoma, whereas increased supporting tissue indicates reticuloendotheliosis and acromegaly. Increased vein size occurs in obstruction of the portal vein as in cirrhosis, thrombosis of the portal vein, and CHF. If the artery has a local increase in size, an aneurysm forms, compressing the splenic veins.

A differential is at hand, but it is still incomplete. Now think of **physiology**. The spleen is a reserve for blood storage. It is also able to form red cells and other components of the blood when the bone marrow is atrophied, as in extramedullary erythropoiesis. More important, it is involved in the destruction of old or damaged red cells and platelets. Finally, it hypertrophies to fight infection just like the lymph glands. Extramedullary erythropoiesis recalls the splenomegaly of aplastic anemia and myeloid metaplasia, just as destruction or sequestration of cells brings to mind the splenomegaly of hemolytic anemias (e.g., hereditary spherocytosis, malaria, and lupus erythematosus) and thrombocytopenic purpura. The hypertrophy to fight infection or diffuse inflammation of the body should suggest the splenomegaly of bacterial endocarditis, kala azar, infectious mononucleosis, miliary tuberculosis, and rheumatoid arthritis. Almost anything that causes generalized lymphadenopathy can cause splenomegaly.

Only one category of splenomegaly is not brought to mind by this approach, but it is easily remembered because it is an exception—infiltration of inert material. Thus, in gargoylism there is a foreign mucopolysaccharide in the spleen. Numerous mucopolysaccharidoses are now described in the literature. There is a buildup of lipids in the reticuloendotheliosis of Gaucher disease, Niemann–Pick disease, and Hand–Schüller–Christian disease, but these are intracellular. Amyloid may infiltrate the spleen. Metastatic carcinoma of the spleen is rare.

Table 52 summarizes the above discussion and gives additional causes of splenomegaly to consider in the differential. One final diagnosis to consider is traumatic splenomegaly.

● Approach to the Diagnosis

How does one go about pinning down the diagnosis? There are several clinical clues. One looks during the physical examination for jaundice, lymphadenopathy, a rash, sore throat, hepatomegaly, and a positive Rumpel–Leede test. The combination of symptoms and signs will eliminate certain causes and make others more plausible. For example, splenomegaly with jaundice but no hepatomegaly suggests hemolytic anemia. The size of the spleen is also an important differential feature. If the spleen is very large, it should suggest myeloid metaplasia, chronic myelogenous leukemia, Gaucher disease, and kala azar.

The laboratory is the principal aid from this point on. Smears for red cell morphology, malaria, and other parasites are invaluable. Blood cultures and a lymph node and bone biopsy may be useful. If a specific disease is strongly suspected, consult Appendix A for appropriate tests.

● Other Useful Tests

1. CBC and differential (anemia, leukemia)
2. Blood smear for morphology (anemia)
3. Reticulocyte count (hemolytic anemia)
4. Platelet count and clot retraction (thrombocytopenia)
5. Radioactive chromium–tagged red cell (hemolytic anemia)
6. Serum haptoglobins (hemolytic anemia)
7. Bone marrow examination (aplastic anemia)
8. Blood cultures (SBE)
9. Febrile agglutinins (infectious disease)
10. Heterophil antibody titer (infectious mononucleosis)
11. Brucellin agglutinins (brucellosis)
12. Blood smear for parasites (malaria, trypanosomiasis)
13. Liver function studies (cirrhosis, Banti syndrome)
14. Rheumatoid arthritis test (Felty syndrome)
15. ANA test (collagen disease)
16. Serum protein electrophoresis (lymphoma, collagen disease)
17. Hemoglobin electrophoresis (hemolytic anemia)
18. Esophagram (esophageal varices) (portal cirrhosis)
19. X-ray of long bones (Gaucher disease, metastasis)
20. Flat plate of abdomen for spleen size (splenomegaly)
21. Lymph node biopsy (Hodgkin lymphoma)
22. Liver biopsy (cirrhosis)

TABLE 52 **Splenomegaly**

	Increased Production	Neoplasia	Increased Destruction	Obstruction	Infiltration
Red Cells	Aplastic anemia Myelophthisic anemia	Polycythemia	Hemolytic anemia Lupus erythematosus Pernicious anemia		
White Cells	Myeloid metaplasia Infection	Leukemia	Agranulocytosis		
Platelets			Idiopathic thrombocytopenic purpura		
Lymph Tissue	Infectious mononucleosis	Hodgkin lymphoma Lymphangioma			
Supporting Tissue		Metastatic carcinoma (rare)	Lupus erythematosus Collagen disease		Hemochromatosis Reticuloendotheliosis Hurler disease Amyloidosis Sarcoidosis
Arteries				Embolism Aneurysm	
Veins		Hemangioma		Congestive heart failure Cirrhosis Thrombosis Banti disease Carcinoma of the tail of the pancreas	

23. Splenic aspirate (lymphoma, leukemia)
24. Splenoportogram and splenic pulp pressure (portal cirrhosis)
25. Purified protein derivative (PPD) test, intermediate, and skin tests for various fungi (see Table 36)
26. Skin biopsy (hemochromatosis)
27. Muscle biopsy (collagen disease, trichinosis)
28. Diagnostic ultrasound (cyst, splenic aneurysm)
29. CT scan (malignancy)
30. Liver–spleen scan (splenomegaly)

SPUTUM

The approach to obtaining a differential is simply to visualize the various anatomic components as one travels down the respiratory tree and then to consider the etiologies of each. A nonbloody discharge is almost invariably due to inflammation, infection, or allergy, but a few important exceptions are worth mentioning here.

CHF from any cause (see page 85) produces frothy sputum that is occasionally bloodstained. Many toxic substances can produce severe acute inflammation or moderate-to-severe chronic inflammation and fibrosis. Most notable of these are pneumoconiosis, silicosis, berylliosis, and asbestosis. Lipoid pneumonia is mentioned in most textbooks of differential diagnosis but is seldom seen. Adult respiratory distress syndrome may result from injection of heroin, shock, and septicemia. This condition is associated with frothy sputum also. A few additional exceptions are mentioned as the respiratory tree is traversed.

In diseases of the **larynx** and **trachea**, sputum production is usually scanty, but several viruses (e.g., influenza) and bacteria *(Haemophilus influenzae*, pertussis, and diphtheria) may cause a productive sputum. Allergic laryngotracheitis does not usually produce sputum.

The **bronchi** may be inflamed by viruses (e.g., influenza and measles), bacteria, and particularly by bronchial asthma. In bacterial infection, the sputum is usually yellow, whereas in bronchial asthma it is white, thick, and mucoid. Chronic bronchitis is usually associated with cigarette smoking or exposure to some other irritating inhalant (such as silicon dioxide). Bronchiectasis may result from acute or chronic bronchitis, or from a congenital lesion (e.g., cystic fibrosis). The sputum in this condition is especially copious (1 cup [240 mL] or more per day) and separates into three layers: a frothy layer (saliva); a greenish layer (white cells and bacteria); and a brown layer (yellow bodies, elastic fibers, or Dittrich plugs).

The **bronchioles** and **alveoli** are the seat of numerous forms of pneumonia. The most common are bacterial, particularly *Streptococcus pneumoniae*, but staphylococcal,

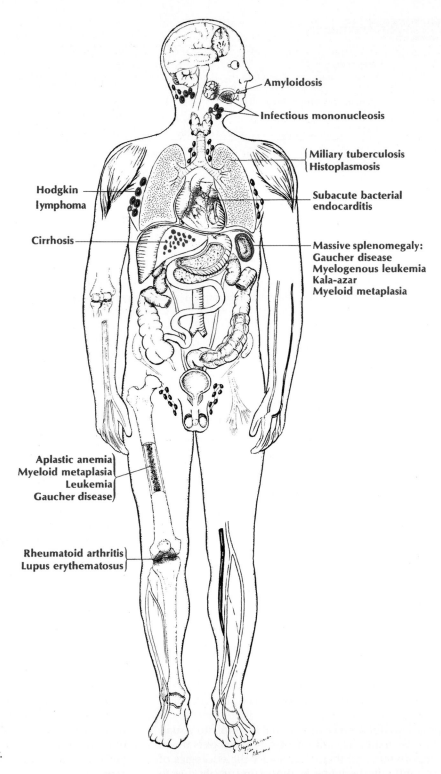

Amyloidosis

Infectious mononucleosis

Miliary tuberculosis
Histoplasmosis

Hodgkin
lymphoma

Subacute bacterial
endocarditis

Cirrhosis

Massive splenomegaly:
Gaucher disease
Myelogenous leukemia
Kala-azar
Myeloid metaplasia

Aplastic anemia
Myeloid metaplasia
Leukemia
Gaucher disease

Rheumatoid arthritis
Lupus erythematosus

● **FIGURE 9** Splenomegaly.

Klebsiella, and *H. influenzae* forms are not unusual. Gram-negative pneumonia is more common in hospitalized patients, especially those who are debilitated or those who have preexisting lung disease or malignancy. Viral pneumonias are also frequent and include psittacosis, mycoplasma, and even influenza or measles.

One cannot bypass either the miliary or the cavitary form of tuberculosis as a frequent cause of a chronic persistent cough that produces grayish yellow sputum. Lung abscesses are important causes of nonbloody sputum; the sputum is usually foul smelling (one can barely stand to walk in the room) because of the many anaerobes in the abscess. Histoplasmosis and other fungi must be looked for.

Allergic and autoimmune diseases that involve the alveoli and may produce nonbloody sputum include Loeffler pneumonitis, Wegener granuloma, rheumatoid arthritis, scleroderma, and lupus erythematosus. Even rheumatic fever can produce a pneumonitis. A more extensive display of the conditions that may produce nonbloody sputum is demonstrated in Table 53.

● Approach to the Diagnosis

Obviously, the approach to the diagnosis begins with examination of the sputum. In acute cases, a Gram stain often shows pneumococci or other bacteria. The laboratory should examine a 24-hour sputum for Curschmann spirals (of bronchial asthma), eosinophils, and elastic fibers, but so should the physician (to differentiate bronchiectasis and lung abscess).

The chest x-ray (posterior anterior and both laterals) plus proper examination of the sputum and culture (routine and acid-fast bacillus [AFB]) are usually all that are necessary. Spirometry and a circulation time will help rule out CHF. Bronchoscopy, bronchography, and lung scans may be necessary in chronic or subacute cases. Repeated cultures and smears are often rewarding. Lung aspiration and biopsy may also be necessary.

● Other Useful Tests

1. CBC (pneumonia, abscess)
2. Sedimentation rate (abscess)
3. Tuberculin test
4. Anaerobic cultures (pneumonia, abscess)
5. Culture for fungi
6. Coccidioidin skin test
7. Blastomycin skin test
8. Histoplasmin skin test
9. Kveim test (sarcoidosis)
10. Cold agglutinins (mycoplasma pneumonia)
11. Sputum for cytology (neoplasm of the lung)
12. Apical lordotic views (tuberculosis)
13. Pulmonary function tests (emphysema, fibrosis, CHF)
14. CT scan of the lung (bronchiectasis, neoplasm)

STOOL COLOR CHANGES

What may be black and white and red all over? The answer is not the newspaper but the pathologic changes in the stool. A **black stool** is usually melena (see page 208), but do not be fooled by iron ingestion or the bismuth in a commonly used antacid. A **white** or **light-colored stool** is most commonly found following the ingestion of a barium test meal, but the clay-colored stool of obstructive jaundice suggests the most important disease to be considered. The stool is light yellow to foamy in celiac disease. In mucous colitis, a large cast of white mucus (sometimes 6 to 10 in [15.2 to 25.4 cm] long) may be described as a white "stool." A **red stool** signifies blood from the lower bowel (see page 367) in most cases, but ingestion of red beets is not an uncommon cause.

The riddle mentioned above forms a key to remembering the causes of aberrations in stool color. Another method is to apply biochemistry. The normal color of the stool is due to the pigment urobilinogen. Color changes may result from a decrease in or absence of this pigment (obstructive jaundice), from an increase (hemolytic anemia) or the addition of another pigment (hemoglobin in melena), and finally from the addition of another substance such as mucus in mucous colitis, fat in celiac disease, and bismuth in antacid ingestion.

● Approach to the Diagnosis

The workup for changes in stool color includes most of the tests for either melena (see page 208) or jaundice (see page 271). The workup of celiac disease can be found in Appendix A.

STRABISMUS

This is the improper alignment of the eyes. It may be paralytic, in which case it is due to paralysis of one or more extraocular muscles, or nonparalytic, in which case it is congenital and usually inherited. Paralytic strabismus is covered under "double vision" (page 135). Nonparalytic strabismus is usually concomitant (the alignment does not change with extraocular movements) and prompts a referral to an ophthalmologist for possible surgical correction.

STRANGURY

This is the constant or almost constant desire to urinate. The differential diagnosis may be developed around the mnemonic **MINT**.

M—Malformations include urethral stricture, retroverted uterus, and prolapse of the uterus and bladder.
I—Inflammatory conditions include bacterial cystitis, urethritis, Bilharziasis, intestinal cystitis, gonorrhea, inflamed hemorrhoids, and anal fissure.
N—Neoplasms include carcinoma of the bladder or prostate, uterine fibroids or carcinoma, and carcinoma of the rectum extending into the bladder. **N** also helps to recall **neurologic conditions** that cause strangury, especially tabes dorsalis and chronic anxiety states or hysteria.
T—Trauma would help to recall contusion or laceration of the bladder, rectum, or urethra.

● Approach to the Diagnosis

A CBC, urinalysis, urine culture, and sensitivity and chemistry panel will routinely be ordered. It is well to do a smear and culture of any vaginal or urethral discharge. If these tests are negative, a urologist needs to be consulted for a cystoscopic examination possibly with retrograde pyelography. A vaginal and rectal examination must be done in all cases but is often neglected.

STRETCH MARKS

Stretch marks in women are usually related to obesity or past or present pregnancies. However, if they are purple (purple striae), they may indicate Cushing syndrome. This

TABLE 53 Sputum

	V Vascular	I Inflammatory	N Neoplasm	D Degenerative and Deficiency	I Intoxication	C Congenital	A Autoimmune Allergic	T Trauma	E Endocrine
Larynx and Trachea		Laryngotracheitis Viral or bacterial infection Diphtheria			Aspiration Alcohol Tobacco	Tracheoesophageal fistula	Allergic laryngitis and epiglottitis		
Bronchi		Bronchitis, acute and chronic	Carcinoma of the lung Bronchial adenoma		Turpentine aspiration Pneumoconiosis Tobacco Poisonous gas	Bronchiectasis Cystic fibrosis α_1-antitrypsin deficiency	Asthmatic bronchitis		
Alveoli	Pulmonary infarct (rarely) Congestive heart failure	Pneumonia (viral, bacterial) Tuberculosis Fungus Parasite Rickettsia	Alveolar carcinoma Metastasis	Pulmonary emphysema Pulmonary fibrosis	Lipoid pneumonia	Alveolar proteinosis	Wegener granuloma		
Capillaries			Hemangioma				Goodpasture syndrome Vasculitis Lupus		

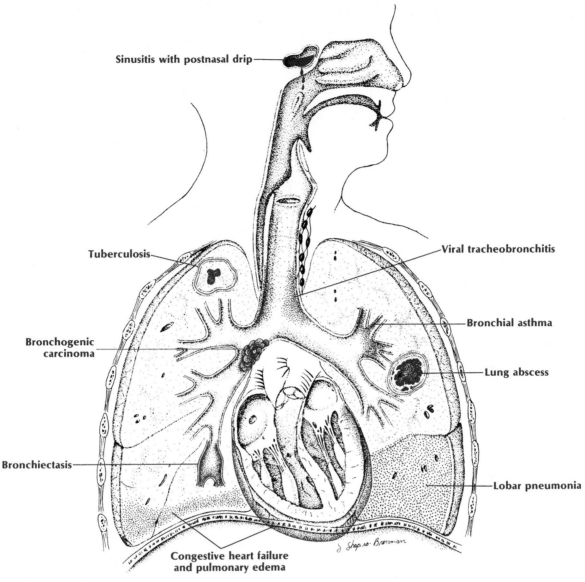

Sinusitis with postnasal drip

Tuberculosis

Viral tracheobronchitis

Bronchial asthma

Bronchogenic carcinoma

Lung abscess

Bronchiectasis

Lobar pneumonia

Congestive heart failure and pulmonary edema

● **FIGURE 10** Sputum.

holds true for purple striae in men also. In these cases one should look for moon faces, a buffalo hump, centripetal obesity, and hirsutism. To help confirm the diagnosis, one can order a serum cortisol or 24-hour urine ketosteroid or hydroxysteroid test to pin down the diagnosis. If these are positive, an endocrinologist should be consulted.

STRIDOR AND SNORING

Both these symptoms are the result of the same pathophysiologic mechanism: obstruction in the upper air passages. That obstruction may be due to any one of the etiologies recalled by the mnemonic **MINT**.

M—Malformations that may cause snoring or stridor include a large tongue, large tonsils and adenoids, a large soft palate, a cleft palate, congenital webs of the glottis, and malformation of the epiglottis (causing the well-known congenital laryngeal stridor). Foreign bodies must be considered here, as well as laryngeal stenosis.

I—Inflammatory conditions obstructing the upper airway include purulent sputum, acute laryngitis of diphtheria, acute tonsillitis, epiglottitis as in *H. influenzae*, rhinitis, hay fever, acute laryngotracheitis (usually of viral origin), Ludwig angina, and angioneurotic edema. Whooping cough should also be remembered here.

N—Neoplasms and neurologic disorders causing stridor or snoring include laryngeal polyps and carcinomas and bulbar or pseudobulbar palsy from basilar artery occlusions or hemorrhage, poliomyelitis or encephalitis, myasthenia gravis, and tabes dorsalis.

T—Traumatic disorders include the passage of an endotracheal tube, tracheotomies, and karate chops to the larynx.

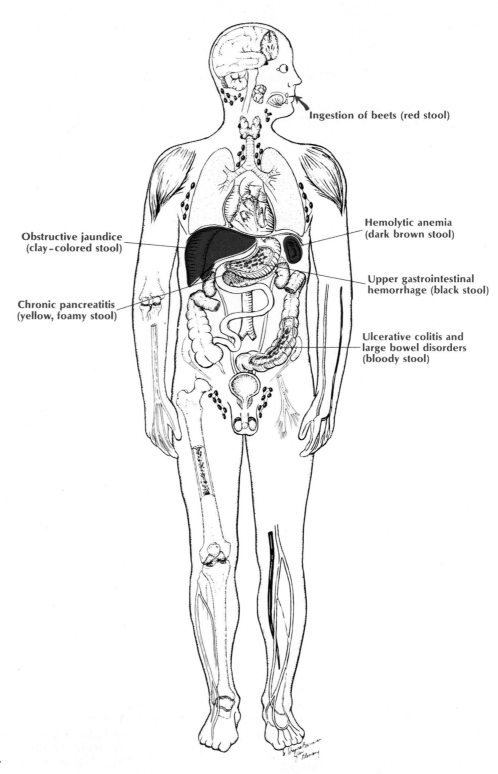

Ingestion of beets (red stool)

Hemolytic anemia
(dark brown stool)

Obstructive jaundice
(clay-colored stool)

Upper gastrointestinal
hemorrhage (black stool)

Chronic pancreatitis
(yellow, foamy stool)

Ulcerative colitis and
large bowel disorders
(bloody stool)

● **FIGURE 11** Stool color changes.

● Approach to the Diagnosis

The approach to the diagnosis involves a careful examination of the air passage with the laryngoscope and bronchoscope (if necessary, under anesthesia). If these have negative findings, a thorough neurologic examination should be performed and a Tensilon test may be indicated. Laryngismus stridulus in children may be terminated by putting the child in a steam bath; this helps to establish the diagnosis. Skin testing for allergies may be necessary. A sleep study is often necessary to rule out neurogenic or obstructive sleep apnea.

● Other Useful Tests

1. CBC (secondary polycythemia)
2. Nose and throat culture (chronic rhinitis or sinusitis)
3. Nasal smear for eosinophils (allergic rhinitis)
4. Acetylcholine receptor antibody (myasthenia gravis)
5. X-ray of the sinuses (sinusitis)
6. Otolaryngology consult
7. Neurology consult

SWOLLEN GUMS AND GUM MASS

The number of conditions causing focal or diffuse swelling of the gums is far out of proportion to the size of this organ and the fact that physicians frequently pay little attention to it unless the patient mentions it. The best approach is to apply the mnemonic **VINDICATE** to the gums, and the list of possible causes will quickly come to mind.

V—Vascular disorders are not a significant cause of swollen gums.

I—Inflammatory lesions include gingivitis, whether viral (aphthous stomatitis), fusospirochetal ("trench mouth"), or monilial. Focal abscesses of the gums are common. Alveolar abscesses also cause focal swelling of the gums.

N—Neoplasms remind one of monocytic leukemia and multiple myeloma, which are associated with diffuse hypertrophy, and local tumors such as a sarcoma, papilloma, odontoma, and squamous cell carcinoma.

D—Deficiency diseases include scurvy and most vitamin deficiencies.

I—Intoxication suggests the common diffuse hyperplasia in patients with epilepsy taking diphenylhydantoin and related drugs, including barbiturates.

C—Congenital or acquired malformations remind one of the gingivitis secondary to malocclusion, poor-fitting

S

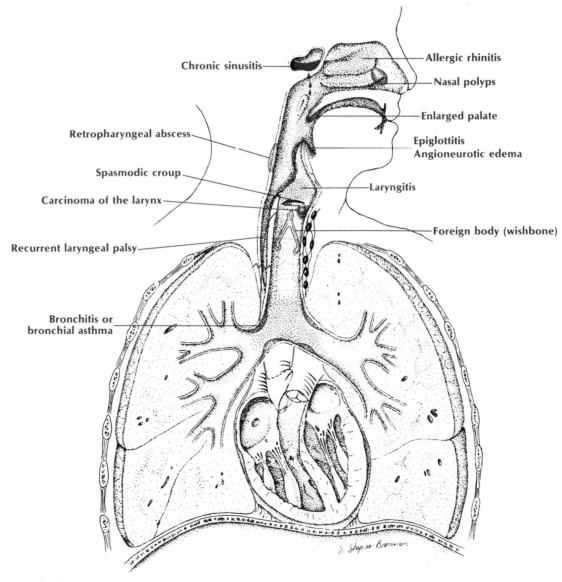

● **FIGURE 12** Stridor and snoring.

crowns or orthodontal appliances, and periodontal cysts, secondary to chronic periapical granuloma.

A—**Autoimmune** and **allergic** diseases include the hypertrophy of thrombocytopenic purpura and the contact gingivitis from dentures, mouthwashes, and toothpastes.

T—**Trauma** to the gums may cause local hematomas and fractures.

E—**Endocrine** disorders suggest several conditions that may cause gum hypertrophy. Gingival hyperplasia in pregnancy, the giant cell granulomas of hyperparathyroidism, juvenile hypothyroidism, pituitary dysfunction, and diabetes mellitus are the most important.

● Approach to the Diagnosis

The approach to the diagnosis is to rule out systemic disease by checking other organs by physical examination and laboratory tests (see other useful tests below). After this is complete, refer the patient to a periodontist. When making a referral, it is wise to have the patient return or call back with the results of the examination after seeing the specialist. In this way, one can be ready to do a further diagnostic workup should the periodontal examination be negative.

● Other Useful Tests

1. CBC (leukemia)
2. Sedimentation rate (dental abscess)
3. Chemistry panel (hyperparathyroidism)
4. Blood smear (leukemia)
5. X-ray of the teeth (dental abscess, hyperparathyroidism)
6. Thyroid profile (hypothyroidism, pituitary adenoma)
7. Skull x-ray (screen for pituitary adenoma)
8. Drug history (phenytoin)
9. Platelet count (thrombocytopenic purpura)

SWOLLEN TONGUE

Swollen tongue (macroglossia) is an uncommon complaint, yet on examination, it is occasionally found. Is it possible to think of more than two or three causes? In most instances this is difficult, yet there is a key to recalling the many causes.

This symptom affords the opportunity to introduce yet another method of arriving at a differential diagnosis—the **histopathologic** method. First, analyze the tissues of the tongue and then decide what can happen to enlarge them. These tissues are the mucosa, submucosal tissue, muscle, supporting tissue, blood vessels, and nerves. What pathologic process can enlarge each of these? Increase in size and number of the cells; infusion of serous fluids, pus, or blood; infiltration of a foreign protein or fat; and infiltration of foreign cells could cause such enlargement. These are all included in Table 54.

The **mucosa** can increase the number of cells in carcinoma of the tongue. It is swollen with a serous fluid in reaction to things put in the mouth such as hot food, mercury, and aspirin. Other less-well-understood sources of fluid in the mucosa are erythema multiforme and pemphigus. The **submucosal** and **supporting tissue** may be enlarged by serous fluid in angioneurotic edema, by purulent fluid in acute diffuse glossitis (usually caused by *Streptococcus* organisms), or by hemorrhagic fluid in leukemia, scurvy, and other hemorrhage disorders. The **subcutaneous** and **supporting tissue** can also be infiltrated by a mucoprotein in myxedema and cretinism and by amyloid in primary amyloidosis. There may be infiltration of neoplastic cells in leukemia and lymphoma.

The **muscle** hypertrophies in acromegaly. Distention of the **blood vessels** may cause macroglossia in CHF and pulmonary emphysema. A few conditions may be left out by this approach. The tongue, for example, seems large in

TABLE 54 Swollen Tongue

	Serous Fluid	Pus	Blood	Foreign Protein	Increase in Cells	Hypertrophy
Mucosa	Mercury Aspirin Burn Erythema multiforme Pemphigus				Carcinoma of the tongue	
Submucosa and Supporting Tissue	Angioneurotic edema Insect bite	Acute diffuse glossitis Ludwig angina	Leukemia Scurvy Thrombocytopenia	Myxedema Cretinism Primary amyloidosis	Lymphoma Leukemic infiltrate	Acromegaly
Muscle						Acromegaly
Blood Vessels	Dermatomyositis		Congestive heart failure Pulmonary emphysema			

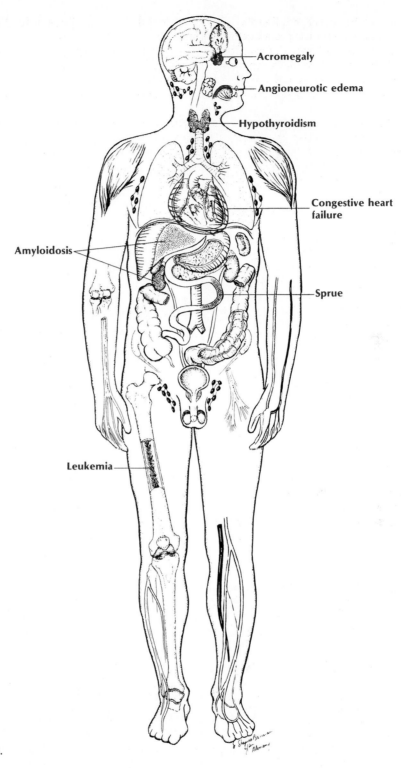

Acromegaly
Angioneurotic edema
Hypothyroidism
Congestive heart failure
Amyloidosis
Sprue
Leukemia

S

● **FIGURE 13** Swollen tongue.

Down syndrome, but this is caused by the fact that it hangs out and appears larger than it really is. The tongue is large and smooth in riboflavin deficiency and sprue.

If the clinician prefers, an excellent differential can be achieved by using the mnemonic **VINDICATE**.

● Approach to the Diagnosis

The diagnosis of macroglossia depends on the presence of other physical findings (almost invariably present) associated with the disorders mentioned above, and, in most

TABLE 55 Syncope

	V Vascular	I Inflammatory	N Neoplasm	D Deficiency or Degenerative	I Intoxication	C Congenital	A Autoimmune Allergic	T Trauma	E Endocrine
Hypoglycemia			Insulinoma Oat cell carcinoma	Cirrhosis of liver	Hypoglycemic drugs and insulin				Insulinoma Addison disease Hypopituitarism
Lungs	Pulmonary embolism	Pneumonia Chronic bronchitis		Pulmonary fibrosis Emphysema	Pneumoconiosis	Cystic fibrosis	Sarcoidosis Anemia	Pneumothorax	
Blood		Chronic anemia Septicemic shock	Leukemia	Aplastic anemia	Drug-induced anemia	Sickle cell anemia	Hemolytic anemia Idiopathic thrombocytopenic purpura	Blood loss	
Heart	Myocardial infarction Ball valve thrombus	Syphilitic aortitis	Atrial myxoma	Myocardiopathy	Cardiac arrhythmias from drugs and alcohol		Rheumatic valvular disease		
Carotid Arteries	Thrombosis Embolism			Atherosclerosis	Drug-induced postural hypotension	Anomalous circle of Willis			
Arteriole	Thrombosis	Subacute bacterial endocarditis				Migraine	Vasculitis Purpura		

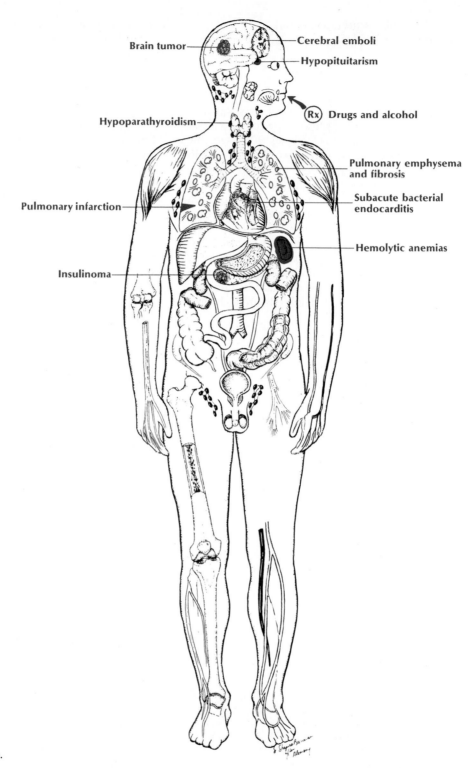

Brain tumor

Cerebral emboli

Hypopituitarism

Hypoparathyroidism

Rx Drugs and alcohol

Pulmonary emphysema
and fibrosis

Subacute bacterial
endocarditis

Pulmonary infarction

Hemolytic anemias

Insulinoma

S

● **FIGURE 14** Syncope.

cases, the results of a systematic workup. A lingual biopsy is valuable in primary amyloidosis.

● Other Useful Tests

1. CBC (leukemia)
2. Sedimentation rate (glossitis)
3. Culture and sensitivity (abscess, glossitis)
4. VDRL test (gumma)
5. Thyroid profile (hypothyroidism)
6. Growth hormone assay (acromegaly)
7. Skull x-ray (screen for pituitary adenoma)
8. Blood smear (leukemia)
9. Circulation time (CHF)
10. Tests for vitamin deficiency

11. Coagulation studies (scurvy, leukemia)
12. Lingual biopsy (amyloidosis)

SYNCOPE

The differential of syncope or a brief loss of consciousness is best developed with the use of **physiology** and, to a lesser extent, **anatomy**. Like convulsions (see page 108), syncope is due to a diminished supply of oxygen and glucose in the brain cell. Anything that produces hypoglycemia (see page 247) may lead to episodes of syncope, but the most common cause is overdose of insulin. It is also important to include insulinomas and overdose of oral hypoglycemic agents (Table 55).

Reduced delivery of oxygen to the brain cell accounts for most cases of syncope. Oxygen must get into the body through the lungs with adequate ventilation. It must then be absorbed through the alveolar–capillary membrane, picked up by an adequate number of red cells, and delivered to the brain by a good functioning heart and unobstructed carotid and vertebral–basilar system. Retracing the above physiology and anatomy will develop the disease entities that must be considered in the differential diagnosis of syncope.

Thus, mechanical obstructions of the larynx (foreign body), the bronchi, bronchioles (asthma and emphysema), or alveolar–capillary membrane (pulmonary fibrosis, sarcoidosis, or pulmonary embolism) may cause anoxia and syncope. Severe anemia prevents the adequate transport of oxygen. Oxygen transport from the heart to the brain may be obstructed mechanically or functionally. It is functionally obstructed by CHF of Stokes–Adams syndrome (heart block) and other arrhythmias, particularly ventricular tachycardia and sick sinus syndrome. Functional obstruction may result from a drop in blood pressure from carotid sinus syncope, postural hypotension (see page 253), and vasovagal syncope. True vertigo (see page 131) may lead to syncope by way of the latter mechanism.

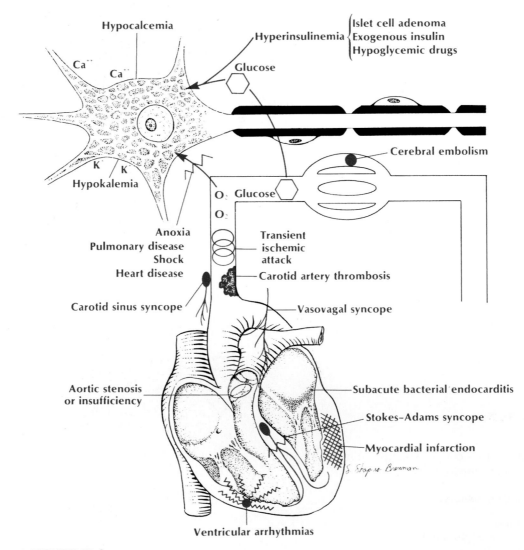

● **FIGURE 15** Syncope.

Mechanical obstruction may occur at the aortic valve (aortic stenosis or insufficiency), at the carotid arteries (thrombi or plaques), or focally in the smaller arteries from ischemia due to arterial thrombi or emboli. Less commonly, mechanical obstruction may occur from ball–valve thrombi in the mitral or tricuspid valve, large pulmonary emboli, or cough syncope in which poor venous return to the heart is the cause.

● Approach to the Diagnosis

Clinical differentiation of the various forms of syncope is made by combinations of symptoms. Thus, syncope with marked sweating and tachycardia is more likely due to hypoglycemia. Syncope with sweating and bradycardia is more likely due to vasovagal syncope. Syncope induced by exercise suggests long QT syndrome. There is often a family history of sudden death. Focal neurologic signs during the attack suggest transient ischemia attack (TIA) and prompt a search for sources of emboli or thrombosis (sickle cell disease, polycythemia, or macroglobulinemia). Transesophageal echocardiography is the procedure of choice to find a cardiac source. A family history of syncope suggests migraine, epilepsy, or vasovagal attacks. Epilepsy is a strong possibility in the young, whereas heart block is more likely in the aged. Consequently, an EEG and Holter monitoring are useful in the workup.

● Other Useful Tests

1. CBC (anemia)
2. Chemistry panel (hypoglycemia, hypocalcemia)
3. Serum and urine osmolality (dehydration)
4. Upright-tilt table test (postural hypotension)
5. ECG (cardiac arrhythmia)
6. Carotid sinus massage (carotid sinus syndrome)
7. ECG (CHF, valvular heart disease)
8. Carotid scans (TIA)
9. Four-vessel cerebral angiogram (TIA)
10. Exercise tolerance test (coronary insufficiency)
11. Signal-averaging ECG (ventricular arrhythmia)
12. 72-hour fast with glucose monitoring (insulinoma)
13. Drug screen (drug abuse)
14. 24-hour ambulatory blood pressure monitoring (postural hypotension)
15. Neurology consult
16. Continuous-loop ECG recording (cardiac arrhythmia)
17. Psychiatric consult
18. Electrophysiologic study (cardiac arrhythmia)
19. MRI or MRA of the brain (cerebrovascular insufficiency)

Case Presentation #81

A 68-year-old mayor's wife suffered sudden attacks of syncope for several years. The attacks occurred without warning, and she would fall to the floor in a stupor for a minute or two, only to recover with no postictal confusion or other symptomatology. It was rare that she suffered any injuries from the attacks. She had been evaluated by several multispecialty clinics without a definitive diagnosis.

Question #1. Utilizing your knowledge of physiology, what is your differential diagnosis?

Complete physical examination was within normal limits. An ECG showed first-degree heart block, but 24-hour Holter monitoring was unremarkable. Echocardiography was normal. Electrophysiologic studies were not available at this time.

Question #2. What is your diagnosis now?

(See Appendix B for the answers.)

T

TACHYCARDIA

Tachycardia, like dyspnea, is usually a sign that the tissues are not getting enough oxygen to meet their demands. To recall a list of causes, **pathophysiology** is applied. If tachycardia results from anoxia, then the causes can be developed on the basis of the causes for anoxia, which may result from a decreased intake of oxygen, a decreased absorption of oxygen, and inadequate transport of oxygen to the tissues. Tachycardia also results when the tissues' demand for oxygen increases. Another cause is peripheral arteriovenous shunts. In addition, anything that stimulates the heart directly, such as drugs, electrolyte imbalances, or disturbances in the cardiac conduction system, will cause tachycardia. Let us review the conditions that may fall into each of these categories.

1. **Decreased intake of oxygen:** Anything that obstructs the airway and prevents oxygen from getting to the alveoli should be recalled in this category. Bronchial asthma, laryngotracheitis, chronic bronchitis, and emphysema are most important to recall. In addition, if the "respiratory" pump (thoracic cage, intercostal and diaphragmatic muscles, and respiratory centers in the brainstem) is affected by disease, especially acutely, there will be tachycardia. Poliomyelitis, myasthenia gravis, barbiturate intoxication, and intoxication by other central nervous system (CNS) depressants are examples of disorders in this category. Finally, the intake of oxygen may decrease if there is a low atmospheric oxygen tension. High altitude is an obvious cause, but hazardous working conditions must also be considered.
2. **Decreased oxygen absorption:** This may result from three mechanisms.
   A. **Alveolar–capillary block** in sarcoidosis, pneumoconiosis, pulmonary fibrosis, congestive heart failure (CHF), alveolar proteinosis, and shock lung.
   B. **Diminished perfusion of the pulmonary capillaries** in pulmonary emboli and pulmonary and cardiovascular arteriovenous shunts.
   C. **Disturbed ventilation/perfusion ratio** in which alveoli are perfused but not well ventilated, in alveoli that are not well ventilated, or in alveoli that are ventilated but not well perfused. This is typical of pulmonary emphysema, atelectasis, and many chronic pulmonary diseases.
3. **Inadequate oxygen transport:** Severe anemia, shock, and CHF (regardless of the cause) fall into this category, as do methemoglobinemia and sulfhemoglobinemia.
4. **Increased tissue oxygen demands:** Fever, hyperthyroidism, leukemia, metastatic malignancies, polycythemia, and certain physical or emotional demands fall into this category.

5. **Peripheral arteriovenous shunts:** These shunts may occur in the popliteal fossa following a gunshot wound, in the sellar area following the rupture of a carotid aneurysm into the cavernous sinus, and in Paget disease.
6. **Disorders that directly affect the heart:** Stimulants of the heart such as caffeine, adrenalin (pheochromocytomas), thyroid hormone (hyperthyroidism), amphetamines, theophylline, and other drugs fall into this category. Nervous tension and neurocirculatory asthenia may be the cause. Electrolyte disturbances such as hypocalcemia and hypokalemia may precipitate ventricular tachycardia. Excessive amounts of digitalis may also provoke atrial or ventricular tachycardia.

Tachycardia of various types may occur from disturbances in the conducting system of the heart. Digitalis has already been mentioned, but the Wolff–Parkinson–White syndrome, focal myocardial anoxia from emboli or infarction, and distention of various chambers of the heart (atria in mitral stenosis, ventricles in essential hypertension and cor pulmonale) are also etiologies of this mechanism. Anticholinergic drugs such as atropine block the ability of the vagus to slow the heart and may cause or contribute to tachycardia. All of the above categories are outlined in Table 56 where a few diseases that are more specific are mentioned.

● Approach to the Diagnosis

The association of other clinical signs and symptoms will often help to pinpoint the diagnosis. Tachycardia with tremor and an enlarged thyroid suggests hyperthyroidism. Tachycardia with respiratory wheezes suggests bronchial asthma. Tachycardia with a black stool suggests a bleeding peptic ulcer. If the blood pressure is low, the workup will proceed as that of shock (see page 252). In contrast, tachycardia with a normal blood pressure should prompt thyroid function studies, pulmonary function studies, arterial blood gases, and a venous pressure and circulation time. Electrolyte determinations, a drug screen, and 24-hour urine for catecholamine determinations may be indicated if there is hypertension as well.

● Other Useful Tests

1. Complete blood count (CBC) (anemia)
2. Sedimentation rate (infection)
3. Chemistry panel (liver disease, uremia)
4. Antinuclear antigen (ANA) (collagen)
5. Antistreptolysin O (ASO) titer (rheumatic fever)
6. Blood cultures (subacute bacterial endocarditis [SBE])
7. Febrile agglutinins (fever of unknown origin)
8. Serial electrocardiograms (ECGs) and cardiac enzymes (myocardial infarction)

TABLE 56   Tachycardia

	V Vascular	I Inflammatory	N Neoplasm	D Degenerative	I Intoxication	C Congenital	A Allergic and Autoimmune	T Trauma	E Endocrine
Decreased Intake of Oxygen	Aortic aneurysm with compression of bronchi	Laryngitis Bronchitis	Carcinoma of the lung	Pulmonary emphysema	Pneumoconiosis	α_1-trypsin deficiency Cystic fibrosis	Bronchial asthma	Pneumothorax	
Increased Oxygen Absorption	Pulmonary embolism	Pneumonia	Hemangioma Carcinoma of the lung	Pulmonary emphysema Fibrosis	Nitrofurantoin Pneumoconiosis Shock lung Lipoid pneumonia	Congenital cyst	Scleroderma Wegener granulomatosis	Shock lung	Fat emboli
Inadequate Oxygen Transport	Shock from myocardial infarction Congestive heart failure	Septicemic shock		Aplastic anemia	Drug-induced shock Methemoglobinemia	Sickle cell anemia Cooley anemia	Hemolytic anemia (autoimmune)	Hemorrhagic shock	
Peripheral Arteriovenous Shunts				Paget disease		Carotic–cavernous shunt		Popliteal aneurysm	
Increased Tissue Demands for Oxygen		Septicemia Fever of any infection	Leukemia Hodgkin lymphoma Polycythemia vera						Hyperthyroidism
Disorders Affecting the Heart Directly	Myocardial infarction Essential hypertension	Myocarditis Tuberculosis Pericarditis	Rhabdomyosarcoma	Muscular dystrophy	Caffeine Amphetamines Alcohol Hyperkalemia Digitalis	Wolff–Parkinson–White syndrome Glycogen storage disease	Lupus erythematosus	Traumatic aneurysm	Hyperthyroidism Pheochromocytomas

T

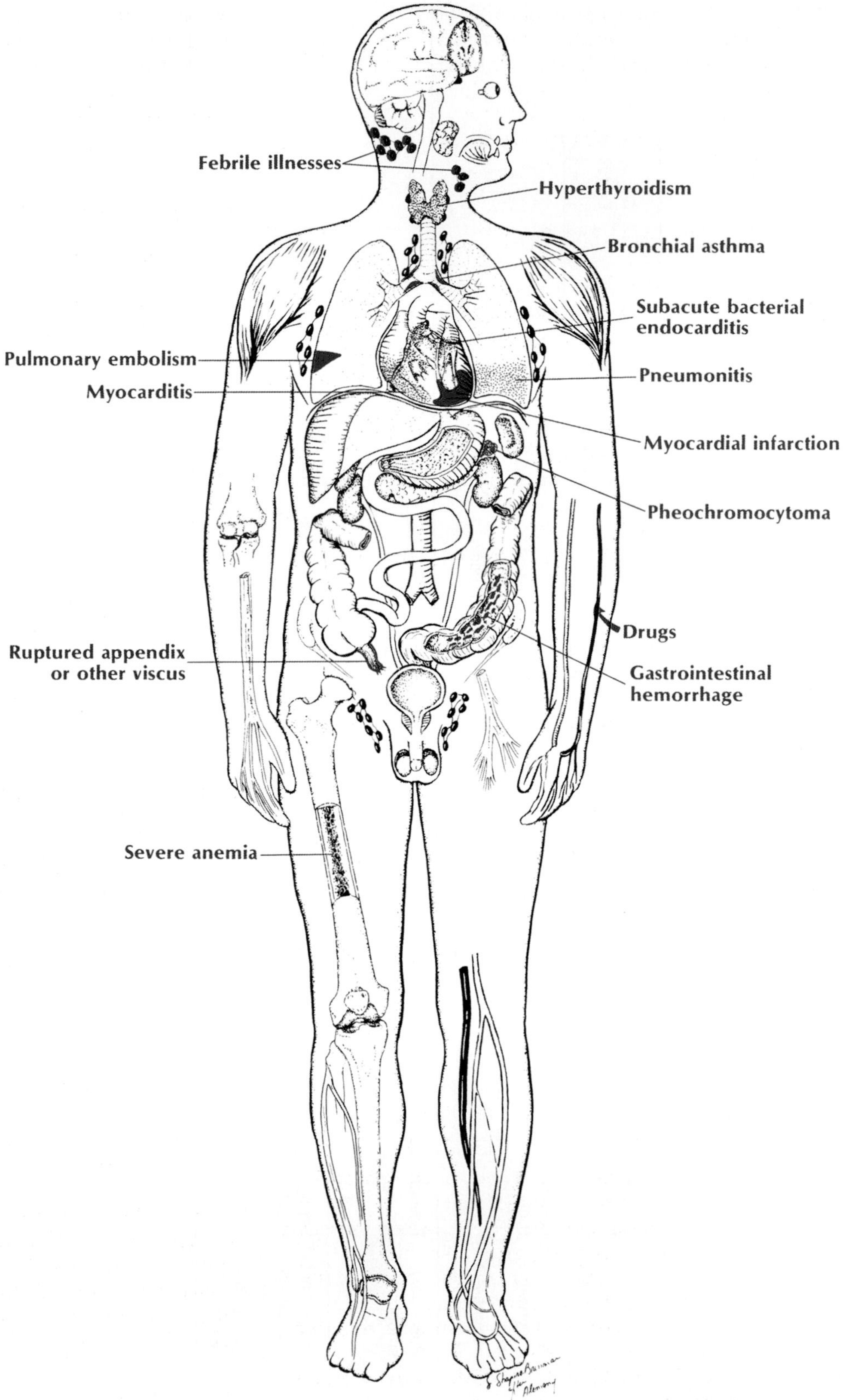

Febrile illnesses

Hyperthyroidism

Bronchial asthma

Subacute bacterial
endocarditis

Pulmonary embolism

Pneumonitis

Myocarditis

Myocardial infarction

Pheochromocytoma

Ruptured appendix
or other viscus

Drugs

Gastrointestinal
hemorrhage

Severe anemia

● **FIGURE 1** Tachycardia.

9. Lung scan (pulmonary embolism)
10. Holter monitoring (cardiac arrhythmia)
11. Echocardiography (CHF, valvular heart disease)
12. 5-hour glucose tolerance test (insulinoma)
13. Temperature chart (fever of unknown origin)
14. Sleeping pulse rate (anxiety neurosis)
15. Psychiatric consult

TASTE ABNORMALITIES

The causes of taste abnormalities can be recalled simply by visualizing the various structures around the tongue, mainly the nose, throat, teeth, gums, joints, and nerves. It is wise to start our discussion with the tongue.

Tongue—Glossitis, stomatitis
Nose—Rhinitis, sinusitis, and hay fever
Throat—Tonsillitis and pharyngitis
Teeth—Dental cases, alveolar abscess
Gums—Gingivitis
Joints—Temporomandibular joint syndrome
Nerves—Bell palsy, brainstem lesions, uncinate fits (epilepsy)

Unfortunately, this method would fail to help recall the drugs and poisons that cause taste abnormalities such as penicillamine, bismuth, iodine, bromide, and mercury.

● Approach to the Diagnosis

Careful examination of the nose and throat ought to reveal most of the above conditions. A neurologic examination should reveal Bell palsy and brainstem lesions. X-ray of the teeth will demonstrate dental cases and abscess. A wake-and-sleep electroencephalogram (EEG) with nasopharyngeal electrodes will be necessary to diagnose uncinate fits. Laboratory studies include a urine drug screen, CBC, chemistry panel, and venereal disease research laboratory (VDRL) test. A psychiatrist should be consulted if there are no objective findings and these studies are negative.

TESTICULAR ATROPHY

The causes of this sign can best be recalled by using the mnemonic **VINDICATE**.

V—Vascular conditions bring to mind varicoceles, which cause atrophy on the side of the dilated veins.
I—Inflammation recalls the atrophy following mumps, orchitis, and other causes of epidydimoorchitis.
N—Neoplasms suggest the atrophy that occurs in the estrogen treatment of prostatic carcinoma.
D—Degenerative disorders suggest the atrophy resulting from aging.
I—Intoxication should remind one of the atrophy resulting from chronic alcoholism, Lannec cirrhosis, and hemochromatosis. X-ray exposure may also produce atrophy.
C—Congenital disorders recall undescended testes and torsion.

A—Autoimmune and **allergic** disorders suggest nothing.
T—Trauma reminds one of the atrophy following vasectomy and accidental ligation of the blood supply during hernia repair.
E—Endocrine disorders suggest the atrophy of hypopituitarism, Klinefelter syndrome, and other eunuchoidal states.

● Approach to the Diagnosis

The workup of testicular atrophy may require a chromatin analysis, serum testosterone, follicle-stimulating hormone (FSH) and luteinizing hormone (LH) levels, and biopsy, but referral to an endocrinologist is the best way to get this accomplished with accuracy.

● Other Useful Tests

1. Sperm count
2. VDRL (syphilis)
3. Serum iron and iron-binding capacity (hemochromatosis)
4. Liver biopsy (hemochromatosis)
5. Electromyogram (EMG) (myotonic dystrophy)
6. Urology consult
7. Computed tomography (CT) scan of the brain (pituitary insufficiency)

TESTICULAR MASS

Like that of most masses, the differential diagnosis of testicular masses is best analyzed by the **anatomic** and **histologic** approach (Table 57). The **skin** may be involved by many inflammatory conditions leading to swelling, including carbuncles, cellulitis, and dermatitis of various types. Edema of the skin and subcutaneous tissue is found in cirrhosis, CHF, nephrosis, and filariasis. The tunica vaginalis is involved with hernias and hydroceles, which may be differentiated by using transillumination. The **venous plexus** of the scrotum and testes is involved by varicoceles and phlebitis (usually of the left venous plexus), and a varicocele may be the sign of a carcinoma of the kidney when the left spermatic vein is obstructed. Thus, one readily sees how frequently obstruction is a pathophysiologic mechanism in tumors here or elsewhere.

The **testis** is swollen in carcinomas (e.g., seminomas, choriocarcinomas, teratomas, Leydig cell tumors) and in orchitis (secondary to mumps, bacterial diseases, syphilis, or tuberculosis). The **epididymis** is frequently inflamed and swollen when there is orchitis and only rarely is inflamed by itself. It may also be enlarged from a spermatocele or from a vas deferens obstruction caused by prostatic disease (inflammation or neoplasm). Finally, **arterial occlusion** caused by torsion of the testicle may cause a testicular mass.

● Approach to the Diagnosis

Testicular masses may be differentiated by **transillumination** (hydroceles and spermatoceles transilluminate, whereas hernias and tumors do not). Hernias may also be differentiated by reducing them (some will not reduce,

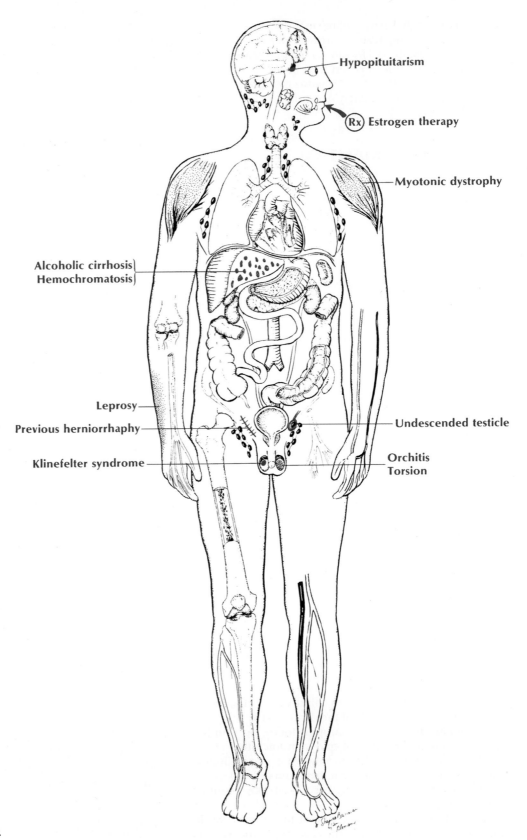

● **FIGURE 2** Testicular atrophy.

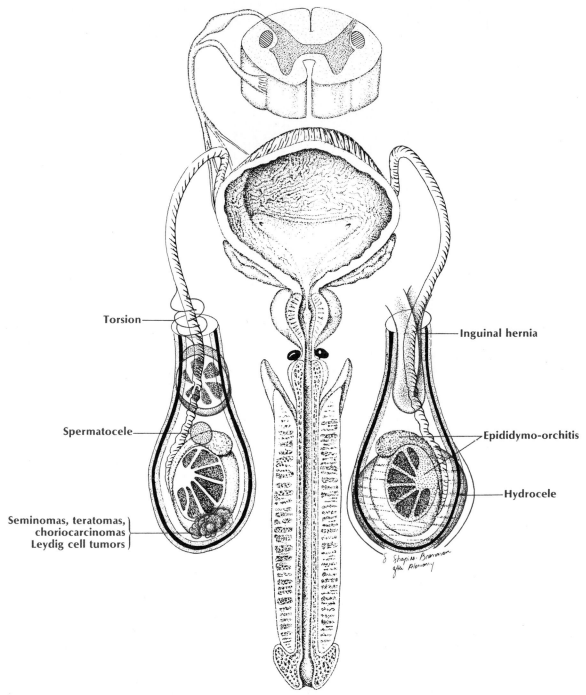

Torsion

Spermatocele

Seminomas, teratomas,
choriocarcinomas
Leydig cell tumors

Inguinal hernia

Epididymo-orchitis

Hydrocele

● **FIGURE 3** Testicular mass.

however, if they are incarcerated), and auscultation may reveal bowel sounds. In noncommunicating hydroceles and testicular tumors, one may get above the swelling, whereas in torsion and hernias one cannot. In torsion, the tenderness is decreased by elevation of the testicle, whereas in orchitis the tenderness is not relieved unless elevation is done for an hour or more. Ultrasonography will easily distinguish between torsion and orchitis because of the significant decrease in blood supply to the testicle in torsion. Serum alpha-fetoprotein beta-human chorionic gonadotropin (HCG) or lactic dehydrogenase (LDH) will

be elevated in testicular tumors. Surgery may be the only way to differentiate the cause of the mass.

● **Other Useful Tests**

1. CBC (orchitis)
2. Sedimentation rate (orchitis)
3. Urinalysis (urinary tract infection [UTI])
4. Urethral smear (infection)
5. Urine culture (UTI)
6. Urine gonadotropin (testicular tumor)

TABLE 57   Testicular Mass

	V Vascular	I Inflammatory	N Neoplasm	D Degenerative	I Intoxication	C Congenital	A Allergic and Autoimmune	T Trauma	E Endocrine	O Obstruction
Skin		Carbuncle	Carcinoma				Urticaria	Contusion		Sebaceous cyst
Subcutaneous Tissue		Cellulitis						Direct inguinal hernia		
Tunica Vaginalis						Indirect inguinal hernia Hydrocele		Hematoma		
Venous Plexus		Phlebitis	Obstruction from renal carcinoma			Varicocele				
Testis		Orchitis Syphilis	Seminoma Chorioepithelioma			Teratoma Hydatid cyst of Morgagni				
Epididymis		Bacterial epididymitis Tuberculosis				Cyst				Spermatocele
Artery	Torsion					Torsion				
Vas Deferens			Secondary to obstruction by carcinoma of prostate							Prostate disease
Lymphatics		Filariasis								

7. Prostatic fluid smear and culture (prostatitis)
8. Mumps skin test and serology (mumps orchitis)
9. Small-bowel series (hernia)
10. CT scan of the abdomen and pelvis (metastatic tumor)
11. Urology consult
12. Sonogram (torsion, hydrocele)
13. Radionuclide scan (torsion)
14. Prostate-specific antigen (PSA) (prostatic carcinoma)

TESTICULAR PAIN

It is helpful but unnecessary to do an anatomic breakdown in developing this differential diagnosis. The mnemonic **MINT** brings the most important causes to mind instantly.

M—Malformation suggests hernias, varicocele, and torsion of the testicle.
I—Inflammation recalls epididymitis and epididymoorchitis.
N—Neoplasms of the testicles may be virtually painless, but the mass will give them away. Tuberculosis is also unlikely to cause significant pain.
T—Traumatic lesions are common in contact sports, but occasionally a boy will deny a history of trauma.

Referred pain from renal calculi is a significant cause of testicular pain. Any condition that irritates the T12 nerve root (e.g., osteoarthritis and herniated disc) and the course of the peripheral portion of this nerve (appendicitis) may cause testicular pain, but these are uncommon causes.

● Approach to the Diagnosis

The approach to the diagnosis of testicular pain involves searching for a mass; if it is present, certain questions must be answered. Does it transilluminate (hydrocele)? Can one get above the swelling (testicular mass)? Is it reducible (hernia)? Does supporting the testicle relieve the pain (orchitis)? Ultrasonography is done to distinguish torsion from orchitis. A search for prostatic hypertrophy or prostatitis should be made, particularly in older men. Smears of urethral discharge, urinalysis and urine culture, cystoscopy, and an intravenous pyelogram (IVP) may be indicated in selected cases. An exploration for torsion or hernia may be the only way to establish these diagnoses.

THROMBOCYTOPENIA

The mnemonic **VINDICATE** is very useful to develop a list of causes of thrombocytopenia.

V—Vascular disorders should help the recall of disseminated intravascular coagulation (DIC).
I—Inflammation: Infectious diseases that may be associated with thrombocytopenia include malaria, rickettsia, toxic shock syndrome, typhoid fever, cytomegalovirus (CMV), and septicemia.
N—Neoplasms that may be associated with thrombocytopenia include leukemia, lymphoma, and myeloma; however, any tumor that may invade the bone marrow can cause thrombocytopenia.

D—Deficiency disorders include vitamin B_{12} and folic acid deficiencies.
I—Intoxication. This category will prompt the recall of thrombocytopenia associated with gold salts, alcohol, chemotherapy, chloramphenicol, phenylbutazone, radiation, thiazides, sulfonamides, and quinidine.
C—Congenital. This category promotes the recall of Wiskott–Aldrich syndrome, Fanconi anemia, maternal drug ingestion, and congenital viral infections.
A—Autoimmune. The most important disorders brought to mind by this category are idiopathic autoimmune thrombocytopenia purpura and collagen diseases.
T—Trauma. Although trauma does not directly induce thrombocytopenia, this category should help to recall transfusion reactions and DIC.
E—Endocrine. This category prompts the recall of hyperthyroidism and thyroiditis.

● Approach to the Diagnosis

The laboratory workup will provide the best means of diagnosing the cause of thrombocytopenia. If there is pancytopenia, the most likely cause is aplastic anemia or bone marrow invasion. Collagen disorders such as lupus erythematosus would paint a similar picture. If only the platelets are affected, autoimmune disorders would be more likely the cause. The initial workup should include a CBC, blood smear for morphology, sedimentation rate, serum B_{12} and folic acid levels, chemistry panel, ANA, serum haptoglobins, red cell survival, and protein electrophoresis. A hematologist should be consulted.

● Other Useful Tests

1. Bone marrow examination (aplastic anemia)
2. Liver–spleen scan (splenomegaly, disease of the spleen)
3. CT scan of the abdomen (neoplasm, Hodgkin lymphoma, splenomegaly)
4. Bone scan (metastasis)
5. Platelet antibody titer (thrombocytopenia)

TINNITUS AND DEAFNESS

If one dissects the **anatomy** of the external, middle, and internal ear one can obtain an excellent list of conditions to be considered in the differential diagnosis of tinnitus and deafness (Table 58).

Beginning in the **external canal**, impacted cerumen and foreign bodies are occasionally the cause. Next, visualizing the **drum**, one is reminded of otitis media, herpes zoster oticus, myringitis bullosa, and traumatic rupture of the drum. Behind the drum are the **auditory ossicles**; these little bones should prompt the recall of otosclerosis. The **chordae tympani nerve** passes behind the drum on its way to the jaw and tongue. This structure should suggest the tinnitus of Costen temporomandibular joint syndrome. The **eustachian tube** should remind one of the aerotitis connected with flying and the serous otitis connected with blockage of the tube from upper respiratory infections and

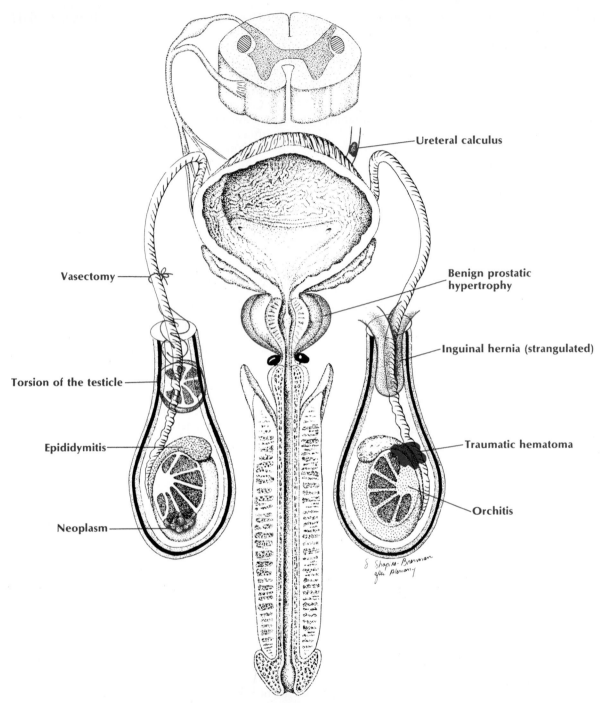

● **FIGURE 4** Testicular pain.

allergies. Behind the middle ear, the connecting passages of the **mastoid bones** suggest mastoiditis.

Moving deeper to the **inner ear**, one is reminded of toxic labyrinthitis from salicylates, quinine, streptomycin, gentamycin, and a host of other drugs. Classified here is also the "toxic" labyrinthitis of uremia, anemia, and leukemia. Syphilis, typhoid, and other bacteria may occasionally invade the inner ear, but most infections here are viral. The

chronic granulomatous cholesteatoma should be recalled. In visualizing the **labyrinth**, one cannot help but recall Ménière disease, a prominent cause of tinnitus and deafness. Severe head injuries may cause tinnitus and traumatic labyrinthitis.

Connecting the auditory apparatus to the brain is the **auditory nerve**, and acoustic neuromas are quickly brought to mind in the differential diagnosis. The **nerve**,

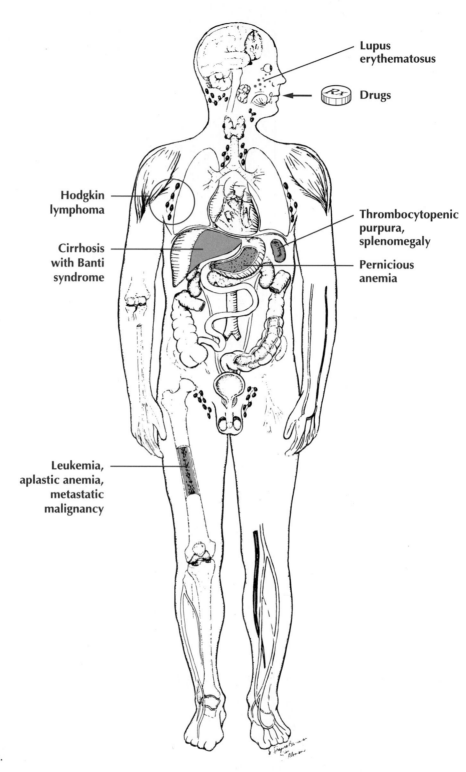

Lupus
erythematosus

Drugs

Hodgkin
lymphoma

Thrombocytopenic
purpura,
splenomegaly

Cirrhosis
with Banti
syndrome

Pernicious
anemia

Leukemia,
aplastic anemia,
metastatic
malignancy

● **FIGURE 5** Thrombocytopenia.

brainstem, and **brain**, however, are affected by numerous conditions, and it would be well to recall them with the mnemonic **VINDICATE**.

V—Vascular lesions include aneurysms and occlusions of the vertebral–basilar or internal auditory arteries. Hypertension and migraine may cause intermittent spasms of these arteries with tinnitus and occasional deafness.

I—Inflammatory lesions include syphilis, tuberculous and bacterial meningitis of other organisms, and many febrile illnesses that may lead to transient tinnitus and deafness. Viral encephalitis, rubella in utero, and mumps may cause tinnitus and deafness.

TABLE 58   Tinnitus and Deafness

	V Vascular	I Inflammatory	N Neoplasm	D Degenerative	I Intoxication	C Congenital	A Allergic and Autoimmune	T Trauma	E Endocrine
External Canal		Otitis externa	Papilloma			Congenital obstruction or absence of canal		Impacted cerumen and/or foreign body	
Middle Ear		Otitis media		Otosclerosis			Serous otitis media	Rupture of drum	
Inner Ear	Spasm of internal auditory artery (migraine)	Petrositis Labyrinthitis or cochleitis	Cholesteatoma	Senile deafness Ménière disease	Streptomycin Gentamycin Isoniazid Other toxins		Ménière disease	Skull fracture Contusion	Myxedema
Acoustic Nerve	Aneurysm		Acoustic neuroma					Skull fracture	Diabetic neuropathy
Brainstem	Basilar artery insufficiency and occlusion	Syphilis Viral encephalitis	Glioma Meningioma	Syringomyelia			Multiple sclerosis	Hemorrhage	

N—**Neoplasms** include acoustic neuromas, meningiomas, and occasional gliomas or metastatic carcinomas and sarcomas.

D—**Degenerative** disorders remind one of the idiopathic symmetric tinnitus and deafness in the aged population (presbycusis) and the dominant progressive nerve deafness diseases considered under the congenital category. Paget disease might also be considered here.

I—**Intoxication:** It is uncertain whether drugs and certain poisons such as lead, phosphorus, mercury, and aniline dyes affect the nerve or cochlea more, but it is well to remember them here also.

C—**Congenital** disorders that may cause tinnitus and deafness include maternal rubella and all the hereditary causes of sensorineural deafness. Hallgren disease, Alström syndrome, Refsum disease, and Treacher–Collins syndrome are only a few of these. Some of these disorders are associated with lesions in other organs. For example, Alport syndrome is the combination of hereditary deafness and nephritis. The aura of tinnitus in epilepsy should be recalled here.

A—**Autoimmune** diseases that cause involvement of the acoustic nerve and its tributaries include multiple sclerosis and postinfectious encephalomyelitis.

T—**Traumatic** conditions include skull fractures and the postconcussion syndrome. The occupational tinnitus and deafness of continuous noise must also be considered here.

E—**Endocrine** diseases include hypothyroidism, acromegaly, and diabetic neuritis.

● Approach to the Diagnosis

When a patient complains of tinnitus and deafness, a good occupational history is essential. Gradual onset of unilateral deafness should be considered an acoustic neuroma until proven otherwise. Look for café au lait spots on the skin (Von Recklinghausen disease). The combination of other symptoms and signs is the key to a clinical diagnosis. Thus tinnitus, deafness, and vertigo suggest Ménière disease. Almost total unilateral deafness (sudden in onset in a diabetic) suggests diabetic neuritis. A similar episode can occur in syphilis, but vertigo is also often present. Tinnitus and vertigo following a head injury suggest traumatic myringitis, labyrinthitis, or postconcussion syndrome. If there is total deafness with the tinnitus and vertigo, a basilar skull fracture should be considered. Tinnitus and headache suggest migraine.

Diagnostic studies that should be done in all cases are audiograms, caloric tests, and x-rays of the skull, petrous bones, and mastoids. If an acoustic neuroma is suspected, tomography of the petrous bones, a CT scan or magnetic resonance imaging (MRI), and basilar myelography may be indicated. Syphilis and multiple sclerosis require a spinal tap to assist in diagnosis. Angiography (especially if there is pulsatile tinnitus) and EEGs may be required in selected cases.

● Other Useful Tests

1. Electronystagmogram (acoustic neuroma, Ménière disease)
2. Tympanogram (otitis media)

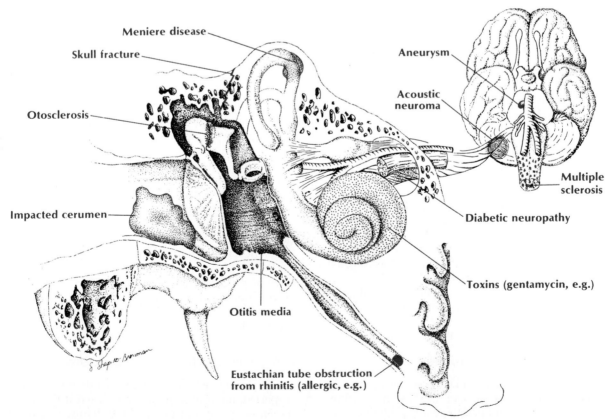

● **FIGURE 6** Tinnitus and deafness.

3. MRI of the brain and auditory canals (acoustic neuroma, multiple sclerosis)
4. Brainstem evoked potentials (multiple sclerosis)
5. Magnetic resonance angiogram (vertebral–basilar artery insufficiency)
6. Neurology consult
7. Otolaryngology consult

Case Presentation #82

A 32-year-old white man complained of increasing high-pitched ringing in his left ear for years. He denied deafness or vertigo. However, he failed the whisper test in his left ear and the Weber test lateralized to the right ear. A Rinné test was 2:1 in both ears.

Question #1. Utilizing your knowledge of anatomy and the mnemonic **VINDICATE**, what is your differential diagnosis?
   Neurologic examination was unremarkable except for diminished left corneal reflex. He had several subcutaneous tumors on his trunk and extremities.

Question #2. What is your diagnosis now?

_____

(See Appendix B for the answers.)

TONGUE PAIN

Examination of the tongue is a time-honored important diagnostic aid, but in my experience, it is unusual for patients to present with pain in the tongue. Nevertheless, there is a plethora of causes. The mnemonic **VINDICATE** lends itself best to prompting the recall of these causes.

V—Vascular disorders suggest pernicious and iron deficiency anemia.
I—Inflammation recalls Vincent stomatitis, herpes simplex, tuberculosis, and syphilis. The referred pain from gingivitis and abscessed teeth should also be considered here.
N—Neoplasms remind one that carcinoma of the tongue often presents with pain.
D—Degenerative and **deficiency** diseases remind one of pellagra and other avitaminoses.
I—Intoxication and **idiopathic** disorders call to mind tobacco, plumbism, mercurialism, and glossopharyngeal or trigeminal neuralgia.
C—Congenital anomalies of the tongue are rare.
A—Allergic and **autoimmune** diseases, in contrast, suggest dermatomyositis and angioneurotic edema.
T—Trauma suggests the numerous times we bite our tongues and may prompt a search for epilepsy when a patient presents with syncope.
E—Endocrine disorders remind one of hypothyroidism.

● Approach to the Diagnosis

The approach to the diagnosis includes a CBC, sedimentation rate, serum B_{12} and folic acid levels, serum ferritin, serology, tuberculin test, and perhaps biopsy of the lesion. A trial of vitamin therapy may be indicated.

TONGUE ULCERS

The mnemonic **MINT** will help the recall of the important causes of tongue ulcers.

M—Malformation suggests malocclusion, which can cause repetitive trauma to the tongue. Also dental prostheses can promote ulceration.
I—Inflammation provokes the recall of herpes simplex, Vincent stomatitis, herpes zoster, syphilis, and tuberculosis. This reminds one of chickenpox, smallpox, and pemphigus.
N—Neoplasm suggests leukoplakia and carcinoma of the tongue.
T—Trauma is probably the major cause of ulcerations. Repetitive trauma from a sharp, broken, or carious tooth produces painful ulceration.

● Approach to the Diagnosis

Herpes simplex and herpes zoster can be diagnosed by the Tzanck tests, viral isolation, or serologic tests. A fluorescent treponemal antibody absorption (FTA–ABS) test will diagnose syphilis. A biopsy will be necessary to diagnose carcinoma. It is best to refer these patients to an oral surgeon if the ulcers do not clear up with observation and conventional treatment.

TOOTHACHE

Toothache is included here not only because dentists might read this book but also because physicians are occasionally called on to manage toothache until a dentist can be reached. A **histologic analysis** of the tooth and surrounding structures will supply the differential diagnosis. Most commonly, the **pulp** may be exposed by dental caries, but then the pain is intermittent. When the pulp is infected (pulpitis) the pain is continuous, and the pulp may subsequently become abscessed. The **periapical tissue** may be inflamed, and an alveolar abscess may ensue. Finally, **osteomyelitis** of the **jaw** or **maxillary bones** may occur. The **gingiva** may be inflamed, and pyorrhea will result. What is often not appreciated by physicians is that the tooth can be sore and inflamed without objective evidence on examination. A common cause of this situation is a filling that is close to or in apposition with the pulp.

Referred pain is as important here as it is in other structures of the head. Thus, sinusitis, otitis media, and temporomandibular joint disease may cause pain in the tooth. Trigeminal neuralgia and other neurologic disorders must occasionally be considered.

● Approach to the Diagnosis

This is simple. Refer the patient to a dentist. If infection is suspected, an antibiotic may be started if there is a delay in getting an appointment. If the dentist cannot find the cause, referral to a neurologist is appropriate.

TORTICOLLIS

Torticollis is relatively infrequent; when seen in the adult it is thought to be "supratentorial." There are, however, organic diseases that actually may be responsible. The best approach to recalling these instantly is **anatomic**, beginning with the muscle and proceeding along the nerve pathways to the brain and "supratentorium."

1. **Muscle:** These may be divided into intrinsic and extrinsic lesions.

   A. **Intrinsic:** Hematomas of the sternocleidomastoid muscle follow trauma, but congenital torticollis is thought to be due to injury or hematoma of the muscle at birth. Another intrinsic lesion is cervical fibromyositis. In this condition, the head is usually held in one position.

   B. **Extrinsic:** Cervical ribs, scars of the neck, tonsillitis, dental abscess, or cervical adenitis may cause torticollis.

2. **Nerve and nerve root:** Conditions of the spinal column such as cervical spondylosis, tuberculosis of the cervical vertebrae, dislocation or fracture of the cervical spine, and cord tumors can cause this disorder.

3. **CNS:** Tumors of the brainstem and cerebellum can cause torticollis. Some cases are due to postinfectious encephalitis and cerebral palsy. Drugs such as phenothiazines and L-dopa may be the culprits.

4. **Supratentorium:** Spasmodic torticollis would seem to fall into this category. I have seen cases begin while a patient is under the pressure of litigation for an occupational injury, especially if he or she is wearing a cervical collar. Hysteria may also cause torticollis.

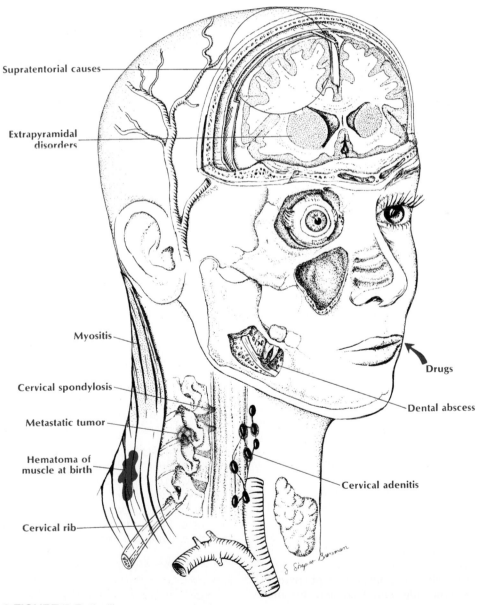

Supratentorial causes

Extrapyramidal disorders

Myositis

Cervical spondylosis

Metastatic tumor

Hematoma of muscle at birth

Cervical rib

Drugs

Dental abscess

Cervical adenitis

● **FIGURE 7** Torticollis.

● Approach to the Diagnosis

A radiograph of the cervical spine and a thorough neurologic examination are axiomatic before one considers the problem to be psychogenic. A Minnesota Multiphasic Personality Inventory (MMPI) will help to support the diagnosis of psychoneurosis, depression, and even malingering. Referral to a psychiatrist may be best if the patient is willing.

TREMOR AND OTHER INVOLUNTARY MOVEMENTS

Anatomy can assist one greatly in formulating a differential diagnosis of tremor of hepatic coma, Wilson disease, and alcoholism. The **thyroid** brings to mind the tremor of Graves disease. The **kidneys** signify the tremor of uremia and electrolyte disturbances. The **heart** suggests the choreiform movements of rheumatic fever (Sydenham chorea). Finally, the CNS indicates a host of other causes that can be further differentiated by considering the tracts and nuclei of the brain. The substantia nigra and globus pallidus are the sites of Parkinson disease and other related diseases, especially chlorpromazine toxicity. The putamen is the site of gross cavitation and atrophy in Wilson disease. The red nucleus may be involved in the syndrome of Benedikt, a vascular occlusion of a branch of the basilar artery. The thalamic syndrome produces a unilateral tremor in the extremities and is caused by an occlusion of the thalamogeniculate artery. Manganese, carbon monoxide poisoning, cerebral palsy, and general paresis all affect the brain and basal ganglia leading not only to a tremor but also to an organic brain syndrome in many cases. Huntington chorea produces bizarre choreiform movements; it can be recalled by its association primarily with atrophy of the caudate nucleus.

Intention tremor is associated primarily with cerebellar disease. The tremor of cerebellar ataxia, olivopontocerebellar atrophy, multiple sclerosis, phenytoin (Dilantin) toxicity, and cerebellar neoplasms can be recalled in this fashion.

Considering the entire **brain** and **brainstem** will bring to mind viral encephalitis and postinfectious encephalitis. If one includes the spinal cord and peripheral nerves, Jakob–Creutzfeldt disease will be recalled. Other rare causes of tremor can be recalled by visualizing the tracts or nuclei of the brain that are most significantly involved.

A second method to recall quickly the causes of tremor is to apply the mnemonic **VINDICATE.**

V—Vascular disorders suggest thalamic syndrome and arteriosclerosis.
I—Inflammatory disorders signify encephalitides.
N—Neoplasms signify neoplasms of the cerebellum and brainstem.
D—Degenerative disorders bring to mind Parkinson disease, Wilson disease, Friedreich ataxia, and a host of other CNS disorders.
I—Intoxication recalls alcoholism; manganese, phenytoin (Dilantin), carbon monoxide, and lead toxicity; and hepatic and renal coma with tremors.
C—Congenital disorders suggest dystonia musculorum deformans and cerebral palsy. Familial tremor should be recalled here.
A—Autoimmune disorders suggest Sydenham chorea.
T—Trauma suggests the tremor in posttraumatic and postconcussion syndrome and in posttraumatic necrosis.
E—Endocrine disorders bring to mind hyperthyroidism.

● Approach to the Diagnosis

The workup of tremor and other involuntary movements involves most of all a good history. A family history may identify familial tremor. Look for exposure to lead, manganese, and various drugs. The neurologic examination is important as it will determine the type of tremor. Rapid fine tremors (8 to 20 per second) are suggestive of hyperthyroidism and emotional disorders. Coarser tremors at rest suggest Parkinsonism, whereas a flapping tremor of 4 to 8 per second suggests Wilson disease. The association of other neurologic signs helps to pin down the diagnosis. Spasms of pain suggest a thalamic syndrome, ataxia suggests Friedreich ataxia, and loss of memory suggests manganese toxicity. Laboratory tests will be useful in selected cases. Blood lead, manganese, copper, and ceruloplasmin levels may be necessary. A triiodothyronine (T_3), thyroxine (T_4), and free T_4 index will confirm the diagnosis of Graves disease. Other tests that may be helpful may be found in Appendix A or listed below.

● Other Useful Tests

1. Drug screen (alcohol or drug abuse)
2. Chemistry panel (hypocalcemia, uremia, other electrolyte disorders)
3. EMG (timing of tremor)
4. MRI of the brain (multiple sclerosis, Wilson disease, cerebellar tumor, etc.)
5. Neurology consult
6. Therapeutic trial of beta blockers (familial tremor)

Case Presentation #83

A 36-year-old white man complained of gradually increasing tremor of his hands for the past 2 years. His wife has noted that his head is occasionally affected also. There is no history of trauma, encephalitis, or drug use.

Question #1. Utilizing your knowledge of anatomy and physiology, what is your differential diagnosis?

Neurologic examination reveals that the tremor is precipitated by movement and disappears at rest. There is no rigidity, speech abnormalities, or focal neurologic signs. His wife notes that the tremor improves after a few cocktails. His mother had a similar tremor.

Question #2. What is your diagnosis now?

(See Appendix B for the answers.)

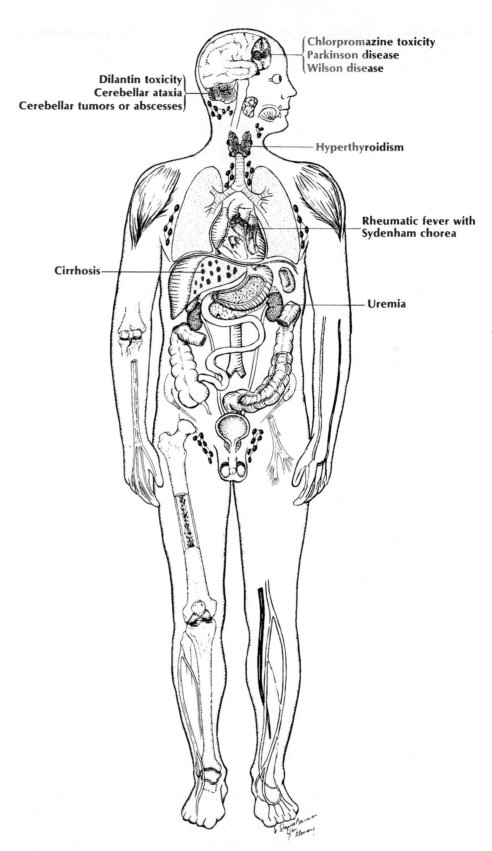

Chlorpromazine toxicity
Parkinson disease
Wilson disease

Dilantin toxicity
Cerebellar ataxia
Cerebellar tumors or abscesses

Hyperthyroidism

Rheumatic fever with
Sydenham chorea

Cirrhosis

Uremia

● **FIGURE 8** Tremor and other involuntary movements.

TRISMUS (LOCK JAW)

Recall of the causes of trismus is facilitated by the mnemonic **MINT**.

M—**Malformation** includes impacted wisdom teeth and temporomandibular joint syndrome.

I—**Inflammation** brings to mind tetanus, rabies, and trichinosis. **I** also signifies **intoxication**, helping one to recall strychnine poisoning.

N—**Neuropsychiatric** disorders call to mind mental conditions such as malingering or hysteria and epilepsy.

T—**Trauma** suggests fracture or contusion of the jaw which will cause pain on opening the jaw but is not a true trismus.

● Approach to the Diagnosis

A careful search for infected wounds, especially needle injection sites in cases of possible drug addiction, is important if tetanus is suspected. X-ray of the teeth, jaw, and temporomandibular joints may be helpful. Trichinosis is diagnosed by a high eosinophil count, serologic tests, and muscle biopsy. A wake-and-sleep EEG should be ordered if epilepsy is suspected. If organic causes are ruled out, a psychiatrist should be consulted.

U

UNEQUAL PULSES

To develop a list of causes of unequal pulses, let's trace the arterial system from its origin in the heart to its termination in the extremities.

Heart: Here is the source of arterial emboli from a mural thrombus in auricular fibrillation or myocardial infarction and subacute bacterial endocarditis (SBE).

Aorta: This will bring to mind a coarctation of the aorta and/or dissecting aneurysm (thrombosis of the terminal aorta).

Proximal arteries: These suggest thoracic outlet syndrome, subclavian steal syndrome, and femoral artery thrombosis or embolism.

Distal arteries: These bring to mind peripheral arteriosclerosis, Buerger disease, arterial embolism, and arteriovenous fistula. A fracture may involve the distal arteries causing pulse inequality.

● Approach to the Diagnosis

If there is a history of sudden onset of unequal pulses in either the upper or lower extremity, a diagnosis of arterial embolism or dissecting aneurysm must be ruled out with immediate angiography. If there is a history of trauma, fracture must be ruled out with plain films of the extremity. When the patient complains of ischemic symptoms (e.g., intermittent claudication) or the pulse inequality is discovered on a routine physical examination, Doppler studies can be used to determine the cause before proceeding with angiography. If you suspect an arterial embolism, order serial electrocardiograms (EKGs) and cardiac enzymes. An EKG may also diagnose auricular fibrillation. If SBE is a possibility, order blood culture. A cardiologist or cardiovascular surgeon may need to be consulted early in the course.

● Other Useful Tests

1. Coagulation studies (disseminated intravascular coagulation [DIC])
2. Echocardiography (valvular stenosis)

UREMIA

In developing a list of possible causes of uremia, the first thing to do is to divide them into three categories: prerenal causes, renal causes, and postrenal causes.

Prerenal causes: These include congestive heart failure (CHF), hypovolemic shock, starvation, trauma, gastrointestinal (GI) hemorrhage, severe dehydration, septic shock, and transfusion reaction.

Renal causes: It is best to further subdivide these using the mnemonic **VINDICATE** to vindicate yourself.

V—Vascular includes renal vein thrombosis, dissecting aneurysm, renal artery embolism, and thrombosis. Malignant hypertension would also fit into this category.

I—Inflammatory disorders include glomerulonephritis, pyelonephritis, and SBE.

N—Neoplasms include multiple myeloma and leukemia.

D—Degenerative disorders are not usually a cause of uremia.

I—Intoxication should bring to mind a host of toxins and drugs including aminoglycosides, sulfanil-amides, cephalosporins, arsenic, mercury, and lead.

C—Congenital disorders should prompt the recall of polycystic kidneys and Henoch–Schönlein purpura.

A—Allergic and **autoimmune** will help one to recall the collagen diseases, serum sickness, Goodpasture syndrome, Wegener granulomatosis, and thrombotic thrombocytopenic purpura.

T—Trauma should help to recall crush syndrome, hemolytic transfusion reactions, burns, and massive hemorrhage as possible causes.

E Endocrine disorders, other than diabetes mellitus, are not associated with a high blood urea nitrogen (BUN) level.

Postrenal causes: This category includes the causes of uremia that are most likely to be treatable. They are bladder neck obstruction from prostatic hypertrophy, a median bar or interureteric bar, urethral stricture, stones, and neoplasms.

● Approach to the Diagnosis

In most cases of prerenal azotemia, the clinical picture is very revealing. Signs of shock, CHF, or GI blood loss will be evident. In more subtle cases, the BUN/creatinine ratio is typically 20:1 or more in prerenal azotemia, whereas it is 10:1 or less in renal cases. The serum and urine osmolality will also be helpful. The next step is to rule out postrenal causes by ultrasonography of the bladder or bladder catheterization. If there is a large volume of urine in the bladder, a urologist needs to be consulted before further workup is done. If not, a nephrologist should be consulted.

● Other Useful Tests

1. Complete blood count (CBC) (anemia, infection)
2. Urinalysis (pyelonephritis, renal azotemia)
3. Urine culture and colony count (pyelonephritis)
4. Chemistry panel (hypercalcemia, other electrolyte imbalance)
5. Sedimentation rate (infection)
6. Blood cultures (SBE)

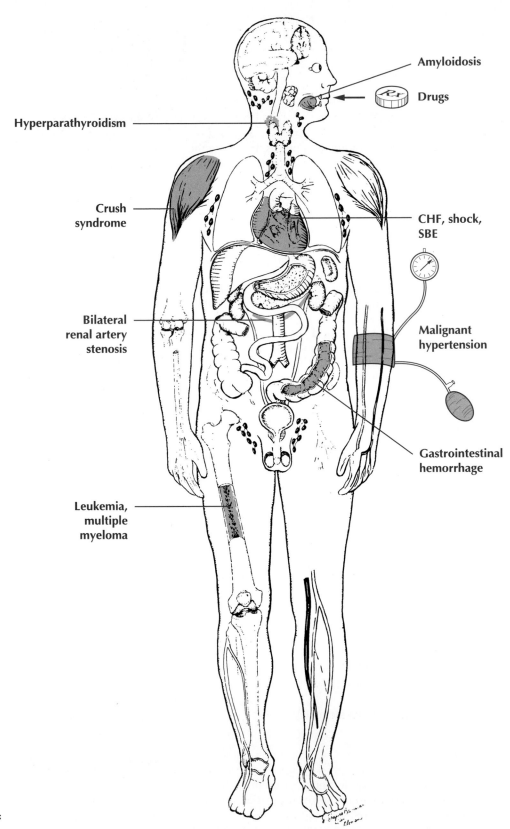

● **FIGURE 1** Uremia, systemic causes.

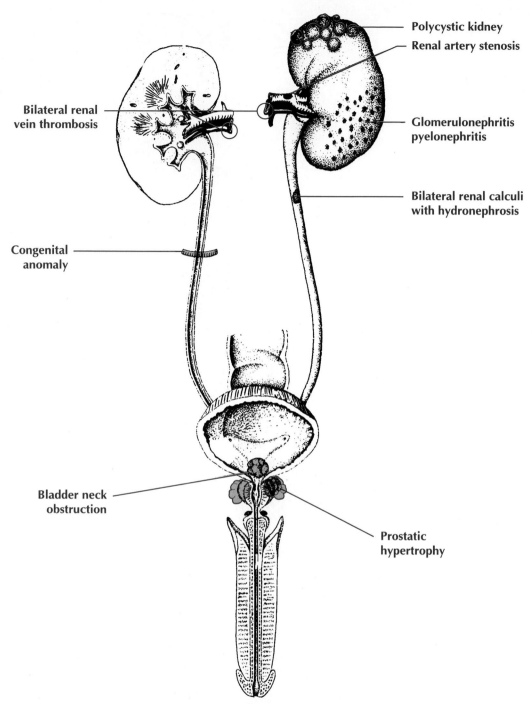

● **FIGURE 2** Uremia, local causes.

7. Arterial blood gas analysis (CHF, shock)
8. Blood volume (CHF, shock)
9. Cystoscopy (bladder neck obstruction)
10. Retrograde pyelogram (obstructive uropathy)
11. Antinuclear antibody (ANA) analysis (collagen disease)
12. Antistreptolysin O (ASO) titer (acute glomerulonephritis)
13. Computed tomography (CT) scan of abdomen (neoplasm, abscess, polycystic kidney)
14. Renal biopsy (glomerulonephritis, interstitial nephritis)

URETHRAL DISCHARGE

A significant purulent urethral discharge invariably signals the diagnosis of gonorrhea and, until a Gram stain is done, little consideration is given to the other causes of a non-bloody urethral discharge. However, one should also consider other etiologic agents *(Staphylococcus, Escherichia coli,* herpes, mima polymorpha, and, particularly, *Chlamydia trachomatis).* Furthermore, the **anatomy** of the urogenital

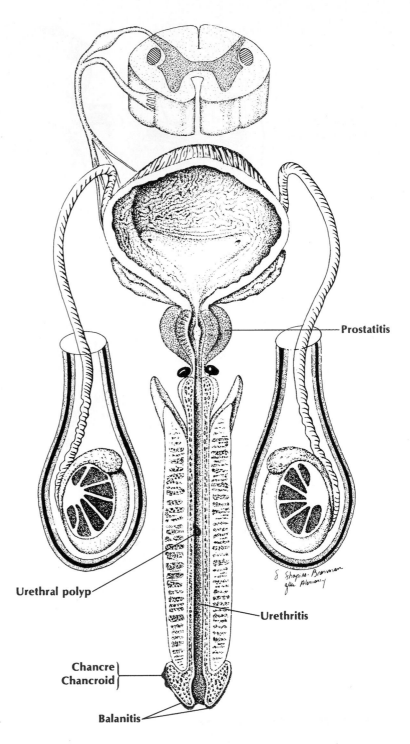

● **FIGURE 3** Urethral discharge.

Labels on figure:

Prostatitis

Urethral polyp

Urethritis

Chancre
Chancroid

Balanitis

tree should be visualized so that inflammation of all the components can be carefully considered in the resistant case.

Beginning with the **prepuce**, the physician should consider balanitis of either infectious or autoimmune origin (e.g., Reiter disease). An ulcer from lues, chancroid, or lymphogranuloma inguinale or venereum must be looked for. The **urethra** suggests urethritis of gonorrhea, *Chlamydia*, and numerous other organisms, whereas autoimmune disorders like Reiter disease precipitate a nonspecific urethritis and nonbloody discharge. Again, chancres, chanchroids, and herpes may involve the anterior urethra. *Trichomonas* organisms rarely produce a discharge in the male. In the female, the Skene glands may be infected by gonorrhea or other organisms. A urethral caruncle can easily be recognized as a small, cherry-red mass at the urethral orifice.

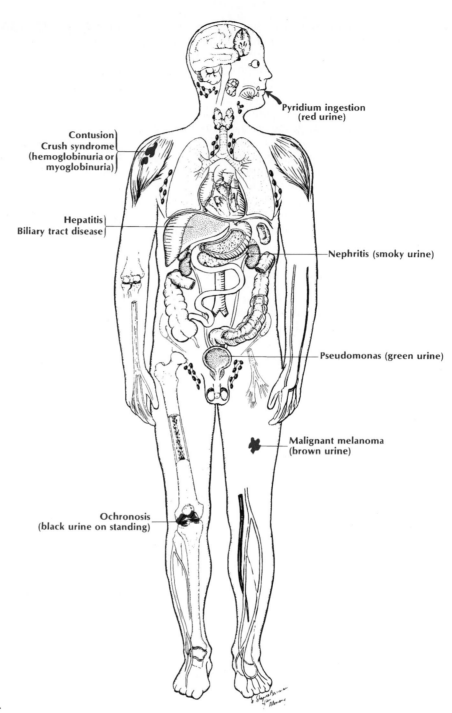

Pyridium ingestion
(red urine)

Contusion
Crush syndrome
(hemoglobinuria or
myoglobinuria)

Hepatitis
Biliary tract disease

Nephritis (smoky urine)

Pseudomonas (green urine)

Malignant melanoma
(brown urine)

Ochronosis
(black urine on standing)

● **FIGURE 4** Urine color changes.

Further up, the **prostate** is encountered, and acute and chronic prostatitis and prostatic abscess are immediately suggested. Inflammation of Cowper glands or of the seminal vesicles should be remembered as a possible cause of a discharge in resistant cases. In the female, urethrovaginal fistula (most frequently from surgery or cervical carcinoma) should be considered.

As elsewhere, a purulent discharge does not necessarily signify inflammation alone. There may be a foreign body, a papilloma, and occasionally a carcinoma that precipitates a superimposed infection.

● Approach to the Diagnosis

The association of other symptoms and signs is helpful in narrowing the list of possibilities. The discharge of acute urethritis is usually associated with severe pain on micturition, whereas the discharge of prostatitis is often not. The discharge of chronic prostatitis is usually painless and occurs most frequently on arising. Urethral caruncles, papillomas, and carcinomas frequently have a bloody discharge, at least intermittently. On examination, the physician can detect induration of a urethral chancre, and the erythema of a balanitis is obvious when the prepuce is retracted. The presence of arthritis or conjunctivitis makes Reiter syndrome a distinct possibility, although gonorrhea may do the same. The boggy prostate of prostatitis and the increase of the discharge on massage will assist greatly in this diagnosis.

In the laboratory, a smear and culture are axiomatic in diagnosis, and one must massage the prostate and milk the urethra if little discharge is found on simple inspection. After massaging the prostate, the first portion of a voided specimen should be examined, smeared, and cultured if no discharge is apparent. Culture for *Chlamydia* if routine cultures are negative. Cystoscopy and cystograms may be necessary, but the indications for these will be at the discretion of the urologist, who should be consulted if routine treatment is ineffective.

● Other Useful Tests

1. CBC (systemic infection)
2. Sedimentation rate (collagen disease, systemic gonorrhea)
3. Venereal disease research laboratory (VDRL) test (chancre)
4. Frei test (lymphogranuloma venereum)
5. Urine culture and sensitivity (cystitis)
6. Chancroid skin test (chancroid)
7. Human leukocyte antigen (HLA)-B27 antigen (Reiter syndrome)
8. Smears for cytology (carcinoma)
9. Cystoscopy (bladder neck obstruction, neoplasm)
10. Intravenous pyelogram (IVP) and cystogram (malformation, obstructive uropathy, neoplasm)
11. DNA probe testing, rapid antigen testing (gonorrhea, Chlamydia)
12. Therapeutic trial of doxycycline (Chlamydia)

URINE COLOR CHANGES

Apart from hematuria, **red urine** may signify hemoglobinuria or myoglobinuria, suggesting the various hemolytic anemias, the march hemoglobinuria, paroxysmal "cold" hemoglobinuria and nocturnal hemoglobinuria, and the Crush syndrome. Red urine is also found in acute porphyria, especially the erythropoietic type. Ingestion of beets and purple cabbage may cause red urine. Phenazopyridine hydrochloride (Pyridium), a urinary tract anesthetic, will turn the urine a reddish orange color. A **dark, yellow-brown** urine usually signifies jaundice (see page 271), but the chartreuse yellow from riboflavin ingestion should be remembered. Urobilinogen may make the urine yellow. A **brown or smoky urine** may be found in nephritis and is usually due to hemoglobinuria or red cells discolored by an acidic pH. A malignant melanoma may present with a brown urine. **Black urine** is characteristic of alkaptonuria but this usually occurs on standing (as the urine turns from acid to alkaline). Melanuria will also turn black on standing but may even be voided black. The **green urine** of *Pseudomonas* infections and the blue-green urine of methylene blue dye should be remembered.

How can these causes of urine discoloration be remembered? One method is to group them into endogenous and exogenous causes (e.g., beets, phenazopyridine hydrochloride [Pyridium], and methylene blue). The endogenous causes are invariably related to the metabolism of a body pigment. Hemoglobin metabolism will suggest porphyria and hemoglobinuria, whereas melanin metabolism will suggest melanuria and alkaptonuria. The other method is to apply the mnemonic **VINDICATE**. I suggest that the reader use this as an exercise.

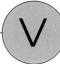

VAGINAL BLEEDING

As with most hemorrhages from body orifices, vaginal bleeding is best approached by the **anatomic** method. Thus, the important structures of the female genital tract are cross-indexed with etiologic categories as in Table 59. In all bleeding symptoms, one must include blood vessels and the blood as part of the anatomic breakdown. Histologic breakdown is of little importance anywhere except in the uterus, and in making certain that one does not forget the many types of ovarian tumors (e.g., fibromas, polycystic ovaries, corpus luteum, follicular cysts, and arrhenoblastoma). In the uterus, histology reminds one of endometriosis, adenomyosis, and fibroids.

Physiology should bring to mind the most common cause of uterine bleeding—dysfunctional bleeding. Thus, when the normal sequence of follicle-stimulating hormone (FSH) stimulating estrogen production and luteinizing hormone (LH) stimulating progesterone production from the corpus luteum is interrupted, by whatever cause, the resulting poorly formed endometrium will bleed at an inappropriate time (metrorrhagia) or excessively during the appropriate time (menorrhagia). Aside from the many neoplasms, cysts, and inflammatory conditions of the ovary (listed in Table 59), one must consider other endocrine disorders such as adrenal neoplasms, hyper- and hypothyroidism, hypopituitarism, and acromegaly.

Although the differential diagnosis is developed adequately in Table 59, a description of the most important causes is provided here. The most important vaginal conditions are a ruptured hymen, atrophic vaginitis, and carcinoma. Cervical carcinoma is the most important cause of bleeding of the cervix. Fibroids may be a more common cause of uterine bleeding than endometrial carcinoma, but both are superceded by pregnancy and dysfunctional uterine bleeding. Proceeding to the fallopian tubes, one must not forget ectopic pregnancy and pelvic inflammatory disease (PID) as causes of vaginal bleeding. Ovarian cysts and tumors are common causes of dysfunctional bleeding, but the serous cystadenoma and carcinomas present that way only infrequently.

● Approach to the Diagnosis

The differential diagnosis of vaginal bleeding depends on the clinical picture. The most common cause of unexpected bleeding in all women is dysfunctional uterine bleeding due to imbalance of estrogen and progesterone during the menstrual cycle. Nevertheless, vaginal bleeding in a postmenopausal woman must be considered a malignancy until proven otherwise. An endometrial biopsy should be done. Vaginal bleeding in the prepubertal female should prompt an investigation for child abuse or incest as well as

neoplasm. There is also the possibility of vaginal carcinoma due to diethylstilbestrol ingestion by the mother.

A careful vaginal examination with the patient fully relaxed is most important. A rectovaginal examination must be performed to palpate masses in the cul-de-sac. If an adequate vaginal examination is impossible (as in the case of obesity), then proceed with ultrasonography. Any vaginal discharge must be cultured for gonococci and *Chlamydia* organisms to rule out PID. A biopsy is done of any suspicious lesion of the vagina or cervix, and a Pap smear is performed. If the diagnosis is uncertain at this point, a gynecology consult is in order. A dilation and curettage (D & C) or endometrial biopsy must be done if uterine carcinoma is suspected. In women of childbearing age, a routine pregnancy test should be done, but if an ectopic pregnancy is suspected a serum radioimmunoassay (RIA) for the beta-human chorionic gonadotropin (β-hCG) subunit pregnancy test will be more definitive. Ultrasonography will often determine if a pelvic mass is an ectopic pregnancy. Ultrasonography will also be helpful in diagnosing ovarian cysts and tumors, but a computed tomography (CT) scan of the pelvis can be more definitive.

Dysfunctional uterine bleeding is most often physiologic. However, a granulosa cell tumor of the ovary can be the cause. Ultrasonography or a CT scan may be able to reveal such a tumor, but culdoscopy or laparoscopy may be required. If the dysfunctional bleeding is thought to be due to hypothyroidism or hyperthyroidism, a thyroid profile may be done. If it is believed to be due to a pituitary adenoma, a magnetic resonance imaging (MRI) of the brain and serum LH and FSH assays should be done. Anemia and systemic disease must be ruled out also (see tests listed below).

If pathologic causes of dysfunctional uterine bleeding are excluded, normal cyclic bleeding may be reestablished by a course of cyclic estrogen and progesterone or progesterone alone (a "medical D & C"). If this is unsuccessful, a surgical D & C is required.

● Other Useful Tests

1. Complete blood count (CBC) (anemia)
2. Sedimentation rate (PID)
3. Venereal disease research laboratory (VDRL) test (chancre, gumma)
4. Tuberculin test (pelvic tuberculosis)
5. Coagulation profile (see page 423)
6. Antinuclear antibody (ANA) analysis (collagen disease)
7. Coombs test (lupus)
8. Serum estradiol and progesterone levels (ovarian cyst or tumor)
9. Urinary gonadotropins (choriocarcinoma)

TABLE 59 Vaginal Bleeding

	V Vascular	I Inflammatory	N Neoplasm	D Degenerative	I Intoxication	C Congenital Malformation	A Allergic or Autoimmune	T Trauma	E Endocrine Disorders
Introitus	Varicosities	Syphilitic ulcer Wart	Granulomatous polyp					Intercourse Trauma to hymen	
Vagina		Vaginitis	Carcinoma Extension of rectal carcinoma	Atrophic vaginitis				Foreign body	
Cervix		Chronic cervicitis Herpes	Carcinoma Polyp			Placenta previa		Laceration	
Uterus		Endometritis Carcinoma Polyps Fibroids Pregnancy	Endometriosis	Menopause Scurvy Vitamin K deficiency	Birth control pills Estrogens and other hormones	Anteversion of uterus Retroversion or flexion of uterus	Idiopathic thrombocytopenic purpura	Foreign body Abortion, induced	Menopause Dysfunctional bleeding Abruptio placenta
Fallopian Tubes		Pelvic inflammatory disease	Ectopic pregnancy						
Ovaries		Oophoritis Tuberculosis	Carcinoma and adenoma Corpus luteum cyst						Hypopituitarism Hypothyroidism Stein–Leventhal ovaries
Blood Vessels and Blood		Leukemia		Anemia Aplastic anemia	Toxic suppression of platelets Heparin Warfarin		Lupus erythematosus	Surgery	
Others			Hydatidiform mole						

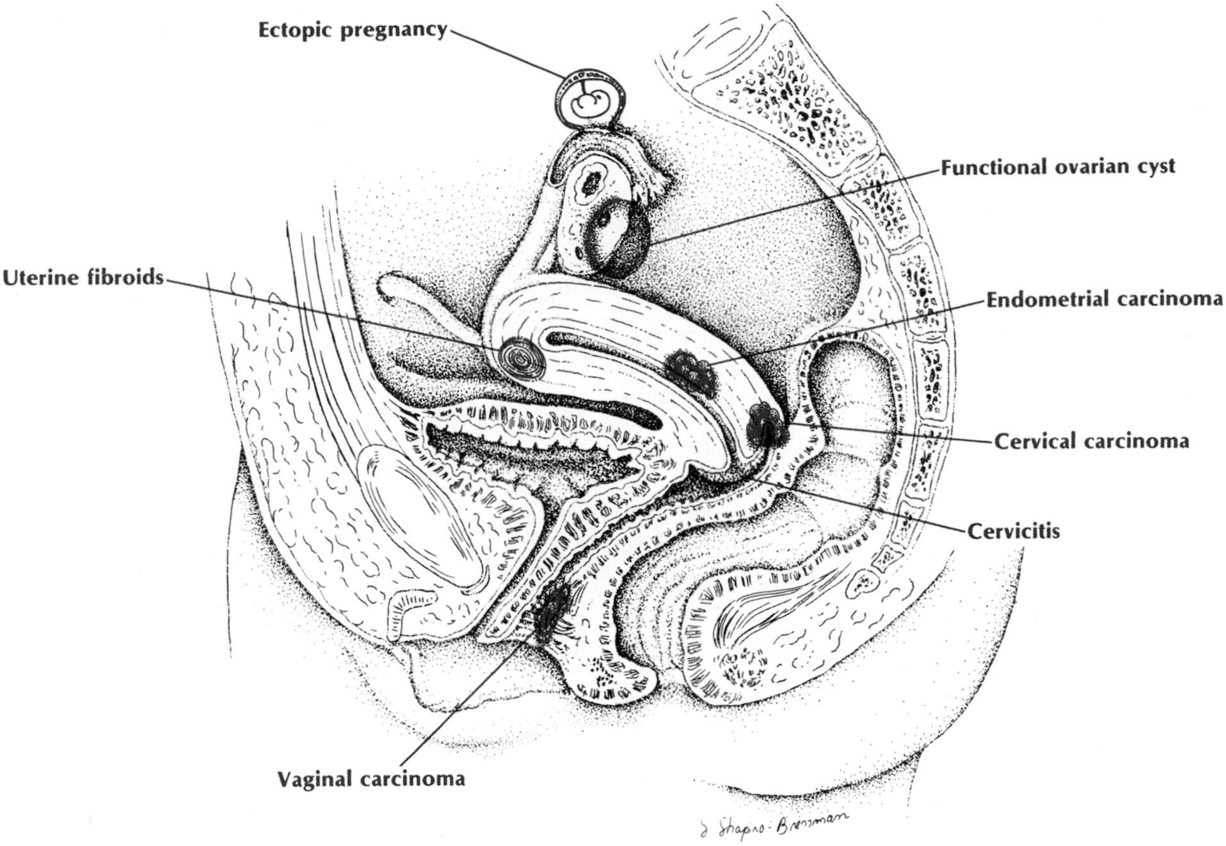

● FIGURE 1 Vaginal bleeding.

10. Cancer antigen 125 (CA125) test (metastatic endometrial carcinoma)
11. Serum iron and ferritin (iron deficiency anemia)

Case Presentation #84

A 54-year-old white woman complained of light vaginal bleeding occasionally with clots for several months. She denies pain, weight loss, or fever. Her last period was 10 years ago.

Question #1. Utilizing your knowledge of anatomy and physiology, what is your list of diagnostic possibilities?

Vaginal examination reveals a mild diffuse enlargement of the uterus but no other abnormalities. General physical examination and laboratory studies are normal.

Question #2. What is the most likely diagnosis now?

(See Appendix B for the answers.)

VAGINAL DISCHARGE

Again, the female genital tract can be infected by all sizes of organisms; thus a useful method for recalling the causes of a purulent vaginal discharge is to work from the smallest to the largest organism. Thus, we begin with herpes progenitalis and proceed to gonorrhea and nonspecific bacterial infection (now known as *Gardnerella vaginalis*), trichomoniasis, and, finally, moniliasis. This, however, does not cover all the causes of a nonbloody vaginal discharge. Consequently, **anatomy** is applied as well.

At the **vulva**, one encounters vulvitis, bartholinitis, and vulval carcinoma. In the **vagina**, the conditions mentioned above are formed in addition to senile vaginitis, foreign bodies, and vaginal carcinomas. One should also not forget vesicovaginal, rectovaginal, and enteric fistulas. At the **cervix**, cervicitis and endocervicitis (gonorrheal or nonspecific), cervical polyps, and carcinomas need to be mentioned. In the uterus, endometritis, polyps, and carcinomas are recalled, but the latter two conditions are usually associated with a bloody discharge. Finally, salpingitis produces a mucopurulent discharge.

● Approach to the Diagnosis

To workup a vaginal discharge, simply examining a fresh wet saline and potassium hydroxide (KOH) (10%) preparation will expose the most common offenders, namely *Trichomonas* and *Candida*. Some physicians treat all patients with negative findings on these examinations as a nonspecific bacterial vaginitis, but this is not a particularly scientific procedure. It is best to do a smear and culture (especially for gonococci). Cultures are also available for *Trichomonas*

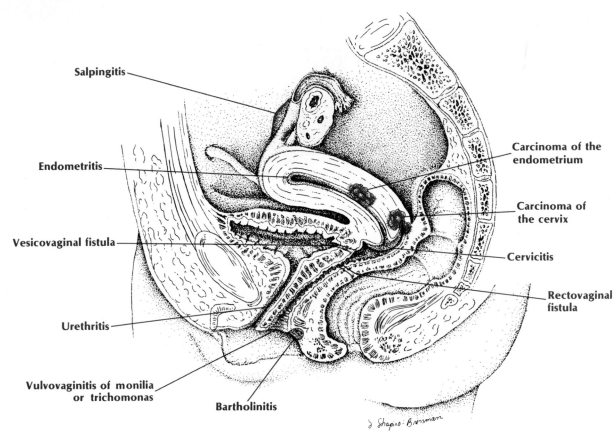

● **FIGURE 2** Vaginal discharge.

and *Candida*. If gonorrhea is suspected, material from the endocervix should be cultured. *Chlamydia* cultures are routinely done in some clinics. DNA probe or rapid antigen testing of urine may pick up these conditions as well.

Obviously, if the cervix is eroded and the discharge seems to be coming from there, biopsy and conization may be indicated. Referral to a gynecologist is preferred if this procedure is deemed necessary; however, the primary physician may prefer to cauterize the superficial lesions. Patients with discharges thought to be due to lesions beyond the cervix should probably be referred.

● Other Useful Tests

1. CBC (PID)
2. Sedimentation rate (PID)
3. VDRL test
4. Tuberculin test (pelvic tuberculosis)
5. Rectal culture (gonorrhea)
6. Vaginal and cervical cytology after infection subsides (carcinoma of the cervix or endometrium)
7. D & C and biopsy (endometrial carcinoma)
8. Sonogram (PID)
9. Laparoscopy (PID)
10. Trial of systemic antibiotics
11. Herpes simplex virus (HSV) antibody titer (bacterial vaginitis)
12. Tzanck smear (herpes progenitalis)
13. Therapeutic trial (nonspecific vaginitis)

Case Presentation #85

A 28-year-old black woman complained of a chronic vaginal discharge and lower abdominal pain for several months. She admits to promiscuous sexual behavior.

Question #1. Utilizing the size of organisms in recalling various causes of vaginal discharge, what is your differential diagnosis?

Vaginal examination revealed tender adnexal masses and a mucopurulent discharge.

Question #2. What is your diagnosis now?

(See Appendix B for the answers.)

VISIBLE PERISTALSIS

This is almost invariably a sign of gastric outlet or intestinal obstruction. The various causes can be recalled using the mnemonic **MINT**.

M—Malformation should bring to mind congenital pyloric stenosis, malrotation, hernias, and volvulus.
I—Inflammation should alert one to peptic ulcer causing gastric outlet obstruction or Crohn disease, ulcerative colitis, and diverticulitis causing internal obstruction.

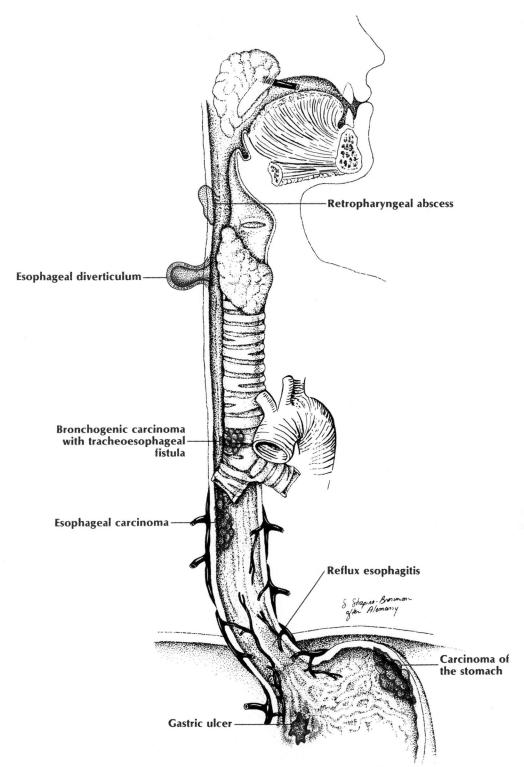

● **FIGURE 3** Vomitus.

N—Neoplasm should help recall gastric outlet obstruction caused by a leiomyoma or gastric carcinoma, intestinal obstruction caused by neoplasms of the large and small intestine, and pancreatic carcinoma.

T—Trauma would help to recall intestinal obstruction caused by adhesions from previous abdominal surgery.

● Approach to the Diagnosis

Congenital pyloric stenosis presents with projectile vomiting, dehydration, and a small right upper quadrant mass. The peristaltic waves are in the upper abdomen progressing downward from right to left. The peristalsis of small intestinal obstruction is also transverse, whereas the peristalsis of large intestinal obstruction is often vertical.

The diagnostic workup includes a stat CBC, electrolytes, chemistry panel, and flat plate of the abdomen. A general surgeon must see the patient immediately as an exploratory laparotomy is usually indicated.

VOMITUS

The numerous causes of vomiting are discussed under functional changes (see page 310). It is worthwhile, however, to discuss a few of the important causes of nonbloody vomitus here. Like other "discharges," simply by visualizing the anatomy of the "tree" one can assimilate the causes of nonbloody vomitus.

In the posterior **pharynx** and **larynx**, mucus may be regurgitated from a postnasal drip of sinusitis or material that cannot be swallowed because of a stricture, myasthenia gravis, or bulbar palsy. There may also be drainage from a retropharyngeal abscess. In the **upper esophagus**, a foreign body, diverticulum stricture, or web of Plummer–Vinson syndrome may cause regurgitation of food, mucus, and saliva. In the **lower esophagus**, lye strictures, esophagitis, cardiospasm, and carcinomas are responsible for regurgitation of food and mucus. Extrinsic pressure and the resulting obstruction from an aneurysm, cardiomegaly, or a mediastinal tumor may also cause a nonbloody "discharge."

Nonbloody vomitus from the **stomach** is usually due to gastritis, ulcer, pyloric obstruction, or carcinoma of the stomach. When intestinal obstruction occurs beyond the pyloris or when there is ulceration or obstruction because of a gastrojejunostomy, the vomitus is often bile stained. The many other causes of intestinal obstruction may produce a nonbloody vomitus. If there is a gastrocolic fistula, the vomitus may be feculent.

Extrinsic causes of vomiting such as migraine, labyrinthitis, or glaucoma usually cause a nonbloody vomitus with or without bile stain. If it becomes bloody, one should consider a complicating Mallory–Weiss syndrome. The approach to the diagnosis of vomiting is discussed on page 313.

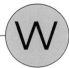

WALKING DIFFICULTIES

When a patient complains of difficulty walking, visualize the **anatomic** components of the leg: skin, muscle, arteries, veins, bones, joints, and peripheral nerves. Going one step further, follow the peripheral artery to its origin (femoral artery, aorta, and so forth) and the peripheral nerve to its origin in the spinal cord, and then follow its secondary connections to the cerebellum and cerebrum. Now it is possible to recall the causes of difficulty walking as the patient is being examined.

1. **Skin:** Look for calluses, infectious ulcers, and deformities of the feet.
2. **Muscle:** Check for possible myositis, contusions, and muscular atrophy or dystrophy. The gait of muscular dystrophy is slapping and waddling, and there is a pelvic tilt forward.
3. **Arteries:** Peripheral arteriosclerosis and Buerger disease will often be detected by palpation of the dorsalis pedis and tibialis pulses. However, do not forget to feel the femoral arteries (to rule out Leriche syndrome) and popliteal arteries. Listening to the heart may determine a cause for a peripheral embolism.
4. **Veins:** Dilated varicose veins will be obvious, but checking for a positive Homan sign will be necessary to rule out deep vein phlebitis.
5. **Bones:** Osteomyelitis and sarcomas or metastatic disease of the bone will usually present with significant pain and make the patient extremely reluctant to walk. A mass or deformity in the bone is usually palpable.
6. **Joints:** Osteoarthritis, gout, and rheumatoid arthritis of the knee are not hard to detect. The gait in diseases in any joint in the leg is a limp. The cause of pain in the other joints may be more difficult to appraise even with an x-ray film. Nevertheless, these and a full joint disease workup will help (see page 274). An osteoarthritic spur of the heel may be found. Bursitis in numerous areas should be looked for. Congenital lesions such as slipped epiphysis, dislocation of the hip, and aseptic necrosis should be considered in children.
7. **Peripheral nerves:** A peripheral neuropathy from alcohol or diabetes will cause a steppage gait (due to moderate or severe foot drop), and traumatic or lead neuropathy may cause an overt foot drop. The atrophy of the muscles without fasciculations will help in the diagnosis of these as well as of Dejerine–Sottas hereditary neuropathy and Charcot–Marie–Tooth disease. Sensory changes (glove and stocking anesthesia and analgesia) are also useful.
8. **Spinal cord:** These diseases present with different types of gaits. There may be a wide-based ataxic gait with a positive Romberg sign in dorsal column and dorsal root involvement, suggesting tabes dorsalis and pernicious anemia. There may be a wide-based reeling ataxia with a negative Romberg sign, suggesting cerebellar disease such as Friedreich ataxia. A spastic gait suggests amyotrophic lateral sclerosis, multiple sclerosis, and diseases with diffuse spinal cord involvement such as anterior spinal artery occlusion. A spastic ataxic gait is typical of multiple sclerosis. Other causes of a spastic gait are compression by tumors, cervical spondylosis, or disks; transverse myelitis; traumatic conditions such as fractures; hematomas; and epidural abscesses. The gait of herniated disks of the lumbosacral spine is usually a list to the left or right or a limp. Loss of the ankle or knee jerk, dermatomal sensory loss, and erector spinae muscle spasm will help in this diagnosis. If there is a cauda equina tumor or poliomyelitis, bladder symptoms are usually present as well. Other conditions of the lumbosacral spine disturb the gait (limp) and include osteoarthritis, rheumatoid spondylitis, spondylolisthesis, metastatic tumors, tuberculosis, and multiple myeloma.
9. **Secondary connections to the brain:** Involvement of the pyramidal tracts in the brain often produces a hemiplegic gait where the weak or spastic leg is dragged along the floor. The gait of vestibular disease is ataxic and reeling during an attack. Cerebellar disease has already been discussed. Tumors or abscesses here and alcoholic and phenytoin sodium toxicity may cause a cerebellar ataxia. Multiple sclerosis is another condition that may result in this type of a gait. Bilateral cerebral involvement in cerebral arteriosclerosis or presenile and senile dementia produces the short-stepped gait of marche à petit pas. Cerebral palsy may cause a scissor gait. The spastic, shuffling gait of parkinsonism with propulsion and retropulsion is not easily missed.

● Approach to the Diagnosis

The clinical picture can help to pinpoint the diagnosis in many cases. If the difficulty develops after walking a block or a certain distance, the patient may have neurogenic or vascular claudication, and spinal stenosis or peripheral arteriosclerosis is suspected. If there is swelling and crepitus of the knee joints, an arthritic condition is likely. Muscular atrophy and fasciculations suggest progressive muscular atrophy, whereas atrophy with sensory changes suggests peripheral neuropathy. A spastic ataxic gait with blurred vision or scotomata suggests multiple sclerosis.

WALKING DIFFICULTIES

The initial workup of a patient with walking difficulties will depend on the clinical picture. If there is possible peripheral vascular disease, Doppler studies and possible femoral

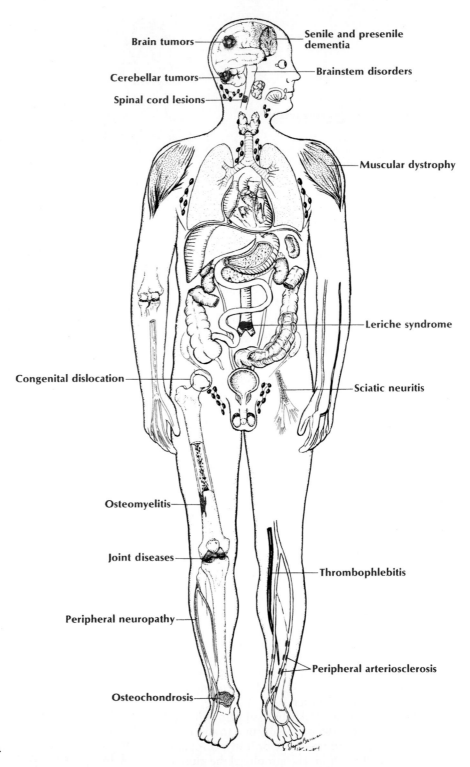

● **FIGURE 1** Walking difficulties.

angiography or aortography need to be done. If a patient is suspected of having a deep vein thrombosis, he or she should be hospitalized and Doppler studies, impedance plethysmography, or contrast venography will be done. If the patient has clinical radiculopathy, a computed tomography (CT) scan or magnetic resonance imaging (MRI) of the lumbar spine will be done to rule out a herniated disk. If multiple sclerosis is suspected, an MRI of the brain or spinal cord will be done depending on the level of the involvement clinically.

● **Other Useful Tests**

1. Complete blood count (CBC) (pernicious anemia)
2. Drug screen (drug abuse)
3. Sedimentation rate (inflammation)

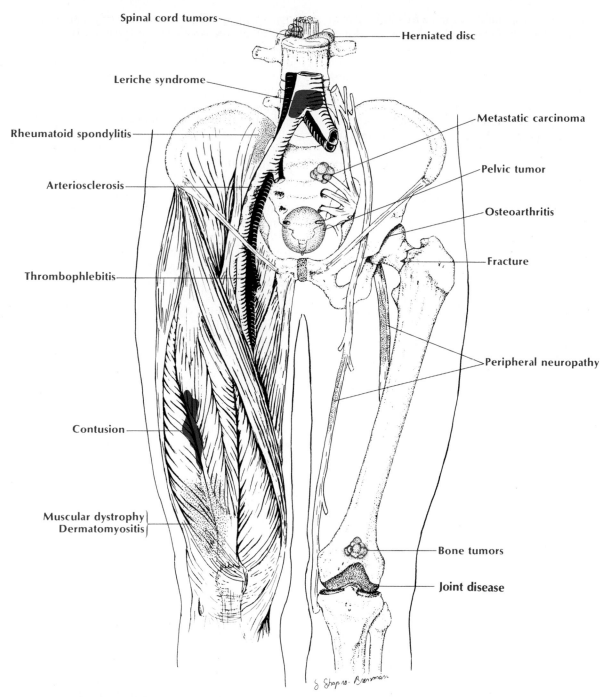

Spinal cord tumors

Herniated disc

Leriche syndrome

Metastatic carcinoma

Rheumatoid spondylitis

Pelvic tumor

Arteriosclerosis

Osteoarthritis

Fracture

Thrombophlebitis

Peripheral neuropathy

Contusion

Muscular dystrophy
Dermatomyositis

Bone tumors

Joint disease

● **FIGURE 2** Walking difficulties.

4. Blood lead level (lead neuropathy)
5. Glucose tolerance test (diabetic neuropathy)
6. Antinuclear antibody (ANA) analysis (collagen disease)
7. Chemistry panel (cirrhosis of the liver, muscle disease)
8. Schilling test (pernicious anemia)
9. Electromyogram (EMG) (muscle dystrophy, peripheral neuropathy)
10. Spinal tap (tumor, multiple sclerosis, neurosyphilis)
11. Urine porphobilinogen (porphyria)
12. X-ray of joints (arthritis)
13. Bone scan (osteomyelitis, neoplasm)
14. Neurology consult
15. Orthopedic consult

WEAKNESS AND FATIGUE, GENERALIZED

The analysis of the causes of weakness depends on a knowledge of both **anatomy** and **biochemistry**. Strength depends on an intact healthy muscle, peripheral nerve, and lower and upper motor neuron pathways and a functioning myoneural junction. Thus, general weakness may develop in **muscle disease** (analyzed according to etiologic categories in Table 60), **myoneural junction disease** (myasthenia gravis and Eaton–Lambert syndrome), **peripheral neuropathies** (Table 60), **anterior horn disease** (poliomyelitis, lead poisoning, and spinal muscular atrophy), and **diffuse disease of the pyramidal tracts**, such as multiple sclerosis. Parkinson disease fatigues the muscles by the tremor and spasticity it induces.

However, this is only half the story. A muscle cannot be strong unless there is adequate intake and absorption of glucose or proper tissue use of glucose (insulin action). Malnutrition and malabsorption syndrome are excellent examples of the former, whereas diabetes mellitus, acromegaly, Cushing disease, and insulinomas are good examples of the latter. The muscle must also have an adequate supply of oxygen. Thus chronic lung disease (see page 112) of any cause, congestive heart failure (CHF) of any cause, and chronic anemia may all produce weakness because of decreased supply of oxygen to the muscles. It is also vital to have the proper minerals surrounding the muscle fiber. Most important are proper sodium, potassium, and calcium balance. Thus, any condition causing a low-sodium syndrome (CHF or diuretics), a high- or low-potassium syndrome (Addison disease, diuretics, aldosterone tumors), or a high or low calcium balance (hyperparathyroidism, metastatic carcinoma of the bone, and hypoparathyroidism) may produce weakness. It is well known that vitamin B deficiency causes fatigue and neuropathy. Recent research indicates that vitamin D deficiency is also a cause of fatigue.

Weakness develops in liver disease because of intermittent hypoglycemia or inability to dispose of toxins. In uremia, the problem is not only poor ability to get rid of toxins, but the altered electrolyte media of sodium, potassium, calcium, and magnesium. In hypermetabolic states, there may be a breakdown of muscle to release protein for nutrition when intake is not adequate to meet demands of vital organs. Thus, in hyperthyroidism, chronic inflammatory and febrile diseases, and diffuse neoplastic disease, weakness is a common manifestation.

No discussion of weakness would be complete without mentioning the psychogenic causes of weakness such as depression and chronic anxiety states. Finally, smoking and chronic ingestion of caffeine, toxins, and various proprietary drugs (e.g., aspirin) are, of course, related to psychogenic disturbances and should always be considered in the differential diagnosis.

● Approach to the Diagnosis

The association of other symptoms and signs with generalized weakness and fatigue is very important in pinning down a diagnosis. Generalized lymphadenopathy and fatigue suggest infectious mononucleosis, lymphoma, or tuberculosis or other chronic infection such as acquired immunodeficiency syndrome (AIDS). Weakness, weight loss, and polyphagia with polyuria and polydipsia would suggest hyperthyroidism or diabetes mellitus. Generalized weakness with polyuria and no significant weight loss suggests

hyperparathyroidism. Weakness with pallor suggests some type of anemia. Weakness and weight loss without polyuria or polyphagia suggest malignancy or malabsorption syndrome. Weakness with other significant neurologic signs and symptoms prompts the consideration of muscular dystrophy, amyotrophic lateral sclerosis, or multiple sclerosis. Weakness with drug or alcohol use prompts the investigation of drug or alcohol abuse. Caffeine, especially in large quantities, can also cause significant weakness and chronic fatigue.

The initial workup of weakness and fatigue requires a CBC, sedimentation rate, drug screen, chemistry panel, thyroid profile, ANA, chest x-ray, and echocardiogram. If muscular dystrophy or dermatomyositis is suspected, urine tests for creatinine, creatine, and myoglobin can be done. Ultimately, a muscle biopsy may be indicated. If myasthenia gravis is suspected, serum for acetylcholine receptor antibody may be done. If Addison disease is suspected, a serum cortisol test before and after ACTH stimulation may be done. A 24-hour urine aldosterone level may be done to exclude primary aldosteronism. Serum parathyroid hormone (PTH) may be done to exclude hyperparathyroidism.

It would be wise to consult an infectious disease specialist before ordering an expensive workup. It would also be wise to consult an oncologist when searching for a malignancy before ordering an expensive workup.

When all tests have negative findings, many clinicians have been tempted to make a diagnosis of chronic fatigue syndrome. It is questionable whether this is truly a disease or not.

● Other Useful Tests

1. Serum luteinizing hormone (LH), follicle-stimulating hormone (FSH), and growth hormone levels (hypopituitarism)
2. Febrile agglutinins (infectious disease)
3. Brucellin antibody titer (brucellosis)
4. Monospot test (mononucleosis)
5. Serial blood cultures (septicemia, subacute bacterial endocarditis [SBE])
6. Tuberculin test (tuberculosis)
7. Human immunodeficiency virus (HIV) antibody titer (AIDS)
8. D-Xylose absorption test (malabsorption syndrome)
9. Bone scan (metastatic malignancy)
10. CT scan of abdomen (malignancy)
11. X-ray of long bones and skull (metastasis)
12. Urine porphobilinogen (porphyria)
13. Polysomnogram (sleep apnea)
14. Neurology consult
15. Endocrinology consult
16. Psychiatry consult
17. Myositis specific antibodies (polymyositis)
18. 1, 25-dihydroxyvitamin D_3*
19. Urine drug screen

---

*Doud JE, et al. *The Vitamin D Cure*. Hoboken, NJ: John Wiley and Sons, Inc. 2008.

TABLE 60 Weakness and Fatigue—Generalized

	V Vascular	I Inflammatory	N Neoplasm	D Degenerative	I Intoxication	C Congenital	A Allergic and Autoimmune	T Trauma	E Endocrine
Muscle	Congestive heart failure	Epidemic myalgia		Malnutrition	Diuretics	McArdle syndrome	Dermatomyositis	Multiple contusion	Diabetes mellitus Acromegaly Cushing disease Insulinoma Addison disease Hyperthyroidism
Myoneural Junction			Eaton–Lambert syndrome		Cholinergic drugs	Familial periodic paralysis	Myasthenia gravis		
Peripheral Nerve			Metastatic carcinoma	Pellagra Beriberi	Lead arsenic Alcohol Porphyria	Hypertrophic polyneuritis Charcot–Marie–Tooth disease	Periarteritis nodosa		Diabetic neuropathy Hypothyroidism
Spinal Cord	Anterior spinal artery occlusion	Poliomyelitis Epidural abscess	Spinal cord tumor	Progressive muscular atrophy			Multiple sclerosis		
Brain	Carotid or basilar insufficiency or occlusion	Encephalitis Meningitis	Brain tumor (primary and metastatic)	Parkinson disease Amyotrophic lateral sclerosis Senile dementia	Manganese intoxication Tranquilizers	Wilson disease	Lupus erythematosus Multiple sclerosis	Concussion Postconcussion syndrome	Hypopituitarism

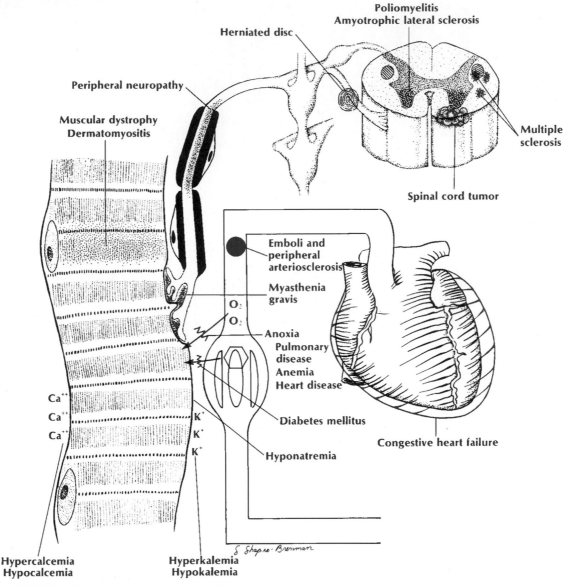

● **FIGURE 3** Weakness and fatigue, generalized.

Case Presentation #86

A 62-year-old black man complained of generalized weakness and fatigue and a chronic cough. He had smoked two packs of cigarettes a day for several years.

Question #1. Utilizing anatomy and biochemistry, what would be your list of possible causes of this man's problem?

Physical examination revealed sibilant and sonorous rales over the right lower lobe, and chest x-ray revealed consolidation in the right lower lobe. A Tensilon test was weakly positive.

Question #2. What is your most likely diagnosis?

(See Appendix B for the answers.)

WEAKNESS OR PARALYSIS OF ONE OR MORE EXTREMITIES

This symptom, as opposed to generalized weakness and fatigue (see page 437), is almost invariably due to a neurologic disorder. Consequently, a comprehensive list of causes is developed using **neuroanatomy**. Muscle weakness or paralysis may be due to disease of the muscle, myoneural junction, peripheral nerve, nerve roots and anterior horn cells, and pyramidal tract involvement in the spinal cord, brainstem, or cerebrum. Table 61 has been constructed with these anatomic components cross-indexed with the various etiologies suggested by the mnemonic **VINDICATE**. The most important of these will be covered in the following discussion.

1. **Muscle:** This should suggest muscular dystrophy, polymyalgia rheumatica, and dermatomyositis.

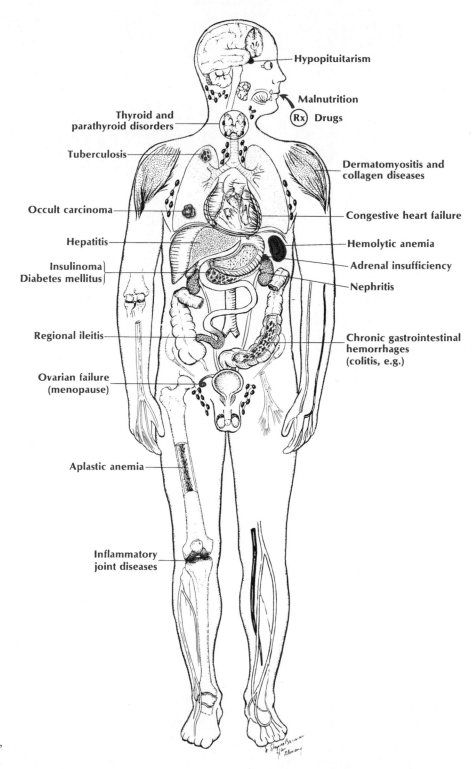

Hypopituitarism

Malnutrition

(Rx) Drugs

Thyroid and
parathyroid disorders

Tuberculosis

Dermatomyositis and
collagen diseases

Occult carcinoma

Congestive heart failure

Hepatitis

Hemolytic anemia

Insulinoma
Diabetes mellitus

Adrenal insufficiency

Nephritis

Regional ileitis

Chronic gastrointestinal
hemorrhages
(colitis, e.g.)

Ovarian failure
(menopause)

Aplastic anemia

Inflammatory
joint diseases

W

● **FIGURE 4** Weakness and fatigue,
generalized.

2. **Myoneural junction:** Primary and symptomatic myasthenia gravis are promptly brought to mind here. The toxic effects of succinylcholine chloride (Anectine), aminoglycosides, cholinergic drugs, and antispasmodics should also be mentioned. Myasthenia gravis is also associated with thyrotoxicosis, lupus, and rheumatoid arthritis.
3. **Nerve:** The many causes of peripheral neuropathy should be recalled here. The most important are diabetic neuropathy, alcoholic and nutritional neuropathies, Guillain–Barré syndrome, Buerger disease, periarteritis nodosa, porphyria, peroneal muscular atrophy, and lacerations or contusions from blunt trauma or surgery.
4. **Nerve root or anterior horn:** Poliomyelitis, postpolio syndrome (occurring 15 to 30 years after the initial attack), lead neuropathy, and progressive muscular atrophy are a few diseases that specifically attack the anterior

Table 61 Weakness or Paralysis of One or More Extremities

	V Vascular	I Inflammatory	N Neoplasm	D Degenerative	I Intoxication	C Congenital	A Allergic and Autoimmune	T Trauma	E Endocrine
Muscle	Peripheral vascular disease	Trichinosis	Rhabdomyosarcoma Wasting of carcinoma	Muscular dystrophy		Muscular dystrophy Familial periodic paralysis	Dermatomyositis	Contusion	Hypothyroid myopathy
Myoneural Junction			Myasthenia of Eaton–Lambert syndrome Thymoma		Cholinergic antispasmodic drugs Aminoglycosides		Myasthenia gravis		
Nerve	Buerger disease Ischemic neuropathy Leriche syndrome	Diphtheria Infectious mononucleosis Leprosy Leptospirosis	Neuroma Neurofibroma Metastasis		Lead and alcoholic neuropathy Furadantin and other drugs	Peroneal muscular atrophy Hypertrophic neuritis Porphyria	Periarteritis nodosa Thrombotic thrombocytopenia purpura	Contusion laceration surgery Carpal tunnel syndrome	Diabetic neuropathy
Spinal Cord	Anterior spinal artery occlusion Aortic aneurysm	Epidural abscess Transverse myelitis Syphilis	Primary and metastatic tumors Myeloma	Syringomyelia Amyotrophic lateral sclerosis	Spinal anesthesia Radiation	Friedreich ataxia	Multiple sclerosis	Epidural hematoma Fracture Ruptured disk Decompression sickness	
Brainstem	Basilar artery occlusion and aneurysm	Syphilis Tuberculosis Viral encephalitis Arachnoiditis	Primary and metastatic tumors	Syringobulbia Amyotrophic lateral sclerosis		Platybasia	Multiple sclerosis Lupus erythematosus		
Cerebrum	Embolus Thrombus Hemorrhage Aneurysm Atrioventricular anomaly	Syphilis Encephalitis Cerebral abscess Venous sinus thrombosis Tuberculosis	Primary and metastatic tumors	Senile and presenile dementia	Bromism Lead intoxication Alcoholism	Schilder disease Cerebral palsy Lipoidosis	Multiple sclerosis Lupus erythematosus	Concussion Epidural and subdural hematoma Cerebral hemorrhage	

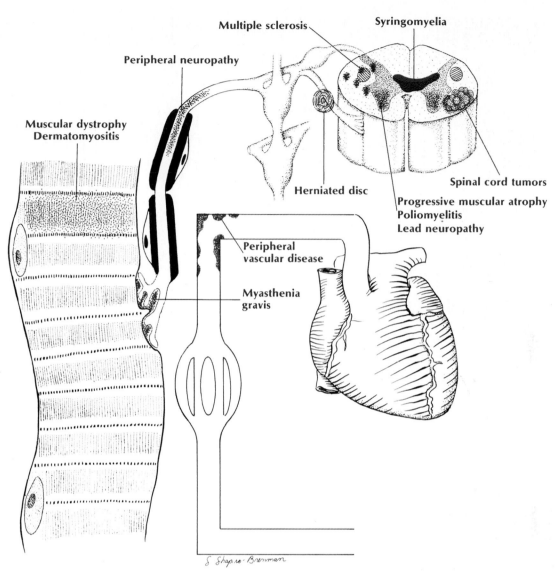

● **FIGURE 5** Weakness or paralysis of one or more extremities.

horn and roots; the roots may also be compressed by herniated disks, fractures, tuberculosis, or metastatic carcinomas of the spine. The spinal cord is often involved in the compression, too. Cervical spondylosis and spondylolisthesis may also compress the nerve root.

5. **Spinal cord:** The pyramidal tracts are involved in **malformations** such as syringomyelia, arteriovenous anomalies, and Friedreich ataxia; in **inflammatory** diseases like syphilis, tuberculosis of the spine, and transverse myelitis; in **neoplasms** (both primary and metastatic); and in **traumatic** lesions such as fractures, herniated discs, and hematomas. Thus, the mnemonic **MINT** is helpful in recalling these lesions. Cervical spondylosis, amyotrophic lateral sclerosis, syringomyelia, pernicious anemia, and multiple sclerosis may be forgotten, however, if only this mnemonic is used.

6. **Brainstem:** Brainstem gliomas and multiple sclerosis are important causes of pyramidal tract disease, but vascular occlusions of the basilar artery and its branches far exceed these in number.

7. **Cerebrum:** Any space-occupying lesions such as neoplasms, cerebral abscesses, subdural hematomas, and large aneurysms may cause focal monoplegia, hemiplegia, or paraplegia (parasagittal meningioma). Occlusions and hemorrhages of the cerebral arteries, however, are much more common causes of focal paralysis. Diffuse paralysis may result from the toxic and inflammatory encephalitides, presenile dementia, lipoidosis, and diffuse sclerosis. Multiple sclerosis and lupus erythematosus may also attack the cerebral peduncles. Tick paralysis affects the central nervous system (CNS) and is associated with incoordination, nystagmus, and flaccid paralysis.

● **Approach to the Diagnosis**

The site of weakness is determined by associated symptoms and signs. Fasciculations suggest nerve root or anterior horn cell involvement, whereas sensory changes suggest peripheral nerve or spinal cord involvement. A combination of spasticity in the lower extremities and flaccid and

TABLE 62 Weight Loss

	Physiologic Analysis			Physiologic Analysis				
Decreased Intake	Decreased Absorption	Decreased Circulation	Impaired Storage	Increased Utilization	Impaired Utilization	Decreased Excretion	Increased Excretion
Oxygen					*Oxygen*		
Asthma Emphysema Central nervous system hypoventilation	Sarcoidosis Pulmonary fibrosis of other causes	Anemia of various causes Congestive heart failure			Cyanide poisoning and other exogenous toxin Electrolyte disorders	Pulmonary disease, chronic obstructive	
Food and Drink					*Food and Drink*		
Vomiting of various causes Kwashiorkor Obstruction by carcinoma of esophagus or stomach cardiospasm Anorexia nervosa Cerebral arteriosclerosis or degeneration Chronic alcoholism	Sprue Nontropical sprue Intestinal parasite Scleroderma Blind loop syndrome Pancreatitis		Cirrhosis Glycogen storage disease Hypopituitarism	Hyperthyroidism Fever due to infection or neoplasm Hypermetabolism in malignancy, chronic infection (e.g., tuberculosis) Chronic inflammation of rheumatoid arthritis	Decreased utilization Various muscle and central nervous system diseases	Jaundice	Aminoaciduria/renal glycosuria Hypocalcemia of various causes Hypokalemia Diabetes insipidus Albuminuria
Vitamin							
Scurvy Pellagra Alcoholism	*Diphyllobothrium latum* Regional ileitis Gastric atrophy Pernicious anemia Sprue						

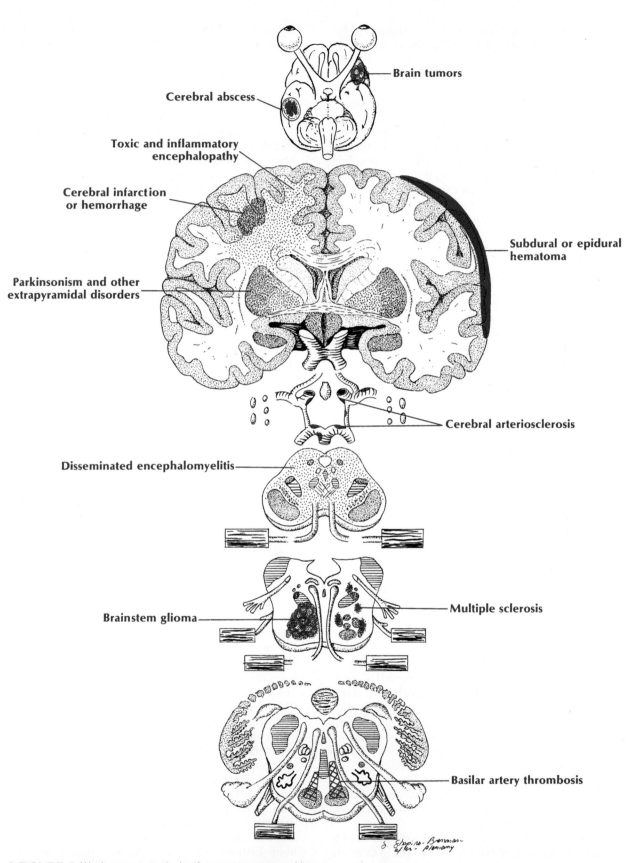

● **FIGURE 6** Weakness or paralysis of one or more extremities.

atrophic weakness in the upper extremities suggests cervical cord involvement. Cranial nerve lesions in association with paraplegia or quadriplegia usually indicate a brainstem lesion.

The workup will depend on the site in which the pathology is suspected to be located. If muscle is the site, then an EMG or biopsy is indicated. If the myoneural junction is involved, a Tensilon test is done. Peripheral nerve lesions require a more extensive workup, including a glucose tolerance test, blood lead level, urine for porpholbilinogens, EMG, nerve conduction velocity (NCV) test, and possibly a muscle biopsy. Spinal cord lesions may require x-ray of the spine, CT scan or MRI, myelography, discography, and spinal fluid analysis. Brainstem and cerebral lesions are best screened with a skull x-ray, MRI, or CT scan before a spinal tap or arteriogram is considered.

● Other Useful Tests

1. CBC (pernicious anemia with neurologic involvement)
2. Chemistry panel (muscle disease, liver or kidney disease with neurologic involvement)
3. ANA analysis (collagen disease with neuropathy or myopathy)
4. Acetylcholine receptor antibody titer (myasthenia gravis)
5. Urine creatine and creatinine levels (muscular dystrophy)
6. Spinal fluid analysis (Guillain–Barré syndrome, multiple sclerosis)

WEIGHT LOSS

As noted in Table 62, the diagnostic analysis of weight loss is best accomplished by applying **physiology**. Food and oxygen must be properly and regularly brought into the body (intake), properly absorbed and circulated to the cells, and properly used; the waste products must then be excreted in order for weight to be maintained. The storage of food is essential to maintain weight when food is not being regularly ingested. Finally, there must be minimal excretion of sugar, protein, electrolytes, and water to maintain weight. Let us explore each of these physiologic functions for possible alterations.

Decreased intake of food results from any disease associated with vomiting, upper intestinal obstruction (e.g., carcinoma of the pyloris), and esophageal obstruction (cardiospasm and carcinoma of the esophagus). Starvation is not uncommon even today, particularly in the elderly population trying to stretch their Social Security checks. Depression, anorexia nervosa, and other psychiatric disturbances may cause weight loss by decreased intake. CNS diseases such as cerebral arteriosclerosis may cause disinterest in food and poor chewing and swallowing. Chronic alcoholics do not eat. The absence of one vitamin, as in scurvy or pellagra, may cause weight loss.

Decreased intake of oxygen occurs in asthma, emphysema, and other respiratory disorders as well as in CNS diseases that may cause hypoventilation (poliomyelitis).

Decreased absorption of food and electrolytes are common in malabsorption syndrome, pancreatitis,

intestinal parasites, and blind loop syndrome. Regional ileitis and tapeworms reduce the absorption of vitamins. The **decreased circulation of oxygen** is probably the main cause of wasting in CHF, but certainly congestion of the liver and decreased excretion of waste products may play a role. Severe anemia of various causes will inevitably decompensate the delivery of oxygen to the tissues.

The weight loss of cirrhosis (numerous etiologies) is probably due to **impaired storage of fat and sugar** for use when it is most needed, but the ability to convert protein to sugar and vice versa is also impaired. In glycogen storage and lipid storage diseases, a one-way trip of sugar or fat into the liver is a prominent factor contributing to weight loss. Probably the most common causes of weight loss today are due to the **increased use of food** in hyperthyroidism and malignancies, but the hypermetabolism of fever and any inflammatory condition (rheumatoid arthritis) is also common. The increased metabolism secondary to opportunistic infections in AIDS should not be forgotten.

Neurologic and muscular diseases cause wasting and thus **decrease the use of sugar. Impaired use of sugar** in diabetes mellitus and other endocrinopathies is a significant cause of weight loss. Various toxins and electrolyte disorders may block the tissue uptake of oxygen (cyanide poisoning and so forth) and cause weight loss. **Disorders of excretion** also commonly play a role; thus, one should always look for uremia, pulmonary emphysema, and jaundice.

Finally, there are many disorders already mentioned associated with albuminuria and glycosuria that may be classified under increased excretion of metabolic substances; these, of course, contribute to weight loss. The numerous aminoacidurias and diabetes insipidus should be remembered in this regard.

● Approach to the Diagnosis

Weight loss rarely occurs as the only symptom. When it seems to be the only symptom, there is almost invariably a psychiatric disorder such as depression, bulimia, or anorexia nervosa to explain it. More often the diagnosis of weight loss can be made by the other associated symptoms. For example, weight loss with a good appetite, polyuria, and polydipsia should point to hyperthyroidism and diabetes mellitus. Weight loss with weakness and polydipsia but no increase of appetite points to diabetes insipidus. Weight loss, weakness, and loss of appetite suggest the possibility of a malignancy, chronic infectious disease, or endocrine disorder. Weight loss with significant local or generalized lymphadenopathy suggests chronic leukemia, lymphoma, sarcoidosis, or a chronic infectious disease process. Weight loss with hyperpigmentation of the skin suggests Addison disease or hemochromatosis. Weight loss with significant pallor of the skin and mucus membranes suggests a diagnosis of anemia, malabsorption syndrome, and malignancy. Weight loss with jaundice suggests alcoholic cirrhosis, chronic hepatitis, primary or metastatic neoplasm of the liver, or biliary cirrhosis. Weight loss in patients with high-risk sexual behavior should suggest AIDS. The initial workup of weight loss should include

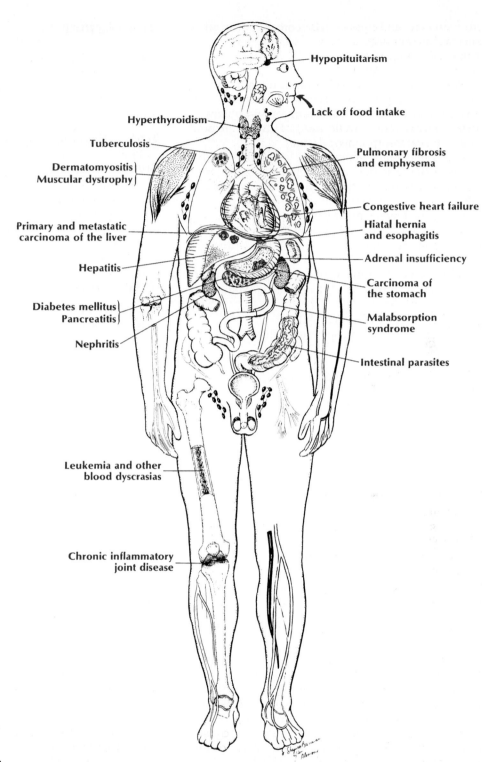

Hypopituitarism

Lack of food intake

Hyperthyroidism

Tuberculosis

Dermatomyositis
Muscular dystrophy

Pulmonary fibrosis
and emphysema

Congestive heart failure

Primary and metastatic
carcinoma of the liver

Hiatal hernia
and esophagitis

Adrenal insufficiency

Hepatitis

Carcinoma of
the stomach

Diabetes mellitus
Pancreatitis

Malabsorption
syndrome

Nephritis

Intestinal parasites

Leukemia and other
blood dyscrasias

Chronic inflammatory
joint disease

● **FIGURE 7** Weight loss.

a CBC, sedimentation rate, chemistry panel, thyroid profile, urinalysis, stool test for occult blood, chest x-ray, and flat plate of the abdomen. If these tests are normal, maybe abdominal ultrasound could be done. If there is fever, the workup of this symptom can be pursued (see page 171). Other tests may be ordered depending on which disease is suspected. Before ordering a battery of tests, it may be wise to get a psychiatric consult and make sure there is not a "supratentorial" cause for the problem. If a trial of a nutritional supplement (3000 to 4000 calories/day) halts the weight loss, depression is most likely a factor.

● **Other Useful Tests**

1. Tuberculin test (tuberculosis)
2. Glucose tolerance test (diabetes mellitus)

3. Serum amylase and lipase levels (chronic pancreatitis, pancreatic neoplasm)
4. Drug screen (drug abuse)
5. HIV antibody titer (AIDS)
6. Stool for fat and trypsin (malabsorption syndrome)
7. Stool for ova and parasites (parasites infestation)
8. D-Xylose absorption test (malabsorption syndrome)
9. Urine 5-hydroxyindole acetic acid (5-HIAA) (carcinoid syndrome, malabsorption syndrome)
10. Bone scan (metastatic malignancy)
11. CT scan of the abdomen (malignancy, abscess)
12. Lymphangiogram (Hodgkin lymphoma, metastatic malignancy)
13. CT scan of the brain (pituitary tumor)
14. Lymph node biopsy (lymphoma, malignancy)
15. Serum antidiuretic hormone (ADH) level (diabetes insipidus)
16. Serum cortisol level (Addison disease, hypopituitarism)
17. Serum growth hormone, LH, or FSH (Simmonds disease)
18. HIV antibody titer, CD4 count (AIDS)
19. Gastroscopy or colonoscopy (gastrointestinal [GI] malignancy)

Case Presentation #87

A 26-year-old singer in a rock band complained of losing 32 pounds over the past year. She denies weakness, polyuria, polydipsia, or diarrhea. Her physical examination is unremarkable except for pale conjunctiva.

Question #1. Utilizing your knowledge of physiology and biochemistry, what is your differential diagnosis?

Stool analysis for fat content, ovum and parasites, and occult blood was normal. A GI series and barium enema were normal. Complete laboratory studies revealed only a microcytic hypochromic anemia.

Question #2. What is your diagnosis now?

(See Appendix B for the answers.)

WHEEZING

The causes of wheezing may be recalled by following the air passages from the larynx to the alveoli.

Larynx: Laryngitis may obstruct the inspiration of air causing wheezing. This is typically respiratory wheezing, especially with epiglottitis.

Trachea: This brings to mind tracheobronchitis and foreign bodies.

Bronchi: This prompts the recall of bronchitis, bronchiolitis, and bronchial asthma. It should also remind one of pulmonary emphysema, pneumoconiosis, sillo-filler's disease, and bronchogenic carcinoma. Hereditary angioedema may cause wheezing.

Alveoli: This suggests pulmonary edema with associated cardiac asthma.

● Approach to the Diagnosis

CBC, chest x-ray, sputum smear, and cultures will help to diagnose infectious causes of wheezing. Bronchial asthma can be diagnosed by sputum for eosinophils and pulmonary function testing. Cardiac asthma (due to CHF) can be diagnosed by a venous pressure and circulation time, BNP, electrocardiogram (EKG) and echocardiography. Bronchoscopy may be necessary if a foreign body is suspected. Hereditary angioedema is diagnosed by a deficiency of C1 esterase inhibitor.

Diseases that are Symptoms of Other Diseases

INTRODUCTION

The author is sure that on numerous occasions, experienced clinicians have diagnosed a common disorder and begun treatment only to find that either the patient does not recover as expected or the condition turns out to be something else. This section has been added to this edition to serve as a warning to inexperienced clinicians that things are not always what they seem to be. Physicians always need to maintain a healthy degree of skepticism when they treat a patient for a common disease; there may be an underlying condition or cause that is being overlooked. Where do physicians turn to find out what they could be missing? It is hoped that this section will provide the answer for a lot of cases. It is not intended to include all the possibilities for each condition—just the most common ones.

ACNE VULGARIS

A 28-year-old obese white female with a history of seizures has developed a rash on both cheeks. You diagnose acne vulgaris and treat her with a benzyl peroxide preparation and oral tetracycline with poor results. She could have

1. Cushing syndrome
2. Reaction to phenytoin
3. Polycystic ovary syndrome
4. Impetigo
5. Sebaceous hyperplasia
6. Chronic use of oral corticosteroids
7. Lupus erythematosus
8. Acne rosacea

ASTHMA

A 43-year-old white male comes to you with recurrent attacks of shortness of breath, cough, and wheezing for 6 months. You treat him with bronchodilators and corticosteroid nebulizers and he fails to improve. He could have

1. Congestive heart failure
2. α-1 trypsin deficiency
3. Cystic fibrosis
4. Chronic obstructive pulmonary disease (COPD)
5. Gastroesophageal reflux disease
6. Tuberculosis
7. Pneumoconiosis
8. Coccidiomycosis
9. Periarteritis nodosa
10. Sarcoidosis
11. Acquired immunodeficiency syndrome (AIDS)
12. Parasite infestation

ATRIAL FIBRILLATION

A 37-year-old white female comes to you for recurrent palpitations. On examination, you find that she has a rapid irregular heart rate and her heart sounds are irregular in intensity also. You should look for

1. Hyperthyroidism
2. Alcohol abuse
3. Hypertensive cardiovascular disease
4. Collagen disease
5. Atrial myxoma
6. Drug toxicity
7. Cardiomyopathy
8. Rheumatic heart disease
9. Coronary artery disease
10. Drug abuse (e.g., cocaine)
11. Mitral valve prolapse

BELL PALSY

A 29-year-old black female wakes on the morning of her visit to your office with weakness of the left side of her face and inability to close her left eye. You diagnose Bell palsy and start her on valacyclovir and corticosteroids. What else should you rule out?

1. Cholesteatoma
2. Acoustic neuroma
3. Ramsey–Hunt syndrome
4. Guillain–Barré syndrome
5. Mastoiditis
6. Petrositis
7. Cerebrovascular accident
8. Sarcoidosis
9. Multiple sclerosis

CARPAL TUNNEL SYNDROME

A 42-year-old female comes to you because of recurrent weakness and tingling of both hands, worse on the right. Her nerve conduction studies are unremarkable. Nevertheless, you inject lidocaine and corticosteroids into her right carpal tunnel with good results. What else could she have?

1. Rheumatoid arthritis
2. Amyloidosis
3. Acromegaly
4. Multiple myeloma
5. Cervical radiculopathy
6. Menopause syndrome
7. Hypothyroidism
8. Collagen disease

ASTHMA

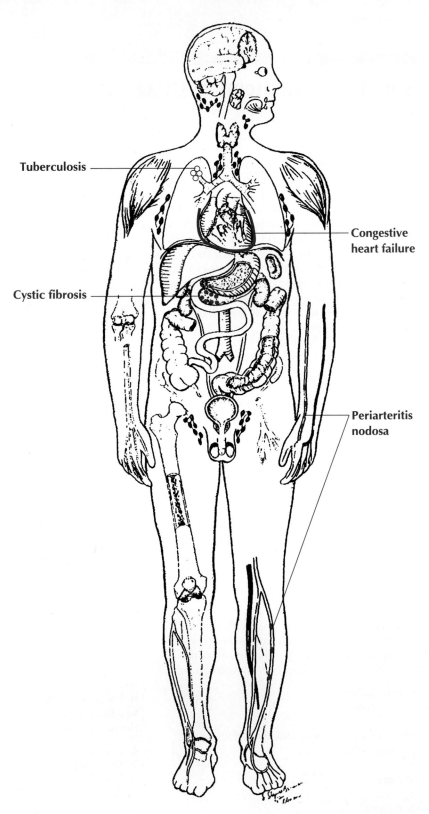

Tuberculosis

Congestive
heart failure

Cystic fibrosis

Periarteritis
nodosa

● **FIGURE 1** Asthma.

ATRIAL FIBRILLATION

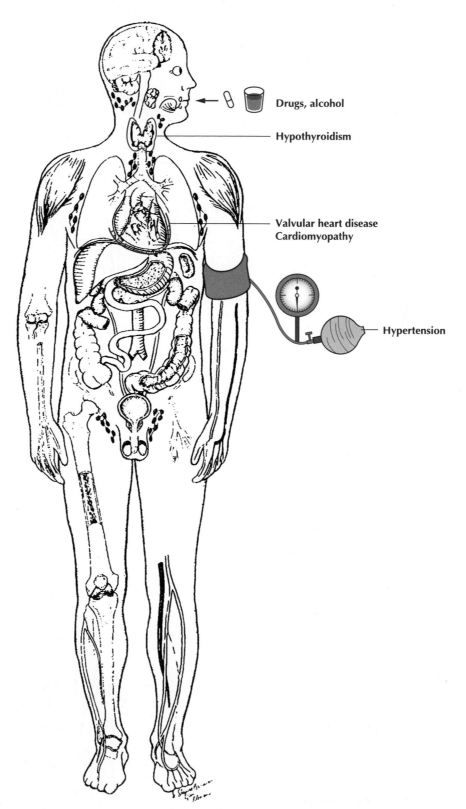

Drugs, alcohol

Hypothyroidism

Valvular heart disease
Cardiomyopathy

Hypertension

● **FIGURE 2** Atrial fibrillation.

CARPAL TUNNEL SYNDROME

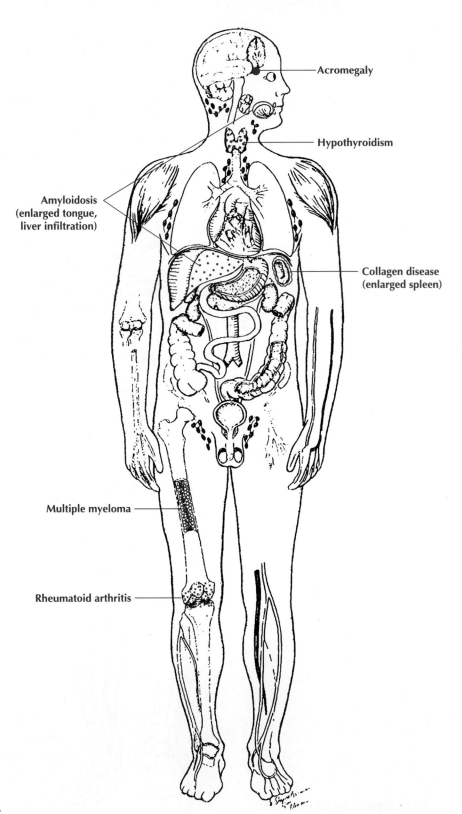

● **FIGURE 3** Carpal tunnel syndrome.

CATARACTS
A 52-year-old white male comes to you for gradual onset of reduced visual acuity in both eyes. You diagnose bilateral cataracts. What else could he have?

1. Diabetes mellitus
2. Myotonic dystrophy
3. Galactosemia
4. Acromegaly
5. Lawrence–Moon–Biedel syndrome

CHOLELITHIASIS
A 12-year-old black female develops acute colicky right upper quadrant pain radiating to her right scapula with nausea and vomiting. Ultrasonography shows several gallstones one of which is blocking the cystic duct. What else could she have?

1. Sickle cell anemia
2. Diabetes mellitus
3. Pancreatitis
4. Congenital anomaly of the biliary tree
5. Hyperlipemia

CHRONIC OBSTRUCTIVE LUNG DISEASE
A 48-year-old white male comes to you with a history of heavy smoking and working in the coal mines for 25 years because of increasing shortness of breath and cough, which is no longer responding to bronchodilators and home oxygen. You diagnose COPD. What else could he have?

1. α-1 trypsin deficiency
2. Bronchial asthma
3. Pneumoconiosis
4. Congestive heart failure
5. Cystic fibrosis
6. Bronchogenic carcinoma
7. Pulmonary embolism
8. Pneumonia
9. Tuberculosis
10. Bronchiectasis
11. Collagen disease
12. Pulmonary fibrosis

CIRRHOSIS OF THE LIVER
A 52-year-old Hispanic male presents to the emergency room in a semiconscious state. Liver function studies show an elevated aspartate aminotransferase, alanine aminotransferase, and serum bilirubin. His prothrombin time and blood ammonia are elevated. You diagnose hepatic coma. What else could he have?

1. Chronic active hepatitis
2. Wilson disease
3. Hemochromatosis
4. Biliary cirrhosis
5. Sclerosing cholangitis
6. Common duct stone with ascending cholangitis

7. Hepatoma
8. Collagen disease
9. Amebic abscess

CONGESTIVE HEART FAILURE
You have just sat down for dinner when you receive a call from an old patient of yours. The man asks if you could "call in" an antibiotic for a "cold" he has had for a week, which is not clearing up. You can tell he is short of breath on the phone, so you decide to make a house call. When you arrive at his home, you note that he is very short of breath and is coughing up frothy, blood-tinged sputum. On examination, he has bilateral crepitant rales, jugular venous distension, and 4+ pitting edema. You diagnose congestive heart failure and arrange for immediate hospitalization. What else should you look for?

1. Pulmonary embolism
2. Bronchopneumonia
3. Hyperthyroidism
4. Hypothyroidism
5. Beriberi heart disease
6. Acute myocardial infarction
7. Acute respiratory distress syndrome
8. Cardiomyopathy
9. Cardiac arrhythmia
10. Rheumatic heart disease
11. COPD

DIABETES MELLITUS
A 34-year-old obese white female comes to your office to initiate a weight loss program. Routine blood work shows a fasting blood sugar of 256/mg%. What else could she have?

1. Cushing syndrome
2. Pheochromocytoma
3. Pituitary tumor
4. Chronic pancreatitis
5. Hemochromatosis
6. Glucagonoma
7. Drug reaction (e.g., diuretic)

FRACTURES
A 55-year-old white male fractured his right femur in a fall. An orthopedic surgeon does an open reduction and fixation. Six weeks later, the fracture fails to show adequate healing. You should look for:

1. Osteoporosis
2. Avitaminosis D
3. Hyperparathyroidism
4. Metastatic or primary neoplasm of the bone
5. Osteomyelitis
6. Paget disease
7. Multiple myeloma
8. Malabsorption syndrome
9. Chronic renal failure
10. Medication induced osteoporosis

CHOLELITHIASIS

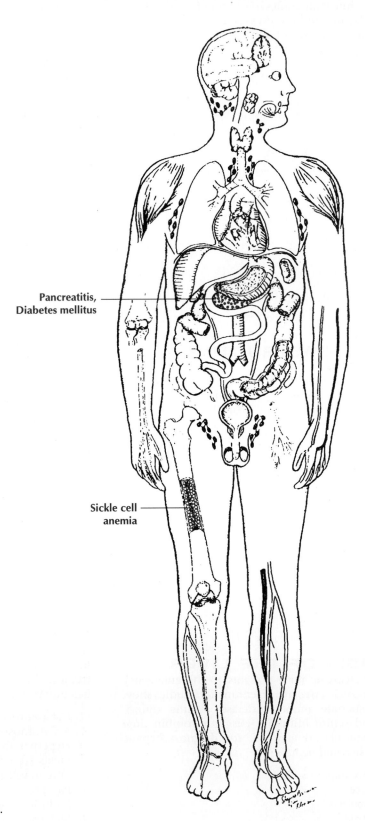

Pancreatitis,
Diabetes mellitus

Sickle cell
anemia

● **FIGURE 4** Cholelithiasis.

CHRONIC OBSTRUCTIVE LUNG DISEASE

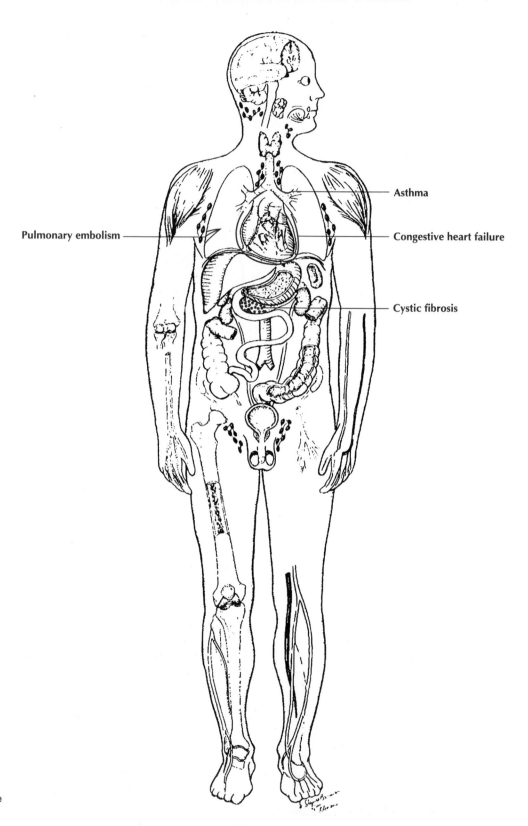

● **FIGURE 5** Chronic obstructive
lung disease.

CIRRHOSIS OF THE LIVER

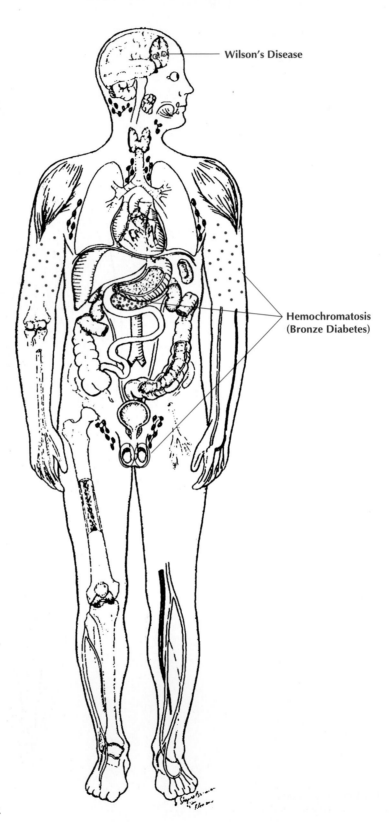

● FIGURE 6 Cirrhosis of the liver.

CONGESTIVE HEART FAILURE

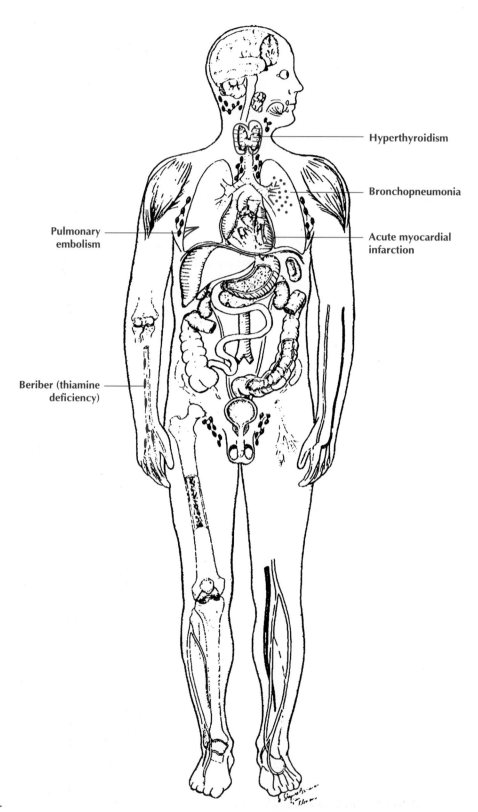

Hyperthyroidism

Bronchopneumonia

Pulmonary embolism

Acute myocardial infarction

Beriber (thiamine deficiency)

● FIGURE 7 Congestive heart failure.

DIABETES MELLITUS

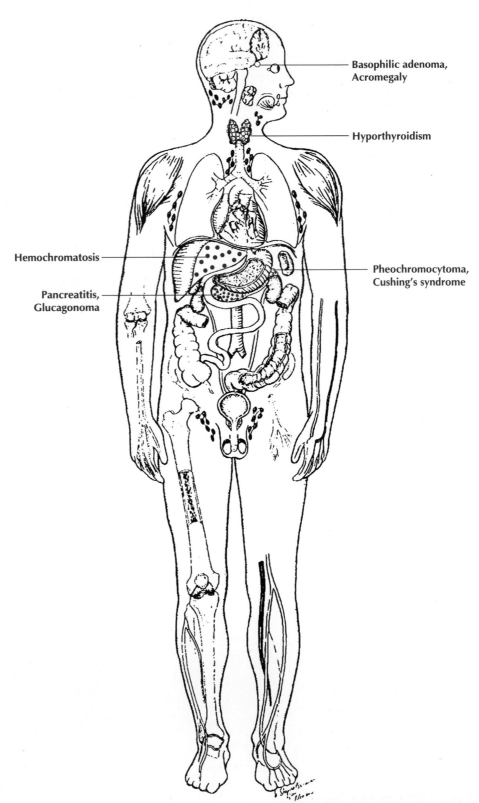

Basophilic adenoma,
Acromegaly

Hyporthyroidism

Hemochromatosis

Pheochromocytoma,
Cushing's syndrome

Pancreatitis,
Glucagonoma

● **FIGURE 8** Diabetes mellitus.

11. Cushing syndrome
12. Corticosteroid use
13. Thyrotoxicosis
14. Hypogonadism

MALABSORPTION SYNDROME

A 38-year-old white male comes to you because of chronic diarrhea and weight loss. A quantitative stool fat is elevated, a D-xylose absorption test is positive, and his urine 5-hydroxyindoleacetic acid (5-HIAA) is increased. You diagnose malabsorption syndrome. What else could he have?

1. Chronic pancreatitis
2. Carcinoid syndrome
3. Whipple disease
4. Celiac disease
5. Crohn disease
6. Post-gastrectomy malabsorption
7. Small bowel resection
8. Amyloidosis
9. Abetalipoproteinemia
10. Intestinal lymphangiectasia
11. Tropical sprue
12. Pancreatic cancer
13. Cystic fibrosis
14. Intestinal parasites (e.g., *Diphyllobothrium latum*)
15. Drug toxicity

PANCREATITIS

A 54-year-old white female comes to the emergency department because of sudden onset of midepigastric pain, nausea, and vomiting. Examination shows severe diffuse abdominal tenderness, rebound, and guarding most marked in the epigastrium. Laboratory studies show an amylase of 2,250 units and an elevated lipase. You diagnose acute pancreatitis and admit her to the hospital. What other conditions should you consider?

1. Common duct stone
2. Pancreatic pseudocyst
3. Mumps
4. Hyperparathyroidism
5. Hypertriglyceridemia
6. Pancreatic carcinoma
7. Alcoholism
8. Drug toxicity
9. Peptic ulcer perforating into the pancreas
10. Cystic fibrosis
11. Carcinoma of the ampulla of Vater

PARKINSON DISEASE

A 44-year-old white male presents to your office with the history of tremor of both hands gradually increasing over the past 8 months. Examination shows tremor, cogwheel rigidity, monotonous speech, masked face, and a short-stepped gait. You diagnose Parkinson disease. You should also consider the possibility of

1. Wilson disease
2. Manganese toxicity
3. Phenothiazine toxicity
4. Other drug toxicity
5. Hyperthyroidism
6. Encephalopathy
7. Essential tremor
8. Diffuse Lewy body disease
9. Corticobasilar degeneration
10. Postinfectious parkinsonism

PEPTIC ULCER

A 42-year-old back male smoker for 25 pack years who consumes one to two beers a day comes to you for right upper quadrant pain and is found to have a duodenal ulcer on endoscopy. You treat him with diet, antacids, and H2 blockers, but he fails to improve. What do you look for?

1. Zollinger–Ellison syndrome
2. Chronic use of nonsteroidal anti-inflammatory drugs
3. Use of potassium preparations
4. More alcohol consumption than he admits
5. Heavy ingestion of caffeinated beverages
6. *Helicobacter pylori* ulcer disease

PERIPHERAL ARTERIOSCLEROSIS

A 62-year-old black male complains that when he goes for his morning walk he repeatedly gets severe cramps in his legs on walking one block. Examination shows his dorsalis pedis and tibialis pulses are diminished in both lower extremities. You diagnose peripheral arteriosclerosis and put him on pentoxifylline (Trental). What other conditions should you consider?

1. Leriche syndrome
2. Buerger disease
3. Spinal stenosis
4. Hyperlipemia
5. Diabetes mellitus
6. Hyponatremia
7. Hypocalcemia
8. Hypoparathyroidism

PLEURAL EFFUSION

A patient has a right pleural effusion on a routine x-ray of the chest. What diseases should you consider in the differential diagnosis?

1. Pneumonia with pleurisy
2. Tuberculosis
3. Fungal disease
4. Congestive heart failure
5. Lupus erythematosus
6. Pulmonary embolism
7. Carcinoma of the lung
8. Mesothelioma
9. Subphrenic abscess
10. Pancreatitis

PEPTIC ULCER

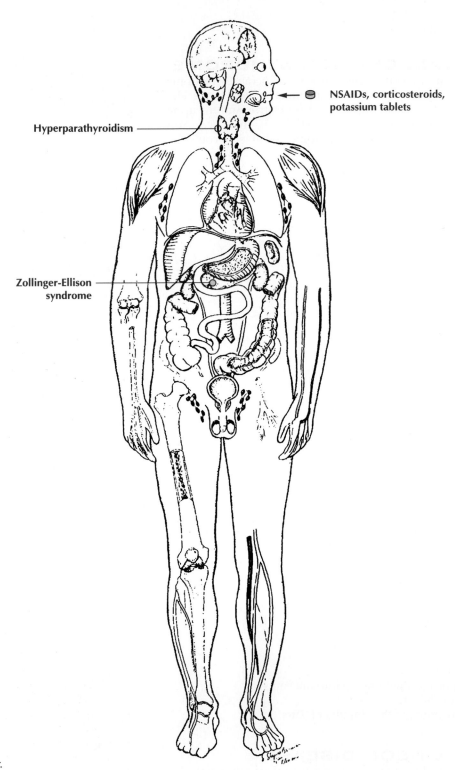

NSAIDs, corticosteroids, potassium tablets

Hyperparathyroidism

Zollinger-Ellison syndrome

● **FIGURE 9** Peptic ulcer.

PLEURAL EFFUSION

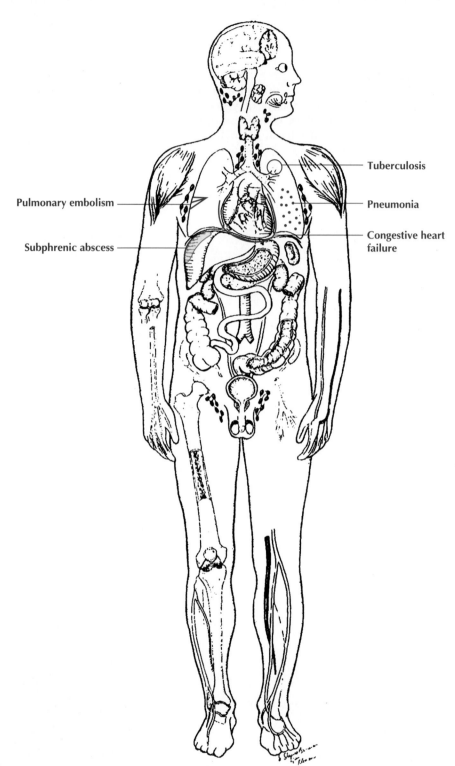

● FIGURE 10 Pleural effusion.

11. Meigs syndrome
12. Other collagen disease
13. Metastatic neoplasm
14. Drug-induced pleural disease
15. Parasitic infestation (e.g., *Echinococcus*)

PNEUMONIA

A 36-year-old white man comes to the office complaining of fever, chills, and cough productive of yellow sputum for 3 days. On examination, there is dullness, diminished tactile fremitus, and crepitant rales at the right base. You start him on amoxicillin 500 mg T.I.D. and expectorants. He returns in 4 days and is no better. What do you look for now?

1. COPD
2. Bronchiectasis
3. Bronchogenic carcinoma
4. Tuberculosis
5. Mycoplasma pneumonia
6. Viral pneumonia
7. Coccidiomycosis and other fungal disease
8. *Pneumocystis jiroveci*
9. AIDS
10. Sarcoidosis
11. Hypersensitivity pneumonitis
12. Parasitic pneumonia
13. Foreign body
14. Legionnaire disease
15. Reflux esophagitis

POLYNEUROPATHY

A 45-year-old white man known alcoholic complains of weakness, numbness, and tingling of both hands and feet for several months. On examination, he is found to have glove and stocking hypesthesia, bilateral foot drop, and steppage gait. You diagnose alcoholic polyneuropathy, but what other conditions should be considered?

1. Nutritional neuropathy
2. Pellagra
3. Pernicious anemia
4. Malabsorption syndrome
5. Porphyria
6. Guillain–Barré syndrome
7. Lead neuropathy
8. Diabetic neuropathy
9. Drug toxicity (e.g., isoniazid)
10. Lyme disease
11. Hereditary sensory motor neuropathy
12. Collagen disease

RENAL CALCULUS

A 47-year-old white male develops acute left flank pain and hematuria. A helical computer tomography scan of the abdomen shows a renal calculus in the proximal ureter. What else should you look for?

1. Hyperparathyroidism
2. Hypercalcemia of other causes

3. Hypervitaminosis D
4. Milk–alkali syndrome
5. Gout, primary
6. Gout, secondary (e.g., polycythemia vera, leukemia)
7. Thyrotoxicosis
8. Renal tubular acidosis
9. Congenital anomaly of the urinary tract
10. Chronic pyelonephritis
11. Drug toxicity
12. Neoplasm of the kidney
13. Obstructive uropathy

SOLITARY PULMONARY NODULE

A 56-year-old black male comes to the office for a routine yearly physical. His examination and laboratory studies are unremarkable, but a chest x-ray shows a 3-cm nodule in his right upper lobe. What possibilities should be considered in the differential diagnosis?

1. Bronchogenic neoplasm
2. Metastatic cancer
3. Bronchial adenoma
4. Tuberculosis
5. Lymphoma
6. Amyloidosis
7. Hemartoma
8. Histoplasmosis or other fungal disease
9. Rheumatoid nodule
10. Wegener granulomatosis
11. Sarcoidosis
12. Pulmonary embolism
13. Collagen disease
14. Parasite infestation

STREPTOCOCCAL PHARYNGITIS

A 16-year-old white male presents with a sore throat. He has definite exudates of his tonsils, and they are swollen and red. He also has prominent cervical adenopathy. You diagnose streptococcal tonsillitis and treat him with appropriate antibiotics but a week later, he is no better. You should look for

1. Infectious mononucleosis
2. Agranulocytosis from drugs he may be taking
3. Leukemia
4. Diphtheria
5. Gonococcal pharyngitis
6. Candidiasis
7. Vincent angina

STROKE

A 68-year-old black female presents to the emergency department with sudden onset of aphasia and right hemiparesis that began 6 hours ago. A computed tomography scan demonstrated a left frontal lobe infarct. What other conditions could this patient have?

1. Myocardial infarction with mural thrombus and cerebral embolism

STREP PHARYNGITIS

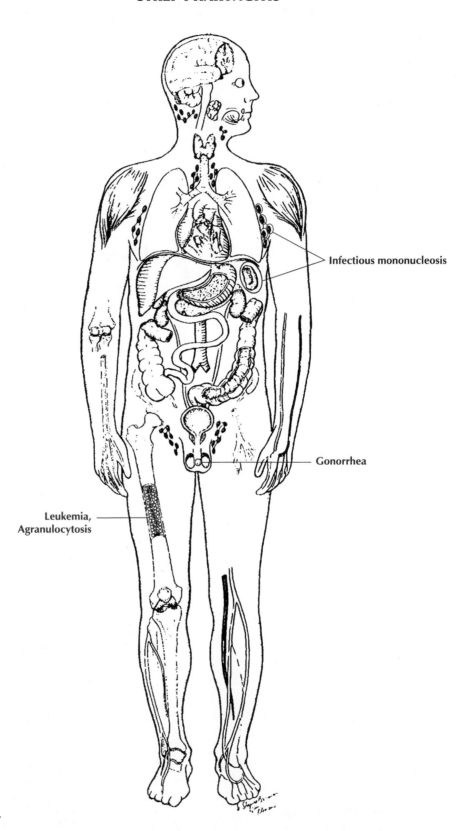

Infectious mononucleosis

Gonorrhea

Leukemia,
Agranulocytosis

● **FIGURE 11** Streptococcal pharyngitis.

STROKE

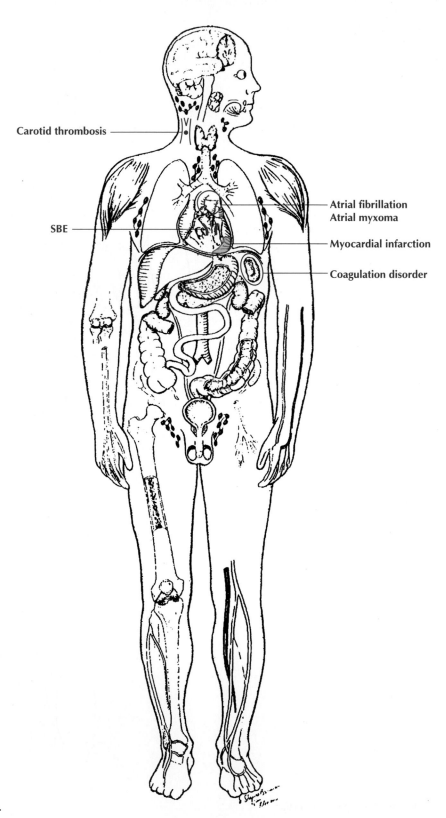

Carotid thrombosis

SBE

Atrial fibrillation
Atrial myxoma

Myocardial infarction

Coagulation disorder

● **FIGURE 12** Stroke.

2. Atrial fibrillation with cerebral embolism
3. Left carotid artery stenosis or atherosclerotic plaque
4. Subacute bacterial endocarditis
5. Lupus cerebritis
6. Left atrial myxoma
7. Coagulation disorder

SYNDROME OF INAPPROPRIATE SECRETION OF ANTIDIURETIC HORMONE (SIADH)

A 68-year-old white male complains of oliguria and generalized fatigue. He had a lobectomy for carcinoma of the lung 6 months prior to admission. Laboratory studies show hyponatremia and decreased serum osmolality with increased urine osmolality. You make a diagnosis of SIADH and treat him with hypertonic saline in low doses and fluid restriction. What other conditions could he have?

1. Congestive heart failure
2. Adrenal insufficiency
3. Recent head trauma or neurosurgery
4. Acute renal failure
5. Cirrhosis
6. Nephrotic syndrome

THYROID NODULE

A 32-year-old Hispanic female complains of a painless lump in her neck that has gradually increased in size over the past few months. On examination, you find a 2.5-cm mass in the upper pole of the right lobe of the thyroid. There is no bruit over the mass. What are the possible causes of this mass?

1. Toxic nodular goiter
2. Thyroid carcinoma
3. Riedel struma
4. Endemic goiter
5. Thyroglossal duct cyst
6. Bronchial cleft cyst
7. Parathyroid adenoma or carcinoma

URINARY TRACT INFECTION

A 13-year-old adolescent female complains of frequency of urination and dysuria. Urinalysis demonstrates 20 to 30 white blood cells per high-power field on a drop of unspun urine and a culture is positive for *Escherichia coli*. She has had three similar episodes in the past 2 years. What other conditions should be ruled out at this time?

1. Congenital anomaly of the urinary tract
2. Neoplasm of the urinary tract
3. Renal calculi
4. Obstructive uropathy
5. Child abuse
6. Urethritis (gonococcal, chlamydial)
7. Vaginitis
8. Vesicoureteral reflux
9. Neurogenic bladder

The Laboratory Workup of Disease

A

Abortion, threatened: serum B–human chorionic gonadotropin (hCG), serum progesterone levels, urine, hCG, pregnanediol, sonogram

Achalasia: barium swallow, mecholyl test, esophagoscopy, and esophageal manometry

Acoustic neuroma: skull x-ray, computed tomography (CT) scan, posterior fossa myelogram, magnetic resonance imaging (MRI)

Acquired Immunodeficiency Syndrome (AIDS): human immunodeficiency virus (HIV) antibody titer, enzyme-linked immunosorbent assay (ELISA), western blot, viral load, CD4 count

Acromegaly: skull x-ray, CT scan, serum growth hormone, MRI

Actinomycosis: smear for sulfur granules, culture skin lesions

Addison disease: serum cortisol before and after corticotrophin, CT scan of abdomen, metapyrapone test

Adrenogenital syndrome: serum cortisol, hydroxyprogesterone, 11-deoxycortisol, urine 17-ketosteroids and pregnanetriol, dexamethasone suppression test, CT scan of the abdomen

Adult respiratory distress syndrome: chest x-ray, sputum culture, blood culture, Swan–Ganz catheterization, arterial blood gases (ABGs)

Agammaglobulinemia: serum electrophoresis and immunoelectrophoresis, blood type, lymph node biopsy, B-lymphocyte and T-lymphocyte counts

Agranulocytosis, idiopathic: complete blood count (CBC), bone marrow examination, spleen scan

AIDS: see Acquired Immunodeficiency Syndrome

Albright syndrome: x-ray of long bones, bone biopsy

Alcaptonuria: urinary homogentisic acid, x-ray of spine

Alcoholism: blood alcohol level, liver function tests, liver biopsy

Aldosteronism, primary: electrolytes before and after spironolactone, plasma renin, 24-hour urine aldosterone, CT scan, exploratory laparotomy

Allergic rhinitis: nasal smear for eosinophils, serum immunoglobulin E (IgE) antibody, radioallergosorbent test (RAST), skin test

Alveolar proteinosis: luteinizing hormone (LH), sputum for periodic acid-Schiff-positive material (PSP), lung biopsy

Alzheimer disease: CT scan or MRI

Amebiasis: stool for ova and parasites, rectal biopsy, hemagglutinin inhibition test

Amyloidosis: Congo red test, rectal biopsy, liver biopsy, gingival biopsy, subcutaneous fat aspiration and stain

Angina pectoris: graded exercise tolerance test (GXT), thallium 201 scintigraphy, coronary angiogram, trial of nitroglycerin

Angineurotic edema: C'1 esterase inhibitor

Ankylosing spondylitis: human leukocyte antigen (HLA) B-27 tissue antigen

Anthrax: smear and culture of lesion, skin biopsy, serologic test

Antitrypsin deficiency: serum protein electrophorosis

Aortic aneurysm: sonogram, CT scan, aortogram

Aortic valvular disease: echocardiogram, CT scan, MRI, cardiac catheterization

Appendicitis: CBC, flat plate of abdomen, CT scan

Aplastic anemia: bone marrow, lymph node biopsy, immunoelectrophoresis

Ascaris lumbricoides: cathartic stool for ova and parasites, eosinophil count

Asthma: spirometry, sputum for eosinophils, serum IgE antibodies, RAST, skin test

Attention deficit disorder: clinical diagnosis

Atrial arrhythmias: free thyroxine (FT$_4$) index, electrocardiogram (ECG), Holter monitoring, His bundle study

Atypical pneumonia, primary: see Mycoplasma pneumoniae

B

Bacillary dysentery: stool smear (for leukocytes) and culture, febrile agglutinins

Balantidiasis: stool for ova and parasites

Banti syndrome: liver function tests, liver–spleen scan, bone marrow examination, hepatic vein catheterization

Barbiturate poisoning: blood or urine for barbiturates, electroencephalogram (EEG)

Basilar artery insufficiency: four-vessel cerebral angiogram, magnetic resonance angiogram

Bell palsy: CT scan of mastoids and petrous bones, electromyogram (EMG)

Beriberi: transketolase activity coefficient, urine thiamine afterload, therapeutic trial

Bilharziasis: stool or urine sediment for eggs, rectal biopsy

Biliary cirrhosis: liver function tests, mitochondrial antibodies, serum bile acids, endoscopic retrograde cholangiopancreatography (ERCP), liver biopsy

Blastomycosis: potassium hydroxide (KOH) prep, culture, chest x-ray, skin test, serologic test

Boeck sarcoid: chest x-ray, transbronchial lung biopsy, lymph node biopsy, Kveim test, liver biopsy, angiotensin-converting enzyme liver, gallium scan

Botulism: culture of food and stool, mouse assay of toxin

Brain tumor: CT scan, MRI

Brill–Symmer disease: lymph node biopsy

Bromide poisoning: blood bromide level

Broncheictasis: bronchogram, bronchoscopy, CT scan of lung

Bronchitis: sputum culture, chest x-ray

Bronchopneumonia: sputum smear and culture, chest x-ray, CBC, cold agglutinins

Brucellosis: blood cultures, serologic tests, skin test

Bubonic plague: culture of bubo, blood, or sputum; animal inoculation; serologic test

Buerger disease: phlebogram, arteriogram, biopsy of affected vessels, ultrasonography

Carbon monoxide poisoning: carboxyhemoglobin determination

Carbon tetrachloride poisoning: liver function tests, infrared spectrometry, liver biopsy, blood carbon tetrachloride

Carcinoid syndrome: serum serotonin, urine 5-hydroxyindoleacetic acid (5-HIAA), exploratory laparotomy, bronchoscopy

Carcinoma of the breast: mammogram, sonogram, fine-needle aspiration, biopsy

Carcinoma of the cervix: Papanicolaou (Pap) smears, cervical biopsy, colposcopy

Carcinoma of the colon: stool for occult blood, sigmoidoscopy, barium enema, colonoscopy, carcinoembyonic antigen (CEA), CT scan

Carcinoma of endometrium: Pap smear, dilatation and curettage (D & C)

Carcinoma of the esophagus: barium swallow, esophagoscopy, biopsy

Carcinoma of the lung: chest x-ray, CT scan, sputum Pap smears, brochoscopy and biopsy, needle biopsy, open lung biopsy, scalene node biopsy

Carcinoma of the pancreas: sonogram, CT scan of abdomen, liver function tests, ERCP, exploratory laparotomy, cancer antigen (CA) 19-9

Carcinoma of the stomach: gastrointestinal (GI) series, gastroscopy and biopsy, gastric cytology

Cardiac arrhythmias: ECG, Holter monitoring, echocardiogram, electrophysiologic study

Cardiomyopathy: see Mycarditis/Myocardiopathy

Carpal tunnel syndrome: nerve conduction velocity (NCV) study, MRI

Cat-scratch disease: skin test, lymph node biopsy

Celiac disease: D-xylose absorption, mucosal biopsy, urine 5-HIAA, small bowel series, tissue transglutinase autoantibody titer by Elisa

Cellulitis: smear and culture of wound exudates, antistreptolysin O (ASO) titer

Cerebellar ataxia: CT scan, MRI

Cerebral abscess: CT scan, MRI

Cerebral aneurysm: CT scan, MRI, arteriogram

Cerebral embolism: CT scan, blood culture, echocardiogram, carotid scan, four-vessel cerebral angiogram, ECG

Cerebral hemorrhage: CT scan, MRI

Cerebral thrombosis: CT scan, MRI, carotid scan, digital subtraction angiogram, four-vessel cerebral angiogram

Cerebral spondylosis: x-ray of cervical spine, EMG, MRI of myelogram with simultaneous CT scan

Chagas disease: blood smear and culture, cerebrospinal fluid (CSF) smear and culture, bone marrow or tissue biopsy, animal inoculation, serologic tests

Chancroid: smear and culture of lesion, skin biopsy, serology tests

Child abuse: skeletal survey, chest x-ray, vaginal smear and culture

Chlamydia pneumonia: chest x-ray, serologic tests

Cholangioma: liver function tests, transhepatic cholangiogram, ERCP, CT scan of abdomen, exploratory laparotomy

Cholangitis: liver function tests, transhepatic cholangiogram, ERCP, exploratory laparotomy

Cholecystitis: sonogram, cholecystogram, liver function tests, hepatobiliary iminodiacetic acid scan (HIDA) test

Choledocholithiasis: liver function tests, duodenal drainage, ERCP, transhepatic cholangiogram, sonogram

Cholelithiasis: sonogram, cholecystogram, liver function tests, ERCP

Cholera: stool smear and culture, dark field microscopy

Choriocarcinoma: plasma B-subunit hCG, urine chorionic gonadotropin, D & C

Cirrhosis: liver function tests, liver scan, CT scan, liver biopsy

Coarctation of the aorta: chest x-ray, clinical evaluation, aortograms rarely required

Coccidioidomycosis: smear, animal inoculation, serology, skin test, chest x-ray

Concussion: CT scan, MRI, EEG, evoked potentials, psychometric tests

Congestive heart failure: ECG, test x-rays, spirometry, circulation time, arterial blood gases (ABG), echocardiogram, B-type naturetic peptide (BNP)

Coronary insufficiency: see Angina pectoris

Costochondritis (Tietze syndrome): lidocaine infiltration

Craniopharyngioma: skull x-ray, CT scan, MRI

Cretinism: FT_4 index, thyrotropin, radioactive iodine (RAI) uptake and scan, x-ray for bone age

Crigler–Najjar syndrome: see Gilbert disease

Cryoglobulinemia: serum protein electrophoresis and immunoelectrophoresis, (SIA) water test, cold agglutinins, rheumatoid arthritis (RA) test, hepatitis C antibody titer

Cryptococcosis: spinal fluid smear and culture, sputum or blood cultures, CSF cryptococcal antigen

Cushing syndrome: 24-hour urine free cortisol, plasma cortisol, single-dose overnight dexamethasone suppression test, CT scan of brain or abdomen

Cystic fibrosis: quantitative pilocarpine iontophoresis, sweat test

Cysticercosis: serologic test, CT scan of brain, MRI, biopsy of subcutaneous cysticerci

Cystinosis: slit-lamp examination, liver biopsy

Cystinuria: serum and urine cystine and arginine, Cyanide–nitroprusside test, thin-layer chromatography

Cytomegalic inclusion disease: blood smear for atypical lymphs, cytomegalovirus (CMV), IgM antibody titer, human fibroblastic cell culture innoculation, immunofluorescence technique for viral demonstration

Dehydration: intake and output of fluid, electrolytes, blood urea nitrogen (BUN) to creatinine ratio, serum/urine osmolality

Dengue: viral isolation from blood, serology test

Dermatomyositis: Antinuclear antibody (ANA), aspartate aminotransferase (AST), lactate dehydrogenase (LDH), creatine phosphokinase (CPK), aldolase, EMG, muscle biopsy

Diabetes insipidus: Hickey–Hare test, serum/urine osmolality intake and output before and after pitressin, CT scan, serum antidiuretic hormone (ADH)

Diabetes mellitus: glucose tolerance test, cortisone glucose tolerance test, glycosylated hemoglobin (HbAlc)

Digitalis intoxication: serum digoxin level, ECG

Di Guglielmo disease: bone marrow, peripheral blood study

Diphtheria: Nose and throat culture

Diphyllobothrium latum: stool for ova and parasites, serum B_{12} level

Dissecting aneurysm: chest x-ray, CT scan or MRI of aorta, aortogram

Disseminated intravascular coagulation (DIC): decreased fibrinogen, increased fibrin degradation products, D-Dimer assay

Diverticulosis: sigmoidoscopy, barium enema, colonoscopy, CT scan of abdomen, gallium scan, sonogram, exploratory laparotomy

Down syndrome: chromosome study, urinary B-aminoisobutyric acid

Dracunculiasis: noting presence of worms in subcutaneous tissues, serum IgE, antifilarial antibody titer

Dubin–Johnson syndrome: liver function tests, liver biopsy

Ductus arteriosus, patent: cardiac catheterization, angiocardiogram, echocardiogram

Duodenal ulcer: see Peptic ulcer

Dwarfism: x-ray of bones; endocrine, renal and GI function tests

Dysfunctional uterine bleeding: D & C, endometrial biopsy, progesterone challenge

Eaton–Lambert syndrome: EMG, Tensilon test, muscle biopsy, chest x-ray

Echinococcosis: CT scan, x-ray of long bones, Casoni skin test, serologic tests, liver biopsy

Eclampsia: uric acid, renal function tests, renal biopsy

Ectopic pregnancy: serum β-hCG by immunoassay, sonogram, laparoscopy, culdocentesis, exploratory laparotomy, serum progesterone levels

Eczema: serum IgE levels

Ehlers–Danlos syndrome: capillary fragility test, bleeding time, skin biopsy

Emphysema: pulmonary function tests, ABGs, α-antitrypsin level, single breath diffusing capacity for carbon monoxide

Empyema: chest x-ray, sputum cultures, gallium scan, thoracentesis

Encephalitis: viral isolation from brain tissue and spinal fluid, MRI, serologic tests

Encephalomyelitis: viral isolation from brain tissue and spinal fluid, MRI, serologic tests

Endocardial fibroelastosis: ECG, chest x-ray, echocardiogram, angiocardiogram

Endocarditis: see Subacute bacterial endocarditis

Epilepsy: wake-and-sleep EEG, CT scan or MRI, positron emission tomography (PET) scan, ambulatory EEG monitoring

Erectile dysfunction: penile blood pressure nocturnal tumescence testing, sonogram

Erythema multiforme: skin biopsy, patch test

Erythroblastosis fetalis: bilirubin, direct Coombs test, amniocentesis

Esophageal varices: esophagoscopy, sphlenovenogram, ultrasonography

Esophagitis: Bernstein test, esophagoscopy and biopsy, esophageal manometry, ambulatory pH monitoring

Extradural hematoma: skull x-ray, CT scan, MRI

Endometriosis: sonogram, CA125 levels

Epididymitis: sonogram, radionuclide scan

Fanconi syndrome: x-ray (pelvis, scapula, femor, ribs), urinary amino acids, glucose, electrolytes, serum uric acid, alkaline phosphatase, renal biopsy

Filariasis: blood smear for microfilariae, skin test, complement-fixation test

Folic acid deficiency: serum folic acid, therapeutic trial

Friedlander pneumonia: sputum smear and culture, blood cultures, lung puncture, serial chest x-rays

Friedreich ataxia: clinical diagnosis

Galactosemia: Paigon assay of blood galactose, red blood cell (RBC) assay of (GAL-1-PUT) transferase

Gallstone: see Cholelithiasis

Gargoylism: urinary chondroitin sulfuric acid, serum assay of α-L-iduronidase, tissue culture, enzyme assay

Gastric ulcer: see Peptic Ulcer

Gastritis: serology for *Helicobacter pylori*, gastroscopy, biopsy

Gastroenteritis: stool for culture, smear, and ova and parasites

Gaucher disease: assay of leukocytes for β-glucosidase, bone marrow examination, x-ray of long bones

General paresis: blood and spinal fluid fluorescent treponemal antibody absorption (FTA–ABS) test

Giardia lambia: cathartic stool for ova and parasites, duodenal analysis, Giardia antigen, string test

Gigantism: CT scan or MRI of brain, serum growth hormone

Gilbert disease: liver function tests, liver biopsy

Gilles de la Tourette syndrome: urinary catecholamines

Glanders: culture of skin lesion, skin test, serologic tests, animal inoculation

Glanzmann disease: platelet counts, clot retraction, prothrombin time, bleeding time, capillary fragility test, see also Thrombocythemia

Glaucoma: tonometry, gonioscopy, visual fields

Glomerulonephritis: serum complement, streptozyme test, ANA, renal biopsy

Glossitis: culture, biopsy, therapeutic trial of vitamins and iron

Glycogen storage disease: glucose tolerance test, epinephrine test, liver biopsy and analysis for glucose-6-phosphatase

Goiter: FT_4 index, RAI uptake and scan, thyrotropin, serum antibodies

Gonorrhea: urethral, rectal, vaginal, or throat smear and cultures; DNA probes and polymerase chain reaction (PCR)

Good pasture's syndrome: circulating antiglomerular antibodies, chest x-ray, renal biopsy

Gout: serum uric acid, synovial fluid analysis, x-ray of bones and joints

Granuloma inguinale: Wright stain of scrapings from lesion and biopsy

Graves disease: see Hyperthyroidism

Guillain–Barré syndrome: EMG, spinal fluid analysis

Gumma: FTA–ABS

Haemophilus influenzae: nose, throat, and sputum culture or spinal fluid smear and culture

Hamman–Rich syndrome: chest x-ray, pulmonary function tests, lung biopsy

Hand–Schuller–Christian disease: x-ray of skull, bone biopsy, bone marrow examination

Hansen disease: see Leprosy

Hartnup disease: urinary amino acid, indican, and indoleacetic acid; FT_4 index; thyrotropin

Hashimoto disease: FT_4 index, thyrotropin, serum thyroglobulin antibodies

Haverhill fever: agglutination titer, aspiration of affected joint or abscess for *Streptobacillus moniliformis*

Hay fever: see Allergic rhinitis

Heart failure: see Congestive heart failure

Helminth infections: stool for ova and parasites, serologic tests, skin tests, liver function tests

Hemangioblastoma: CT scan or MRI

Hemochromatosis: serum ferritin, serum iron and iron binding capacity, liver or skin biopsy

Hemoglobin C disease: blood smear for target cells, hemoglobin electrophoresis

Hemoglobinuria, paroxysmal cold: CBC, Coombs test, Donath–Landsteiner test, FTA-ABS, serum haptoglobins

Hemoglobinuria, paroxysmal nocturnal: CBC, Ham test, sucrose hemolysis test

Hemolytic anemia: serum haptoglobins, radioactive chromium–tagged red cell survival, urine and fecal urobilinogen, Coombs test, blood smear

Hemophilia: coagulation profile, thromboplastin generation test, assay of factors VIII, IX, XI

Hepatitis: liver function test, hepatitis profile, IgM, anti–hepatitis A virus (HAV), hepatitis B surface antigen (HBsAG), liver biopsy, anti–hepatitis C virus (HCV)

Hepatitis, chronic active: HBsAG, liver function tests, ANA, liver biopsy, anti–smooth muscle antibody

Hepatolenticular degeneration: see Wilson disease

Hepatoma: ultrasonography, CT scan, α-fetoprotein, liver biopsy, arteriogram, MRI

Hernia, diaphragmatic: see Hiatal hernia

Herniated disc: EMG, MRI, CT scan, myelogram, discogram

Herpangina: serologic tests, viral isolation

Herpes genitalis: examination of skin scrapings, Tzanck test, culture, serologic tests

Herpes simplex: serologic tests, viral isolation, Tzanck test

Herpes zoster: Tzanck test, serologic tests

Hiatal hernia: Bernstein test, esophogram, esophagoscopy and biopsy, esophageal manometry, therapeutic trial

Hirschsprung disease: rectal or colonic biopsy

Histamine cephalgia: test trial of histamine subcutaneously, response to sumatriptin

Histoplasmosis: sputum culture, bone marrow culture, animal inoculation, skin test, serologic tests, chest x-ray

HIV infections: see Acquired Immunodeficiency Syndrome

Hodgkin lymphoma: lymph node biopsy, bone marrow lymphangiogram, CT scan, liver–spleen scan, exploratory laparotomy

Huntington chorea: clinical diagnosis, genetic markers, CT scan

Hurler syndrome: see Gargoylism

Hydronephrosis: intravenous pyelogram (IVP), sonogram

Hyperaldosteronism: see Aldosteronism, primary

Hypercholesterolemia, familial: lipoprotein electrophoresis, lipid profile

Hyperlipemia, idiopathic: lipoprotein electrophoresis, ultracentrifugation

Hypernephroma: IVP or retrograde pyelogram, CT scan, angiogram

Hyperparathyroidism: serum calcium, phosphorus, and alkaline phosphatase; urine calcium; serum parathyroid hormone (PTH); 1,25-(OH)2D; phosphate reabsorption test; exploratory surgery

Hyperprolactinemia: CT scan, MRI of brain

Hypersplenism: CBC, blood smear, red cell survival, spleen/liver ratio, bone marrow, epinephrine test, exploratory laparotomy

Hyperthyroidism: thyroid-stimulating hormone (TSH), free T_3, FT_4 index, free T_4

Hypoparathyroidism: serum calcium and phosphorus, 24-hour urine calcium, skull x-ray, phosphate reabsorption, therapeutic trial, PTH assay, urine cyclic adenosine monophosphate (AMP)

Hypopituitarism: serum cortisol, serum thyroxine, serum growth hormone, serum corticotrophin, thyrotropin, follicle-stimulating hormone (FSH), LH, CT scan, MRI

Hypotension, idiopathic postural: clinical observation, response to vasopressin injection (Pitressin), tests to rule out causes of secondary hypotension

Hypothermia: EKG [J waves (Osborn waves)]

Hypothyroidism: FT_4 index, thyrotropin-sensitive assay, thyroid microsomal antibodies, therapeutic trial

Idiopathic hypertrophic subaortic stenosis: EKG, echocardiography

Ileitis: see Regional enteritis

Inappropriate ADH secretion: plasma and urine osmolality, spot urinary sodium, serum ADH

Infectious mononucleosis: monospot test, heterophil antibody titer, smear for atypical lymphocytes, liver function tests, repeat tests, Epstein-Barr virus (EBV) antibody titer

Influenza, viral: culture of nasopharyngeal washing, complement-fixation tests

Insulinoma: see Islet cell tumor

Interstitial cystitis: cystoscopy and biopsy

Intestinal obstruction: flat plate of the abdomen with lateral decubitus films, double enema, sonogram, CT scan, GI series with diatrizoate maglumine and diatrizoate sodium (Hypague), exploratory laparotomy

Iron deficiency anemia: serum ferritin, serum iron and iron binding capacity, free erythrocyte protoporphyrins (FEP), bone marrow, therapeutic trial

Irritable bowel syndrome: clinical diagnosis

Islet cell tumor: glucose tolerance test 72-hour fast, plasma insulin, C-peptide, tolbutamide tolerance test, pancreatic arteriogram, exploratory laparotomy

Kala azar: blood smear, bone marrow or splenic aspirate for parasites, culture, serologic tests (ELISA)

Kaposi sarcoma: Human Herpes Virus 8 (HHV8) antibody titer, biopsy

Klinefelter syndrome: sex chromatin pattern, testicular biopsy, serum FSH and LH

Kwashiorkor: serum albumin, CBC

Lactase deficiency: lactose tolerance test, mucosal biopsy, hydrogen breath test

Laennec cirrhosis: see Cirrhosis

Larva migrans, visceral: eosinophil count, serum globulin, skin testing, serologic tests, liver biopsy

Laryngeal carcinoma: laryngoscopy

Laryngitis: nose and throat culture, washings for viral studies, laryngoscopy

Lead intoxication: serum and urine lead content, urine for γ-aminolivulinic acid (ALA), coproporphyria FEP, test dose of diaminoethanetetraacetic acid (EDTA), x-ray of long bones

Legionnaire disease: sputum culture, serology, urinary Ag assay

Leishmaniasis: CBC, blood spleen and bone marrow smears for parasites, biopsy, serologic tests

Leprosy: Wade scraped incision procedure, culture of lesion, biopsy of skin nerves, x-ray of hands and feet, histamine tests, lepromin skin test

Leptospirosis: see Weil disease

Lettere–Siwe disease: x-ray of bones, bone marrow, lymph node biopsy

Leukemia: blood smear, bone marrow, uric acid, serum B_{12} concentration, iron binding capacity, Philadelphia chromosome

Listeriosis: blood or spinal fluid smear and spinal fluid agglutination titer, bone marrow biopsy

Liver abscess: liver scan with technetium or gallium, liver aspiration and biopsy, CT scan, amebic hemagglutinin inhibition titer, cathartic stool for ova and parasites

Loeffler syndrome: eosinophil count, sputum for eosinophils, stool for ova and parasites

Lung abscess: chest x-ray, tomogram, CT scan, sputum culture, bronchoscopy, sputum cytology, needle aspiration, biopsy, and culture

Lupoid hepatitis: see Hepatitis, chronic active

Lupus erythematosus: ANA, anti–double-stranded DNA antibody titer (not usually positive in drug-induced lupus), Coombs test, lupus erythematosus prep, coagulation profile, biopsy of skin, muscle, lymph node, or kidney

Lyme disease: serologic tests

Lymphangitis: CBC, sedimentation rate

Lymphogranuloma inguinale: lygranum test, Giemsa-stained smear, serologic tests, tissue or lymph node biopsy

Lymphogranuloma venereum: serologic tests, lymph node biopsy, aspiration of bubo for culture

Lymphoma: see Hodgkin disease

Lymphosarcoma: CT scan, x-rays of chest and abdomen, lymphangiogram

Macroglobulinemia: serum electrophoresis and immunoelectrophoresis, ultracentrifugation, Sia water test, bone marrow

Malabsorption syndrome: D-xylose absorption test, urine 5-HIAA, mucosal biopsy, small-bowel series

Malaria: blood smear for parasites, bone marrow, serologic tests

Mallory–Weiss syndrome: esophagoscopy

Marfan syndrome: x-ray of long bones and ribs, slit-lamp examination of eyes, IVP, urinary hydroxyproline, CT scan of aorta

Marie–Strumpell spondylitis: x-ray of lumbosacral spine, bone scan, HLA typing

Mastocytosis: skin biopsy, Darier sign, long bone x-ray, bone marrow biopsy

Mastoiditis: x-ray of mastoid, CT scan

McArdle syndrome: liver biopsy, enzyme assay of muscle phosphorylase, muscle biopsy, urine myoglobin

Measles: smear of nasal secretions for giant cells, serologic tests

Meckel diverticulum: technetium scan, exploratory laparotomy

Mediastinitis: CT scan or MRI of chest, mediastinoscopy, exploratory surgery

Medullary sponge kidney: IVP, CT scan

Medulloblastoma: CT scan, MRI

Megaloblastic anemia: see Pernicious anemia

Meig syndrome: thoracentesis, culdoscopy, laparoscopy, exploratory laparotomy, sonogram

Melanoma: serum or urinary melanin, biopsy

Ménière disease: CT scan, audiogram, caloric tests, electronystagmography (ENG)

Meningioma: CT scan, MRI, x-ray of skull or spine, myelogram

Meningitis: spinal fluid examination, smear and culture, serum for viral serologic studies, blood culture

Meningococcemia: blood culture spinal fluid examination, smear and culture, Gram stain of punctured petechiae

Menopause syndrome: serum LH, FSH, serum estradiol, vaginal smear for estrogen effects, therapeutic trial

Mental retardation: CT scan or MRI, EEG, psychometric testing, skull x-ray, phenylketonuria (PKU), FT_4 index, thyrotropin, urinary amino acids, chromosomal analysis

Methemoglobinemia: erythrocyte methemoglobin, ABG, blood diaphorase 1, spectrophotometry

Migraine: nitroglycerin test, histamine test, sedimentation rate to rule out temporal arteritis

Mikulicz disease: CBC, bone marrow, tuberculin test, biopsy of lesion, ANA, lymph node biopsy

Milk–alkali syndrome: serum calcium, phosphorus, alkaline phosphatase, urinary calcium and phosphates

Milroy disease: clinical diagnosis

Mitral insufficiency or stenosis: ECG, chest x-ray, echocardiogram, phonocardiogram, cardiac catheterization

Moniliasis: vaginal smear or culture, skin scrapings with KOH prep, biopsy

Mononucleosis, infectious: see Infectious mononucleosis

Mucormycosis: nose and throat culture, biopsy

Mucoviscoidosis: see Cystic fibrosis

Multiple myeloma: serum protein, electrophoresis, 24-hour urine electrophoresis, bone marrow, x-ray of skull and spine, MRI

Multiple sclerosis: somatosensory evoked potentials, (SSEP), visual evoked potential (VEP), spinal fluid globulin (IgG), and myelin basic protein, MRI

Mumps: skin test, serologic tests, viral isolation from throat washings

Muscular dystrophy: EMG, muscle biopsy, urine creatine, chromosome analysis, serum enzyme (creatine kinase, and so forth)

Myasthenia gravis: EMG, Tensilon test, acetylcholine receptor antibody titer, CT scan of chest to rule out thymoma

Mycoplasma pneumoniae: cold agglutinins, (MG) streptococcal agglutinins, culture

Mycosis fungoides: skin biopsy

Myeloid metaplasia, agnogenic: red cell morphology, CBC, bone marrow, leukocyte alkaline phosphatase, urine and serum erythropoietin

Myelophthisic anemia: CBC, bone marrow, bone scan, lymph node biopsy

Myocardial infarction: serial enzymes ([MB], creatine phosphokinase [CPK]), and so forth), serial ECGs serum troponin-1, thallium 201 scintigraphy, pyrophosphate imaging, echocardiogram

Myocarditis/Myocardiopathy: echocardiogram, endomyocardial biopsy, cardiac catheterization

Myotonia atrophica: EMG, urine creatinine and creatine, muscle biopsy

Myxoma, cardiac: echocardiogram, angiocardiogram

Narcolepsy: sleep study, EEG, HLA-DR2

Nematodes: gastric analysis, muscle biopsy, eosinophil count, skin test, serologic tests, stools for ova and parasites, duodenal aspiration for ova and parasites, GI series, rectal swabs with Scotch tape

Nephritis: see Glomerulonephritis

Nephrocalcinosis: serum PTH, serum calcium, phosphorus and alkaline phosphatase, IVP, renal biopsy

Nephrotic syndrome: urinalysis serum complement, sedimentation rate, serum protein electrophoresis, renal function tests, ANA, renal biopsy

Neurinoma, acoustic: see Acoustic neuroma

Neuritis, peripheral: see Neuropathy

Neuroblastoma: urinary vanillylmandelic acid (VMA) and homovanillic acid acid (HVA), CT scan, bone marrow, exploratory laparotomy

Neurofibromatosis: biopsy, skeletal survey, CT scan, spinal fluid analysis, myelogram

Neuropathy: glucose tolerance test, blood lead level, urine porphobilinogen, blood and urine arsenic levels, urine N-methylnicotinamide, ANA, serum B_{12} and folic acid, spinal fluid examination, NCV, EMG, serum transketolase activity coefficient, nerve biopsy

Neurosyphilis: blood and spinal fluid FTA–ABS

Niacin deficiency: see Pellagra

Niemann-Pick disease: demonstration of sphingomyelin in reticuloendothelial cells, bone marrow biopsy, tissue biopsy, skeletal survey, culture of skin fibroblasts

Nocardiosis: sputum smear and culture, spinal fluid examination, smear and culture

Nonketotic hyperosmolar coma: blood sugar, plasma osmolality

Normal pressure hydrocephalus: CT scan, nuclear flow study (radioactive iodinated albumin [RISA])

Nutritional neuropathy: see Neuropathy

Ochronosis: urinalysis (Benedict solution, isolation of homogentisic acid), x-ray of spine

Oppenheim disease: EMG, muscle biopsy

Optic atrophy: CT scan of brain and orbits, visual fields, spinal tap, serum B_{12}, x-ray of skull and optic foramina

Optic neuritis: FTA–ABS antibody titer, visual fields, MRI of the brain

Osteitis deformans: serum calcium, phosphorus, alkaline phosphatase, skeletal survey, bone scan, bone biopsy, urine hydroxyproline

Osteoarthritis: x-ray of spine and joints, exclusion of other forms of arthritis

Osteogenic sarcoma: alkaline and acid phosphatase, x-ray of bone, bone scan, bone biopsy

Osteomalacia: serum calcium phosphorus, alkaline phosphatase, x-ray of long bones, response to vitamin D and calcium, serum vitamin D levels

Osteomyelitis: sedimentation rate, blood culture, culture of bone biopsy, x-ray of bone, bone scan, teichoic acid antibody titer (TAAB)

Osteopetrosis: bone marrow, x-ray of bones, bone biopsy

Osteoporosis: serum, calcium, phosphorus, alkaline phosphatase, bone biopsy, x-ray of spine, quantitative computerized tomogram, bone mineral density (BMD), bone densitometry

Otitis media: nasopharyngeal or aural smear and culture, CBC, sedimentation rate, tympanometry, audiogram

Otosclerosis: audiometry

Ovarian cancer: serum CA125, pelvic sonogram, CT scan of abdomen and pelvis

Paget disease: see Osteitis deformans

Pancreatic carcinoma: see Carcinoma of the pancreas

Pancreatitis, acute: serum amylase and lipase, blood sugar, serum calcium, paracentesis, flat plate of abdomen, 2-hour urinary amylase

Pancreatitis, chronic: serum and urinary amylase and lipase before and after secretin, glucose tolerance test, duodenal analysis for bicarbonate and enzyme concentration, CT scan, ERCP, fecal fat, triolein iodine 131 (^{131}I) uptake

Panniculitis: bone marrow, skin and subcutaneous tissue biopsy

Paralysis agitans: clinical diagnosis

Pediculosis: Woods lamp, microscopic examination of hair shafts

Pellagra: urine *N*-methylnicotinamide, urine niacin after loading dose

Pelvic inflammatory disease (PID): laparoscopy, culture of cervical mucus, exploratory laparotomy

Pemphigus: skin biopsy, Tzanck test, immunofluorescence studies

Penicillin allergy: skin testing with penicilloyl polylysine

Peptic ulcer: upper GI series, stool for occult blood, gastroscopy and duodenoscopy, gastric analysis, serology for *H. pylori*

Periarteritis nodosa: ANA; eosinophil count; CBC; urinalysis; muscle, skin, subcutaneous tissue, and testicular biopsy; nerve biopsy; angiography

Pericarditis: ECG, echocardiogram, chest x-ray, angiocardiogram, pericardial tap, CT scan or MRI

Periodic paralysis, familial: serum potassium, ECG, EMG, response to glucose

Peritonitis: CBC, flat plate of abdomen, CT scan, sonogram, peritoneal tap, exploratory laparotomy

Pernicious anemia: CBC, blood smear, serum B_{12} and folic acid, Schilling test, gastric analysis with histamine, bone marrow

Pertussis: CBC, nasopharyngeal smear and culture

Petit mal: sleep EEG, CT scan

Peutz–Jeghers syndrome: small bowel series, exploratory laparotomy

Pharyngitis: nose and throat culture, rapid agglutination test of throat swab (Abbott test pack strep A, Abbott Laboratries, Abbott Park, IL), streptozyme test

Phenylpyruvic oligophrenia: urine for PKU and phenylalanine, Guthrie test, serum phenylalanine

Pheochromocytoma: plasma and urine catecholamines, 24-hour urine VMA, CT scan, MRI

Phlebitis: see Thrombophlebitis

Phlebotomus fever: serologic tests

Pickwickian syndrome: pulmonary function tests, ABG, sleep study

Pinealoma: CT scan or MRI

Pinworms: Scotch tape swab of perianal area with microscopic examination for eggs

Pituitary adenoma: CT scan, MRI, serum thyrotropin, corticotrophin, LH and FSH, FT_4 index, serum cortisol, growth hormone

Placenta previa: ultrasonography

Plague: see Bubonic plague

Platyhelminthes: stool for ova and parasites, serologic tests, skin test, urine sediment for eggs, eosinophil count

Pleurisy: chest x-ray, thoracentesis, pleural biopsy, bronchoscopy, CT scan, ultrasonography

Pleurodynia, epidemic: serologic tests, stool and throat cultures for Coxsackie B virus

Pneumococcal pneumonia: see Pneumonia

Pneumoconiosis: chest x-ray, pulmonary function tests, ABG, sputum smear, lung biopsy, lung scan, scalene node biopsy

Pneumonia: stat sputum smear, culture, blood cultures, chest x-ray

Pneumothorax: chest x-ray, ABG, CT scan

Poliomyelitis: viral isolation from stool, serologic tests, spinal fluid analysis

Polyarteritis: see Periarteritis nodosa

Polycystic kidney: sonogram, CT scan

Polycystic ovary: see Stein–Leventhal syndrome

Polycythemia vera: CBC, platelet count, uric acid, ABG, pulmonary function tests, serum erythropoietin, bone marrow

Polymyalgia rheumatica: sedimentation rate

Polyneuritis: see Neuropathy

Porphyria: urine porphyrins and porphobilinogen

Portal cirrhosis: see Cirrhosis

Pott disease: x-ray of the spine, aspiration and culture of synovial fluid, synovial or bone biopsy, purified protein derivative (PPD)

Preeclampsia: see Eclampsia

Pregnancy: blood or urine test for pregnancy

Prostate carcinoma: serum acid and alkaline phosphatase, prostate-specific antigen (PSA) skeletal survey, bone scan, biopsy of prostate

Prostatic hypertrophy: sonogram cystoscopy, IVP

Protein-losing enteropathy: I^{131} polyvinylpyrrolidone test, serum protein electrophoresis

Pseudogout: synovial analysis

Pseudomembranous colitis: *Clostridium difficile* toxin B

Pseudohypoparathyroidism: serum calcium, phosphorus, alkaline phosphatase, urine calcium, Ellsworth–Howard test, parathyroid tissue biopsy

Pseudotumor cerebri: CT scan, MRI, spinal tap

Psittacosis: chest x-ray, serologic test, virus isolation

Pulmonary embolism: see Pulmonary infarction

Pulmonary emphysema: see Emphysema

Pulmonary fibrosis: diffusion capacity, bronchoscopy, lung biopsy, CT scan

Pulmonary hypertension, idiopathic: ABG, pulmonary function test, cardiac catheterization, pulmonary angiogram

Pulmonary infarction: ABG, lung scan, pulmonary angiogram, impedance plethysmogram, helical CT scan, rapid D-dimer assay

Pyelonephritis: urine culture, colony count, IVP, cystoscopy, renal biopsy

Pyloric stenosis: GI series, gastroscopy, sonogram

Pyridoxine deficiency: serum iron and iron binding capacity, blood pyridoxine, urine pyridoxic acid

Q fever: serologic tests

Rabies: autopsy of infected animals, isolation of virus from saliva, serum and CSF antibody titer, fluorescent antibody stain of corneal or skin cells

Rat-bite fever: dark field examination, culture of lesion, aspiration and culture of regional lymph node, animal inoculation, serologic tests

Raynaud disease: ANA, lupus erythematosus prep, immunoelectrophoresis, cold agglutinins, cryoglobulins, skin or muscle biopsy, cold challenge

Reflux esophagitis: see Esophagitis

Regional enteritis: sedimentation rate, small bowel series, sigmoidoscopy or colonoscopy and biopsy, surgical exploration

Reiter disease: HLA typing, bone scan, synovial analysis

Relapsing fever: peripheral blood smear for Borrelia organisms, animal inoculation, serologic tests, total leukocytes, spinal tap

Renal calculus: IVP, noncontrast helical CT scan, cystoscopy, retrograde pyelogram, sonogram, stone analysis

Renal tubular acidosis: serum electrolytes, calcium, phosphorus, alkaline phosphatase, urine calcium, phosphatase and bicarbonate, urine pH after ammonium chloride load

Respiratory distress syndrome: Ratio PaO_2 to FiO_2, pulmonary artery catheterization

Reticuloendotheliosis: x-ray, CBC, tissue cholesterol content, biopsy of skeletal lesion, bone marrow, or lymph nodes

Reticulum cell sarcoma: alkaline phosphatase, lymph node biopsy, x-ray of chest, skeletal survey, GI series, IVP, cytologic examination of pleural or ascitic fluid

Rheumatic fever: throat culture, streptozyme test, C-reactive protein (CRP), sedimentation rate, ECG, echocardiogram, serial ASO titer

Rheumatoid arthritis: RA test, sedimentation rate, ANA, x-ray of joints, synovial fluid analysis

Riboflavin deficiency: activity coefficient of erythrocyte glutathione reductase

Rickets: serum calcium, phosphorus, alkaline phosphatase, urine calcium, x-ray of bones, serum PTH, serum 25-OHD, bone biopsy

Rickettsialpox: serologic tests

Rocky Mountain spotted fever: specific serologic tests, Weil–Felix test, fluorescent antibody staining of skin lesions

Rubella: viral isolation, latex agglutination card assay, other serologic tests

Rubeola: see Measles

Saddle embolus of aorta: oscillometry, Doppler flow study, aortogram

Salicylate intoxication: serum or urine salicylates, electrolytes

Salmonellosis: stool culture, febrile agglutinins

Salpingitis: vaginal smear and culture, sonogram, laparoscopy, exploratory surgery

Sarcoidosis: chest x-ray, Kveim test, lymph node biopsy, elevated angiotensin converting enzymes, gallium scan

Scabies: KOH prep

Scalenus anticus syndrome: x-ray of cervical spine, arteriogram

Scarlet fever: nose and throat culture, streptozyme test, Schultz–Charlton reaction

Schilder disease: EEG, CT scan, MRI, spinal tap, brain biopsy

Schistosomiasis: stool or urine for ova, rectal biopsy, liver biopsy, serologic tests

Schönlein–Henoch purpura: urinalysis, platelet count, coagulation profile, bleeding time, capillary fragility

Schuller–Christian disease: see Hand–Schuller–Christian disease

Scleroderma: ANA, RA test, anticentromere antibody titer, skin biopsy, esophagram, malabsorption workup

Scurvy: serum ascorbic acid, capillary fragility, x-ray of bones, therapeutic trial

Seminoma: urine hCG, sonogram, exploratory surgery, α fetoprotein

Septicemia: blood culture

Sexual precocity: skull x-ray, CT scan, urine 17-ketosteroids and 17-hydroxysteroids, plasma cortisol, metyrapone test, exploratory surgery

Shigellosis: stool examination for leukocytes, stool culture

Sickle cell anemia: CBC, blood smear, sickle cell preparation, hemoglobin electrophoresis

Silicosis: chest x-ray, pulmonary function tests, ABG, lung biopsy, CT scan

Silo-filler's disease: chest x-ray, clinical observations

Simmond disease: see Hypopituitarism

Sinusitis: x-ray of sinuses, CT scan of sinuses, nose and throat culture, erythrocyte sedimentation rate (ESR), CRP

Sjogren syndrome: Schirmer test for tear production, ANA, RA titer, HLA typing, thyroglobulin antibody titer, anti-Sjogren syndrome B (La) antibody titer

Smallpox: smear of vesicular fluid for virus particles, viral isolation, serologic test

Spherocytosis, hereditary: CBC, blood smear, red cell fragility test, reticulocyte count, serum haptoglobins, bilirubin

Spinal cord tumor: x-ray of spine, CT scan of spine, MRI

Spinal stenosis: CT scan, MRI, myelogram

Sporotrichosis: cultures of exudates from ulcer, serologic tests, skin tests, chest x-ray

Staphylococcal pneumonia: sputum smear and culture, chest x-ray

Steatorrhea: see Celiac disease

Stein–Leventhal syndrome: culdoscopy, laparoscopy, serum LH, urine 17-ketosteroids, sonogram, exploratory surgery, biopsy of ovaries

Stevens–Johnson syndrome: streptozyme test, nose and throat culture

Still disease: RA test, sedimentation rate, CRP, synovianalysis

Stokes–Adams syndrome: ECG, Holter monitoring, event monitoring, electrophysiologic testing

Streptococcal pharyngitis: see Pharyngitis

Strongyloidiasis: stool or duodenal aspirate for ova and parasites

Sturge–Weber syndrome: skull x-ray, CT scan, MRI

Subacute bacterial endocarditis: blood culture, bone marrow cultures, echocardiogram, RA test, FTA–ABS, transesophageal echocardiography

Subarachnoid hemorrhage: CT scan of brain, spinal tap, arteriogram

Subdiaphragmatic abscess: chest x-ray, gallium scan, indium scan, CT scan, needle aspiration, exploratory surgery

Subdural hematoma: CT scan, MRI, arteriogram

Subphrenic abscess: see Subdiaphragmatic abscess

Substance abuse: blood alcohol level, urine drug screen, CAGE questionnaire

Sulfhemoglobinemia: shaking of venous blood in test tube, spectroscopic examination of blood

Syphilis: blood and spinal fluid venereal disease research laboratory (VDRL) test or FTA–ABS, dark field microscopy

Syringomyelia: CT scan, myelogram, MRI

Tabes dorsalis: blood and spinal fluid, FTA–ABS

Takayasu disease: CT scan of aorta, aortogram, serum protein electrophoresis

Tapeworm infections: stool for ova and parasites, serology, sonogram, CT scan

Tay-Sachs disease: cortical biopsy

Temporal arteritis: sedimentation rate, biopsy of temporal artery

Tetanus: clinical diagnosis, positive culture does not establish diagnosis

Thalassemia: CBC, blood smear, reticulocyte count, serum haptoglobin, hemoglobin electrophoresis

Thromboangiitis obliterans: see Buerger disease

Thrombocythemia (thrombasthenia): platelet count, bleeding time, clotting time, clot retraction, capillary fragility

Thrombocytopenic purpura, idiopathic: coagulation profile, platelet count, platelet antibody titer, bone marrow, liver–spleen scan, capillary fragility

Thrombophlebitis: impedance plethysmography, compression ultrasonography, fibrinogen I 125 scan, venogram, thermogram, ultrasonography

Thymoma: chest x-ray, CT scan of mediastinum, mediatinoscopy, exploratory thoracotomy

Thyroiditis, subacute: FT_4 index, RAI uptake and scan, sedimentation rate, antithyroid autoantibodies

Thyroid carcinoma: serum calcitonin, RAI uptake and scan, CT scan of the neck

Thyroid nodule: RAI uptake and scan, fine-needle aspiration, biopsy, FT_4 index, sonogram, trial of thyroid suppression therapy

Tonsilitis: see Pharyngitis

Torsion of testicle: ultrasonography, radionuclide scintigraphy

Tourette syndrome: clinical diagnosis

Torulosis: see Cryptococcosis

Toxemia of pregnancy: see Eclampsia

Toxoplasmosis: indirect fluorescent antibody (IFA) titer, passive hemogglutination test (PHA), skin test, animal inoculation

Trachoma: smear of conjunctival scrapings, culture for *Chlamydia*, tears for microimmunofluorescent antibodies

Transfusion reaction: serum hemoglobins and methemalbumin, Coombs test

Transient ischemic attack (TIA): carotid scan, digital subtraction angiogram, CT scan, four-vessel cerebral angiogram, MRI

Trichinosis: eosinophil count, skin test, serologic tests, muscle biopsy

Trypanosomiasis: smears and culture of blood, CSF, lymph node aspirate for parasites, animal inoculation, serology

Tuberculosis: smear and culture of sputum and gastric washings, Guinea pig inoculation, skin test, chest x-ray, CT scan

Tuberosclerosis: skull x-ray, CT scan, skin biopsy, cortical biopsy, EEG

Tularemia: smear and culture of ulcer, lymph nodes, or nasopharynx; Foshay skin test; serologic tests

Turner syndrome: buccal smear for chromatins (Barr bodies), chromosome analysis

Typhoid fever: culture of stool, blood, or bone marrow; febrile agglutinins

Typhus, epidemic: serologic tests, Weil–Felix reaction

Typhus scrub: isolation from blood, serologic tests, Weil–Felix reaction

Ulcer: see Peptic ulcer

Ulcerative colitis: barium enema, sigmoidoscopy or colonoscopy, biopsy

Urethritis: urethral smear and culture, vaginal smear and culture, urine culture, *Chlamydia* culture, cystoscopy

Uterine fibroids: sonogram, CT scan, MRI

Urticaria: RAST, allergic skin testing, elimination diet, C'I esterase inhibitor

Uveitis: slit-lamp examination, ANA, HLA-B27 typing, VDRL, lyme serology

Varicella: serologic tests

Varicose veins: phlebogram, thermogram

Variola: see Smallpox

Ventricular septal defects: ECG, echocardiogram, cardiac catheterization

Visceral larva migrans: blood typing, serologic tests, biopsy

Vitamin A deficiency: serum vitamin A or carotene, skin biopsy

Vitamin B deficiency: see Beriberi

Vitamin C deficiency: see Scurvy

Vitamin D deficiency: see Rickets

Vitamin K deficiency: coagulation profile including prothrombin time

Von Gierke disease: see Glycogen storage disease

Von Willebrand disease: coagulation profile, thromboplastin-generation test, factor VIII assay

Waterhouse-Friderichsen syndrome: blood cultures, spinal fluid examination, nose and throat culture, plasma cortisol

Wegener granulomatosis: x-ray of nose, sinuses, and chest; urinalysis; renal biopsy; lung biopsy; nasal biopsy; antineutrophil cytoplasmic antigen(ANCA)

Weil disease: dark field examination of blood, Guinea pig inoculation, serologic tests, spinal tap

Wernicke encephalopathy: response to intravenous thiamine

Whipple disease: small-bowel series, lymph node biopsy, jejunal biopsy, malabsorption tests

Whooping cough: see Pertussis

Wilson disease: urine copper and amino acids, serum copper and ceruloplasmin, liver biopsy, slip-lamp examination of cornea, uric acid

Yaws: dark field examination, serologic tests

Yellow fever: viral isolation, serologic tests, liver biopsy

Zollinger–Ellison syndrome: 12-hour quantitative and basal gastric acid output (BAO) gastric analysis, serum gastrin, GI series, gastroscopy, exploratory laparotomy

Answers to Questions on Case Presentations

Case #1

Question #1

1. Gall bladder hydrops
2. Courvoisier gall bladder with pancreatic carcinoma
3. Duodenal diverticulum
4. Hepatitis
5. Cirrhosis of the liver
6. Metastatic carcinoma
7. Pancreatic pseudocyst
8. Hypernephroma
9. Colon, carcinoma
10. Hernia
11. Cholangioma
12. Other causes of hepatomegaly

Question #2

1. Courvoisier gall bladder with pancreatic carcinoma
2. Carcinoma of the common duct
3. Carcinoma of the ampulla of Vater
4. Common duct stone
5. Cholangioma

Final Diagnosis: Ultrasonography confirmed that the mass indeed was an enlarged gall bladder, and CT scan demonstrated a carcinoma of the head of the pancreas.

Case #2

Question #1

1. Appendiceal abscess
2. Meckel diverticulum
3. Intussusception
4. Regional ileitis
5. Incarcerated inguinal hernia
6. Contusion of the abdominal wall
7. Ptosis of kidney

Question #2

1. Ruptured appendiceal abscess
2. Ruptured Meckel diverticulum
3. Peritonitis

Final Diagnosis: Exploratory laparotomy revealed a ruptured appendiceal abscess with peritonitis.

Case #3

Question #1

1. Chronic pancreatitis
2. Pancreatic pseudocyst
3. Pyloric ulcer with walled off perforation
4. Omental cyst or hernia
5. Pancreatic carcinoma
6. Ventral hernia
7. Retroperitoneal sarcoma
8. Aortic aneurysm
9. Carcinoma of the stomach
10. Liver abscess
11. Other causes of hepatomegaly

Question #2

1. Pancreatic pseudocyst
2. Chronic pancreatitis
3. Carcinoma of the pancreas

Final Diagnosis: CT scan and ultrasonography confirmed a diagnosis of pancreatic pseudocyst.

Case #4

Question #1

1. Acute cholecystitis
2. Acute pancreatitis
3. Peptic ulcer
4. Acute hepatitis
5. Myocardial infarction
6. Pyelophlebitis
7. Porphyria
8. Black widow spider bite
9. Pneumonia
10. Pyelonephritis
11. Common duct stone
12. Renal colic
13. Retrocecal appendicitis

Question #2

1. Acute cholecystitis
2. Common duct stone
3. Acute pancreatitis

Final Diagnosis: Ultrasonography confirmed the presence of gall stones, and endoscopic retrograde cholangiography revealed a stone in the common duct.

Case #5

Question #1

1. Ruptured ectopic pregnancy
2. Salpingitis
3. Ruptured or twisted ovarian cyst
4. Diverticulitis
5. Urethral calculus
6. Incarcerated femoral or inguinal hernia
7. Intestinal obstruction
8. Mesenteric thrombosis
9. Porphyria
10. Mittelschmerz

Question #2

1. Ruptured ectopic pregnancy
2. Salpingitis
3. Ruptured or twisted ovarian cyst

Final Diagnosis: Ultrasonography and an exploratory laparotomy confirmed the diagnosis of a ruptured ectopic pregnancy.

Case #6

Question #1

1. Coronary insufficiency
2. Herniated cervical disc
3. Cervical spondylosis
4. Thoracic outlet syndrome
5. Pancoast tumor
6. Brachial plexus neuritis
7. Thalamic syndrome
8. Subacromial bursitis
9. Space-occupying lesion of the spinal cord
10. Sympathetic dystrophy
11. Rheumatoid arthritis or osteoarthritis of the shoulder joint
12. Torn rotator cuff

Question #2

1. Herniated cervical disc
2. Cervical spondylosis
3. Compression fracture of the cervical spine
4. Space-occupying lesion of cervical spine

Final Diagnosis: MRI of the cervical spine revealed a herniated disc at C5–C6.

Case #7

Question #1

1. Thrombocytopenia purpura
2. Meningococcemia
3. Subacute bacterial endocarditis
4. D I C

5. Henoch–Schönlein purpura
6. Collagen disease
7. Rocky Mountain spotted fever
8. Acute leukemia
9. Weil disease
10. Scurvy

Question #2

1. Meningococcemia with meningococcal meningitis
2. Rocky Mountain spotted fever
3. D I C
4. Other coagulation disorders with subarachnoid hemorrhage

Final Diagnosis: A spinal tap revealed 1100 **WBC**/cubic centimeter, elevated CSF pressure, and smear and cultures were positive for *Neisseria meningitidis*.

Case #8

Question #1

1. Retinal artery occlusion
2. Glaucoma
3. Optic neuritis
4. Iridocyclitis
5. Vitreous hemorrhage
6. Retinal vein thrombosis
7. Migraine
8. Retinal detachment
9. Diabetic retinopathy
10. Internal carotid artery thrombosis

Question #2

1. Internal carotid artery
2. Thrombosis or embolism

Final Diagnosis: Magnetic resonance angiography confirmed the diagnosis.

Case #9

Question #1

1. Chest wall trauma
2. Tietze syndrome
3. Pericarditis
4. Myocardial infarction
5. Coronary insufficiency
6. Reflux esophagitis and hiatal hernia
7. Pneumothorax
8. Pulmonary embolism
9. Dissecting aneurysm
10. Gastric ulcer
11. Pancreatitis
12. Cholecystitis

Question #2

1. Reflux esophagitis
2. Gastric ulcer
3. Cholecystitis
4. Pulmonary embolism
5. Coronary insufficiency

Final Diagnosis: The pain was relieved by Xylocaine viscus. A Bernstein test and esophagoscopy confirmed a diagnosis of reflux esophagitis.

Case #10

Question #1

1. Brain abscess
2. Cerebral hemorrhage, thrombosis, or embolism
3. Other space-occupying lesion of the brain
4. Meningitis
5. Viral encephalitis
6. Epilepsy in the postictal state
7. Thyroid crisis
8. Collagen disease
9. Thrombotic thrombocytopenic purpura
10. D I C

Question #2

1. Subacute bacterial endocarditis (SBE) with cerebral embolism
2. Collagen disease
3. D I C
4. Thrombotic thrombocytopenic purpura

Final Diagnosis: Blood cultures were positive for alpha hemolytic streptococci, and MRI demonstrated an infarction in the left middle cerebral artery distribution, confirming the diagnosis of SBE with a cerebral embolism.

Case #11

Question #1

1. Pancoast tumor
2. Carotid thrombosis
3. Migraine
4. Thoracic outlet syndrome
5. Spinal cord tumor
6. Aortic aneurysm
7. Mediastinal tumor
8. Basilar artery insufficiency

Question #2

1. Thoracic outlet syndrome
2. Subclavian Steal syndrome
3. Pancoast tumor

Final Diagnosis: Adson tests and four-vessel cerebral angiography confirmed the diagnosis of thoracic outlet syndrome due to hypertrophied scalenus anticus muscle.

Case #12

Question #1

1. Space-occupying lesion of the brain
2. Post-traumatic epilepsy
3. Cerebral hemorrhage

4. Lead encephalopathy
5. Cerebral aneurysm
6. Arteriovenous malformation
7. Migraine
8. Viral encephalitis
9. Collagen disease
10. Porphyria
11. Toxic or metabolic encephalopathy

Question #2

1. Metastatic carcinoma in the parasagittal area of the brain
2. Other space-occupying lesion
3. Anterior cerebral artery aneurysm or thrombosis
4. Arteriovenous malformation
5. Collagen disease

Final Diagnosis: Metastatic carcinoma

Case #13

Question #1

1. Toxic encephalopathy due to drugs
2. Viral encephalitis
3. Bacterial meningitis
4. Early diabetic acidosis
5. Postictal state of epilepsy
6. Cerebral concussion

Question #2

1. Toxic encephalopathy due to drugs
2. Cerebral concussion
3. Postictal state of epilepsy

Final Diagnosis: A urine drug screen demonstrated phencyclidine, confirming the diagnosis of toxic encephalopathy due to drugs.

Case #14

Question #1

1. Presenile dementia
2. Pellagra
3. Pancreatic carcinoma
4. Apathetic hyperthyroidism
5. Tuberculosis
6. Cerebral arteriosclerosis
7. Chronic alcoholism or drug abuse
8. Porphyria
9. Hyperparathyroidism
10. Adrenal insufficiency
11. Hypopituitarism

Question #2

1. Apathetic hyperthyroidism

Final Diagnosis: Laboratory studies revealed an increased free T4 and low TSH confirming the diagnosis of apathetic hyperthyroidism.

Case #15

Question #1

1. Chronic pancreatitis
2. Chronic cholecystitis
3. Regional ileitis
4. Irritable bowel syndrome
5. Overuse of antacids
6. Pernicious anemia
7. Pellagra
8. Amebiasis
9. Zollinger–Ellison syndrome
10. Lactose intolerance

Question #2

1. Zollinger–Ellison syndrome
2. Regional enteritis
3. Amebiasis

Final Diagnosis: Serum gastrin was elevated significantly, confirming the diagnosis of Zollinger–Ellison syndrome.

Case #16

Question #1

1. Cavernous sinus thrombosis
2. Sphenoid ridge meningioma
3. Syphilitic meningitis
4. Space-occupying lesion of the brain with tentorial herniation
5. Diabetic neuropathy
6. Multiple sclerosis
7. Aneurysm of the circle of Willis
8. Weber syndrome
9. Brainstem glioma
10. Tuberculous meningitis

Question #2

1. Aneurysm of the circle of Willis
2. Syphilitic meningitis
3. Tuberculous meningitis

Final Diagnosis: Cerebral angiography confirmed the diagnosis of a large aneurysm of the right internal carotid artery. CT scan demonstrated a subarachnoid hemorrhage.

Case #17

Question #1

1. Otitis media
2. Acute labyrinthitis
3. Toxic labyrinthitis
4. Benign positional vertigo
5. Cholesteatoma
6. Acoustic neuroma
7. Méniére disease
8. Multiple sclerosis
9. Basilar artery insufficiency
10. Vestibular neuronitis

Question #2

1. Multiple sclerosis
2. Basilar artery insufficiency
3. Aneurysm of the basilar artery or its tributaries

Final Diagnosis: An MRI of the brain and brainstem confirmed a diagnosis of multiple sclerosis.

Case #18

Question #1

1. Myasthenia gravis
2. Ophthalmoplegic migraine
3. Basilar artery insufficiency
4. Multiple sclerosis
5. Cerebral aneurysm
6. Wernicke encephalopathy
7. Drug intoxication

Question #2

1. Myasthenia gravis

Final Diagnosis: A Tensilon test revealed the symptoms, and a high titer of acetylcholine receptor antibodies confirmed the diagnosis of myasthenia gravis.

Case #19

Question #1

1. Congestive heart failure
2. Pulmonary emphysema
3. Bronchial asthma
4. Pulmonary fibrosis
5. Pulmonary embolism
6. Foreign body
7. Methemoglobinemia
8. Acute respiratory distress syndrome
9. Pneumothorax
10. Anemia

Question #2

1. Congestive heart failure with uncontrolled auricular fibrillation due to a myocardial infarction
2. Acute respiratory distress syndrome
3. Congestive heart failure with auricular fibrillation due to hyperthyroidism

Final Diagnosis: An EKG and test of cardiac enzymes confirmed the diagnosis of a recent myocardial infarction with auricular fibrillation causing the congestive heart failure.

Case #20

Question #1

1. Acute prostatitis
2. Acute pyelonephritis
3. Reiter syndrome

4. Cystitis
5. Hypernephroma complicated by pyelonephritis
6. Renal or vesical calculus complicated by pyelonephritis
7. Tuberculosis
8. Gonorrhea with systemic complications

Question #2

1. Acute prostatitis
2. Acute pyelonephritis
3. Gonorrhea with systemic complications

Final Diagnosis: Rectal examination revealed an enlarged tender and boggy prostate, confirming the diagnosis of acute prostatitis.

Case #21

Question #1

1. Congestive heart failure due to alcoholic cardiomyopathy
2. Cirrhosis of the liver
3. Nephrotic syndrome due to diabetes mellitus
4. Beriberi heart disease
5. Collagen disease

Question #2

1. Congestive heart failure due to alcoholic cardiomyopathy aggravated by the use of a beta blocker.

Final Diagnosis: The pitting edema resolved upon discontinuing the timolol, confirming the above diagnosis.

Case #22

Question #1

1. Schmincke tumor
2. Tuberculosis
3. Chronic rhinitis
4. Coagulation disorder
5. Symptomatic or essential hypertension
6. Pulmonary emphysema

Question #2

1. Pulmonary emphysema
2. Bronchial asthma

Final Diagnosis: Pulmonary function studies and arterial blood gas confirmed the diagnosis of chronic pulmonary emphysema.

Case #23

Question #1

1. Hyperthyroidism
2. Islet cell adenoma
3. Functional hypoglycemia
4. Pheochromocytoma
5. Infectious disease

6. Caffeine or other drug use or abuse
7. Chronic anxiety neurosis
8. Cardiac arrhythmia
9. Occult neoplasm

Question #2

1. Pheochromocytoma
2. Migraine

Final Diagnosis: A 24-hour urine vanillylmandelic acid was elevated, confirming the diagnosis of pheochromocytoma.

Case #24

Question #1

1. Migraine
2. Glaucoma
3. Temporal arteritis
4. Acute sinusitis
5. Cavernous sinus thrombosis
6. Space-occupying lesion of the brain
7. Cluster headaches

Question #2

1. Glaucoma
2. Temporal arteritis
3. Migraine
4. Acute sinusitis

Final Diagnosis: Tonometry revealed increased ocular pressure in the right eye, confirming the diagnosis of glaucoma.

Case #25

Question #1

1. Acute maxillary sinusitis
2. Temporal arteritis
3. Cluster headaches
4. Trigeminal neuralgia
5. Temporomandibular joint syndrome
6. Abscessed tooth
7. Orbital cellulitis
8. Herpes zoster

Question #2

1. Acute maxillary sinusitis

Final Diagnosis: X-rays of the sinuses confirmed a diagnosis of acute maxillary sinusitis.

Case #26

Question #1

1. Bell palsy
2. Multiple sclerosis
3. Myasthenia gravis
4. Mastoiditis

5. Basilar artery insufficiency
6. Acoustic neuroma
7. Herpes zoster

Question #2

1. Guillain–Barré syndrome
2. Poliomyelitis
3. Muscular dystrophy
4. Myasthenia gravis

Final Diagnosis: Spinal fluid analysis revealed a marked elevation of protein but normal cell count, confirming the diagnosis of Guillain–Barré syndrome.

Case #27

Question #1

1. Scarlet fever
2. Drug reaction
3. Rheumatic fever
4. Infectious mononucleosis
5. Acute leukemia
6. Measles
7. Cytomegalovirus
8. Diphtheria
9. Viral tonsillitis

Question #2

1. Infectious mononucleosis
2. Drug reaction
3. Acute leukemia

Final Diagnosis: A heterophil antibody titer confirmed the diagnosis of infectious mononucleosis.

Case #28

Question #1

1. Hydronephrosis
2. Hypernephroma
3. Polycystic kidneys
4. Benign renal cyst
5. Pheochromocytoma
6. Adrenocortical adenoma or carcinoma
7. Neuroblastoma
8. Tuberculosis
9. Retroperitoneal sarcoma

Question #2

1. Hypernephroma
2. Renal tuberculosis
3. Hydronephrosis
4. Benign renal cyst

Final Diagnosis: A CT scan of the abdomen confirmed the diagnosis of a hypernephroma.

Case #29

Question #1

1. Renal calculus
2. Pyelonephritis
3. Perinephric abscess
4. Renal tuberculosis
5. Renal artery embolism
6. Renal vein thrombosis
7. Renal neoplasm
8. Contusion or laceration
9. Herpes zoster

Question #2

1. Herpes zoster
2. Herniated thoracic disc
3. Tabes dorsalis
4. Epidural abscess
5. Compression fracture of the spine

Final Diagnosis: The following day the patient developed a vesicular rash in the left T12 dermatome, confirming the diagnosis of herpes zoster.

Case #30

Question #1

1. Reflux esophagitis
2. Gastric ulcer
3. Chronic gastritis
4. Gastric carcinoma
5. Pancreatic carcinoma
6. Plummer–Vinson syndrome
7. Pernicious anemia
8. Esophageal carcinoma
9. Cholecystitis
10. Malabsorption syndrome

Question #2

1. Pernicious anemia
2. Malabsorption syndrome
3. Iron deficiency anemia

Final Diagnosis: A Schilling test confirmed the diagnosis of pernicious anemia.

Case #31

Question #1

1. Menopause
2. Chronic alcoholism
3. Primary or secondary polycythemia
4. Carcinoid syndrome
5. Systemic mastocytosis
6. Medullary carcinoma of the thyroid
7. Cushing syndrome

Final Diagnosis: Urine 5-hydroxyindole acetic acid was significantly elevated, confirming the diagnosis of a carcinoid tumor with liver metastasis.

Case #32

Question #1

1. Gout
2. Arterial embolism
3. Cellulitis
4. Osteomyelitis
5. Fracture
6. Other forms of arthritis
7. Ingrown toenail
8. Phlebitis
9. Metatarsalgia
10. Peripheral arteriosclerosis
11. Herniated lumbar disc

Question #2

1. Gout
2. Cellulitis
3. Osteomyelitis
4. Other forms of arthritis

Final Diagnosis: Serum uric acid was elevated, and the patient responded to a therapeutic trial of colchicine, confirming the diagnosis of gout.

Case #33

Question #1

1. Neurogenic bladder
2. Cystitis
3. Bladder neck obstruction
4. Bladder calculus
5. Polyuria
6. Extrinsic lesions of the bladder (salpingitis, ectopic pregnancy, e.g.)

Question #2

1. Multiple sclerosis
2. Space-occupying lesion of the spinal cord
3. Syphilitic meningomyelitis

Final Diagnosis: Magnetic resonance imaging of the thoracic spine confirmed a diagnosis of multiple sclerosis.

Case #34

Question #1

1. Parkinson disease
2. Muscular dystrophy
3. Peripheral neuropathy
4. Cervical spondylosis
5. Hereditary cerebellar ataxia
6. Multiple sclerosis

7. Space-occupying lesion of high cervical cord
8. Chronic demyelinating neuropathy

Question #2

1. Muscular dystrophy
2. Diabetic neuropathy

Final Diagnosis: Myotonic dystrophy was confirmed by electromyography and muscle biopsy.

Case #35

Question #1

1. Inguinal hernia
2. Femoral hernia
3. Lymphadenopathy
4. Cellulitis
5. Aneurysm
6. Varicose vein
7. Undescended testicle
8. Hypertrophic osteoarthritis
9. Lipoma
10. Neurofibroma

Question #2

1. Direct or indirect inguinal hernia

Final Diagnosis: Surgery confirmed a diagnosis of indirect inguinal hernia.

Case #36

Question #1

1. Osteoarthritis of the hips
2. Osteomyelitis
3. Renal colic
4. Regional ileitis
5. Sliding hernia
6. Herniated lumbar or thoracic disc
7. Phlebitis
8. Postherpetic neuralgia
9. Meralgia paresthetica

Question #2

1. Herniated thoracic or lumbar disc
2. Diabetic neuropathy
3. Postherpetic neuralgia

Final Diagnosis: MRI revealed a herniated disc at the T12–L1 level of the spine.

Case #37

Question #1

1. Hemochromatosis
2. Pituitary tumor
3. Klinefelter syndrome

4. Alcoholic cirrhosis liver
5. Adrenocortical tumor or hyperplasia
6. Hyperthyroidism

Question #2

1. Hemochromatosis
2. Alcoholic cirrhosis
3. Other liver disorder plus chronic pancreatitis

Final Diagnosis: Elevated serum iron, iron binding capacity, and liver biopsy confirmed the diagnosis of hemochromatosis.

Case #38

Question #1

1. Bilateral carpal tunnel syndrome
2. Raynaud phenomena
3. Rheumatoid arthritis
4. Thoracic outlet syndrome
5. Herniated cervical disc
6. Cervical spondylosis

Question #2

1. Bilateral carpal tunnel syndrome

Final Diagnosis: Carpal tunnel syndrome was confirmed by nerve conduction velocity testing.

Case #39

Question #1

1. Migraine
2. Space-occupying lesion of the brain
3. Subarachnoid hemorrhage
4. Cerebral hemorrhage
5. Meningitis
6. Hypertensive encephalopathy
7. Encephalitis
8. Muscle traction headache
9. Concussion
10. Postspinal tap headache

Question #2

1. Subarachnoid hemorrhage
2. Meningitis

Final Diagnosis: Subarachnoid hemorrhage due to a ruptured aneurysm of the anterior communicating artery.

Case #40

Question #1

1. Reflux esophagitis
2. Coronary insufficiency
3. Pericarditis
4. Gastritis
5. Peptic ulcer

6. Cholecystitis
7. Chronic pancreatitis
8. Mediastinitis

Question #2

1. Coronary insufficiency

Final Diagnosis: Thallium scans and coronary angiography confirmed a diagnosis of coronary insufficiency.

Case #41

Question #1

1. Acute hemorrhagic gastritis
2. Gastric ulcer
3. Duodenal ulcer
4. Gastric carcinoma
5. Reflux esophagitis
6. Mallory–Weiss syndrome
7. Hereditary telangiectasis
8. Coagulation disorder

Question #2

1. Mallory–Weiss syndrome

Final Diagnosis: Esophagoscopy confirmed the diagnosis of Mallory–Weiss syndrome.

Case #42

Question #1

1. Renal calculus
2. Renal artery embolism
3. Pyelonephritis
4. Glomerulonephritis
5. Contusion or laceration of the kidney
6. Coagulation disorder

Question #2

1. Malingering

Final Diagnosis: Malingering (The patient was found to have a history of narcotic addiction.)

Case #43

Question #1

1. Bronchiectasis
2. Tuberculosis
3. Bronchogenic carcinoma
4. Chronic bronchitis and emphysema
5. Cystic fibrosis
6. Bronchial adenoma
7. Collagen disease
8. Sarcoidosis
9. Fungal disease
10. Congestive heart failure

Question #2

1. Bronchiectasis
2. Early bronchogenic carcinoma

Final Diagnosis: High resolution computed tomography confirmed the diagnosis of bronchiectasis.

Case #44

Question #1

1. Alcoholic cirrhosis
2. Chronic active hepatitis
3. Hemochromatosis
4. Metastatic carcinoma
5. Gaucher disease
6. Myeloid metaplasia
7. Leukemia
8. Tuberculosis
9. Parasitic infection
10. Collagen disease

Question #2

1. Schistosomiasis
2. Chronic active hepatitis
3. Other parasitic disease

Final Diagnosis: Schistosomiasis was confirmed by liver biopsy and stools for ovum and parasites.

Case #45

Question #1

1. Wilson disease
2. Alcoholic cirrhosis
3. Hepatic encephalopathy
4. Chronic pancreatitis
5. Pancreatic carcinoma
6. Hepatoma
7. Hodgkin lymphoma
8. Amebic abscess of the liver
9. Reflux esophagitis
10. Chronic gastritis

Question #2

1. Subphrenic abscess
2. Amebic abscess of the liver

Final Diagnosis: Subphrenic abscess was confirmed by transthoracic aspiration of the subdiaphragmatic space.

Case #46

Question #1

1. Metastatic carcinoma
2. Osteoarthritis
3. Rheumatoid arthritis
4. Multiple myeloma

5. Herniated lumbar disc
6. Fracture of the hip
7. Greater trochanter bursitis
8. Osteomyelitis
9. Tuberculosis
10. Avascular necrosis

Question #2

1. Greater trochanter bursitis
2. Early rheumatoid or osteoarthritis

Final Diagnosis: Greater trochanter bursitis was confirmed by complete relief of the pain and restricted range of motion by a lidocaine and steroid injection into the greater trochanter bursa.

Case #47

Question #1

1. Arrhenoblastoma
2. Cushing syndrome
3. Adrenocortical carcinoma
4. Polycystic ovary syndrome
5. Ectopic adrenocorticotropin hormone syndrome

Question #2

1. Adrenocortical carcinoma or adenoma

Final Diagnosis: Adrenocortical carcinoma was confirmed at surgery.

Case #48

Question #1

1. Laryngeal carcinoma
2. Tuberculosis
3. Syphilis
4. Chronic sinusitis
5. Reflux esophagitis
6. Singer nodes
7. Hypothyroidism
8. Myasthenia gravis
9. Thyroid carcinoma

Question #2

1. Hypothyroidism

Final Diagnosis: Hypothyroidism was confirmed by low T4 and high TSH levels.

Case #49

Question #1

1. Iron deficiency anemia
2. Hypothyroidism
3. Endometriosis
4. Pelvic inflammatory disease

5. Granulosa cell tumor of the ovary
6. Retained placenta
7. Choriocarcinoma
8. Coagulation disorder

Question #2

1. Lupus erythematosus
2. Thrombocytopenia purpura

Final Diagnosis: Lupus erythematosus was confirmed by a positive antinuclear antibody and anti–double-stranded DNA antibody titer.

Case #50

Question #1

1. Chronic pyelonephritis
2. Hypernephroma
3. Renal artery stenosis
4. Adrenocortical hyperplasia or tumor
5. Pheochromocytoma
6. Polycystic kidney
7. Coarctation of the aorta
8. Collagen disease
9. Toxic nephritis

Question #2

1.Primary aldosteronism

Final Diagnosis: Primary aldosteronism was confirmed by a plasma renin and a CT scan of the abdomen.

Case #51

Question #1

1. Space-occupying lesion of the cervical spinal cord
2. Amyotrophic lateral sclerosis
3. Neurosyphilis
4. Pernicious anemia
5. Friedreich ataxia
6. Syringomyelia
7. Cervical spondylosis

Question #2

1. Cervical spondylosis
2. Space-occupying lesion of the cervical spinal cord

Final Diagnosis: Cervical spondylosis was confirmed by magnetic resonance imaging of the cervical spine.

Case #52

Question #1

1. Anorexia nervosa
2. Arrhenoblastoma
3. Granulosa cell tumor
4. Hypopituitarism

5. Hyperthyroidism
6. Addison disease
7. Bilateral ovarian carcinoma
8. Prolactinoma

Question #2

1. Hypopituitarism (Sheehan syndrome)

Final Diagnosis: Hypopituitarism was confirmed by low urine follicle-stimulating hormone levels even after gonadotropin-releasing factor was administered.

Case #53

Question #1

1. Addison disease
2. Hypopituitarism
3. Anemia
4. Malabsorption syndrome
5. Chronic nephritis
6. Anorexia nervosa
7. Mitral stenosis
8. Myocardiopathy
9. Drug or alcohol abuse

Question #2

1. Addison disease
2. Hemochromatosis

Final Diagnosis: Addison disease was confirmed by a low serum cortisol that failed to respond to adrenocorticotropin hormone. The cause of the adrenocortical insufficiency was tuberculosis.

Case #54

Question #1

1. Alzheimer disease
2. Cervical arteriosclerosis
3. Korsakoff syndrome
4. Normal pressure hydrocephalus
5. Chronic cystitis
6. Bladder neck obstruction with overflow incontinence
7. Stress incontinence
8. General paresis

Question #2

1. Normal pressure hydrocephalus

Final Diagnosis: Normal pressure hydrocephalus was confirmed by radioactive cisternography.

Case #55

Question #1

1. Diabetic neuropathy
2. Peripheral arteriosclerosis

3. Chronic anxiety neurosis
4. Cerebral arteriosclerosis
5. Hemochromatosis
6. Cushing disease

Question #2

1. Leriche syndrome

Final Diagnosis: Leriche syndrome was confirmed by aortography.

Case #56

Question #1

1. Chronic cholecystitis and cholelithiasis
2. Reflux esophagitis
3. Chronic gastritis
4. Peptic ulcer
5. Chronic pancreatitis
6. Congestive heart failure
7. Pernicious anemia
8. Chronic hepatitis
9. Gastric carcinoma
10. Chronic intestinal obstruction
11. Urinary tract infection

Question #2

1. Chronic cholecystitis and cholelithiasis

Final Diagnosis: Chronic cholecystitis and cholelithiasis

Case #57

Question #1

1. Pelvic inflammatory disease
2. Retroverted uterus
3. Polycystic ovary syndrome
4. Chronic cervicitis
5. Hormone-secreting ovarian tumor
6. Hypopituitarism
7. Hypothyroidism
8. Adrenocortical tumor or hyperplasia
9. Emotional stress

Question #2

1. Chronic cervicitis
2. Carcinoma of the cervix

Final Diagnosis: Chronic cervicitis was confirmed by biopsy. The patient got pregnant after the cervicitis was successfully treated.

Case #58

Question #1

1. Endogenous depression
2. Hyperthyroidism

3. Occult neoplasm
4. Drug abuse
5. Chronic alcoholism
6. Pre-senile dementia
7. Physiologic or environmental causes

Question #2

1. Cirrhosis of the liver

Final Diagnosis: Cirrhosis of the liver was confirmed by liver function tests and liver biopsy.

Case #59

Question #1

1. Viral hepatitis
2. Toxic hepatitis
3. Hemolytic anemia
4. Infectious mononucleosis
5. Weil disease
6. Ascending cholangitis
7. Malaria
8. Dubin–Johnson syndrome
9. Pyelophlebitis

Question #2

1. Toxic hepatitis due to ranitidine hydrochloride

Final Diagnosis: Toxic hepatitis due to ranitidine hydrochloride

Case #60

Question #1

1. Gout
2. Pseudogout
3. Septic arthritis
4. Gonorrhea
5. Torn meniscus
6. Osteoarthritis
7. Rheumatoid arthritis
8. Collagen disease

Question #2

1. Pseudogout
2. Gout
3. Osteoarthritis

Final Diagnosis: Pseudogout was confirmed by finding calcium pyrophosphate crystal in the synovial fluids.

Case #61

Question #1

1. Rheumatoid arthritis
2. Lupus erythematosus
3. Gonorrhea
4. Lyme disease

5. Rheumatic fever
6. Reiter syndrome
7. Brucellosis
8. Sickle cell anemia
9. Viral hepatitis

Question #2

1. Gonorrhea
2. Lupus erythematosus
3. Reiter syndrome
4. Rheumatic fever

Final Diagnosis: Gonorrhea was confirmed by a positive vaginal culture.

Case #62

Question #1

1. Deep vein thrombophlebitis
2. Arterial embolism
3. Osteomyelitis
4. Herniated lumbar disc
5. Contusion
6. Cellulitis

Question #2

1. Deep vein thrombophlebitis

Final Diagnosis: Deep vein thrombophlebitis was confirmed by ultrasonography.

Case #63

Question #1

1. Rheumatoid spondylitis
2. Herniated lumbar disc
3. Lumbar spondylosis
4. Spinal cord tumor

Question #2

1. Rheumatoid spondylitis
2. Lumbar spondylosis
3. Alkaptonuria

Final Diagnosis: Alkaptonuria was confirmed by the finding of homogentisic acid in the urine.

Case #64

Question #1

1. Pelvic inflammatory disease
2. Tuberculous peritonitis
3. Metastatic carcinoma
4. Ruptured viscus (appendix, etc.) with peritonitis
5. Lupus erythematosus
6. Hodgkin lymphoma
7. Pancreatitis
8. Lymphatic leukemia

Question #2

1. Tuberculosis peritonitis

Final Diagnosis: Tuberculous peritonitis was confirmed by acid-fast bacillus culture and Guinea pig inoculation of peritoneal fluid.

Case #65

Question #1

1. Alzheimer disease
2. Pick disease
3. Korsakoff syndrome
4. Pellagra
5. Cerebral arteriosclerosis
6. Complex partial seizures
7. Insulinoma with chronic hypoglycemia
8. Normal pressure hydrocephalus
9. Pernicious anemia
10. Cerebral arteriosclerosis

Question #2

1. Pernicious anemia

Final Diagnosis: Pernicious anemia was confirmed by a macrocytic anemia and decreased serum vitamin B12.

Case #66

Question #1

1. Herniated lumbar disc
2. Sciatic neuritis
3. Space-occupying lesion of the spinal cord
4. Compression fracture improved and was rarely seen
5. Spondylolisthesis

Final Diagnosis: Compensation neurosis (The patient improved and was rarely seen at the office after his worker's compensation case was settled.)

Case #67

Question #1

1. Leriche syndrome
2. Peripheral arteriosclerosis
3. Aldosteronism
4. Cramps induced by electrolyte imbalance
5. Spinal stenosis

Question #2

1. Spinal stenosis
2. Aldosteronism
3. Cramps induced by electrolyte imbalance.

Final Diagnosis: Spinal stenosis was confirmed by magnetic resonance imaging of the lumbar spine.

Case #68

Question #1

1. Polymyalgia rheumatica
2. Rheumatoid arthritis
3. Dermatomyositis
4. Myasthenia gravis
5. Cervical spondylosis
6. Hyperthyroidism
7. Malignant neoplasm
8. Collagen disease
9. Epidemic myalgia
10. Trichinosis

Question #2

1. Polymyalgia rheumatica

Final Diagnosis: Polymyalgia rheumatica

Case #69

Question #1

1. Herniated cervical disc at C5–C6
2. Other space-occupying lesion of cervical spine

Final Diagnosis: Herniated cervical disc at C5–C6 was confirmed by MRI.

Case #70

Question #1

1. Idiopathic obesity
2. Insulinoma
3. Klinefelter syndrome
4. Cushing syndrome
5. Pituitary and hypothalamic lesions

Question #2

1. Cushing syndrome

Final Diagnosis: Cushing syndrome was confirmed by an elevated serum cortisol.

Case #71

Question #1

1. Hyperthyroidism
2. Early congestive heart failure
3. Pheochromocytoma
4. Chronic anxiety neurosis
5. Fever of unknown origin
6. Coronary insufficiency
7. Hiatal hernia and esophagitis

Question #2

1. Chronic anxiety neurosis
2. Substance abuse
3. Caffeine intolerance

Final Diagnosis: Caffeine intolerance (All his symptoms subsided upon the elimination of caffeine from his diet.)

Case #72

Question #1

1. Peripheral neuropathy
2. Tumor of the cervical spinal cord
3. Pernicious anemia
4. Multiple sclerosis
5. Basilar artery insufficiency
6. Parasagittal meningioma
7. Brainstem glioma
8. Hypoparathyroidism
9. Neurosyphilis
10. Collagen disease
11. Hyperventilation syndrome

Question #2

1. Multiple sclerosis

Final Diagnosis: Multiple sclerosis was confirmed by MRI of the cervical spine.

Case #73

Question #1

1. Hyperthyroidism
2. Diabetes mellitus
3. Hyperparathyroidism
4. Diabetes insipidus
5. Chronic renal disease
6. Psychogenic polydipsia

Question #2

1. Diabetic acidosis

Final Diagnosis: Diabetic acidosis

Case #74

Question #1

1. Hyperthyroidism
2. Cushing syndrome
3. Islet cell adenoma
4. Diabetic mellitus
5. Pituitary adenoma
6. Tapeworm infestation
7. Chronic anxiety neurosis

Question #2

1. Insulinoma

Final Diagnosis: Insulinoma was confirmed by significant hypoglycemia during a 72-hour fast and exploratory surgery.

Case #75

Question #1

1. Hyperthyroidism
2. Diabetes mellitus
3. Chronic glomerulonephritis
4. Pyelonephritis
5. Diabetes insipidus
6. Primary hyperparathyroidism
7. Aldosteronism
8. Endogenous depression

Question #2

1. Primary hyperparathyroidism

Final Diagnosis: Primary hyperparathyroidism was confirmed by repeatedly elevated serum calcium and parathyroid hormone assays.

Case #76

Question #1

1. Drug eruption
2. Tinea versicolor
3. Typhoid fever
4. Gonorrhea
5. Syphilis
6. Rubella
7. Measles
8. Pityriasis rosea
9. Dermatitis herpetiformis
10. Infectious mononucleosis
11. Collagen disease

Question #2

1. Pityriasis rosea

Final Diagnosis: Pityriasis rosea was confirmed by a dermatology consultation.

Case #77

Question #1

1. Carcinoma of the colon
2. Hemorrhoids
3. Ulcerative colitis
4. Granulomatous colitis
5. Ischemic colitis
6. Pseudomembranous colitis
7. Mesenteric artery occlusion
8. Coagulation disorder

9. Rectal polyp
10. Amebic colitis
11. Diverticulosis

Question #2

1. Carcinoma of the sigmoid colon

Final Diagnosis: Carcinoma of the sigmoid colon was confirmed by colonoscopy.

Case #78

Question #1

1. Foreign bodies
2. Corneal abrasion
3. Keratitis
4. Iritis
5. Glaucoma
6. Scleritis
7. Cavernous sinus thrombosis
8. Conjunctivitis
9. Sinusitis
10. Histamine headache

Question #2

1. Ulcerative colitis with uveitis

Final Diagnosis: Uveitis was confirmed by ophthalmological consultation.

Case #79

Question #1

1. Shoulder–hand syndrome
2. Torn rotator cuff
3. Osteoarthritis
4. Rheumatoid arthritis
5. Gout
6. Subacromial bursitis
7. Sympathetic dystrophy
8. Fracture
9. Collagen disease
10. Herniated cervical disc
11. Osteomyelitis

Question #2

1. Shoulder–hand syndrome

Final Diagnosis: The same

Case #80

Question #1

1. Streptococcal pharyngitis
2. Diphtheria
3. Gonorrhea
4. Infectious mononucleosis
5. *Listeria monocytogenes*

Question #2

1. Infectious mononucleosis
2. Leukemia
3. Agranulocytosis
4. Diphtheria

Final Diagnosis: Infectious mononucleosis was confirmed by a positive monospot test.

Case #81

Question #1

1. Stokes–Adams syndrome
2. Vasovagal syncope
3. Transient cardiac arrhythmia
4. Anemia
5. Valvular heart disease
6. Insulinoma
7. Migraine
8. Epilepsy
9. Conversion hysteria
10. Postural hypotension

Question #2

1. Stokes–Adam syndrome
2. Vasovagal syncope
3. Conversion hysteria

Final Diagnosis: Stokes–Adams syndrome was confirmed by the complete resolution of symptoms after the insertion of a pacemaker.

Case #82

Question #1

1. Acoustic neuroma
2. Ménière disease
3. Postconcussion syndrome
4. Vertebral artery aneurysm
5. Cholesteatoma
6. Neurosyphilis
7. Multiple sclerosis
8. Drug-induced nerve deafness
9. Occupational tinnitus and deafness

Question #2

1. Acoustic neuroma due to neurofibromatosis

Final Diagnosis: Acoustic neuroma due to neurofibromatosis was confirmed by MRI of the brain and tissue biopsy.

Case #83

Question #1

1. Parkinson disease
2. Wilson disease
3. Manganese toxicity
4. Alcohol encephalopathy

5. Familial tremor
6. Hyperthyroidism
7. Multiple sclerosis
8. Caffeine-induced tremor

Question #2

1. Familial tremor

Final Diagnosis: Familial tremor was confirmed by neurologic consultation.

Case #84

Question #1

1. Uterine fibroids
2. Endometrial carcinoma
3. Dysfunctional uterine bleeding
4. Cervical carcinoma
5. Functional ovarian cyst or tumor
6. Endometriosis
7. Coagulation disorder
8. Anemia

Question #2

1. Endometrial carcinoma

Final Diagnosis: Endometrial carcinoma was confirmed by endometrial biopsy.

Case #85

Question #1

1. Pelvic inflammatory disease

Final Diagnosis: Pelvic inflammatory disease due to gonorrhea was confirmed by culture of the cervical mucus.

Case #86

Question #1

1. Tuberculosis
2. Bronchogenic carcinoma with Lambert–Eaton syndrome
3. Addison disease
4. Hyperthyroidism
5. Muscular dystrophy
6. Hyperparathyroidism
7. Collagen disease
8. Myasthenia gravis
9. Polymyalgia rheumatica
10. Peripheral neuropathy

Question #2

1. Small cell carcinoma of the lung with Lambert–Eaton syndrome

Final Diagnosis: Small cell carcinoma of the lung with Lambert–Eaton syndrome was confirmed by lung biopsy and electromyography.

Case #87

Question #1

1. Malabsorption syndrome
2. Bulimia
3. Anorexia nervosa
4. Endogenous depression
5. Diabetes mellitus
6. Hyperthyroidism
7. Addison disease
8. Occult neoplasm
9. Iron deficiency anemia
10. Drug or alcohol abuse
11. Chronic active hepatitis

Question #2

1. Anorexia nervosa
2. Bulimia

Final Diagnosis: Anorexia nervosa was confirmed by psychiatric consult.

Page numbers followed by *f* indicate figures; page numbers followed by *t* indicate tables.